THIS PACK HAS BEEN GENEROUSLY DONATED TO MEDICINE AND
HEALTH PROFESSIONALS BY
DOUG STEAD,
DIRECTOR OF CHILD PROTECTION
RAMAS

*Doug Stead has devoted an extraordinary amount of time and resources for the
protection of children. He also provides assistance to law enforcement agencies in
combating the illegal use of technology to facilitate and hide sexual crimes against
children. Over the years, Doug Stead has frequently been on radio and TV as a
guest speaker and as a presenter at numerous international, national and local
conferences on the subject of child pornography and the adults involved in these
types of crimes. Doug Stead has also developed and funded "Reveal", a free
software application which enables a technologically challenged parent to easily
and quickly scan the family computer for indicators (words and images) that may
be of an unhealthy interest by child users.*

Medical, Legal, & Social
Science Aspects of

# Child Sexual

# Exploitation

A Comprehensive Review of
Pornography, Prostitution,
and Internet Crimes

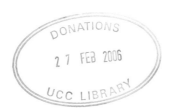
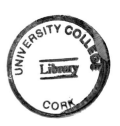
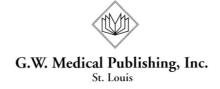

**G.W. Medical Publishing, Inc.**
St. Louis

# Medical, Legal, & Social Science Aspects of

# Child Sexual

# Exploitation

## A Comprehensive Review of Pornography, Prostitution, and Internet Crimes

**Richard J. Estes, DSW, ACSW**
Professor
Chair, Concentration in Social and
    Economic Development
Director, International Programs
University of Pennsylvania School of Social
    Work
Philadelphia, Pennsylvania

**Victor I. Vieth, JD**
Director
APRI's National Child Protection Training
    Center
Winona State University
Winona, Minnesota

**Sharon Cooper, MD, FAAP**
Adjunct Associate Professor of Pediatrics
University of North Carolina School of
    Medicine
Chapel Hill, North Carolina
Clinical Assistant Professor of Pediatrics
Uniformed Services University of Health
    Sciences
Bethesda, Maryland
Chief , Developmental Pediatric Service
    Womack Army Medical Center
Fort Bragg, North Carolina

**Angelo P. Giardino, MD, PhD, FAAP**
Associate Chair – Pediatrics
Associate Physician-in-Chief/
Vice-President, Clinical Affairs
St. Christopher's Hospital for Children
Associate Professor in Pediatrics
Drexel University College of Medicine
Adjunct Professor of Pediatric Nursing LaSalle
University School of Nursing
Philadelphia, Pennsylvania

**Nancy D. Kellogg, MD**
Professor of Pediatrics
University of Texas Health Science Center at
    San Antonio
Medical Director
Alamo Children's Advocacy Center

**G.W. Medical Publishing, Inc.**
St. Louis

Publishers: Glenn E. Whaley and Marianne V. Whaley

Assistant Publisher: Jonathan M. Taylor

Design Director: Glenn E. Whaley

Managing Editors: Karen C. Maurer
Megan E. Ferrell

Associate Editors: Jonathan M. Taylor
Christine Bauer

Book Design/Page Layout: G.W. Graphics
Sudon Choe
Charles J. Seibel, III

Print/Production Coordinator: Charles J. Seibel, III

Cover Design: G.W. Graphics

Color Prepress Specialist: Richard Stockard

Copy Editor: Bonnie F. Spinola

Developmental Editors: Aimee E. Loewe
Laurie Sparks

Proofreader/Indexer: Robert A. Saigh

Printed in Canada.

Publisher:
**G.W. Medical Publishing, Inc.**
**77 Westport Plaza, Suite 366, St. Louis, Missouri, 63146-3124 U.S.A.**
**Phone: (314) 542-4213 Fax: (314) 542-4239 Toll Free: 1-800-600-0330**
**http://www.gwmedical.com**

Library of Congress Cataloging-in-Publication Data

Cooper, Sharon 1952-
Medical, legal, & social science aspects of child sexual exploitation: a comprehensive review of pornography, prostitution, and internet crimes /
Sharon Cooper . . . [et al.] -- 1st ed.
p. cm.
Includes bibliographical references and index.
ISBN 1-878060-70-8 (v. 1, hardcover : alk. paper) -- ISBN 1-878060-71-6 (v. 2, hardcover : alk. paper) -- ISBN 1-878060-37-6 (v. 1 & 2, casebound : alk. paper)
1. Child sexual abuse -- United States -- Prevention. 2. Children -- Crimes against -- United States.
3. Abused children -- Services for -- United States. 4. Child prostitution -- United States. 5. Children in pornography -- United States. 6. Internet pornography -- United States. I. Title: Medical, legal, and social science aspects of child sexual exploitation. II. Title.
HV6570.2.C65 2005
362.76`0973 -- dc22
2005005612

# CONTRIBUTORS

**Mary P. Alexander, MA, LPC**
MA Counseling-Marriage and Family Therapy
MEd Educational Psychology and Special Education
Certified School Counselor
Eagle Nest, New Mexico

**Elena Azaola, PhD**
PhD in Social Anthropology
Psychoanalyst
Professor at the Center for Advanced Studies and Research in
    Social Anthropology
Mexico City, Mexico

**Joseph S. Bova Conti, BA**
Detective Sergeant, Maryland Heights Police Department
Crimes Against Children Specialist
Certified Juvenile Specialist — State of Missouri
Member MPJOA, MJJA, SLCJJA
Lecturer, Author, Consultant
Maryland Heights, Missouri

**Duncan T. Brown, Esq**
Assistant District Attorney
Sex Crimes/Special Victims Bureau
Richmond County District Attorney's Office
Staten Island, New York

**Cormac Callanan, BA, MSc**
Secretary General
Association of Internet Hotline Providers in Europe (INHOPE)

**Lt. William D. Carson, MA, SPSC**
Commander, Bureau of Investigation
Maryland Heights Police Department
Maryland Heights, Missouri

**Michelle K. Collins, MA**
Director, Exploited Child Unit
National Center for Missing & Exploited Children (NCMEC)
Alexandria, Virginia

**Peter I. Collins, MCA, MD, FRCP(C)**
Manager, Forensic Psychiatry Unit
Behavioural Sciences Section
Ontario Provincial Police
Associate Professor, Department of Psychiatry
University of Toronto
Toronto, Canada

**Jeffrey A. Dort, JD**
Deputy District Attorney
Team Leader Family Protection Division
Lead Prosecutor — ICAC: Internet Crimes Against Children
San Diego District Attorney's Office
San Diego, California

**V. Denise Everett, MD, FAAP**
Director, Child Sexual Abuse Team
WakeMed
Raleigh, North Carolina
Clinical Associate Professor, Department of Pediatrics
University of North Carolina at Chapel Hill School of Medicine
Chapel Hill, North Carolina

**Fadi Barakat Fadel**
Director of Programmes of the International Centre to Combat
    Exploitation of Children
Founder of Sexually Exploited Youth Speak Out Network
    (SEYSO)

**James A. H. Farrow, MD, FSAM**
Professor, Medicine & Pediatrics
Director, Student Health Services
Tulane University
New Orleans, Louisiana

**David Finkelhor, PhD**
Director, Crimes Against Children Research Center
Family Research Laboratory
Professor, Department of Sociology
University of New Hampshire
Durham, New Hampshire

**Katherine A. Free, MA**
Program Manager
Exploited Child Unit
National Center for Missing & Exploited Children (NCMEC)
Alexandria, Virginia

**Nadine Grant**
Director of Programs
Save the Children Canada
Toronto, Canada

**Ernestine S. Gray, JD**
Judge
Orleans Parish Juvenile Court
Section "A"
New Orleans, Louisiana

**Donald B. Henley**
Senior Special Agent
US Department of Homeland Security
Immigration and Customs Enforcement (ICE)

**Marcia E. Herman-Giddens, PA, DrPH**
Child Maltreatment Consulting
Senior Fellow, North Carolina Child Advocacy Institute
Adjunct Professor, University of North Carolina School of
 Public Health
Pittsboro, North Carolina

**Nicole G. Ives, MSW**
Doctoral Candidate
University of Pennsylvania, School of Social Work
Philadelphia, Pennsylvania

**Eileen R. Jacob**
Supervisor Special Agent
Crimes Against Children Unit
Federal Bureau of Investigation
Washington, DC

**Terry Jones, BA (Hons), PGCE**
Consultant: Internet Paedophilia Training Awareness
Consultancy (IPTAC)
Former Head Greater Manchester Police Abusive Images Unit
United Kingdom

**Aaron Kipnis, PhD**
Professor — Clinical Psychology
Pacifica Graduate Institute
Carpenteria, California
Psychologist
Santa Barbara, California

**Susan S. Kreston, JD, LLM**
Consultant
New Orleans, Louisiana

**Kenneth V. Lanning, MS**
(Retired FBI)
CAC Consultants
Fredericksburg, Virginia

**Mary Anne Layden, PhD**
Codirector
Sexual Trauma and Psychopathology Program
Director of Education
Center for Cognitive Therapy
Department of Psychiatry
University of Pennsylvania
Philadelphia, Pennsylvania

**Shyla R. Lefever, PhD**
Assistant Professor of Communication
Hampton University
Hampton, Virginia

**Ingrid Leth**
Former Senior Adviser
UNICEF HQ, USA
Associate Professor — Clinical Child Psychology
Department of Psychology
University of Copenhagen
Copenhagen, Denmark

**Elizabeth J. Letourneau, PhD**
Assistant Professor
Department of Psychiatry and Behavioral Sciences
Medical University of South Carolina
Charleston, South Carolina

**L. Alvin Malesky, Jr, PhD**
Assistant Professor, Department of Psychology
Western Carolina University
Cullowhee, North Carolina

**Bernadette McMenamin, AO**
National Director of CHILD WISE
ECPAT in Australia
Director, NetAlert (Internet safety advisory board)
Director, KidsAP (Internet safety advisory board)
Advisor to the Federal Government for the National Plan of
Action on CSEC (Commercial Sexual Exploitation of Children)
South Melbourne, Australia

**Kimberly Mitchell, PhD**
Research Associate — Crimes Against Children Research Center
Assistant Research Professor of Psychology
University of New Hampshire
Durham, New Hampshire

**Thomas P. O'Connor, BA, MA**
Chief of Police, Maryland Heights Police Department
Law Enforcement Instructor, Specialty Crimes Against Persons,
 Criminal Investigation Procedures
Maryland Heights, Missouri

**John Patzakis, Esq**
Vice Chairman and Chief Legal Officer
Guidance Software, Inc.

**David S. Prescott, LICSW**
Treatment Assessment Director,
 Sand Ridge Secure Treatment Center
Mauston, Wisconsin

**Ethel Quayle, BA, MSc, PsychD**
Lecturer
Researcher with the COPINE Project
Department of Applied Psychology
University College Cork
Cork, Ireland

**Erika Rivera Ragland, JD**
Staff Attorney
National Center for Prosecution of Child Abuse
American Prosecutors Research Institute (APRI)
Alexandria, Virginia

**Thomas Rickert**
Attorney at Law
President, Association of Internet Hotline Providers in
    Europe (INHOPE)
Chair, Internet Content Task Force eco
Cologne, Germany

**Migael Scherer**
Director, Dart Award for Excellence in Reporting on Victims of
    Violence
Dart Center for Journalism and Trauma
Department of Communication
University of Washington
Seattle, Washington

**Daniel J. Sheridan, PhD, RN, FAAN**
Assistant Professor
Johns Hopkins University School of Nursing
President, International Association of Forensic Nurses
Baltimore, Maryland

**Linnea W. Smith, MD**
Psychiatrist
Chapel Hill, North Carolina

**Raymond C. Smith**
Assistant Inspector in Charge
Fraud, Prohibited Mailings and Asset Forfeiture
US Postal Inspection Service
Washington, DC

**Max Taylor, PhD, C. Forensic Psychology**
Professor and Head of Department
    of Applied Psychology
University College Cork
Director, COPINE Project
Cork, Ireland

**Govind Prasad Thapa, MA, BL, MPA, PhD**
Additional Inspector General, Nepal Police
Chief — Crime Investigation Department
Police Headquarters
Kathmandu, Nepal

**Phyllis L. Thompson, LCSW**
OUR KIDS Center
Nashville General Hospital
Instructor in the Department of Pediatrics
Vanderbilt University Medical Center
Nashville, Tennessee

**Christopher D. Trifiletti**
Special Agent
Federal Bureau of Investigation
Baltimore, Maryland
Chair, Interpol Specialists Group on Crimes Against Children,
Child Pornography, and Internet Investigations Theme Groups
Lyon, France

**Dawn Van Pelt, BSN, RN**
Graduate Student
Johns Hopkins University School of Nursing
Baltimore, Maryland

**Bharathi A. Venkatraman, Esq**
United States Department of Justice
Civil Rights Division
Washington, DC

**F. Bruce Watkins, MD**
Assistant Clinical Professor of Ob/Gyn
University of Illinois College of Medicine
Medical Director, Women's Health Service
Crusader Clinic
Rockford, Illinois

**Bruce Watson, LLB, CA**
Past President, Enough Is Enough
Fairfax, Virginia

**Neil Alan Weiner, PhD**
Senior Research Investigator
Center for Research on Youth and Social Policy
School of Social Work
University of Pennsylvania
Philadelphia, Pennsylvania

**Cathy Spatz Widom, PhD**
Professor of Psychiatry and University Professor
UMDNJ — New Jersey Medical School
Department of Psychiatry
Newark, New Jersey

**Janis Wolak, JD**
Research Assistant Professor
Crimes Against Children Research Center
University of New Hampshire
Durham, New Hampshire

### G.W. Medical Publishing, Inc.
St. Louis

## OUR MISSION

To become the world leader in publishing and

information services on child abuse, maltreatment

and diseases, and domestic violence. We seek to

heighten awareness of these issues and provide

relevant information to professionals and consumers.

*A portion of our profits is contributed to nonprofit organizations
dedicated to the prevention of child abuse and the care of victims of abuse
and other children and family charities.*

# FOREWORD

In my career as a prosecutor, and now a Congressman, I have seen tremendous improvements in our nation's response to cases of child maltreatment. In most communities today, multidisciplinary teams work together for the benefit of children. Many elected district attorneys, sheriffs, and police chiefs have developed specialized units to respond to cases of child abuse.

Through the work of the American Prosecutors Research Institute's National Center for Prosecution of Child Abuse, the National Child Protection Training Center at Winona State University, Fox Valley Technical College, the National Center for Missing & Exploited Children, and other federally funded programs, thousands of frontline professionals are trained annually in the art and science of handling child protection cases.

Perhaps the most important development is the Children's Advocacy Center program. Children's Advocacy Centers (CACs) are child-friendly facilities where children can be interviewed sensitively and receive medical and psychological services. As a district attorney, I had the privilege of starting the nation's first Children's Advocacy Center. As a member of Congress, I championed support for the National Children's Advocacy Center in Huntsville, Alabama, and the National Children's Alliance, a coalition of CACs from across the nation that is headquartered in Washington, DC. Today there are hundreds of CACs in every part of our country.

We can not, however, rest on our laurels. As detailed in the pages of this book, modern technology poses a new threat to our children. It is increasingly easy for perpetrators to exploit children through the Internet, to create and disseminate child pornography, and to solicit children for illicit purposes.

The commercial exploitation of children is a global problem that impacts every community in the United States. Through the pioneering work of Dr. Richard Estes and other researchers, we know that hundreds of thousands of children are at risk of commercial exploitation. Although more research needs to be done, there is some evidence to suggest these children are just as likely to come from rural and suburban communities as urban centers.

I commend GW Medical Publishing as well as the editors and contributors to this book for producing a treatise that addresses child sexual exploitation from every angle. I am particularly grateful to the survivors of child pornography, commercial exploitation, and online solicitation for sharing their pain with those of us who will read this book. I hope the courage of these survivors spurs all of us to do more to protect children.

Finally, I want to commend the frontline investigators, prosecutors, medical and mental health professionals, and other child advocates who are in the trenches daily trying to spare children from every form of exploitation. You labor long hours for little pay or honor on behalf of someone else's children. Please know that your selfless dedication is not unnoticed. Indeed, your heroism is an inspiration to us all.

**Congressman Robert E. "Bud" Cramer, Jr.**
Member of the US House of Representatives (1991-present)
Founder of the Children's Advocacy Center movement

# FOREWORD

It is common to hear pronouncements from public figures that children are society's most important and treasured assets. To an overwhelming majority, this concept is fundamentally true. To a marginal and deviant minority, however, children are viewed as commodities to be traded, imported, and exported like any other merchandise. Parents and professionals need help combating the alarming growth of child exploitation and this book is a valuable tool in the fight to protect our children from predators who would use them for financial gain or prurient reasons.

Global in scope, these 2 volumes are written by individuals who represent a wide array of backgrounds, disciplines, and perspectives. Some authors are the authentic voices of those who were victimized and forced to navigate a system that was intended to help but found to be less than helpful. Some speak from distant lands that are growing ever closer with the ease of air travel and where the youth are being sold to travelers seeking to indulge their perverse needs with someone else's children. Some voices are actually electronic particles from cyberspace delivering images of unspeakable abuse to our home and office computers.

Some of the highlights of this book that I found interesting include:

— A chapter discussing exploitation in advertising and the need for healthcare providers to be aware of the "slippery slope" that can occur when girls and teens are used in sexualized marketing

— A chapter about the resources of the National Center for Missing & Exploited Children with a focus on their Exploited Child Unit

— A chapter from UNICEF on the global commodification of children for sexual work and exploitation

— A chapter from the University of Washington School of Journalism discussing the importance of addressing child victims of sexual exploitation in an empathetic and nonvictimizing manner in the newspapers; the chapter includes excerpts and photographs from a focused series in the *Atlanta Journal Constitution* called "The Selling of Atlanta's Children," which played an important role in convincing the Georgia State Legislature to change its laws to make the selling of children a felony, as compared to its history of misdemeanor status for over a century

— A chapter from the Association for the Treatment of Sexual Abusers (ATSA) regarding the ethical issues in child sex offender assessments and the benchmarks for parole and probation determinations

— Chapters relating to the medical and surgical complications of prostitution

— A chapter discussing the demographics of girls who are brought into the criminal justice system and recommendations for communities to avoid the incarceration of prostituted children and youths

— A chapter that explains the nuts and bolts of "cloning a computer" when an investigation is conducted in a child pornography case

— A chapter describing other aspects of federal laws that are involved when children and youths are trafficked into the United States for sexual exploitation purposes, including civil rights violations and labor law violations

— A chapter on the AMBER Alert legislation and the several children whose lives contributed to its inception

— A chapter detailing the frequently overlooked concept of child sexual exploitation in rural communities

This book represents the culmination of the efforts of an impressive collection of premier investigators, judicial participants, child protection agency personnel, and clinicians to gather and organize information about child exploitation. It is the most comprehensive text on this subject and it is a welcome addition to the literature on child maltreatment.

**Robert M. Reece, MD**
Clinical Professor of Pediatrics
Tufts University School of Medicine
Visiting Professor of Pediatrics
Dartmouth Medical School
Editor, *The Quarterly Update*

# FOREWORD

In 1981, my worst nightmare became a reality when my 6-year-old son, Adam, was abducted and murdered. The prime suspect in Adam's case was never charged. He died in prison while serving a life sentence for other crimes. With determination to spare other families from enduring a similar tragedy, my wife Revé and I worked to help enact the Missing Children Act of 1982 and the Missing Children's Assistance Act of 1984. We founded the National Center for Missing & Exploited Children (NCMEC) in 1984. In the past 20 years, the rate of recovery of missing children has increased from 62% to 95%.

While the NCMEC is best known for its work in tracking down missing children, the Exploited Child Unit, established in 1997, has also been a primary resource for law enforcement and families in the investigation and prosecution of the sexual exploitation of children. Child sexual exploitation is a worldwide problem, encompassing child pornography, molestation, and prostitution. In recent years, computers and the Internet have become favorite tools of child molesters as they collect and trade pornographic images and solicit new victims online.

*Medical, Legal, & Social Science Aspects of Child Sexual Exploitation: A Comprehensive Review of Pornography, Prostitution, and Internet Crimes* is a 2-volume text that addresses this pervasive problem. Written by physicians, nurses, attorneys, social workers, and law enforcement officials who are leading experts in the field, the text takes a multidisciplinary approach to the medical and legal issues faced by victims of sexual exploitation. The contributions of authors from countries outside the United States help to highlight the international nature of this problem. First-person accounts by adults who were exploited as children and teenagers help to put a human face on the issue. The role of the media is addressed, both as contributors to the problem and as partners in creating and implementing solutions. Other chapters discuss the role of the United States Postal Inspection Service, the investigation of Internet exploitation cases, prosecutorial and judicial issues, the role of the medical expert, and the establishment of criminal liability for groups promoting child sexual exploitation.

It is my sincere belief that this book will be a significant contribution to the literature in this field, and by doing so, will help to combat this worldwide problem.

**John Walsh**
Cofounder, National Center for Missing & Exploited Children
Host, Fox Television's *America's Most Wanted*

# PREFACE

The idea for this work originated from the need to establish a repository of information for multidisciplinary team members who are learning about Internet crimes against children. When the concept of mass communication began with Gutenberg's printing press in the 14th century, the purpose was to disperse information and promote new ideas. Seven centuries later, the Internet has expanded upon the original purpose of the printing press and now includes the deception and entrapment of our most vulnerable resource: children. As methods of victimization have become more innovative, sophisticated, and elusive, professionals are challenged in their efforts to prevent, detect, intervene, and treat children that fall prey to online predators.

Knowledge regarding Internet crimes against children has been primarily limited to media coverage of the topic. This text serves to separate fact from fiction and to dispel several myths and misconceptions, including the belief that prostituted youths typically market themselves by choice and can easily escape from this form of abuse. To the uninformed, it is inconceivable that children and youth are often sold from within their own homes, that the Internet is used in numerous capacities to make such arrangements, and that Internet cafés present a nearly untraceable means of making the deal. Online solicitation has become an increasing threat to children. Many naïve children and youths unwittingly receive unwanted sexual solicitations, and may be enticed to leave their homes and families to meet online predators; such encounters may end tragically in sexual assault, physical assault, abduction, or murder. What was slavery and bondage in the past has now become human trafficking for forced labor and sexual exploitation. These crimes continue to escalate worldwide.

The text begins with the history of child exploitation and proceeds to explain the contemporary and global nature of this form of child victimization. A careful analysis of the acquaintance molester leads the reader to complex types of sexual exploitation, illustrated with online, local, national, and international examples of the scope of these crimes against children. A collage of perspectives is presented, including exploitation in advertising, the role of the journalistic media response to these types of victims of crime, medical evaluation and treatment of victims, offender psychology and victim mental health impact, and social science research in the area of commercial sexual exploitation of children. The reader will experience a judicial and criminal justice view, the perspective of the sexually exploited male, an education regarding the Internet community with respect to offender dynamics, and important aspects of the offender evaluation when potential parole, probation, and public safety is being considered.

From the investigative and prosecuting platform, numerous important issues are discussed: the role of the first responder in an Internet crime against a child; the details of "cloning software" and the best way to present this complex information to a judge or jury; the technology of victim identification from an Internet Web site; the importance of strategy in prostitution cases when the common bias is that the victim is an offender; the recognition of the organized crime aspects of girls domestically trafficked across a country for sexual slavery and prostitution; the international requirements of police agencies in abduction and exploitation cases; and the realization that child pornography production and collection is a highly recidivistic crime. Investigations of high profile cases of sexual exploitation have resulted in an organized response to the sex tourist who travels to exploit young children for sexual purposes. The worst-case scenario of child abduction, sexual assault, and homicide are described, as well as community responses such as the AMBER Alert program, designed to facilitate a rapid and safe recovery of a missing child or youth.

From a child maltreatment perspective, this groundbreaking work provides comprehensive and diverse information for this contemporary, yet misunderstood and daunting, form of child exploitation. It has been an immense honor to work with truly professional contributors, all of whom have been eager and cooperative in providing an international and expert treatise on a subject that all parents and professionals must acknowledge and understand. As the Internet, the "printing press" of the 21st century, has opened new doors for the worldwide exchange of information and ideas, so too has it opened a Pandora's box of opportunities for criminals that victimize children and youths. At present, the knowledge regarding Internet crimes against children is fragmented, scant, and discipline-specific. This text is the first step toward comprehension, effective intervention, and the multidisciplinary coordination of investigations of crimes involving these exploited children. It will open your eyes and your mind to a new dark side of child abuse that we can no longer afford to ignore.

**Sharon W. Cooper, MD, FAAP**
**Richard J. Estes, DSW, ACSW**
**Angelo P. Giardino, MD, PhD, FAAP**
**Nancy D. Kellogg, MD**
**Victor I. Vieth, JD**

# REVIEWS

*As a former Police Chief I know that important policy decisions regarding the establishment of comprehensive child protection strategies are often based upon a tragic case or anecdotal evidence that often ignores the scope and scale of the overall problem. The research conducted by these nationally recognized experts provides important insight into emerging threats to children and serves as a guide for developing an effective national response.*

Brad Russ
ICAC Training & Technical Assistance
Program Director
University of New Hampshire
Internet Crimes Against Children
Research Center
Durham, NH

*The factual information, practical methodologies, and expertise in this book can be used as a practical tool in combating the horror of the commercial sexual exploitation of children. The fact that this text is guided by internationally recognized child rights principles and documents gives one hope that change is possible in a world where exploitation of children is so prevalent. As a survivor and now activist, I encourage the government, professionals, and the public to care about this issue and be practical and humane in their approach to combating exploitation. This book provides us with that template.*

Cherry Kingsley
Special Advisor
International Centre to Combat
Exploitation of Children
Vancouver, Canada

*With the emergence of the Internet and its worldwide expansion as a favored mode of communication, there is an ever-increasing avenue for the sexual exploitation of children. This informative publication, authored by acknowledged leaders in the field of forensic science, provides professionals working with child abuse victims, their families, and the suspected perpetrators with a wide range of forensic techniques and knowledge that will serve as an essential forensic reference.*

Faye Battiste-Otto, RN, SANE
Founder/President of American
Forensic Nurses
Cofounder, International Association
of Forensic Nurses
Palm Springs, CA

*In giving a broad scope of understanding about the sexual exploitation of children, this book delineates familial child sexual abuse and commercial sexual exploitation. Its international perspective suggests that the causes are broader than defined by western countries and therefore prevention foci need to be tailored accordingly. While giving information on offender motives and treatment, it emphasizes the victim as blameless, a view that continues to need reinforcement. The detailed nature of the book and the number of worthy contributors reiterate its use as a text for all manner of helping professionals.*

Jane Rudd, PhD
Associate Professor
Saint Joseph College
West Hartford, CT

*The subject matter is disturbing, but this is a must-read resource book for professionals working in the field of child maltreatment in the 21st century. The contents provide a comprehensive review of research, current programs, and concepts that address intervention, investigation, and prevention.*

Jeanie Ming, CPNP
Forensic Pediatric Nurse Practitioner
Child Abuse Services Team
Orange, CA

*Medical, Legal, & Social Science Aspects of Child Sexual Exploitation is a rare and welcome departure from the "same old, same old" of recent years and is truly new and innovative. This book is the first to provide in-depth coverage of an emerging and serious global issue. The authors and editors are well qualified to address the complex social, psychological, and legal issues presented by child sexual exploitation.*

John E.B. Myers
Distinguished Professor and Scholar
University of the Pacific
McGeorge School of Law
Sacramento, CA

*This text brings to light the necessary role of interagency collaboration in child exploitation cases while providing direct guidance through case study and lessons of necessary considerations, benefits and limitations of emerging tools, and strategies for the investigation, proper assessment, and ongoing management of perpetrators.*

Margaret Bullens
Forensic Psychophysiologist and Sex
Offender Management Consultant
Grapevine, TX

*Very worthwhile and a must-read for law enforcement and other professionals involved in identifying, rescuing, and treating child victims of sexual abuse. This book allows the reader to better understand how and why individuals use the computer to facilitate the sexual exploitation of children.*

Det Sgt Paul Gillespie
Officer In Charge
Child Exploitation Section
Toronto Police Service
Toronto, Canada

*Whether it is child prostitution, trafficking, cyber-enticement, child pornography, or sex tourism, tens of thousands of children suffer irreparable physical and psychological harm from producers and customers of this form of abuse. As a leader in the education of forensic nurses, the International Association of Forensic Nurses supports all efforts to educate healthcare providers, criminal justice and social service professionals about the crimes of child exploitation. Since there is presently a lack of evidence-based information, we look forward to this new professional resource.*

International Association of Forensic
Nurses (IAFN)
Board of Directors, 2005-2006

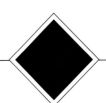

# CONTENTS IN BRIEF

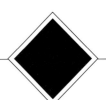

# CONTENTS IN DETAIL

## VOLUME ONE

**CHAPTER 4:** RAPE SURVIVORS: PSYCHOSOCIAL PROBLEMS AND
INVESTIGATION IN SOUTHERN ASIA

**CHAPTER 5:** THE COMMERCIAL SEXUAL EXPLOITATION OF
CHILDREN IN THE UNITED STATES

**CHAPTER 6:** WHAT IT IS LIKE TO BE "SERVED" IN THE "SYSTEM":
A SURVIVOR'S PERSPECTIVE

**CHAPTER 7:** ADULT SURVIVORS OF THE CHILD SEXUAL
EXPLOITATION INDUSTRY: PSYCHOLOGICAL PROFILES

# CHAPTER 16: PSYCHOSOCIAL CONTEXT LEADING JUVENILES TO PROSTITUTION AND SEXUAL EXPLOITATION

# CHAPTER 17: MEDICAL CARE OF THE CHILDREN OF THE NIGHT

## CHAPTER 18: THE MEDICAL IMPLICATIONS OF ANOGENITAL TRAUMA IN CHILD SEXUAL EXPLOITATION

## CHAPTER 22: THE USE OF THE INTERNET FOR CHILD SEXUAL EXPLOITATION

## VOLUME TWO

## CHAPTER 23: ACQUAINTANCE CHILD MOLESTERS: A BEHAVIORAL ANALYSIS

## CHAPTER 31: HUMAN TRAFFICKING FOR SEXUAL EXPLOITATION: THE ROLE OF INTERPOL

## CHAPTER 32: INVESTIGATION AND PROSECUTION OF THE PROSTITUTION OF CHILDREN

## CHAPTER 33: INTERNET PEDOPHILIA

## CHAPTER 34: THE MEDICAL EXPERT AND CHILD SEXUAL EXPLOITATION

## CHAPTER 35: COMPUTER FORENSIC SOFTWARE AND ITS LEGAL VALIDATION

## CHAPTER 36: INTERNET TRAVELERS

## CHAPTER 37: ESTABLISHING CRIMINAL CONSPIRACY AND AIDER AND ABETTOR LIABILITY FOR GROUPS THAT PROMOTE SEXUAL EXPLOITATION OF CHILDREN

## CHAPTER 38: THE HIDDEN TRUTH OF INVOLUNTARY SERVITUDE AND SLAVERY

## CHAPTER 45: SHADOW CHILDREN: ADDRESSING THE COMMERCIAL EXPLOITATION OF CHILDREN IN RURAL AMERICA

## CHAPTER 46: RECOMMENDATIONS FOR ACTION FOR DEALING EFFECTIVELY WITH CHILD SEXUAL EXPLOITATION

# Medical, Legal, & Social Science Aspects of

# Child Sexual

# Exploitation

## A Comprehensive Review of Pornography, Prostitution, and Internet Crimes

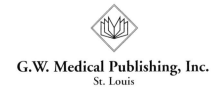

G.W. Medical Publishing, Inc.

St. Louis

# A Brief History of Child Sexual Exploitation

Sharon W. Cooper, MD, FAAP

A discussion of the history of sexual exploitation must include pornography and prostitution; these 2 entities are closely intertwined. It is common for children and youth who have been exploited through one venue to be victimized by the other. In ancient times, images that were drawn, carved, or chronicled were felt to have been reproductions or reminiscent of actual experiences. Consequently, the unfolding of centuries of sexual practices with intermittent travesties crosses cultures, religions, and even the developments of the so-called spoils of war that led to exploitation reserved for enslaved populations.

It is difficult to separate child exploitation historically from that of adults for several reasons:

1. Children were often seen in historical times as chattel with little value to their lives. Consequently, their use as sexual objects was not worthy of close scrutiny and, therefore, was not necessarily worthy of documentation.

2. Many ancient societies were patriarchal, and the position of women and children was far below the needs and desires of men. Because of this, child sexual abuse and exploitation were not acknowledged and were less likely to be documented or seen as illegal.

3. The gradual transition from childhood to adulthood was often heralded by puberty. Because these physiological changes varied in different centuries, cultures, and ethnic groups, exploitation of children is more difficult to define in a historical sense.

For these reasons, historical reviews will often combine adult and child pornography and prostitution, recognizing that many children and youth were included in such sexual practices.

## Ancient Civilizations

Pornography has been present for centuries. The word *pornography* is derived from the Greek words *porni* ("prostitute") and *graphein* ("to write"). In the Greek and Roman era, erotic and obscene themes were readily depicted in literature and art. Dionysus, the Greek god of wine, brought to literature frivolity and resulting drunkenness and the eastern orgies with their associated religious themes. Dionysus, often referred to in Roman mythology as Bacchus, was the source of salacious writings of songs performed at ancient Greek festivals. These writings became some of the first written historical evidences of pornography.

### Ancient Egypt

The ancient Egyptians developed the process of using the papyrus plant to make sails, cords, and paper. Paper made from the papyrus plant, which was the chief writing material in ancient Egypt, was adopted by the Greeks, and was used extensively in the Roman Empire. Used mainly as scrolls for legal documents and as pages for the production of books, it was also used for correspondences. Consequently, the pornographic texts were initially documented on papyrus. Papyrus became unnecessary in the eighth and ninth centuries AD when other plant fibers were introduced.

## THE OLD TESTAMENT

Biblical history described and warned against sexual exploitation primarily regarding the use of prostitutes. Sexual favors, as described in the Old Testament, were often for the purposes of hospitality or for procreation when a wife was infertile. Such was the case when Sarai gave Abram her handmaid, Hagar, who later bore the child Ishmael (Genesis 16:1-16) (Rainbow Studies Inc, 1996). Concubines were considered different from prostitutes in Biblical times because they were mistresses who lived in the homes of their patrons. Concubines may have been girls or women and were housed separately from the wives of the patriarch. Prostitution was not thought to exist in the early Israelite tribes until they came in contact with the Canaanites in the 15th century (Third Millennium Trust, 1890). The Canaanites had fertility cults and worshipped gods in temples, temples which had their own prostitutes. The Israelites began to divide prostitutes into 2 separate categories: the zonah, which were profane prostitutes, and the q'deshah, or the holy prostitutes. The latter, referred to as shrine prostitutes, were derived from those cultures that had polytheistic deities (Larue, 1998).

Hebrew law did not forbid prostitution but confined the practice to foreign women. In the Book of Leviticus, which was written around 1500 BC, Israelites were warned regarding the dangers of prostitution. The 19th chapter was devoted to instructions for holy living. In particular, it was considered a traresty for parents to lead their children to a life of prostitution: "Do not degrade your daughter by making her a prostitute, or the land will turn to prostitution and be filled with wickedness" (Leviticus 19:29) (Rainbow Studies Inc, 1996). In addition, Israelites were warned against becoming prostitutes: "No Israelite man or woman is to become a shrine prostitute. You must not bring the earnings of a female prostitute or of a male prostitute into the house of the Lord your God to pay any vow, because the Lord your God detests them both" (Deuteronomy 23:17) (Rainbow Studies Inc, 1996).

Not all prostitutes in the Bible, however, were seen as evil. In the Book of Joshua in the Old Testament, Rahab was a well-known and respected prostitute who hid 2 spies sent by Joshua to survey the land of Jericho, in exchange for the safety of her family. She let them down by a rope through a window in her house, over the city wall, to escape guards from the king of Jericho (Joshua 2:1-15) (Rainbow Studies Inc, 1996).

## ANCIENT GREECE

In ancient Greece, around the fifth century BC, art and culture reflected the diversified roles of girls and women. Athenian girls were usually married by the age of 14 to 15 years, whereas the Athenian women of Sparta were specifically forbidden to marry before the age of 18 years. Spartan women were thought to have a higher level of respectability and were not to be depicted as showing any flesh. Even in Athenian art depicting marital relations between husbands and wives, the women were completely clothed, while their husbands were nude.

The Greeks sought to establish a "refined" level of prostitution. This embodiment was the *hetaera*, or the groomed prostitute. Greek men had concubines (who would be called mistresses in the current era) for their daily bodily care, wives for legitimate childbearing, and hetaerae for pleasure. Even though the hetaerae were beautifully cared for and coiffed, they were still treated as prostitutes and were beaten and raped at the will of their sponsors. Grecian artwork of the hetaerae occasionally depicted beatings with fists, sticks, and sandals. Though the hetaerae were highly refined and similar to Japanese geishas in their skills as courtesans, they were usually slaves from the poorest classes. Other classes of prostitutes included the streetwalkers, prostitutes who were confined to brothels, and the temple or consecrated prostitutes (**Figure 1-1**).

Brothel prostitutes were sometimes the daughters of Athenians who had sold them as infants to the brothels as an alternative to infanticide (Garrison, 2000).

Homosexual prostitution was also common in ancient Greece. Although described in Greek literature, it was censored from the artwork of that time. In paintings discovered through archeological expeditions, homosexual men were depicted together fully clothed although homosexual male prostitutes were depicted nude (Garrison, 2000).

## ANCIENT ROME

Further pictorial evidence of pornography was found at the ancient Roman city of Pompeii, dating from the first century AD where erotic drawings covered numerous walls recounting sexual orgies. Vase paintings, wall paintings, and sculptured images clearly revealed many forms of sexual practices, not the least of which was pedophilia. Roman art, which depicted the deviant and perverse, provided material for obscene written discourse. Such "art" was often confined to the collections of the Roman elite, and when it depicted child pornographic themes, it was seen as a more liberal sexual view than the norm. This was particularly true, for example, in the circumstance of the silver Warren cup, dating probably from the Augustan period (100 BC to 200 AD), which portrayed on one side of the cup a man-boy couple engaged in sex, and 2 adult men engaged in sex on the other side, a behavior well recognized to be outside the Roman norm for gender and sexuality (Verstraete, 1999).

Written pornography was found in the epigrams of Catullus and Martial in the first century BC. Most of Martial's love poetry was heterosexual, but **pederasty**, or descriptions of homosexual anal intercourse, were certainly present in a finite number of his works. The *Priapea* is a collection of poems in which the phallic god Priapus is the speaker. This work describes the association of erotic stimulation and penile tumescence. Centuries later, the medical term **priapism** was derived to mean persistent erection of the penis, not intentionally associated with sexual stimulation. The writings of the ancient Greco-Roman genre contained what were proposed to be sexual fantasy-like ideations. It was important that the reader understand that the suggested risqué themes were separate from the personal lives of the authors. Martial writes that "my writing is salacious, but my life virtuous" (Verstraete, 1999). This written dismissal of the veracity of the themes as a personal thought process is frequently seen in contemporary Internet-based pornographic "fantasy" writings. These writings are often found in association with child pornography image collections.

Homer's well-known work, the *Iliad*, detailed many of the trysts that Zeus had with mortal women, and there was the suggestion of the comic domestic context of Zeus' troubles with his wife Hera. The *Odyssey* has a more central erotic theme though it is somewhat more subtle. The poetry of Ovid's *Ars Amatoria* (*The Art of Love*) was a treatise on the skill and art of sensual arousal, sexual seduction, and the psychological intrigue associated with the process. This translation of Ovid by Rolfe Humphries (1970) shows the lead-in to its most explicit parts, in which Ovid daringly described and recommended various lovemaking positions:

In our last lesson we deal with matters peculiarly secret;
Venus reminds us that here lies her most intimate care.
What a girl ought to know is herself, adapting her method,
Taking advantage of ways nature equips her to use.

Such poetry dealing with the erotic was meant to be sexually stimulating. Consequently, it was ironic that Ovid warned in the beginning that his work was not to be read by respectable Roman matrons (Verstraete, 1999).

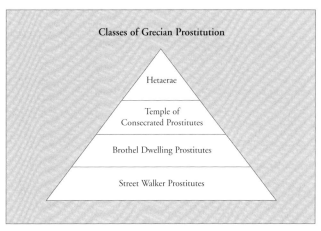

**Figure 1-1.** *Classes of prostitution in ancient Greece.*

Classes of Grecian Prostitution

Hetaerae

Temple of Consecrated Prostitutes

Brothel Dwelling Prostitutes

Street Walker Prostitutes

However, Ovid's *Ars Amatoria*, in conjunction with his political indiscretions, led to his banishment by Augustus to the outskirts of the Roman Empire until his death around 18 AD. Consequently, Ovid was the only author in Greco-Roman times who was severely punished and censored for writing pornographic literature. Ovid had actually encouraged certain readers to avoid his writings so that he could not be accused of advocating adultery, even though in the patriarchal Roman times, adultery was not seen as a huge indiscretion. It was Augustus who outlawed the practice of adultery for the first time. Ovid's warnings seemed insincere and certainly contradicted the tone and content of his erotic poetry.

### ANCIENT CHINA

Written pornography was not limited to the Greek and Roman cultures. In ancient China, during the Chou Dynasty (770 BC to 222 BC), Taoist doctrine began to evolve though Taoism was not yet a formal religion. The philosophy behind the sexual aspects of this religion was based upon the belief that men and women were divided and designated as the yin and the yang (**Figure 1-2**). Women were thought to have a limitless supply of the yin, which was closely linked with orgasms and sexual pleasure, if not ecstasy. The yang essence was the limited supply of male ejaculate and had to be carefully guarded from autoeroticism or masturbation. During this period, prostitution was acceptable because men thought that they could gain more yin from prostitutes than from normal women. However, ancient Chinese medicine began to correctly describe diseases that men would develop after being with prostitutes, and there began to be warnings regarding the yin of prostitutes.

Of course, pornography in the ancient Chinese era was not restricted to heterosexual relationships. The act of sodomy was sanctified by Tcheou-Wang, the god of Sodomy. Therefore, during the Manchu Dynasty (17 BC to 20 BC), classic erotic literature and images often depicted anal sex. During this time, Chin P'ing Mei depicted adult male sex with boys. This encouraged the social acceptance of boy prostitution and propagated the practice of boy sexual companions for the wealthy. This was in the time period that male geisha houses in Japan were recognized as acceptable.

Paper has been traced to the Chinese in about 170 BC. Its use reached central Asia around 750 AD, and by the 14th century paper mills were in several parts of Europe. This development allowed written documents to be duplicated by scores of scribes and disseminated more easily than in ancient Egyptian times, when papyrus required a more lengthy process for paper production.

During the Han Dynasty (25 AD to 220 AD), Taoist doctrine began to be refined and propagated. At this time, pornographic "texts" began to circulate, such as *The Handbook of the Plain Girl* and *The Art of the Bedchamber*. These works referred to a Yellow Emperor who was attempting to live a long and healthy life by obtaining immortality through sex. Part of this immortality arose from a woman's yin essence. Metaphors and symbols became evident in ancient Chinese literature and art, such as the color red for women and white for men. By 600 AD, during the Sui Dynasty, more pornographic sexual literature emerged, which described in great detail unique sexual positions with animal-like names (Golden, 2002).

## THE MIDDLE AGES

During the subsequent centuries, pornography remained entertainment for the upper classes in Eurasia and China. After the Fall of Rome in 410 AD, the rise and spread of Islam began to change societal attitudes toward the light and farcical treatment of sexuality. Following the teachings of the Quran, many restrictive rules were instituted regarding relationships between men and women. The use of women for anything other than procreation and mutual respect was forbidden by the Islamic religion.

Between the second and fifth centuries AD, Hinduism became more prominent in the illustration of sexuality. During this time, the concept of Kama became more main-

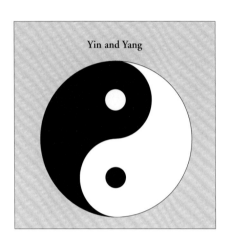

Yin and Yang

**Figure 1-2.** *Ancient Chinese symbol of men and women within the context of sexual symbiosis.*

stream. The most well-known collection of Kama literature was the 10 000 chapters of the *Kamasutra*, initially announced by Nandi, Shiva's companion (Vatsyayana, 1994). In this Hindu text, simplistically stated, there were 3 aims in life:

— *Dharma*, or virtue, which referred to the need for social duty

— *Artha*, or prosperity, which emphasized the need for collection of wealth for the family

— *Kama*, or love, which instructed the art and skill of physical lovemaking

Often referred to as the oldest textbook of erotic love, the *Kamasutra* was composed in Sanskrit, which was the literary language of ancient India. The book was about more than sex, however; it included information on finding a life partner, living with or living as an adult or youth courtesan, using drugs, maintaining power and control in a marriage, committing adultery, and the many positions available to lovers for sexual pleasure. A collection of illustrations of these sexual encounters was created centuries later. Its reception in India and Europe was historically notable, and its impact upon society and sexual mores has continued to promote lively discussion in the 21st century (Vatsyayana, 2002).

During the Middle Ages, pornography remained primarily in the written format, as common jokes, satire, and even riddles. A principal theme of European medieval pornography was the sexual behaviors of monks and clergy in association with their hypocritical public protestations. It is important to recall that during this era, children were thought to have the value of chattel, and because of this, child pornography and prostitution were not seen as human rights violations. Children were often sold to support their family's survival. Female children who were sold into indentured servitude were frequently cast into the dual role of servant and sexual partner.

Once children became older and were no longer the sexual preference of the masters or had run away, they likely had to resort to a life of prostitution out of a dire need, as is the case today. In Europe, attempts were made by church leaders to rehabilitate penitent prostitutes and provide funding for their dowries. However, the revenue produced by the sex trade has historically been so significant that, often in the Middle Ages, this form of sex work was protected, licensed, and regulated by law. Public brothels and bordellos were well established in larger cities and frequently protected by law enforcement as a means of providing safe and sanctioned outlets for physical pleasures.

In Toulouse, France, in the 17th and 18th centuries, the cities and the university shared the profits of government-sanctioned bordellos. In England, the bishops of Winchester and subsequently the Parliament licensed these establishments. Because there was minimal concern during that era for the protection of children, promoting a child into a lifestyle of prostitution was neither forbidden nor punished.

During this same period in India, the tradition of the *mahari* or *devadasi* of the temples became commonplace; these were children who were offered as dancers and as sanctioned, consecrated sexual initiators in the Yellamma cult. The devadasis were usually trained in the art of dance from childhood and would be officially married to the Temple of God at the onset of puberty. The dance form performed by the devasdasis was erotic and spiritual. This tradition was well established by the 10th century AD. Temples were built to honor the goddess Yellamma (also known as Jogamma, Holiyyamma, Renuka, and other names) in the Belgaum district, the Shimoga district, and the district of Karnataka State. Additional regions today devoted to the Yellamma cult include the Maharashtra and Andhra Pradesh.

Female and male children could be dedicated to the goddess Yellamma. Girls were referred to as Jogathis and boys as Jogappa. The ritual of their dedication required total nudity, and these rites were repeated at least twice a year. Controversy remains regarding the attitudes of foreign authorities, particularly the British, who expressed great concern for the plight of these children. The concerns were based on the many reports of corruption and the prostitution of children associated with the temple priests. This concern originates from the role of highly religious followers that serve their deity by attending to the needs of the general public, which includes sexual urges of men. Various state governments have banned the nude parade of worshippers of the goddess Yellamma, and although this tradition continues today, men frequently assume the roles of both the Jogathis and the Jogappa. Many Indian girls and women refuse because they do not wish to be associated with the illusion or reality of prostitution.

This tradition of the devadasi has survived many centuries; although it is illegal, the Indian Health Organization estimates that 1000 girls are dedicated each year, a decrease from 7000 each year in the late 1980s. Those children who are dedicated to the goddess Yellamma and who have not yet reached puberty will return home, but upon their sexual maturational development, they will be sold into the sexual traffic king trade in larger cities such as Bombay (Reuters, 1997a,b).

It is believed that child pornography became more mainstream in the 1400s in China with the sex manual *The Admirable Discourses of the Plain Girl*, in which sexual intercourse and other sexual acts involving children were graphically described (Tannahill, 1980). Printed texts of this type involved engraved woodblocks. Movable type, consisting of individual elements from which texts could be composed and then printed, was devised in China in the 11th century, but the complexity of the language discouraged the further development of the technique.

## THE RENAISSANCE

Printing from carved woodblocks appeared in Europe in the 14th century. Johann Gutenberg brought together the 2 ideas of movable type and woodblocks constituting the invention of modern printing. The use of dies to make individual pieces of type that could be assembled as required and reused, and the use of a press by which sharp impressions could be made many times over, on both sides of a sheet of paper if desired, brought this technology to the forefront. The ability to provide copies of one document in large quantities led to an immense increase in the demand and the supply for written and pornographic imagery. Prior to this time, handmade copies of written and visual images of pornography took significant time to reproduce and distribute. Now, pornography had the potential for a new high-volume medium. It was the printing press, the emergence of the novel as a literary form, and the creation of a middle class along with the changes wrought by the Renaissance, the Enlightenment, and the French Revolution that established pornography as a more distinct and recognized literary category.

The 16th century in Italy revealed that politics played a much greater role than was seen in England, making pornography more politically motivated. In its earliest growth after the end of the Middle Ages in Europe, pornography's main purpose was that of subversion and stimulation of unrest within political boundaries. It was meant to shock the reader. The most celebrated originator of European pornography is thought to have been Pietro Aretino, author of *I Modi*. A resident of Venice, Italy, a journalist, a publicist, an entrepreneur, and an art dealer who made a living writing political tracts and essays, Aretino created and circulated *I Modi* to an increasingly literate audience. Privately printed texts were no longer solely found in possession of the elite aristocrats. The production of *I Modi* involved the collaboration of 3 major artists of the Renaissance: Aretino, Giulio Romano, and Marcantonio Raimondi.

Romano, a great Mannerist painter and former pupil of Raphael, drew 16 scenes of pornographic heterosexual couples in erotic detail on some of the Vatican walls. It was thought that he had a vendetta against Pope Clement VII, who was indebted to Romano.

Raimondo, one of the foremost engravers of the time, made copper plates of Romano's work, which was subsequently named *I Modi* (literally, "postures"). Raimondo printed copies, circulating them among the Roman aristocrats. This outraged the pope to such a degree that he ordered all of the pornographic plates destroyed, with threat of death if prints were made.

Later, Aretino wrote 16 sonnets to accompany the illegal *I Modi* prints from Raimondi's engravings (Beck, 1999). Aretino's actions had 2 purposes: to depict lush sex in vivid terms and to mock the papal court as a repository of corruption. Aretino subsequently wrote of variations in sexual appetites to include pedophilia. Aretino's style of pornographic writing became so popular that many artists and writers borrowed heavily from the Aretinian tradition long after his death in 1556. Throughout Europe, the term "Aretinian postures" became synonymous with the depiction of acrobatic sex (Beck, 1999).

## THE AGE OF ENLIGHTENMENT

Seventeenth-century Europe ushered in the beginning of the Age of Enlightenment, when basic attitudes about authority, religion, science, and society began to change. The propagation of sexual pleasure became almost a new "religion" during this time. Hedonism, or the belief that pleasure is the chief good in life, grew. Hedonism was and is a continuing belief used to rationalize having sex with children. The value of science gained a greater interest in the whole area of sexuality. An example of the overt nature of sexuality was illustrated by condoms becoming available in London in the 1660s, as a scientific response to the need to avoid sexually transmitted diseases and pregnancy.

## PURITANISM

During the late 16th century and 17th century a religious reform movement began in England, which sought to purify the Church of England from remnants of the Roman Catholic Church. Followers of this religious reform movement were called Puritans. The Puritans developed a belief system that moral and religious earnestness would reform the entire nation and bring about a transformation from the lifestyle of debauchery, crime, and exploitation. The Puritan movement brought about a time of punishment for those who were found guilty of a myriad of behaviors. It was Oliver Cromwell who, as the head of state of England, prompted a political agenda based on moral reformations. Prostitution, in particular, or any degree of sexual deviancy, brought such severe physical and social repercussions that the period after Oliver Cromwell's death in 1658 became known as the Great Persecution. This term was rightly applied and to such a degree that civil unrest followed the Great Persecution. Eventually, the Act of Toleration, which allowed for the development of dissenting religious groups, came to define England's religious solution in 1689.

Thomas Dale brought Puritanism to the American colony of Virginia, but its greatest spread in the United States was in New England. The New England Puritans fashioned the civil laws according to the framework of the church. In so doing, sexual impropriety received a significant civil response. Punishment, imprisonment, and even death were common consequences of prostitution. Such consequences began a legal pattern of harshness toward prostitutes which continues today. Prostituted children and adults were often found in brothels referred to as "bawdy houses." During this period, women were regarded as physically weak but were expected to be morally strong. The home was their domain, and such ideology left no room for poor women who had to enter the work force out of necessity.

Unwed mothers, some of whom were youths, were held in such disdain that they were often placed in workhouses for minor criminals. Some women chose to become prostitutes to avoid the work-houses. Such women could not receive any social aid although vagrants could readily attain assistance. Prostituted women and girls were targeted because during the Puritan era, high moral standards were consistent with Boston's reputation and economy, and such women and girls brought a poor impact upon the public image. Eventually, riots broke out when the city did not move swiftly enough to destroy bawdy houses, and rioters destroyed almost all such establishments.

## PORNOGRAPHY AND LITERATURE

The connection between prostitution and pornography continued to be evident as more art and literature of a pornographic nature highlighted the escapades of "happy prostitutes" in the late 1600s. Some of the themes frequently included young schoolgirls or adolescents who were "coming of age" as their sexual development left them with no recourse but to entice and seduce. As Italy made its contribution to the history of pornography, so did France. Many thought that France was the most sexually radical culture in Europe in the late 1600s and in later years.

A preponderance of female characters heralded the early French works, which became landmarks of "Europorn" at that time. *L'Ecole des Filles* (1650) and *L'Academie des Dames* (1680) were written in the Aretinian style. Anonymously penned (although thought to have been written by Michel Millot and Jean L'Ange), *L'Ecole des Filles* idealized sex between 2 adolescents, a 16-year-old and her older cousin. This work was offensive because it represented a significant undermining of the moral teachings of parents and religion. Its language was explicit and its characters enthusiastic. It was also felt to have been written in protest of Louis XIV's climate of political repression (Beck, 1999).

In the 18th century, there emerged a literary form seemingly devoted exclusively to the sexual arousal of the reader. A small underground trafficking group became apparent in England, which both published and sold such pornographic works. An example included John Cleland's book, *Memoirs of a Woman of Pleasure*, which later became known as *Fannie Hill*. This book described the practice of prostitution taught to young girls and is among the most frequently reprinted, translated, and illustrated of all English novels in history. It has been available legally in the United States only since 1963 and in England since 1970 (Sabor, 1985).

In the subsequent years leading to the French Revolution, politically motivated pornography grew tremendously in quantity. Of particular note was the slanderous pornographic writings regarding the wife of King Louis XVI, Queen Marie Antoinette. Pamphlets were written questioning the paternity of her children and accusing her of wild orgies and of presumed lesbian activities. The descriptions of these illicit behaviors were graphically pornographic. The purpose of these attacks was to undermine the monarchy. Degrading the queen had a kind of leveling, democratizing effect, particularly when she was portrayed as having sex with members of the lower classes. These attacks continued until she was beheaded in 1793.

The next lasting mark made in European pornographic history was the writings of Donatien Alphonse Francoise de Sade, known more popularly as the Marquis de Sade. Sade's pornographic writings focused on the annihilation of the body in pursuit of pleasure. All social restrictions, including pedophilia, were ignored. Many of the themes in modern pornography, written and in videography, were touched upon in Sade's novels. Sade's writings were not so much sexually provocative as violent and blasphemous. His was not a written world of men and women but of masters and slaves. He wrote of orgy scenes in *Juliette*, for example, where role reversal took place, and females became aggressive and predatory. This pornographic literature predicted the development of the fictional and eventual real-life dominatrix. Such a woman often provides sadistic sexual pleasure by causing pain and subservience to whomever she seeks to control in a given encounter. Any other form of sexual encounter besides a heterosexual one was preferred in Sade's writings.

*The Misfortunes of Virtue*, which is considered Sade's greatest contribution to 18th-century fiction, was later revised and renamed *The New Justine* in 1797. This book is a story of a young virtuous girl who suffers the whips and branding irons of her persecutors. The destruction of innocence, particularly if the victim was young and female, was a favorite theme of Sade's. He particularly preferred to highlight his "heroes" as those who tortured and murdered their victims. Sade's influence continues well into the 21st century, where themes of sadomasochism predominate in pornography.

Lebegue (1991) reviewed more than 3000 magazine and book titles of pornography so ascertained by the 1985 Attorney General's Commission on Obscenity and Pornography. This research sought to define if the titles suggested a specific and recognized form of paraphilia. Lebegue determined whether the title did infer a clinical paraphilia and then if the content of the materials actually demonstrated what the title suggested. The results of this review revealed that 16.7% of the total titles were consistent with perversions, and 49.9% of the perversion titles were sadomasochistic, more than 4 times more than any other perversion cited. The second most common paraphilia noted was incest (Lebegue, 1991). The results are summarized in **Table 1-1**. These results do not include ***partialism***, the concentration on body parts with sexual significance.

# THE 19TH CENTURY
## GOVERNMENT REGULATION
The Society for the Suppression of Vice was an organization founded in 1802 in London to "check the spread of open vice and immorality, and more especially to preserve the minds of the young from contamination by exposure to the corrupting

### Table 1-1. US Titles Excluding Partialism

| PARAPHILIA | NUMBER OF TITLES | % OF PARAPHILIA TITLES | % OF ALL TITLES |
|---|---|---|---|
| Exhibitionism | 1 | 0.2 | 0.03 |
| Fetishism | 38 | 7.4 | 1.24 |
| Frotteurism | 0 | 0.0 | 0.0 |
| Pedophilia | 25 | 4.9 | 0.81 |
| Sadomasochism | 256 | 49.9 | 8.39 |
| Transvestism | 55 | 10.7 | 1.8 |
| Voyeurism | 5 | 1.0 | 0.16 |
| Telephone scatologia | 0 | 0.0 | 0.0 |
| Necrophilia | 0 | 0.0 | 0.0 |
| Zoophilia | 17 | 3.3 | 0.56 |
| Coprophilia | 0 | 0.0 | 0.0 |
| Klismaphilia | 4 | 0.8 | 0.13 |
| Urophilia | 2 | 0.4 | 0.06 |
| **Total paraphilia titles** | 403 | 78.6% | 13.18% |
| Incest | 110 | 21.4% | 3.6% |
| **Total perversion titles** | 513 | 100.0% | 16.78% |

*Reprinted with permission from Lebegue B. Paraphilias in US pornography titles: "pornography made me do it" (Ted Bundy).* Bull Amer Acad Psychiatry Law. *1991;19(1):43-48.*

influence of impure and licentious books, prints, and other publications" (The Leisure Hour, 1872). The power of the Society for the Suppression of Vice grew with the passing in 1857 of the Obscene Publications Act by Lord Campbell, the Lord Chief Justice. London's Holywell Street was known as the Bookseller's Row because it was full of print shops and bookshops. During Victorian times, it was unregulated, and at one point there were 57 pornography shops on Holywell Street, all with display signs to attract potential shoppers. Pornographic novels, erotic prints, etchings, and catalogs for prostitutes that contained their "specialties" were all sold there. Successful prosecutions took place after the establishment of the Obscene Publications Act, with the most celebrated being that of William Dugdale, a blackmailer, forger, plagiarist, and a most prolific pornographer of the age.

Twenty years after the first laws regarding pornography in England were passed, the United States passed the Comstock Law (1873), named after its strongest advocate, Anthony Comstock. This law made it a felony in the Unites States to deposit mail that was obscene, lewd, or lascivious. This included books, pamphlets, pictures, writings, paper, or other publications. This was to be enforced by the inspector of the United States Postal Service. This was the first documented federal investigative agency with a mission to eradicate the distribution of pornography. The New York Society for the Suppression of Vice was established with a similar goal as that of England (New York Society for the Supression of Vice, 1936).

In 1868, the Hicklin rule was enacted in England, imposing one of the tightest gags ever. It established that the test for obscenity was whether or not material could corrupt those whose minds were open to immoral influences. This rule, though a serious deterrent, caused pornography to become more of an underground publication operation. *The Pearl*, which was published between 1879 and 1880, contained serialized novels and short stories with a heavy interest in flagellation, homosexuality, and bisexuality. It became one of the first secret and outlawed pornographic documents.

## CHANGES IN FAMILY LIFESTYLES

From the 16th century to the 19th century, families gradually began to live apart from the workplace, and their homes, which were initially single great rooms, began to change. Sexual relations began to occur behind closed doors, and as the Puritan era approached, sexuality developed a "sinful" mantle. Children began to be taught that their bodies were something to be ashamed of and that they were not to refer to their "legs" or "bellies" by anything but the proper terms—for example, "limbs" or "lower portions." The 19th century brought about the Victorian era, during which parents were frightened that their children would masturbate, or commit "self-abuse," leading to insanity, tuberculosis, syphilis, impotency, sterility, deformities, and epilepsy. It was during this time that children were viewed in a more humane and even romantic way. Concerns for their protection began to supersede their previous value as a commodity. It was because of this gradual consideration of children that sexual references began to be phrased within the context of "love" (Yates, 1996).

Late-Victorian erotica studies must include *My Secret Life*, a 4000-page prolific, firsthand portrait of Victorian sexuality. "Walter," whom experts believe was in reality Sir Henry Spencer Ashbee, wrote this book. Sir Ashbee was a well-known collector of erotic books who ultimately donated his huge collection to the British Library. *My Secret Life* chronicles Walter's sexual exploits with more than 1200 women. This book describes the exploitation of women and girls with particular attention to prostituted children.

## THE INFLUENCE OF PHOTOGRAPHY

Child pornography was becoming more popular through the development and use of the daguerreotype. This precursor of the camera was invented by a Frenchman, Louis Jacques Mande Daguerre, in 1837. Just 3 years later, the first American patent was issued in photography to Alexander Wolcott for his camera, and during each subsequent decade, the field of photography and eventually videography became more mainstream and refined.

It was during this time that a clergyman of the Oxford University Christ Church College named Charles L. Dodgson (1832-1898) began to keep diaries that referred to his photographing of young girls. His first entries were about photographing a nude girl in which he refers to the child, Beatrice Latham, age 6, as "sans habiliment" (Tyler & Stone, 1985). Though the photographs, which have survived, would not likely be considered obscene by today's standards, in the Victorian era nudity was considered scandalous, shocking, and pornographic (see **Figure 1-3** for an example).

While at least one writer considered Dodgson an "avid collector" (Anson, 1980) of child pornography, many others have defended his reputation, suggesting that children were perceived as asexual during this time in history. In 1880, Dodgson abandoned photography altogether; it is speculated that this was to avoid scandal. Dodgson was also a writer of children's stories. His most well-known publications were *Alice's Adventures in Wonderland* (**Figure 1-4**) and *Through the Looking Glass*, written under the pen name of Lewis Carroll (Tyler & Stone, 1985).

## PORNOGRAPHY AND PROSTITUTION IN THE 20TH AND 21ST CENTURIES

A discussion of child pornography is interwoven into adult pornography literature because of the frequent association of the use of young teenagers in such photographic productions. One of many factors that contributed to the use of children in the production of pornography and subsequent prostitution stems from the tradition of regarding children as asexual objects and marketable commodities. Not until the 20th century did various countries begin to restrict written and visual depictions of youths' sexuality (Mirkin, 1999).

In the first half of the 20th century, child pornography was predominantly found in photographs, books, and magazines. After the 1940s, children were included in the pornographic motion pictures industry. With the advent of videography and the Internet in the early 1960s, propagation of this contraband became infinitely easier. As the Internet became available to the general public by the early 1990s, control of dissemination of still images and videographic pornography became more problematic. Often referred to as "kiddie porn" and "chicken porn," nearly every form of child sexual abuse and perversion was produced, including rape, sadism, bestiality, pedophilia, and even murder.

In the early years of the 20th century, prostitution was seen as mainstream. This was particularly the case in larger cities in the United States. There was less discussion regarding whether or not women and children were voluntarily entrepreneurs or victims of a terrible vice forced by poverty than there was regarding the need to eradicate this business because of the threat to public decency and public health. Between 1907 and 1914, a major concern arose regarding "white slavery," a phenomenon in which girls and women were forced into sexual work through brothels after having been kidnapped and taken far from their homes. This concept became somewhat sensationalized although there was likely some degree of authenticity of the events in American society.

In response to the threat of what would be the precursor to modern-day "traveler cases," a federal law was enacted called the White Slave Traffic Act (Mann Act). Written by Illinois congressman James R. Mann, this law prohibited the transportation of individuals in interstate or foreign commerce for the

*Figure 1-3.* Alice Liddell photographed by Charles Dodgson in 1858 as "The Beggar Maid." Reprinted from Nickel DR. *Dreaming in Pictures: The Photography of Lewis Carroll.* New Haven, Conn: Yale University Press; 2002.

*Figure 1-4.* "Down the rabbit hole" illustration from Lewis Carroll's Alice's Adventures in Wonderland. Reprinted from Carroll L. *Alice's Adventures in Wonderland.* New York, NY: The Macmillan Company; 1898:16.

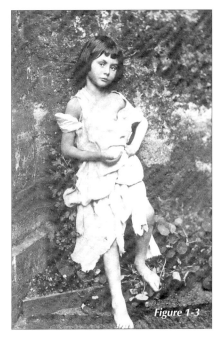

*Figure 1-3*

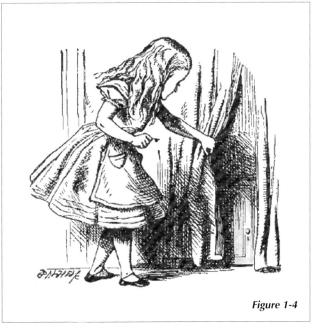

*Figure 1-4*

purpose of engaging in prostitution or any sexual activity. For several years, this act was misused and resulted in prosecution of consenting adults who crossed state lines to engage in sexual relations. Although the spirit of the law was to discourage prostitution, in the era of Prohibition and fundamentalism, the government investigated noncommercial transgressors with zeal.

The phenomenon of white slavery has a disturbingly predictive echo of the modern-day cyber-enticement cases presently being described in many countries. Instead of children being kidnapped from their homes, they are enticed to leave their homes voluntarily, only to be sexually assaulted and used as a commodity for pornography and prostitution. As in the early 1900s, these children fall prey to the false impression that they have met a potential romantic partner, or a young person who has similar interests. At times, adolescents are coerced to travel thousands of miles from their homes (traveler cases) and are subjected to a sadomasochistic sexual slavery scenario from which the only escape is a life of prostitution.

Justification for the use of children as prostitutes has national and international roots. In addition to children being viewed as unreliable witnesses that can be easily intimidated into silence, there are many myths that contribute to the use of children for paid sexual gratification. These are listed in **Table 1-2**.

---

**Table 1-2. Myths That Promote Child Prostitution**

— Children are free from sexually transmitted diseases.

— Children are not at risk for HIV/AIDS.

— Children may cure an individual of HIV/AIDS.

— Children are psychologically more resilient than adults.

— Sex constitutes a compassionate "rite of passage" for children, particularly in same-sex encounters.

— Religious mores lend to the use of virgin children for sexual cleansing.

— Children obtained through sexual slavery are chattel and oblivious to the impact of sexual abuse.

— Young children will not recall the sexual experience.

— If a sexual encounter is consummated in an empathic and kind way, the child will enjoy the sex as much as the provider.

---

The Mann Act was modified eventually to a law in 1978 that targeted those who commercially exploited minors of either sex by involving them in various forms of specifically defined, prohibited sexual conduct. With respect to the prostitution of children, the specific federal statutes were comprehensive. Some of these statutes are summarized in **Table 1-3**.

In the 1970s and 1980s, an effort to study the causal relationship between pornography and antisocial behavior toward females led to the establishment of 2 national commissions. The first, the Attorney General's Commission on Obscenity and Pornography, appointed by President Nixon, exonerated obscenity and erotica from any role in the development of a crime. The commission considered no violent materials and was looking only for violent effects as a result of exposure to obscenity and pornography (*The Report of the Commission on Obscenity and Pornography*, 1970). Based on the findings of this commission, it was recommended that the obscenity laws be abolished except for those concerning minors.

**Table 1-3. Select Federal Statutes Relating to Sexual Crimes Against Children***

SEXUAL ABUSE

| | |
|---|---|
| 2241 | Aggravated sexual abuse |
| 2242 | Sexual abuse |
| 2243 | Sexual abuse of a minor or ward |
| 2244 | Abusive sexual contact |
| 2245 | Sexual abuse resulting in death |

SEXUAL EXPLOITATION AND OTHER ABUSE OF CHILDREN

| | |
|---|---|
| 2251 | Sexual exploitation of children |
| 2251A | Selling or buying of children |
| 2252 | Certain activities relating to material involving the sexual exploitation of minors |
| 2252A | Certain activities relating to material constituting or containing child pornography |
| 2260 | Production of sexually explicit depictions of a minor for importation into the United States |

TRANSPORTATION FOR ILLEGAL SEXUAL ACTIVITY AND RELATED CRIMES

| | |
|---|---|
| 2421 | Transportation generally |
| 2422 | Coercion and enticement |
| 2423 | Transportation of minors |
| 2425 | Use of interstate facilities to transmit information about a minor |
| 2426 | Repeat offenders |
| 2427 | Inclusion of offenses relating to child pornography in definition of sexual activity for which any person can be charged with a criminal offense |

RACKETEER-INFLUENCED AND CORRUPT ORGANIZATIONS ACT

| | |
|---|---|
| 1961 through 1968 | Definitions, prohibited activities, criminal penalties, civil remedies, venue and process, expedition of actions, evidence, and civil investigative demand |

*\* All statutes are from title 18 from US Code.*

Approximately a decade later, a second commission was appointed, which entailed extensive testimonies of survivors of pornographic media production. The commission investigated the effects of violent and nonviolent sexual materials. This second commission was later referred to as the "Meese Commission," named after Attorney General Edwin Meese although the official name of the report was the *Attorney General's Commission on Pornography: Final Report* (1986). The Meese Commission discussed pornography that was violent, involved children, or had domination as a theme, as is seen in sadomasochistic pornography. The commission pointed out that violent versus nonviolent pornography was an important distinction.

The report found that "the harms at which the ordinance is aimed are real and the need for a remedy for those harms is pressing," and that "civil and other remedies ought to be available to those who have been in some way injured in the process of producing these materials" (*Attorney General's Commission on Pornography: Final Report,* 1986). For the first time, the concept of civil rights violations came into the language of sexual exploitation, as the commission found that the civil rights approach "is the only legal tool suggested to the commission that is specifically designed to provide direct relief to the victims of the injuries so exhaustively documented in our hearings throughout the country" (*Attorney General's Commission on Pornography: Final Report,* 1986).

A landmark case in Amsterdam in 1984 began to turn the tide of public attitude regarding the extreme impact of pornography on children. A 6-year-old child, Thea Pumbroek, was found dead of an overdose of cocaine in a hotel where she was being pornographically photographed. This tragic experience sparked a legislative response and revision of laws in the area of child sexual exploitation (CSE) in Holland.

Subsequent child pornographic movies and magazines became more apparent primarily in Europe, and titles such as *Chicken, Wonderboy, Nymph Lovers, Incestuous Love, Lollitots, Sweet Pattie, Sweet Linda, Lolita Color Specials, Joyboy, Prinz, Kim,* and *Kinde Liebe* became more recognized within the quiet communities of consumers. It is important to acknowledge the close relationship between commercial pornographic production and the role of family facilitation. Children are rarely sexually abused with pornography production by strangers except in the circumstances of child sex tourism. In the majority of cases, a family member facilitates exploitation through pornography.

Between 1983 and 1992, civil hearings were held in Minnesota, Indiana, California, and Massachusetts regarding pornography and sexually associated crimes. It was common for discovered pornographic materials to include images of adults and children. In addition, the link between the use of pornography for the grooming of children for sexual abuse was well described by numerous victims (Mackinnon & Dworkin, 1997). During these civil hearings, testimony by Bill Neiman, assistant county attorney in the Hennepin County, Minnesota Attorney's Office, revealed an important association. He cited that in most child sexual abuse cases prosecuted by his office, pornography was present. Neiman noted these pornographic materials were readily seen by investigators who were not intent upon their discovery. He noted the pornographic materials were of "very substantial numbers" and the materials were of adults and children (Mackinnon & Dworkin, 1997).

Included in the civil hearings in Minnesota was testimony by numerous former prostitutes. The following is a poignant illustration of the real-world relationship between pornography and prostitution (Mackinnon & Dworkin, 1997).

I am speaking for a group of women. We all live in Minneapolis, and we all are former prostitutes. All of us feel very strongly about the relationship between pornography and prostitution. Many of us wanted to testify at this hearing but are unable because of the consequences of being identified as a former whore. This is absolutely incredible to me that prostitution is seen as a victimless activity and that many women are rightly terrified of breaking their silence, fearing harassment to themselves and families and loss of their jobs.

We have started to meet together to make sense of the abuse we have experienced in prostitution and how pornography endorses and legitimizes that abuse. These are some of our stories. The following has all happened to real women who are the exception because they have survived both pornography and prostitution. We are all living in Minneapolis, and all of these events happened in Minneapolis. And as we sit here, this abuse is happening right now in the city tonight.

One of the very first commonalities we discovered as a group: We were all introduced to prostitution through pornography. There were no exceptions in our group, and we were all under 18.

Pornography was our textbook. We learned the tricks of the trade by men exposing us to pornography and us trying to mimic what we saw. I could not stress enough what a huge influence we feel this was. Somehow it was okay. These pictures were real men and women who appeared to be happy, consenting adults engaging in human sexuality.

Before I go on—one might make the assumption that if a woman got involved in pornography and prostitution after she was 18, that she is a willing participant. And since the women I speak for were all underage when they began, it is easier to see them as victims. Personally, I feel this to be very dangerous. By talking to women who got involved with prostitution and pornography in their early 20s, the powerlessness and victimization they described and experienced is the same that younger women and children feel.

The last decade of the 20th century brought about the realization that sexual exploitation had become a more significant international problem. This was glaringly apparent due to the growing use of the Internet. Child pornography became fairly ubiquitous on the Internet, and the images were simply spoken, hard-copy child sexual abuse. The images were available in various media forms, including single computer images, video clips on the Internet, or full-length videotapes, which could be ordered, and even audio clips for those who preferred to listen. This contraband was disseminated nationally and internationally. Often the pictures and videos were made by the sexually abused victim's family members. These images were sold or traded to others, including commercial Webmasters who would post graphics on their Web sites that consumers could visit for a fee.

Other sources of child pornography included commercially made images and videotapes of very poor children from indigent countries. Although the identity of the majority of children is still not known, efforts continue to locate and rescue such exploitation victims. The National Center for Missing & Exploited Children (NCMEC), as well as the Federal Bureau of Investigation, the United States Postal Inspection Service, the United States Immigration and Customs Enforcement, and local Internet Crimes Against Children (ICAC) task forces continue to work to identify these children (**Figures 1-5-a** and **b**). The NCMEC dedicates significant manpower to the task of finding and, if possible, rescuing exploited children. Bringing together the public and the private sectors, this agency uses some of the most sophisticated technology to establish a "library" of known children, whose images often appear in the collections of persons who save and treasure child pornography. The effort to identify victims requires and is addressed by multiple international agencies, to include Interpol, New Scotland Yard, the Royal Canadian Mounted Police, and others.

At times, sexual exploitation goes beyond child pornography into the arena of child and juvenile prostitution. In 1984, a study on runaway and homeless youth issued by the Office of the Inspector General of the Department of Health and Human Services reported that one woman posing as a destitute adolescent runaway in the downtown bus station of a large metropolitan area was propositioned by 135 different adults in just 12 hours. It was the conclusion that her experience was the rule more so than an exception (Arenberg, 1984). Further research reported in 2001 by the University of Pennsylvania School of Social Work reveals that child and juvenile prostitution often begins from the home and encompasses more than 100 000 children and youths in the United States (Estes & Weiner, 2001). As cited in the civil hearings on pornography, the link between child pornography and the prostitution of children and juveniles can not be overlooked. The infamous Evans family is an example of how easily youths can be lured into prostitution.

**Case Study 1-1**

In August of 2001, the Federal Bureau of Investigation and the Minneapolis law enforcement authorities arrested 15 members and associates of the Evans family on charges related to the operation of a multimillion-dollar prostitution ring. This ring had been in operation for 17 years and included at least 24 states and Canada as sites for this illegal activity (Clayton, 1996). Girls as young as 14 years of age were recruited at local malls, at nightclubs, from advertisements in the newspaper, and from the street. With the use of physical and mental intimidation, as well as threats of murder, the Evans family trapped these girls into a life of

*Figures 1-5-a and **b**. Logos of the Federal Bureau of Investigation and the United States Postal Inspection Service.* Reprinted with permission from the US Dept of Justice, Federal Bureau of Investigation. The US Postal Inspection Service Seal is a trademark owned by the United States Postal Service. Displayed with permission. All rights reserved.

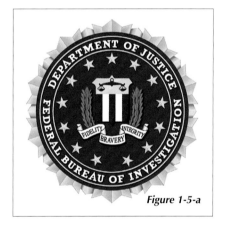

*Figure 1-5-a*

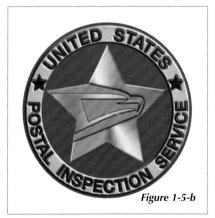

*Figure 1-5-b*

prostitution and cut them off from their family and friends. The violence perpetrated against these young girls was in keeping with that discussed within the context of multiple sexual assaults associated with street prostitution. Victims of such treatment have a high likelihood of suffering depression and posttraumatic stress disorder. Two of the girls involved with the Evans family are missing or dead.

An analysis of the Evans family case reveals that juvenile prostitution in the United States is an underground, highly mobile, and complex network of organized crime. Escort services are another venue through which these youths are marketed, and this type of exploitation is often outside of public view. Children and teens do not "choose" a life of prostitution. Juveniles lack the knowledge, maturity, and awareness to fully understand their actions and make responsible choices (Minnesota Attorney General's Office, 2000).

Other aspects of CSE include the involvement of the gang cultures and juvenile prostitution. In August 1999, a 19-year-old member of a St. Paul, Minnesota, gang called the King Mafia Crips pled guilty to a charge of promoting prostitution. The gang member forced girls aged 14 and 15 to have sex with men in hotels and motels in a specific county in Minnesota. The gang had escalated from "turf" battles to more traditional organized crime including distributing drugs, prostituting youth, and gambling.

Further research on the commercial sexual exploitation of children (CSEC) in the North American Free Trade Agreement (NAFTA) countries reveals that one of the venues of juvenile prostitution is that of gangs. Often, female teens involved with gangs were coerced into prostitution to support the gang economy. Considering the violence inherent in the gang culture, it is no surprise that the addition of prostitution compounds the vulnerability to untold trauma. A study of Oregon women who had exited from prostitution revealed that at least 84% were victims of aggravated assault, 49% were kidnapped, and 53% were victims of sexual torture. Specifically, prostitutes who were tortured reported that they were burned, gagged, hung, bound, or had their body parts mutilated by pinching, clamping, and stapling. Although the study was not limited to juveniles, the majority of women admitted that they became exploited through prostitution when they were still juveniles (Miller & Schwartz, 1995).

USE OF THE INTERNET

Children shown in Internet-based pornography have been seduced or coerced to participate in essentially every sexual perversion cited in the *Diagnostic and Statistical Manual of Mental Disorders,* Fourth Edition, Text Revision under the subcategory of paraphilias. To believe that all such images have been constructed in a "virtual laboratory" would be naïve. Well-known series of child pornography collections reveal that severe child sexual abuse had been occurring over prolonged periods of time in families, and the temptation of profit was too enticing. The Internet is often used to order videotapes of child sexual abuse, which has been documented to be a multi-million-dollar industry (R. Smith, US Postal Inspection Service, oral communication, 2003).

Although child pornography existed long before computers became publically available, the computer hard drive has become the modern day "copper plate" of existing visual pornography, providing the ability to copy and distribute contraband at will. Whereas in centuries past some of the motivation for pornographic images was for political purposes, today the role of pornography is different in that it often has a close association with offending. There are 2 distinct pathways to offending: coercive and noncoercive (Proulx et al, 1999). The latter circumstance was described by 53% of a sample of child molesters who deliberately used pornographic stimuli as part of their planned preparation for offending. Consequently, it is naïve to consider the collection of pornography to be only for acquisition trophies (Quayle & Taylor, 2003).

Victims of commercial child pornography often run away and resort to sexual acts as a survival strategy. The use of extortion, beatings, rape, and illicit substances are implemented at times, as seen with prostituted children and youths. Destitute children in underdeveloped countries are enticed to hotel rooms with food and money; adult pornography is used to stimulate them sexually and prepare them to become subjects of pornography. These indigent children commonly participate in autoerotic pornography production or youth-on-youth sexual encounters for these filming episodes. Many times, such children are involved in street prostitution. Some children are depicted in bondage scenarios or with obvious sadistic sexual abuse. Youth orgies are a common theme, often involving as many as 20 or 30 male and/or female youths in a given scene. These children come from numerous countries as well as the United States. As with prostitution, the victims are poorly paid for their services and are used only for as long as is necessary to capture the specific sexual behaviors for each specific production.

Often so-called taboo themes are depicted in computer-based pornography, such as mother-daughter incest, bestiality, and the use of infants and toddlers in sexually abusive encounters. The development of sophisticated methods of hiding such contraband has occurred over the past 5 to 10 years through such means as password-protected entry links and encryption.

## THE HISTORY OF THE ROLE OF THE INTERNET IN SEXUAL EXPLOITATION

In 1957, as a response to Russia's first artificial earth satellite launch, the Sputnik, the United States formed the Advanced Research Projects Agency (ARPA) within the Department of Defense. The goal of the ARPA was to advance US science and technology for the military. Over the next 10 years, the Department of Defense created the first computer network called ARPANET. At that time there were only 4 computers connected: one each at the University of California at Los Angeles, Stanford University, the University of California Santa Barbara, and the University of Utah. By 1970, the concept of computer-based "resource sharing" was entertained in the developing industry. Within 12 months, the first 4 nodes had grown to 15 sites, two thirds of which were in corporate America. Within a year, the program that gave birth to electronic mail was developed. At about the same time, France began to build its own ARPANET system.

The concept of the Internet, which was a link internationally between existing networks, became a reality in 1973. Although initially restricted to academic institutions, the defense and technology industry's further growth was inevitable. Within 24 months, the Internet had all-inclusive e-mail, with replying, forwarding, and filing capabilities. Over the next 5 years, the realization that colleges and universities would need to begin to educate technology experts in these new applications led to involvement of the National Science Foundation. This collaboration lasted for almost the remainder of the century. Highlights in the development of the Internet are summarized in **Figure 1-6**.

*Figure 1-6. Highlights in the development of the Internet.*

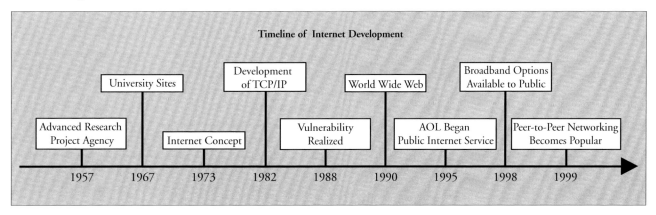

The 1980s saw further growth of the technology and the industry. In 1982, the ARPA established the Transmission Control Protocol (TCP) and Internet Protocol (IP), which led to the first definitions of an "internet" as a connected set of networks, specifically those using TCP/IP (Zakon, 2004). Shortly afterward, the first desktop workstations were designed, allowing for more personal computer activity.

In 1988, the first Internet worm infected the Internet, affecting between 6000 and 60 000 hosts. The realization that the Internet could be sabotaged became apparent.

By 1989, there were more than 100 000 hosts on the Internet. Countries that had connected with the National Science Foundation's Internet site (NSFNET) included Australia, Germany, Israel, Italy, Japan, Mexico, the Netherlands, New Zealand, Puerto Rico, and the United Kingdom.

By 1990, ARPANET ceased to exist, and within a year, the World Wide Web was born in its stead. The brainchild of Tim Berners-Lee, an Englishman with a doctorate in physics who was working at CERN, the European particle physics research center in Switzerland, the Web was the future of comprehensive research and information storage. The Web was software architecture that made it easy to post documents on the Internet (Ferguson, 1999). Within the next 5 years, more information became accessible on the Net. The United States White House came online during the Clinton administration, and the Senate and the House of Representatives began to provide information servers.

In 1995, the largest Internet Service Provider (ISP), America Online (AOL), began to provide Internet access. Domain names were offered for fees, such that certain abbreviations made immediate identification of a source much easier. The ".edu" designation became accepted for an educational institution, and the ".gov" designation meant a government agency. The ".com" suffix meant that the entity was a commercial group. Fees were levied for domain registration. Telephone line dial-up access led ISPs to become more than a $200 billion industry (Lieberman, 2003). During 1995, search engines began to evolve; one could search for information under a description and immediately access almost limitless amounts of data. To the detriment of the industry, computer hackers became more obvious, posing a less severe threat than a worm but still a serious concern for identity-theft crimes.

In 1996, concerns regarding obscenity and pornography on the Internet led to the short-lived US Communications Decency Act, a law that sought to prohibit distribution of indecent materials over the Internet. In only a few months, the Supreme Court ruled that due to the First Amendment to the Constitution of the United States, which upheld the right to free speech, most of the act was unconstitutional.

Within the next 3 years, new entities such as e-commerce and e-auctions began to emerge. Internet CSE links became commonplace. In addition, arrangements for the exchange of children for money entered the realm of electronic mail (e-mail). Scattered reports appeared in the newspapers of parents who were prostituting their children via the Internet. Such reports dispelled the notion that large cities and organized crime were the primary repositories of such illicit commerce. Indeed, many arrangements for child prostitution or cyber-enticement were made on the computers of school libraries.

Catastrophic errors occurred such as the accidental release on the Web of secret British agents' information. By the time the error was discovered and reversed, the information had been replicated. Immense worry about the computer technology transition into the year 2000, aptly abbreviated as "Y2K," brought numerous scientific agencies to the table to attempt to circumvent stock market and financial institutional record keeping crashes. Fortunately, the new millennium arrived with no obvious adverse effects initially although the first year of the new century did bring the first of numerous computer "bugs," the Love Letter virus.

## INTERNET CRIMES AGAINST CHILDREN

Continued growth and development of Internet technology caused the risks to children to increase exponentially. With an estimated 148 million Internet users in the United States and about 377 million users online worldwide, a concerted effort was needed to address the risk of the Internet to children.

The use of Internet chat rooms for sexual abuse and exploitation poses the greatest risk to children. Exploiters share adult and child pornography to desensitize a child or youth to the fearfulness of a sexual encounter. This type of exploitation could be confined to the child's home; without any parental knowledge, a potential offender could invite a child to share pornographic and sexual experiences. The exposure of the child to pornography within the home on the computer serves many functions:

— To normalize the sexual experience and convince the child that other children participate in and enjoy such activities.

— To desensitize the child to the explicit nature of various acts that would otherwise be unacceptable behavior for most children and adults

— To sexually stimulate the child, leading him or her to react in a sexualized manner

— To lure the child into a secret relationship with the exploiter, laying the groundwork for a schism in family allegiance as the child becomes convinced that this romantic relationship has more worth than family moral values

— To facilitate a private and confidential encounter with the child; since computer images can be deleted with an almost instantaneous click of a mouse, nonoffending care providers are generally unaware of the cyber-seduction efforts taking place in their own homes

In the United States, important federal laws have evolved since the concerns for child pornography became evident. These laws are summarized in **Table 1-4**.

In 2002, a Supreme Court decision, *Ashcroft v Free Speech Coalition*, found that 2 of the 4 definitions of child pornography were unconstitutional. One of the 2 definitions, which became internationally recognized, was 18 USC § 2256(8)(B), which defined "child pornography" as including visual depictions that *appear to be* of minors

---

**Table 1-4. Federal Child Pornography Legislation**

1977 — Protection of Children Against Sexual Exploitation Act

1984 — Child Protection Act

1986 — Child Sexual Abuse and Pornography Act

1986 — Child Abuse Victims' Rights Act

1988 — Child Protection and Obscenity Enforcement Act

1996 — Communications Decency Act

1996 — Child Pornography Prevention Act

1998 — Child Online Protection Act

1998 — Protection of Children from Sexual Predators Act

2000 — Children's Internet Protection Act

2003 — Prosecutorial Remedies and Other Tools to end the Exploitation of Children Today Act (PROTECT Act)

---

engaging in sexually explicit conduct. This definition became popularly known as the "virtual child pornography" definition and included computer-generated images as well as images of adults who appeared to be minors. The Court found this definition to be overly broad (Slocum & Waldron, 2004).

In response to this restriction and the subsequent extreme difficulty in prosecuting child pornography cases, the US Congress enacted the Prosecutorial Remedies and Other Tools to end the Exploitation of Children Today Act of 2003 (PROTECT Act). This act included numerous aids to prosecution for child pornography cases and included in the definition of child pornography, images that, to an ordinary observer, could be assumed to be authentic. The act allowed a defendant the protection of escape from conviction if he could establish that the images were clearly produced without the use of a real child (Slocum & Waldron, 2004).

International laws, charters, conventions, and covenants continue to be devised and revised to address the problem of CSE. In 1996, the First World Congress Against Commercial Sexual Exploitation of Children, held in Stockholm, Sweden, ignored a conscientious effort to eradicate this problem worldwide. The congress was organized by End Child Prostitution, Child Pornography and Trafficking of Children for Sexual Purposes International (ECPAT International). This meeting hosted 130 countries with governmental agencies, nongovernmental organizations (NGOs), the United Nations Children's Fund (UNICEF), and other United Nations agencies. All of the parties committed to a global partnership in eradicating this ubiquitous problem. The final outcome was an "Agenda for Action," shown in **Table 1-5**.

This plan of action sparked a response from many organizations across the globe and began to facilitate law enforcement collaboration. To date, investigative agencies such as Interpol, the US Customs Service, and the US Postal Inspection Service have established cooperative efforts.

The year 2001 brought the Second World Congress in Yokahama, Japan. Results of research conducted after the First World Congress were presented, and participants began to attest to the scope of the problem of sexual exploitation in their countries or regions, as well as barriers to resolution of this complex form of abuse. The Second World Congress provided the first phases of actions recommended in its preceding conference, and more documentary resolutions, referred to as "instruments," were suggested and included in the summaries for use by nations. The Second World Congress included far more youths who expressed an immense interest in participating and working on this far-reaching travesty. Their presence sensitized the participants to the devastation of exploitation victims. Instruments noted as useful from an international perspective as means of addressing the legal issues of CSE included but were not limited to the following:

— Convention on the Rights of the Child

— African Charter on the Rights and Welfare of the Child

— The Charter on the Rights of the Arab Child of the League of Arab States

— Convention for the Suppression of the Traffic in Persons and the Exploitation of the Prostitution of Others

— SAARC Convention on Preventing and Combating Trafficking of Women and Children for Prostitution (southern Asia)

— Optional Protocol to the Convention on the Rights of the Child on the Sale of Children, Child Prostitution, and Child Pornography

— Convention Concerning the Prohibition and Immediate Action for the Elimination of the Worst Forms of Child Labour

— Council of Europe: Draft Convention on Cyber-Crime

**Table 1-5  Essential Points From the Agenda for Action Against Sexual Exploitation of Children (First World Congress Against Commercial Sexual Expoitation of Children, 1996)**

COORDINATION AND COOPERATION

**Local and national levels**
— Strengthen strategies and measures, so by the year 2000 national agendas for action and indicators of progress are targeted to reducing the number of children vulnerable to sexual exploitation.

— Develop implementation and monitoring mechanisms so by the year 2000 established databases on sexual exploitation exist.

— Foster close interaction and cooperation between governmental and nongovernmental sectors to plan, implement and evaluate measures against exploitation.

**Regional and international levels**
— Promote better cooperation between countries and international organizations.

— Advocate and support child rights and ensure that adequate resources are available to protect children from sexual abuse.

— Press for implementation of the Convention on the Rights of the Child by State Parties.

PREVENTION

**Education**
— Provide children with education as a means of improving their status.

— Provide relevant health services, education, training, recreation, and a supportive environment to families and children vulnerable to commercial sexual exploitation.

— Maximize education on child rights and incorporate the Convention on the Rights of the Child by State Parties into formal and nonformal education.

— Initiate gender-sensitive communication, media, and information campaigns to raise awareness and educate about child rights and sexual exploitation.

— Establish peer education programs and monitoring networks to counter child exploitation.

**Change social and governmental policies**
— Formulate or strengthen gender-sensitive national, social, and economic policies and programs to assist children vulnerable to sexual exploitation.

— Develop, implement, and publicize relevant laws, policies, and programs to prevent the exploitation of children.

— Review laws and practices that lead to or facilitate exploitation and adopt effective reforms.

**Other**
— Mobilize the business sector, including the tourism industry, against the use of its networks for exploitation.

— Encourage the media to provide quality information concerning all aspects of exploitation.

PROTECTION

**Develop, strengthen, or implement national laws, policies, and programs**
— Prohibit the sexual exploitation of children.

— Establish the criminal responsibility of those who provide the services that promote exploitation.

— Protect child victims of sexual exploitation and human trafficking from being penalized as criminals.

— Criminalize (in the circumstance of sex tourism) the acts of nationals and promote extradition to ensure that a person who exploits a child for sexual purposes in another country is prosecuted.

*(continued)*

**Table 1-5  Essential Points From the Agenda for Action Against Sexual Exploitation of Children (First World Congress Against Commercial Sexual Expoitation of Children, 1996)** *(continued)*

PROTECTION

**Identify and encourage the establishment of national and international networks**
— Counter sexual exploitation of children between law enforcement authorities.

— Protect children from sexual abuse and monitor and report cases to the authorities among the civil society.

RECOVERY AND REINTEGRATION

— Adopt a nonpunitive approach to child victims of sexual exploitation.

— Provide social, medical, and psychological counseling and other supports to child victims and their families.

— Provide gender-sensitive training to those working to help exploitation victims on child development and rights.

— Take effective action to prevent and remove societal stigmatization of child victims and facilitate the recovery and reintegration of child victims in communities and families.

— Promote alternative means of livelihood with adequate support services to child victims and their families.

— Adopt sociomedical and psychological measures to create behavioral changes on the part of the perpetrators.

CHILD PARTICIPATION

— Promote the participation of children in decision making.

— Identify and support child and youth networks as advocates of child rights.

*Adapted from Defence for Children International Web site. An Agenda for Action. Stockholm, Sweden. August 1996. Available at: http://193.73.242.145/ong/DciHome.nsf/0/1ceb345f5905ffaa412564dd005f6802?OpenDocument. Accessed September 24, 2004.*

## CONCLUSION

The history of child pornography and child prostitution is woven over the centuries into the tapestry of anthropology and the study of societies. As children have become more "humanized" in the last few centuries, the realization that this form of abuse has a life-changing impact is becoming more evident. The computer age has facilitated the enticement of children as well as continued prostitution and sex tourism. This most underreported form of child abuse has and continues to affect untold numbers of victims worldwide. It has been suggested that predators who abuse children in these manners are more adroit in their practices than the public could ever recognize. More than 1million images of child sexual abuse have been documented online. For this and many other reasons, this form of abuse requires attention to detail, technological savvy, a realization of the global perspective, and the resolution that eradication will mandate a rigorous response from families, communities, lawmakers, nations, and the world.

## REFERENCES

Anson R. The last porno show. In: Schultz L, ed. *The Sexual Victimology of Youth.* Springfield, IL: Charles Thomas; 1980:275-291.

Arenberg GS, Bartimole CR, Bartimole JE. *Preventing Missing Children: A Parental Guide to Child Security.* Hollywood, Fla: Compact Books; 1984.

*Ashcroft v Free Speech Coalition,* 535 US 234 (9th Cir 2002).

# COMMERCIAL SEXUAL EXPLOITATION OF CHILDREN IN ADVERTISING

Linnea W. Smith, MD
Marcia E. Herman-Giddens, PA, DrPH
V. Denise Everette, MD, FAAP

In a society where in a year an estimated quarter of a million children are sexually exploited for profit in the United States alone (Estes & Weiner, 2001), and 2 to 3 million reports were filed alleging the maltreatment of children, there is a growing movement to determine what may be contributing to this climate of misuse and abuse of children. Applying the public health model that no illness is ever brought under control by treating only the casualties, the health care profession, along with other social scientists and organizations, is examining cultural influences that may contribute to this exploitation. Of primary focus is the content of mass media that may increase the vulnerability of children to victimization or contribute to the demand side of sexual and physical abuse and other sexual exploitation of children.

Though there has been investigation and discussion of certain forms of media violence and television content, advertising has not received as much emphasis as other media forms when looking at the use and portrayal of children in ads and children as consumers of advertising. This chapter will examine the role of advertising in the sexual exploitation of children and what pediatricians, parents, and others are doing and can do to keep children safe and healthy.

This chapter draws on the theories and methods developed in cultural studies, founded in the 1970s by media scholars who were dissatisfied with the traditional approach to the study of media. This approach tended to ignore the ideological impact of popular culture and its role in constructing hegemonic discourse (DeFleur, 1998). The main aim of the cultural studies approach is to explore the long-term effects of living in a culture where individuals are bombarded with images that distort notions of reality (Barker, 2000; Grossberg & Radway, 1997; Lewis, 2002). This contrasts with the more positivist paradigm that posits a somewhat simplistic relationship between images and short-term behavioral change. Cultural studies theorists were critical of quantitative content analysis, arguing that splitting media texts into quantifiable units failed to capture the way that the texts work as a structured whole. For this reason, the research discussed in this chapter utilizes qualitative rather than quantitative content analysis to examine the codes and conventions of the images.

## WHY ADVERTISING?

Advertising is a pervasive and powerful force in American culture (Jhally, 1995). According to the Canadian Advertising Foundation's Code of Advertising Standards (2004), *advertising* is defined as "any paid message communicated by the media with the intent to influence the choice, opinion, or behavior of those addressed by the commercial message." One leader in mass communication research identified advertising as the "most concentrated effort in history to change public consciousness" (Jhally, 1998). More money, more effort, and more thought go into this form of communication than any other. The amount of money spent annually by the advertising industry has been steadily increasing and has now surpassed $200 billion in the US (Kilbourne, 1999). Fifty percent of the total advertising revenue in the US goes into print advertising, while 22% is expended on television advertising (Kellner, 1995). The average individual sees more than 3000 commercial impressions a day; typical Americans will spend 3 years of their life watching TV commercials (Kilbourne, 1999). Advertising makes up 70% of newspaper content and 40% of mail (Kilbourne, 1999). It is the most powerful and widespread way to send a message, and that message is increasingly tuned to teens and children.

Advertising has found a significant source of income: In 2000, the largest US teen population ever, 33 million, spent $100 billion in one year and influenced their parents to spend another $50 billion (Frontline, 2001). Spending by preteens has increased as well. In 1998, 4- to 12-year-olds were responsible for approximately $27 billion in discretionary spending, an amount 4 times that spent by this group a decade earlier. They directly or indirectly influenced some $500 billion in spending by their parents (Steyer, 2002).

In this Information Age, access to information from various media has never been easier, especially for teens and children, yet less than 50% of today's magazines consist of editorial content. So, what are children and teens consuming? Advertising. Ads sell more than just products; they sell values, identities, desires, and dreams, a way of seeing the world—right or wrong. For example, 60% of boys and 44% of girls consider brand names on clothing very or somewhat important. But it is more than just preferring brand names: Until the age of 5, children can not tell the difference between commercials and programming. Only when they reach the age of 8 do children realize that the intent of ads is to sell products. The American Academy of Pediatrics (AAP) believes "advertising directed toward children is inherently deceptive and exploits children under 8 years of age" (Committee on Communications, 1995).

There is nothing benign about the marketing techniques used to influence children. They are designed to exploit the vulnerabilities of children. The president of one California ad agency explained, "[a]dvertising at its best is making people feel without their product you're a loser. Kids are very sensitive to that" (Steyer, 2002).

A European broadcasting executive with perhaps more critical distance describes commercial TV in the United States as a system that trains children to be consumers rather than citizens. "No other major democratic nation in the world has so willingly turned its children over to mercenary strangers this way. No other democratic nation has so willingly converted its children into markets for commercial gain and ignored their moral, intellectual, and social development" (Minow, 1995).

Apart from children being directly targeted by advertising, juveniles live in a culture immersed in advertising with no clear boundary between commercial messages or imagery and the rest of culture. Pop culture media are everywhere and are fast replacing all other venues as a source of information. Children and adults are completely immersed without realizing it. The most effective propaganda is that which is not recognized as such. We are less on guard, less critical, and more desensitized to the unintended effects of advertising, which are more important and difficult to measure. Many in media and advertising like to tell parents that they can turn off the radio or change the TV channel to protect their kids from the negative impact of advertising. "This is like telling us that we can protect children from air pollution by making sure they never breathe. Advertising is our environment. We swim in it as fish swim in water. We cannot escape it" (Kilbourne, 1999). According to Gail Dines (oral communication, March 2003), the job of parents is to socialize their children. Asking parents to keep culture outside of the home is counterintuitive.

Youth are currently confronted with advertising for nude and exotic dancing, strip bars, "gentlemen's clubs," and topless car washes on billboards, in university student directories, and in newspaper ads on sports and entertainment pages, as well as even more sexually explicit ads and personals in free weekly newspapers, especially in metropolitan areas. There were more than 50 pages of listings for escort services and 10 pages for massage parlors in the 2000-2001 Manhattan yellow pages. Free entertainment weeklies feature hundreds of listings for sexual services in their advertising section (Spangenberg, 2001). There are "print commercials and classified advertisements for escorts or modeling agencies recruiting 'innocent' or 'barely legal' teens" (Hecht, 2001).

Although we may not pay direct attention to many of the ads, we continue to be influenced, partly on an unconscious level. Ads are designed in ways so that we do not pay critical or studious attention. Society's public airwaves and public spaces are saturated with unavoidable advertising: from logos on clothing to storefronts and sides of buses and trucks, athletic event scoreboards to unsolicited e-mail spam. The opportunities are endless and continue to expand as new forms of media technology are developed and powerful global conglomerates increasingly influence the content of varied media. Because of this pervasiveness of advertising and the inundation of commercial products, ads, to compete amid the "clutter" to grab the attention of potential consumers, are becoming more novel, bizarre, or explicit. Examples of such advertising campaigns are discussed later in this chapter.

According to children who say they watch TV and surf the Internet without parental supervision, parents are not paying enough attention to the media consumption of their children. "Not only do parents frequently underreport the number of hours that their offspring view (TV) but they also underreport the problematic shows that they view" (Strasburger & Donnerstein, 1999). Parents express feeling overwhelmed and undermined by the impossible task of monitoring and restricting children's access at home and away from home to the increasingly sophisticated and sexually explicit or exploitative media available to younger and younger audiences.

Pediatricians and child development professionals have expressed concern about television being the electronic babysitter. But just what is this surrogate for parent and caregiver interaction teaching children? According to the American Academy of Pediatrics (AAP) policy statement, television may be the "super-peer" for kids, warping their perceptions of real-world sex and, instead, presenting a "fantasy" world where sex happens all the time (Committee on Public Education, 2001). This then has the effect of normalizing and encouraging sexual behavior in teens.

The average child between the ages of 8 and 18 spends 6 hours and 43 minutes a day with media (Rich, 2001). Children ages 9 to 17 years old use the Internet 4 days a week, averaging 2 hours online at a time. By the time they graduate from high school, young people will have watched 15 000 hours of TV, compared with just 12 000 hours spent in school (Committee on Public Education, 2001).

What's even more disturbing than the amount of time spent with the venues is the amount of sexual programming the children are observing. The average American adolescent will view nearly 14 000 sexual references per year; only 165 deal with birth control, abstinence, self-control, risk of pregnancy, or sexually transmitted diseases (STDs). More than half of all television programs, 56%, contain sexual content. Even prime-time TV's family hour averages 8 sexual situations, 4 times more than it did in 1976. Teens rank the media as a leading source of sexual information, second only to school sex education (Committee on Public Education, 2001).

Sixty-one percent of all high school seniors have had sexual intercourse, approximately half are currently sexually active, and 21% have had 4 or more partners (Committee on Public Education, 2001). According to one study, 74% of girls who had intercourse before age 14 and 60% who had intercourse before age 15 did so involuntarily (Committee on Public Education, 2001). Up to two thirds of teen mothers reported sex was forced upon them by adult men when they were younger, according to the Alan Guttmacher Institute's 1994 study *Sex and America's Teenagers.* Sexual assault is one of the fastest growing crimes in America, with acquaintance and date rape making up to 70% to 80% of rape crisis center contacts. With one of the highest teen pregnancy rates in the world, the United States holds the dubious distinction of having people under the age of 25 account for two thirds of all STDs (Committee on Public Education, 2001), and there are 12 million new cases each year (Brownback, 2001).

But what is the media link, especially in advertising? The relationship between advertising and society has been a topic of debate for some time. Some researchers may focus on how advertising influences society while others may concentrate on how it reflects society.

Most serious scholars of advertising take a middle position and the most common metaphor for the relationship between advertising and society is a 'fun-house mirror' with the relationship between popular culture and society as distorted and complex. Advertising imagery often consists of ritualized displays and stereotypes that may offer a window to the belief structure of society, but not depict 'life' or even 'idealized life' (Alexander, 1994).

Condrey goes further in arguing that, "the values of the media are the values of the marketplace. It cannot be a useful source of information for children. ... Indeed it may be a dangerous ... Advertising offers ideas that are false, unreal; it has no coherent value system other than consumerism; it provides little useful information about the self" (Steyer, 2002).

How is this complex relationship evolving over time and what is it today, especially when most agree that we live in a more "image-based world—in an increasingly visual culture" (Schroeder & Borgerson, 1998) in which advertising images play a more central part? Media researchers Schroeder & Borgerson (1998) argue that

[a]dvertising acts as a powerful means of constructing, influencing, and illustrating the consumer vision of the good life, including, in large part, sexual attraction. ... advertising and the mass media contribute to the visual landscape that constructs reality. Advertising shapes identity, particularly gender identity. ... advertising offers an excellent window into cultural values and trends.

They go on to emphasize that, "[t]he more prominent certain images become, the more power they have in the sea of images, whether they are intended to control or manipulate or not. Visual images play an important role in the production and reproduction of gender identities; they do not merely reflect or portray them" (Schroeder & Borgerson, 1998). Unfortunately, while this relationship is inadequately researched and addressed in the academic literature, the question remains: What does this relationship mean to a society consuming child and childlike images that portray adult sexuality? What is the influence on individuals and groups of individuals that include juveniles and increasingly younger and younger children? (Kilbourne, 1995).

## WHAT SEXUAL EXPLOITATION OF CHILDREN IN ADVERTISING LOOKS LIKE

Her hair is stylishly tousled, her make-up heavy. She stares into the camera seductively, clutching a perfume bottle to her chest. She is topless ... and she is 4 or 5 years old. Be it jeans, women's perfume, men's cologne, high-fashion business suits, or luxury bath products, children of all ages are depicted in advertising for adult and juvenile consumers. Why? And what is *really* for sale?

Being a media-savvy society means more than just knowing how to tune through 500 channels and surf the Internet. Today, it means recognizing the impact of the various messages in commercial media—television and "new" media, in the form of video games and Web sites—and teaching parents and children to navigate the slippery slopes of what is and is not healthy.

No organization, even one whose primary focus is the welfare of children, is exempt from the normalization of these portrayals. Although this example did not appear in an ad, there are several important lessons to learn from the cover photo for the June/July 2001 issue of *Healthy Kids* (**Figure 2-1**), a bimonthly parenting magazine from the American Academy of Pediatrics for parents of children aged 2 to 10 years old. Unfortunately, this kind of portrayal of female children is common in print advertising and normalized in our popular culture, in part due to the cumulative effect of frequent pictures like this in the media. Consequently, many of us in society, including child advocates and healthcare professionals, have become desensitized to the overt and underlying messages these powerful images convey.

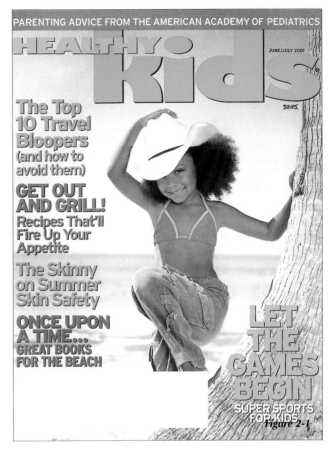

What is the purpose of the image? What unintended communication is *really* happening? The 5- to 7-year-old child model is wearing a contrived costume of a white cowboy hat, pink two-piece bathing suit top, and tan cargo pants (pants perhaps more commonly associated with teen fashion). Her hat is coyly positioned, not as a child would wear it on her own. Her left knee is bent with the left leg in front of the right, holding a nearby tree trunk with her left arm. Her pose is passive, artificial, and in keeping with the traditional female pin-up pose. Her head is positioned downward, an example of Goffman's "head cant" in which the level of the head is lowered or tilted "in a display of ingratiation and submissiveness" (Schroeder, 1998). This is in sharp contrast to the traditional male stance that is taut, rigid, or straining, indicating power and control, or standing on both feet ready to act. Yet she looks up at the camera and reader, as if knowing she is on display.

She is not playing, reading, talking with other children, or doing any of the things appropriate for a child her age. She is doing nothing but being displayed for the pleasure of the viewers. She is submissive and compliant to the photographer's wishes. She is trivialized as an active child who is going swimming, playing on the beach, getting ready to ride horses, or engage in other cowboy activity. Yet her "costume" is not practical, and dress-up games traditionally do not occur on a beach. The cowboy hat seems to sexualize the costume (see also **Figure 2-2**). Her hair is carefully groomed and fluffed. (There are credits to the hairdresser, modeling agency, and fashion companies on the inside front page). Her only value as a female child is the attention she gets and that is based on her physical appearance and groomed beauty. She is eye candy for all viewers. The public would be unlikely to accept a photo of a male child presented in this way.

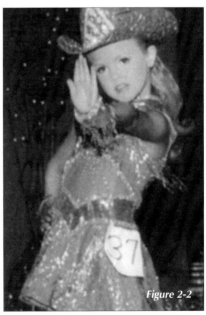

Figure 2-2

In addition to the valid concerns about the female child being presented in a sexualized manner, there are also important issues regarding the social construction of gender. The cover is similar to print advertising today, which has traditionally emphasized sexuality and physical appearance to sell products. In her research, Moog "shows how print advertising communicates immature attitudes about sexuality to young people; consequently, their definitions and perceptions of sexuality and gender identity become 'stunted'" (Fox, 1996).

Because of this conventionalized display of the body, Kuhn (1985) believes that the viewer is more likely to hold the girl responsible for soliciting the spectator's gaze and constructing her own body as an object of scrutiny. This gives an exhibitionistic

**Figure 2-1.** *This child model is in a traditional female pin-up pose, leg bent and head tilted coyly* (Healthy Kids, *cover photo, June/July 2001*).

**Figure 2-2.** *As in its grown-up counterparts, western-theme fashion is an advertising focus, this time for child beauty pageant contestants* (Pageantry, *Summer 2003*).

quality to the depiction and again places more responsibility on the child, relieving the viewer of guilt about voyeurism.

What are the messages to parents and children about female beauty and appearance and value? What was the impact on the young child used as a model for this photo? Her image is hauntingly reminiscent of the media flood of JonBenet Ramsey photos, especially the beauty contest poses and costumes. According to Kilbourne (1999), a major periodical referred to JonBenet as a "*preadolescent* beauty queen." Yet, Ramsey was just 6 years old at the time of her tragic death. Kilbourne (1999) points out that "it is increasingly difficult in such a toxic environment to see children, boys and girls, as children. … When everything and everyone is sexualized, it is the powerless who are most at risk. Young girls, of course, are especially vulnerable."

The photo is especially disturbing because it was on the cover of an AAP publication, an organization often at the forefront of issues involving media and child health and development, including its laudatory "Media Matters" program. The AAP works hard to be especially vigilant in using socially responsible and age-appropriate photos of children. This role is even more important as it is becoming increasingly difficult to persuade mainstream media to set limits or publish critical analyses of corporate-produced commercial images. Popular culture is teaching young girls inappropriate dress and behavior that results in their being more vulnerable to victimization, while continuing to blame them for any victimization.

The fact that the photo was deemed acceptable enough to warrant placement on the cover of the magazine can serve as a needs assessment and a warning bell. Educational programs directed to professionals, as well as parents and children and the general public, continue to be an important and necessary service. Parenting magazines can be useful for general articles on media literacy as well as for healthy media habits for children. Readers must be aware that however well-intentioned these magazines are, they are advertiser-driven and not operating outside the influence of commercial interests.

According to Michele Elliott (1992) in her chapter "Images of children in the media: 'soft kiddie porn,'"* these portrayals of children are contributing to the problem of child sexual abuse in the following ways:

— Condoning the use of children in inappropriate sexual contexts

— Desensitizing the public and setting new standards for what is acceptable

— Strengthening the argument of pedophiles that children are asking for sex

— Exploiting and dehumanizing children without their informed consent

— Glamorizing children as sexual objects

— Implying to children that adults think this sexualization is acceptable by not challenging these portrayals

— Suggesting to other children that this is a desirable way to be depicted

## THE HISTORY OF CHILD SEXUALLY EXPLOITATIVE ADVERTISING

The impact of advertising on children has been studied to a greater extent than the impact of the portrayal of children in advertising targeted to adults. One study examined the changing portrayal of children in magazine advertisements from 1905 through 1990 while contributing to developing methodology for analyzing visual

---

* The authors discourage use of the term "kiddie porn" when referring to child pornography. This slang term often is a kind of sarcastic pet name which can trivialize the seriousness of the effects of child pornography and may even signify for some an acceptance of the genre.

data, which is distinct from textual data. The author looked at the frequency of the appearance of children in ads. There was a positive correlation with the percentage of children in the US population, as well as the periods during which society was considered more "child-centered." As consumerism increased in recent decades, it was felt to be a contributing factor to an increase in images of children (Alexander, 1994).

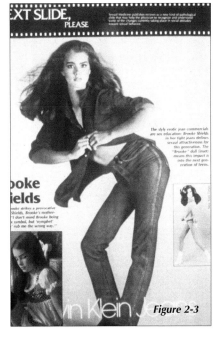

*Figure 2-3*

In her article on public images, Adatto (1995) reminds us that the ideals of childhood often taken for granted have been centuries in the making. Not until the 17th century did childhood come to be understood as a special province of life with special needs for protection from the adult world. There was a clear boundary between childhood and adulthood. The ideals of childhood holding a privileged place in American culture persisted for over a century and, despite society's claims to uphold these ideals, she believes they began to unravel in the 1960s. Looking at the photographic images of children in advertising and art, "[w]e see the soul of the child under siege. There has been a hollowing out of the belief in the innocence and moral agency of the child" (Adatto, 1995). According to her analysis, one of the most disturbing trends in fashion photography was the emphasis on the child-woman as supermodel. Beginning in the late 1960s and early 1970s, this trend was exemplified by the popular, wide-eyed teenage model, Twiggy, with her anorexic-like body and girlish appearance. Twiggy in the 1970s was followed by an adolescent Brooke Shields (**Figure 2-3**) in the early 1980s in provocative ads for Calvin Klein's sexy skintight jeans.

Around the same time, the pornography industry was following a similar path by depicting children or childlike models or poses. According to Carr (2001) in his paper on child pornography, "[p]art of a tradition that stretches back centuries, the consumption of sexualized children for adult pleasure developed quickly in the early 1970s to become a thriving commercial enterprise, in the process becoming increasingly hardcore and pornographic." As the pornography industry expands and becomes more mainstream, it exerts an influence on other media forms. The depiction of children, often sexualized or engaged in sexual activity, in mainstream sexually explicit men's magazines in the United States peaked in frequency between 1971 and 1978 for the 3 top-grossing magazines: *Playboy*, *Penthouse*, and *Hustler* (**Figure 2-4**). A study including extensive content analysis funded by the Office of Juvenile Justice and Delinquency Prevention (OJJDP) researched the images of children in these magazines from 1954 to 1984. Although the project and its findings generated controversy in the media, when the public and the magazine industry became aware of the study, the numbers of children displayed in a sexual context dropped precipitously, a phenomenon that may speak to the importance of this type of research (Reisman, 1994). No subsequent studies regarding the portrayal of children in these or similar magazines have been undertaken.

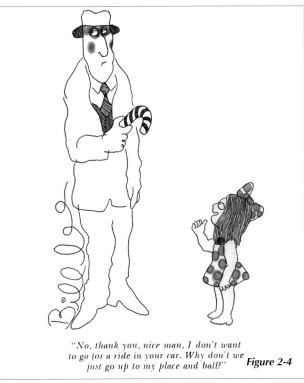

*"No, thank you, nice man, I don't want to go for a ride in your car. Why don't we just go up to my place and ball?"*  **Figure 2-4**

**Figure 2-3.** *Fifteen-year-old Brooke Shields exclaims, "Nothing comes between me and my Calvins..." in this 1981 ad reproduced and critiqued in* Sexual Medicine Today, *April 1982.*

**Figure 2-4.** *Child sexual abuse was trivialized and normalized in Playboy cartoons. Playboy glamorized the distortion used by pedophiles that even very young children desire and initiate sexual encounters with adult men (Playboy, November 1972).*

Using examples of art photography and advertising from print media, Adatto (1995) describes the progression of a transformed view of childhood in public images. Brooke Shields' career as a model began early as the Ivory Snow baby in the 1960s when the emphasis was on innocence. However, when she was 10 years old, suggestive nude photos of her were published in the Playboy Press publication, "Sugar and Spice." In 1978, she rose to stardom cast as a 12-year-old girl initiated into child prostitution with no apparent harm in Louis Malle's movie, *Pretty Baby*, followed by the ads for Calvin Klein.

*Figure 2-5. Kate Moss in a Calvin Klein ad (Vanity Fair, November 1992).*

*Figure 2-6. Kate Moss is more childlike and androgynous for broader appeal in this Calvin Klein ad (Mirabella, December 1993).*

*Figure 2-7. Sexual access to childlike females appears to be an "obsession" for men according to this Calvin Klein ad (Details, June 1995).*

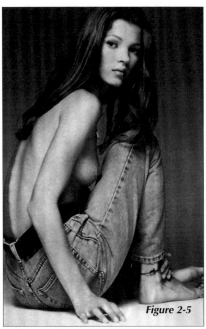

Figure 2-5

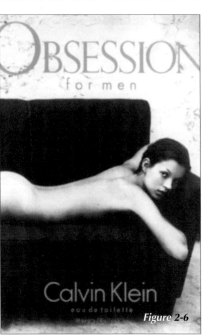

Figure 2-6

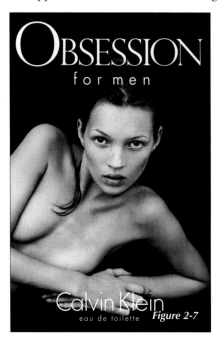

Figure 2-7

The early 1990s saw a more explicit pairing of childhood innocence and adult sexuality with Kate Moss and others in Calvin Klein fashion advertising (**Figure 2-5**). Although Moss was chronologically older than her predecessors, her appearance was that of an even younger, somewhat androgynous, adolescent (**Figure 2-6**). The co-mingling of innocence and eroticism was thought to form the dissonance that caught the attention of viewers.

Media critic Kilbourne recognizes changes in the portrayal of children:

In the past twenty years or so, there have been several trends in fashion and advertising. … One has been the obsession with thinness. Another has been an increase in images of violence against women. Most disturbing has been the increasing sexualization of children, especially girls. Sometimes the little girl is made up and seductively posed. Sometimes the language is suggestive (Kilbourne, 1999).

When comparing earlier photos of the female child to a mid-90s ad for Obsession perfume (**Figure 2-7**), Adatto (1995) noted that the child-woman supermodel not only shed her clothes, but, "[t]here is nothing soulful in her look, no innocence in her provocative stare. Her dead-on look at the camera says, 'You can have me.' Her objectification representing innocence with an overlay of eroticism form the message, 'If you like little girls, you'll love our cologne.'"

A chairman of a university graduate marketing department described the advertising of Calvin Klein without addressing the harm or misuse of children: "Klein's campaigns have been recognized as avant-garde and artistic as well as scandalous. He is one of those leading-edge people who presses at the boundaries of what is acceptable. His ads violate taboos, they use vivid looks at things we are not supposed to see" (Grant, 1992). Calvin Klein and other fashion designers positioned themselves as champions of sexual liberation and artistic freedom. Modesty and innocence became signs of repression and commercial public displays of nudity as acts of personal and political liberation. Critics were trivialized as censors and prudes. The controversy generated free media attention and most likely became an important factor for escalating sexual images in Klein's subsequent advertising campaigns (**Figure 2-8**). See **Appendix 2-1** for an example from a highly criticized clothing store.

The advertising that sexually exploits children knows no boundaries or limits; these ads appear in various mainstream magazines that have a wide readership and are circulated throughout society. It is noteworthy that many of the advertisements were carried in women's magazines and presumably directed toward female readers (including adolescent females). A decade ago, the top 5 best sellers of women's magazines had a combined circulation of more than 7 million. A dominant common thread was to confuse adulthood with childhood (**Figure 2-9**). There was no clear appreciation of the separation between childhood and adulthood. It was implied that sexual themes that may be appropriate for adults were appropriate for children. If a parent is desensitized or worse, confused, regarding which sexual attitudes are appropriate or inappropriate for children, she or he is less likely to provide consistent and clear guidance and protection for children.

Sex and sexualized images of females are used to sell women's fashion magazines as well as fashion, beauty, and other products. Reading the subtitles of magazines at the grocery store check-out counters, in view of all children as well as parents, will substantiate what most shoppers already know. In a recent article about the magazine industry, women's magazine editors expressed concern about too much advertiser influence on editorial content. Many writers, editors, and fact-checkers, without revealing their names, admitted that they have much lower editorial standards for the sex articles published. Stories are embellished, quotes tweaked, ages changed, and composite characters described. Exaggerating to make copy racier and more entertaining to readers was more important than informing them (Featherstone, 2002). This revelation reinforces the concern that this genre is more problematic as a source of sex education for impressionable and inexperienced youth, who regularly read these magazines. Many of the publishers of women's magazines also publish magazines for adolescents.

Sixty-one percent of all teen girls report reading at least one fashion magazine regularly (Elias, 1999). Teenage girls are heavy users of teen magazines; three quarters of white teen girls ages 12 to 14 report reading a teen magazine monthly. Many teens, especially adolescent girls, rely on magazines as a source of information about sex, birth control, and STDs. In one study, teen magazines devoted an average of 2 pages per issue to sexual concerns (Huston et al, 1998).

Popular preteen and teen magazines, in addition to stories about dating, intimate relationships, and grooming, teem with waif-thin models in provocative fashion and make-up ads. For decades, 3 magazines, *Seventeen*, *Teen*, and *YM*, dominated the field. Currently more than 8 magazines compete for teen readers. More publishers, primarily of women's magazines, are directing a version for the preteen and teenage female market. These publications are an effective way for advertisers to attract adolescent consumers with the added goal of keeping them as consumers for years if they maintain brand loyalty into adulthood. Marketers are now looking at even younger girls, choosing not to wait until children become teenagers. Most of these magazines contain frank adult content and treat teens as miniaturized versions of grown-ups with as many pressures and problems as parents. And the trends for clothing are the same: more revealing, hyper-sexualized miniature versions of adult fashion (**Figure 2-10**). The same styles marketed to 16-year-olds are marketed to 6-year-olds: low-rise jeans, tight miniskirts, midriffs, halter tops, and stretch tee shirts with sexually loaded phrases such as "Wild Thing" or "Hottie." There are even lacy black bras for 7-year-olds and G-strings designed for 9-year-olds. One sex educator and author recently exclaimed,

[a]nd when exactly did 'fashion' stop being about getting dressed, and start being about getting—or increasing the chance that you'll be getting—undressed? ... And excuse me, but who was paying attention

*Figure 2-8.* Note the blackened eyes, vulnerable posture, and the childlike doodling in this Calvin Klein ad. Does this depict a child or adult, and why blur the line? (Vanity Fair, March 2002).

*Figure 2-9.* The young girl in this cosmetics ad is portrayed as interchangeable with the adult woman. The ad copy, which reads, "The most unforgettable women in the world," calls her a woman when she is obviously a child (Cosmopolitan, May 1998).

*Figure 2-10.* The mannequins in Abercrombie have children's size 6 clothes, featuring elementary school kids in low rise, midriff bearing slacks and shorts, and shirts with slogans like "red hots" on them.

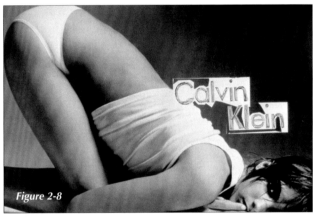

Figure 2-8

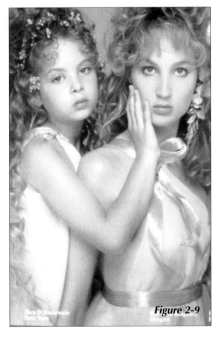

Figure 2-9

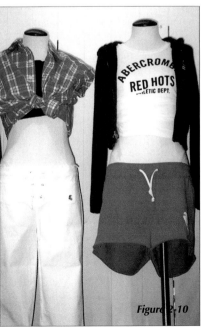

Figure 2-10

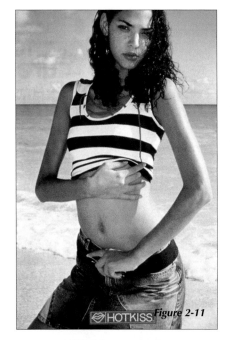

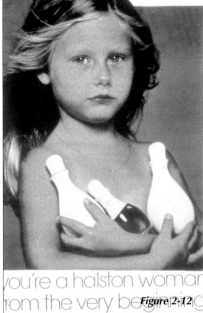

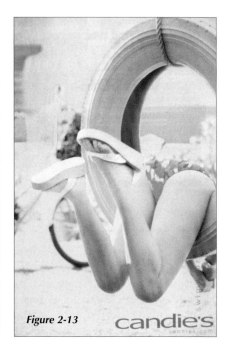

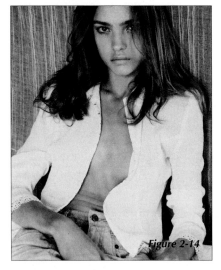

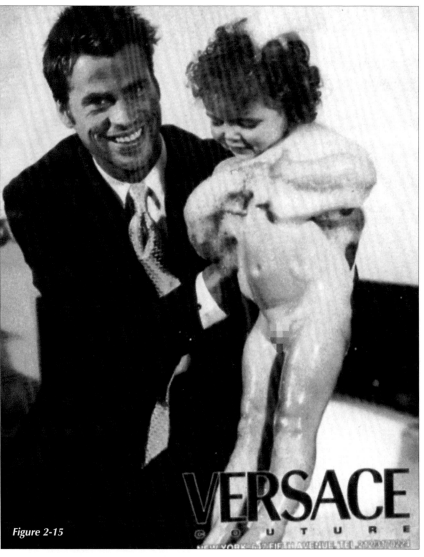

**Figure 2-11.** *This is a Hotkiss fashion ad featuring their provocative clothing line* (Seventeen, *March 2002*).

**Figure 2-12.** *This Halston ad was one of the first examples of mainstream media featuring a young child mimicking a glamorous and sexualized adult female* (New York Times Magazine, *1977*).

**Figure 2-13.** *This ad prominently features buttocks when this apparent child on a playground is actually advertising shoes* (Seventeen, *April 2002*).

**Figure 2-14.** *This ad for Calvin Klein jeans features a childlike model with her shirt unbuttoned and open for viewers* (Jane, *March 2003*).

**Figure 2-15.** *This Versace ad features a nude female toddler being displayed by a father figure* (GQ, *October 1996*).

when the junior streetwalker/sex slave look became the predominant mode of 'dress' among teens and even preteens? Or the wide-midriff, belly-button-baring trend for the seven-year-old crowd? Or short shorts, sporting phrases like 'Hot Stuff' across the buttocks, for first-graders? (Roffman, 2002).

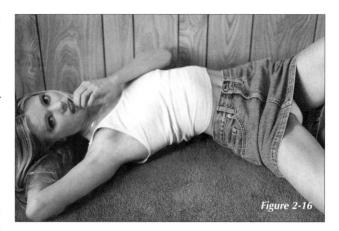

Figure 2-16

The creative director of an advertising firm explains the use of sexual images in order to grab the attention of a youth market shopping for designer jeans: "With the Calvins [Calvin Klein] of the world doing what they're doing, you almost have to stay comfortably close to that edge; otherwise, you're a wimp. You look like you're selling clothes for old people" (Givan, 1996).

One cumulative effect of this type of advertising is an emphasis on appearance as a way to get attention. Preschool girls get the message about dressing to be pretty. In grade school, pretty means sexy like Britney Spears and other youth celebrities. This is not sexy as in wanting or understanding sexual attention, but rather, wanting positive attention and peer approval. As children grow older, clothing becomes more important for communicating identity and being included in a valued peer group. According to a professor of sociology at Manhattan's Fashion Institute of Technology, teen fashion magazines popularized the attitude that sexy dressing equals power and self-confidence. Marketing techniques reinforce that goal of being on display and viewed by others, that titillation equals liberation for those who put their bodies on display for public gaze. The marketing director for Hotkiss (**Figure 2-11**), a fashion line advertised widely in teen magazines, knew exactly what to say: "We appeal to an independent girl with enough self-confidence to wear our body-conscious and provocative clothing" (Stepp, 2003).

Society's challenge is to let children, especially girls, know there are better and healthier ways to get attention. For example, educate children in language they can understand and accept that they are being influenced by industries with products to sell who may not be considering their best interests. Children have a right to express themselves in their dress, but they may not mean what they're saying with their clothes; they may be stereotyped or misunderstood because of their wardrobe.

The following are inappropriate uses of children as sexual objects in advertising:

— Children made or dressed up to invoke adult sexual themes (**Figure 2-12**)

— Preadolescent girls made or dressed up to mimic adults, posed in a sexualized way

— Emphasis on the clothed or unclothed genitals and buttocks of children or adults made to look like children (**Figure 2-13**)

— Confusion of the true age of a childlike model in a sexualized pose or situation (**Figure 2-14**)

— Portrayal of the nudity of a child or childlike model in a sexual or exploitive way, whether the nudity is real or implied (**Figure 2-15**)

— Adult models equipped with childhood props or facial expressions that create a sense of helplessness or vulnerability in a sexual context (**Figure 2-16**)

— A child posed with an adult who is nude or sexualized (**Figure 2-17**)

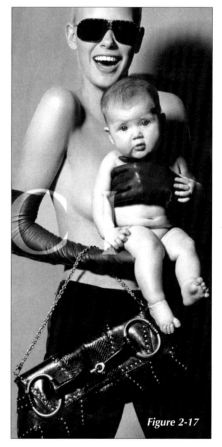

Figure 2-17

***Figure 2-16.*** *This ad, one of a series featured in a Calvin Klein print and TV advertising campaign, was thought to verge on child pornography (Spin, September 1995).*

***Figure 2-17.*** *In an ad for Gucci fashion, the topless mother figure holds the nude infant, which is used as an attention-getting object (Vanity Fair, August 2003).*

## SEX AND VIOLENCE

Katz (1995) contends that "hegemonic constructions of masculinity in mainstream magazine advertising normalize male violence" (**Figure 2-18**). In contemporary ads involving male imagery, often the focus is on big, strong, and well-developed youth-

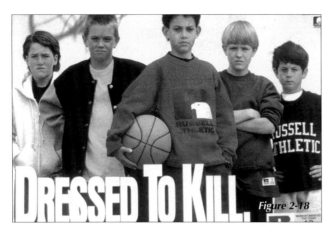

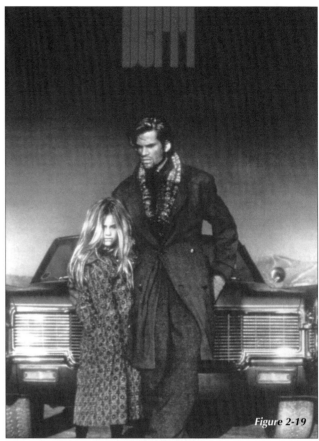

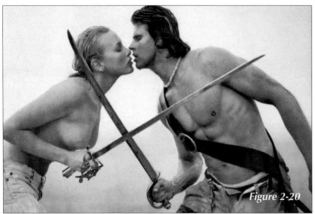

**Figure 2-18.** This ad for boys athletic clothing was headlined, "Dressed to Kill" (Sports Illustrated for Kids, *November 1991*).

**Figure 2-19.** An aggressive-looking adult male is juxtaposed with a vulnerable-looking female child in this ad (Vanity Fair, *September 1995*).

**Figure 2-20.** Sex and violence pair up in this ad (A&F Quarterly, *Summer 2002*).

**Figure 2-21.** Children are on display in a troubling and ambiguous setting for this Calvin Klein ad (Elle Girl, *Fall 2001*).

**Figure 2-22.** This Prada ad sequence appears to feature a young, fearful model as she's stalked (a), and next, lying on the floor injured or possibly dead (b) (Harper's Bazaar, *August 1997*).

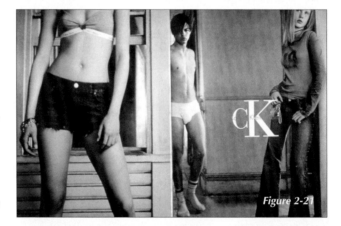

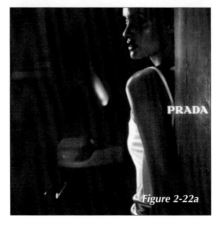

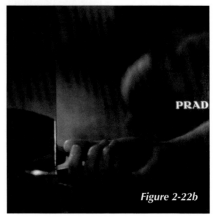

ful males. Hypertrophied muscles are signifiers of masculine power and bodies are to be used as instruments of dominance and control.

Currently, ads contain numerous images of dangerous-looking males and "men who are positioned as sexy because they possess a certain aggressive 'attitude'" (Katz, 2002) (**Figure 2-19**). There is not much of a leap to extend male aggression to the sexual realm. "By helping to differentiate masculinity from femininity, images of masculine aggression and violence—including violence against women—afford young males across class a degree of self-respect and security (however illusory) within the more socially valued masculine role" (Katz, 2002).

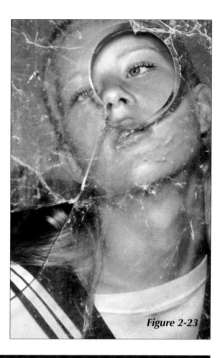

*Figure 2-23*

With the bombardment of so many sexual and violent ads comes desensitization, an acceptance of what is seen as status quo. A blend of sex and violence is becoming a popular marketing tool to help advertisers compete more effectively amid the blur of images and encourage consumers to stop and look. Adatto (1995) describes this trend in fashion photography as a progression of a "hard-edged eroticism ... that suggested illicit sex, violence, and sadomasochism." This trend has become more prevalent and explicit today. Images that threaten violence in a sexual context or the juxtaposing of sex and violence can be explicit (**Figure 2-20**), but, according to sociology professor Chris McCormick, more likely are "a sly, elusive blend of sex and violence. ... The very subtlety of these ads is deceptive and what makes them dangerous" (Roberts, 1994). Violence is "tied to sex, so what it does is sexualize violence. It almost makes violence desirable or at least makes violence acceptable as part of that package of desire and pleasure" (Cobden, 1994). The ambiguity of the ad grabs the attention of the viewer (**Figure 2-21**), making him or her wonder: Is it fear or fun? Is she being stalked by a predator or chased by a lover? Is she in danger or is it the thrill of risk? (**Figures 2-22-a** and **b**) Symbols of pain, torture, and sadomasochism are now glamorized in mainstream advertising, implying that subordination and suffering may result in sexual gratification. Victimization is used to attract attention, yet it is used to exploit the victims without any accompanying outrage or empathy for the victims. In addition to children being exposed routinely to this material, they are not exempt from these techniques, including advertisements directed to children and those portraying children (**Figure 2-23**). Messages within the highly familiar and approved cultural context of mainstream advertising are more likely to make previously unacceptable concepts more acceptable.

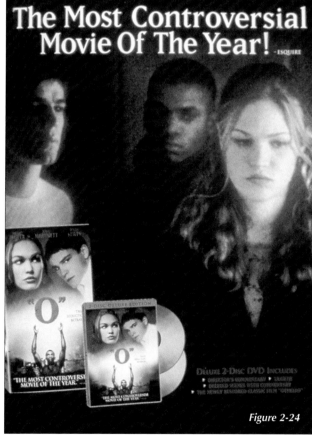

*Figure 2-24*

"There's a lot of really implicit, subtle violence, and it occurs over and over again in these ads. Once you start looking for it, once you educate yourself to see it, you realize it's there all the time," McCormick says (Roberts, 1994). Media literacy studies have shown that the more educated and critical a viewer is, the less influenced by media he or she will be.

Original and follow-up studies by the Federal Trade Commission in 2001 on the marketing of violent entertainment to children found that most of the video games, music, and movies, including those with R ratings (children under 17 must be accompanied by a parent or guardian), were promoted to appeal to children. Some movie companies actually use 9- to 10-year-olds to test-market violent R-rated films (Rosenbaum, 2001). Many more people are exposed to the ads for these movies than actually view the movies themselves (**Figure 2-24**).

**Figure 2-23.** *Suffering is portrayed in this ad with a childlike model (Jalouse, July 2001).*

**Figure 2-24.** *This R-rated movie about sex and violence in the lives of contemporary high school students was advertised in a magazine with a young audience (Seventeen, April 2002).*

# The Impact of Sexually Exploitative Advertising on Children, Adults, and Society

Advertising can play a role for many youth in distorting impressions of sexuality and reinforcing views of sex as a commodity or impersonal recreational activity. According to Brown et al (1993), researchers often can not ethically conduct the kinds of experiments with juveniles needed to establish a relationship between sexual content in the media and a change in behavior. Instead, they investigate what adolescents learn and how they interpret sexual content, with the assumption that learning will affect subsequent sexual behavior.

Music videos on MTV are a form of advertising for the music industry, marketing to a youthful audience. Experimental studies indicate that watching music videos may influence teen attitudes about early or risky sexual behavior. Adolescents who were shown a set of just 10 music videos in one study were more likely to find premarital sex acceptable for teens than adolescents from a comparison group who were not exposed to the videos (Brown et al, 1993).

Greenberg studied high school students who viewed sexual scenes taped from prime-time situation comedies and soap operas and asked them to rate the scenes according to how sexy, funny, enjoyable, and acceptable for TV viewing each was. Subjects rated intercourse between unmarried people as the sexiest, and they ranked prostitution scenes as the funniest and most enjoyable (Greenberg, 1993).

Junior high students who are exposed to more sexual content appear more likely to become involved in sexual activity. A study comparing pregnant versus non-pregnant teens found that the pregnant girls had watched more soap operas before becoming pregnant (a recent analysis found 156 acts of sex in 50 hours of programming on soap operas) and were less likely to think that their favorite characters practiced safe sex. Data from the National Surveys of Children found that boys who watched more TV had higher rates of sexual intercourse, and those who watched television alone had sex 3 to 6 times more than those who watched television with their families (Strasburger & Donnerstein, 1999). In another study, one third of teens surveyed said that entertainment media encourages them to have sex. Several polls have found that 3 out of 4 parents—and sometimes as many as 90% of parents—are worried about the amount of sexual content on television (Brownback, 2001).

Gender stereotyping and sexism in advertising are important concerns. Rudman and Borgida's study with male college undergraduate students pre-tested subjects with the Likelihood to Sexually Harass (LSH) Scale to assess the probability that they would sexually exploit women. In this study, which distinguished between chronic and acute priming effects, subjects were exposed to sexist advertising that consisted of ads that "portrayed women as interchangeable, decorative objects whose sole function is to please (ie, be sexually accessible to) men. For the most part, the ads depicted women as the 'implied reward' for product consumption" (Rudman, 1995). Each participant then interviewed and evaluated a female job candidate. Compared to men who had watched no television, the men who had seen the commercials asked more sexist questions, remembered more about her appearance than her personal background, and rated her as friendlier and more hirable but less competent. The female interviewee and observers deemed the men's behavior more sexualized. The study, using examples of routinely available and culturally sanctioned ads, found that even normally nonsexist subjects were influenced by the institutionalized sexism that sexist advertising represents (Rudman, 1995; Ward, 2002).

In Villani's 10-year review of the research on the impact of media on children and adolescents, she includes advertising as a distinct category of media. While acknowledging that advertising has not been studied as extensively as television programming, she states, "[t]he studies of the past decade document in a compelling fashion the influence of advertising media on the attitudes of young children and adolescents in ways that ultimately shape later behaviors" (Villani, 2001). During this decade (1990-2000), research focused on the areas of tobacco and alcohol advertising. She concludes that children's media consumption, especially of violent, gender-stereotyped, sexually explicit, or drug- or alcohol-influenced media, skews children's world view, including the frequency of sexual activity, the number of sexual partners, and beliefs about sexual norms in the real world. Consumption is correlated with increases in high-risk behavior and accelerates the onset of sexual activity (Villani, 2001).

The AAP was firm in its assessment of advertising, claiming it contains a significant amount of sexual imagery, including the inappropriate use of children in provocative poses. Advertising uses sexualized female bodies to sell everything from jeans to hotel rooms, shampoos to cars, yet, the AAP observes, when youth follow advertising's cues and become sexually active too soon, society seems to point a finger at the children instead of the advertisers. The AAP policy statement is clear: While early sexual activity may be caused by any number of factors, experts believe the media play a significant role (AAP, 2004).

In his theme paper for the Second World Congress Against the Commercial Sexual Exploitation of Children, Hecht (2001) addresses the role of the media. He emphasizes that in the advertising sub-sector, the portrayal of children in exploitative manners in conjunction with popular market products creates an additional layer of potential harm. The explicit and subtextual messages embedded in the commercials (**Figure 2-25**) can be further disseminated and legitimized by consumers buying the products, especially if peers and significant others are wearing, using, and/or valuing these products.

The strength of advertising messages can be enhanced by their repetitive nature. "Children learn patterns of behavior in what researchers refer to as 'stalagmite effects'—cognitive deposits built up almost imperceptibly from the drip-drip-drip of repeated exposure over time" (Steyer, 2002). Advertising functions as a legitimizing agent in subtle and complex ways. "In a post modern image culture, individuals get their very identity from these figures. Thus advertising becomes an important and overlooked mechanism of socialization as well as manager of consumer demand" (Kellner, 1995).

While the link between media and attitudinal and behavioral changes is evident, what may not be as clear are the *physical* effects on children exposed to sexual material in the media. It is well known that visual stimuli can have physiological effects on the body; for example, Pavlov's work with dogs or the common human response of salivation upon seeing a grapefruit cut. Research on adults watching erotica or pornographic material has found that visual stimulation can produce hormonal changes (Exton, 2000). Some professionals have questioned whether this stimulation from widespread highly sexualized mainstream media could be one of the factors in the earlier onset of puberty among children now (Herman-Giddens, 2002; Khadilkar, 2004).

Save the Children Canada conducted vitally important consultations with more than 150 commercially sexually exploited children in communities across Canada. Too often the mainstream media portrays street life and being on the run as exciting and glamorous. "The youth interviewed felt that movies

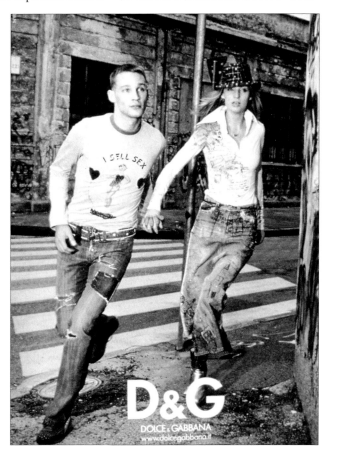

***Figure 2-25.*** *In this D&G Fashion ad, the male model sports a T-shirt with the phrase, "I Sell Sex." Whose, his or hers? If a high school student wears this shirt at social functions, he or she personifies the harmful message of glamorizing pimping and prostitution to peers (Elle, September 2003).*

such as *Pretty Woman*, magazines, and fashion glamorized the idea of the sex trade, and that they did not represent the reality of their lives" (Kingsley & Mark, 2000) (**Figure 2-26**). "Youth who work the streets do not have a glamorous lifestyle. They suffer from extremely high rates of violence and addiction, and many do not survive due to AIDS, overdoses, suicide, and murder. Media glamorization of the sex trade is harmful" (Kingsley & Mark, 2000) (**Figure 2-27**). Psychologist Frederick Matthews said,

[p]aradoxically it is the very desirability of this youthful sexuality that is used in advertising to titillate and sell consumer goods. Perhaps this is an indication that we undervalue our young people, that we are really more interested in their 'youth' as a commodity, with its exchange and use value. Although not intended in the usual sense of the word, the media acts as an advertising agent for prostitution. It does this through advertising escort agencies and in the way media portrays and glorifies prostitution in many pocket novels, in films, on commercial television, and in music videos. When one considers the extent to which cultural images of youthful sexuality permeate our society, it becomes difficult to fathom the difference, if any, between adolescent prostitution and sexual exploitation of young people in the media and in advertising (Kingsley & Mark, 2000).

## BODY IMAGE

An extraordinary amount of media attention is focused on an idealized, flawless female physical appearance, defined by sexual desirability and accessibility, seductiveness, and the ability to attract male attention. The female body type the media has chosen to idealize is that of the stick-thin model who is 13% to 18% below normal weight (Elias, 1999), and in some studies as much as 23% below normal weight (Gilday, 1990) (**Figure 2-28**). For a diagnosis of anorexia, body weight is 15% below normal weight (American Psychiatric Association, 1994). To what extent does media influence the perception of youth regarding ideal body size and shape? What is the cumulative impact of repetitive, stereotypical images reinforced over multiple media forms? An area of significant concern for pediatricians and other health professionals is the link between media, including advertising, and eating disorders. The term "trigger pictures" has been used for commercial photos of extremely slender and emaciated-looking models and celebrities (**Figure 2-29**). This label is also used by anorexic youth who use these images as inspiration and impetus for ongoing starvation and are even posted as "trigger pix" on pro-anorexia Web Sites (Quart, 2003).

It has been noted that "[h]igh school girls who saw 15 commercials that emphasized sex appeal and/or physical attractiveness were more likely than girls who saw a set of neutral commercials to say that beauty characteristics were important for them to feel good about themselves and to be popular with men" (Brown et al, 1993). Author Philip Myers states, "[a]nother experimental study found that exposure to just 30 minutes of television programming and advertising that included ideal body images altered college women's perceptions about the shape of their bodies" (Brown et al, 1993). Studies have shown a link between reading fashion magazines and body dissatisfaction in girls. Among surveyed 5th- through 12th-grade girls, 7 in 10 say magazine pictures influence their ideas of perfect body shape, and nearly half report wanting to lose weight because of magazine photos. Only 29% of girls in the study were overweight (Field et al, 1999).

Higher scores on a factor of preoccupation with a thin body and social pressures, measuring concerns with weight, shape, and eating (including media modeling, social eating, dieting, and weight teasing), significantly predicted the onset of eating disorders in girls in middle and high school. This study proposes consideration of prevention programs before 6th grade (McKnight, 2003).

The oppressive focus on the "perfect" body is not limited to the female form; it has influenced male imagery. In addition to the portrayals of male power and aggression, some images of males in ads became more "objectified" in the late 1980s and early

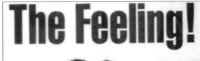

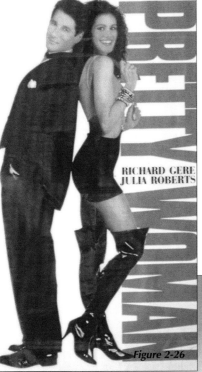

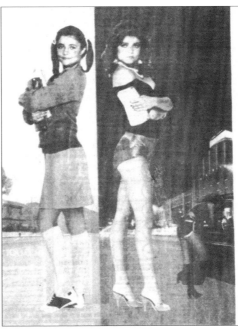

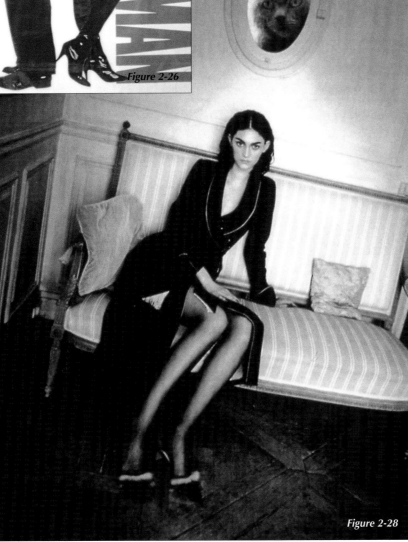

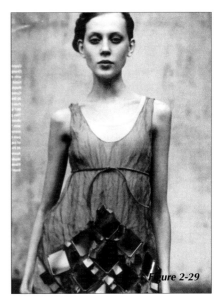

**Figure 2-26.** *This poster advertising the movie* Pretty Woman *features a famous actress as a prostituted young woman in a Cinderella-like story.*

**Figure 2-27.** *The copy in this ad promoting a movie about juvenile prostitution reads: "High school honor student by day. Hollywood hooker by night. … It's her choice. Her chance. Her life." This movie is currently available on DVD in mainstream department stores (New York Times, January 6, 1984).*

**Figure 2-28.** *This fashion ad features a profoundly thin female model (New York Times Magazine, August 23, 1998).*

**Figure 2-29.** *This ad is a possible example of a "trigger pix," used to inspire young women to become anorexic (New York Times Magazine, Spring 1999).*

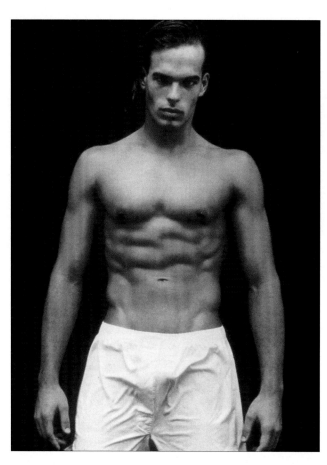

**Figure 2-30** *A male model in Calvin Klein underwear displays his muscles for the viewers* (Spin, *December 1995*).

1990s, displaying bodies passively for sexual attractiveness. (Objectification is traditionally associated with the portrayal of females.) Ironically, fashion advertising began featuring more young males wearing less and less and displaying not clothes, but denuded, shaved, buff torsos. This new style of male eroticism had more to do with the increasing commercialization of sexuality and upping the ante for novel stimuli to compete with the advertising clutter. Currently, advertising includes countless, repetitious images of big, barechested, youthful models with well-developed bodies and washboard abdomens (**Figure 2-30**). This marketing approach may help to create a sense of inadequacy among boys about their own bodies and ongoing physical development. Demanding body-building programs with austere diets, nutritional supplements, dubious and sometimes dangerous sports, and performance-enhancing over-the-counter drugs among preteen and adolescent males have become a public health concern (Quart, 2003).

## The Sex Exploiter

Many of those who sexually exploit children are not pedophiles or sadistic, psychopathic criminals. To simplify the problem to a few types of perpetrators removed from what we understand as "normal" is a common but not helpful practice. All kinds of people (advertisers among them) sexually exploit children in many ways and for many reasons. To better protect children, it is imperative to identify and understand the social, political, and economic factors that drive the demand side for child sex.

Davidson (2001), in her paper presented at the Second World Congress Against Commercial Sexual Exploitation, raises this disturbing indictment by stating that "most societies attach a good deal of aesthetic and erotic value to youthful bodies. Adults who seek out younger and more attractive sexual partners, including persons under the age of 18, are not necessarily transgressing the socially agreed perimeters of acceptable sexual desires and therefore cannot be automatically described as sexually 'deviant' or psychologically 'abnormal.'"

In their study on university males' sexual interest in children, Briere & Runtz (1989) published some disturbing statistics. According to their research with university undergraduate men, 21% reported sexual attraction to some small children, 9% described sexual fantasies involving children, 5% admitted having masturbated to such fantasies, and 7% indicated some likelihood of having sex with a child if he could avoid detection and punishment. This is considered by the authors to be an underestimate as it is socially unacceptable to admit sexual interest in a child. Child-focused sexual interest of "normal" college-aged males was most strongly associated with negative early sexual experiences and masturbation to pornography (Briere & Runtz, 1989). This may be one of the effects of "normalizing" children as sexual objects by depicting them inappropriately in more mainstream and legitimized media such as advertising. This study was conducted before the full impact of the Internet. The growth of the Internet has had a profound effect on the number of child pornography images now circulating in the public discourse. This makes the images of sexualized children in advertisements more dangerous, as they are appealing to an audience that may have intentionally or unintentionally seen pornographic images of children and may have masturbated to them.

Media, as a leading sex education resource, teach young males what they want and that their masculinity is demonstrated by sexual access to unlimited, youthful trophy-sex objects, while it teaches girls that physical appearance and sex are their only value and are used as commodities of exchange. If men are socialized to believe that success in sex depends on the domination and conquest of a submissive partner, or even that sexuality is linked with power over another, then children's vulnerability, dependence, and lack of power are effective stimuli, especially for insecure adults. Children make fewer emotional demands and are easier to control. Adding repetitive and dramatic sexualized images of children across multiple media forms can serve as powerful reinforcement for a sexual interest in children.

British and US studies of convicted child sex offenders suggest that they are most likely to respond to the cognitive dissonance associated with child sexual abuse by shifting their attitudes towards adult-child sexual contact and/or towards their victims. Thus, they typically exhibit distorted attitudes and beliefs which allow them to construct children as being in some way responsible for their own abuse, and/or to imagine that children are not harmed by sexual contact with adults, and/or that children are able to consent to, or obtain benefits from, sexual encounters with adults (Davidson, 2001).

More and more experts are making a connection between sexual abuse and the sexual portrayal of children and adolescents in everyday media. When children are glamorized as sexual objects, it condones their use in sexual contexts, which is always inappropriate. It confuses children, leading them to think that this is a good way to behave. Worse, it confuses certain adults into thinking the same thing: in extreme cases, it validates the child sexual abuser's excuse that children are asking for sex (Elliott, 1992).

There is a strong link between child sexual abuse, the production of child pornography, and child prostitution. The adults involved in the sex trade continuum frequently employ manipulative and coercive tactics, and there is considerable movement between the different forms of commercial sexual exploitation of children.

Ron O'Grady, Honorary President of End Child Prostitution, Child Pornography and Trafficking of Children for Sexual Purposes (ECPAT) International, was strong in his stand at the Second World Congress against the Commercial Sexual Exploitation of Children. "Equally apparent at the conclusion of the Congress was the feeling that we must deal more adequately with the 'demand' side of child sex abuse. This is a strong confirmation of the stand which ECPAT has stressed since we began 12 years ago. Our emphasis has always been on trying to end the trade in children and that means dealing with those who cause the problem and changing the behavior of the abusers" (O'Grady, 2002).

## REGULATION OF ADVERTISING TO CHILDREN IN THE UNITED STATES

According to information from the Council of Better Business Bureaus, the Children's Advertising Review Unit (CARU) was established by the National Advertising Review Council to promote responsible advertising to children (defined as those under 12 years of age) and respond to public concerns. Published by the Association of National Advertisers, Inc, in 1972, the Children's Advertising Guidelines encourage truthful and accurate advertising sensitive to the special nature of children. Subsequently, the advertising community established CARU to serve as an independent manager of the industry's self-regulatory program. The latest revisions, in 1999, deal expressly with data collection and privacy on the Internet. The assistance of CARU's Advisory Board, and of other children's advertisers, agencies, and trade associations, has been invaluable.

The National Advertising Review Council is a strategic alliance of the advertising industry and the Council of Better Business Bureaus. The board of directors of this council comprises key executives from the Council of Better Business Bureaus, the American Advertising Federation, the American Association of Advertising Agencies, and the Association of National Advertisers. This board sets the policy for the Children's Advertising Review Unit's self-regulatory program. Administered by the Council of Better Business Bureaus, it is funded directly by members of the children's advertising industry. Advisory boards comprised of experts in education, communication, child development, and industry representatives are supposed to advise on general issues concerning children's advertising and to assist in the revision of the guidelines published by CARU (last revised in 2001). These guidelines can be found at http://www.caru.org/guidelines/index.asp.

CARU's guidelines provide a basis for evaluating child-directed advertising addressed to children under 12 years of age in all media, including print, broadcast and cable television, radio, video, point-of-sale, and online advertising and packaging. These guidelines are based on 7 underlying principles (CARU, 2003):

1. Advertisers should always take into account the level of knowledge, sophistication, and maturity of the audience to which their message is primarily directed. Younger children have a limited capacity for evaluating the credibility of information they receive. They may lack the ability to understand the nature of the information being provided. Advertisers, therefore, have a special responsibility to protect children from their own susceptibilities.

2. Realizing that children are imaginative and that make-believe play constitutes an important part of the growing up process, advertisers should exercise care not to exploit unfairly the imaginative quality of children. Unreasonable expectations of product quality or performance should not be stimulated either directly or indirectly by advertising.

3. Products and content that are inappropriate for use by children should not be advertised or promoted directly to children.

4. Recognizing that advertising may play an important part in educating the child, advertisers should communicate information in a truthful and accurate manner and in language understandable to young children with full recognition that the child may learn practices from advertising that can affect his or her health and well-being.

5. Advertisers are urged to capitalize on the potential of advertising to influence behavior by developing advertising that, wherever possible, addresses itself to positive and beneficial social behavior, such as friendship, kindness, honesty, justice, generosity, and respect for others.

6. Care should be taken to incorporate minority and other groups in advertisements in order to present positive and pro-social roles and role models wherever possible. Social stereotyping and appeals to prejudice should be avoided.

7. Although many influences affect a child's personal and social development, it remains the prime responsibility of the parents to provide guidance for children. Advertisers should contribute to this parent-child relationship in a constructive manner.

CARU's basic activity is to review and evaluate advertising directed to children. When advertisements are found to be misleading, inaccurate, or inconsistent with the industry's self-regulatory guidelines, CARU works with the advertiser on a case-by-case basis to make a change through voluntary cooperation. Complaints may come from individuals, consumer groups, professional or trade associations, government agencies, and other advertisers. However, according to Dominic Lyle, Executive Director of the European Association of Communications Agencies (written communication, June 2002), more than 95% of CARU's inquiries stem from its own monitoring of television, print advertising, and Web sites (132 in 2001). Complaints made to local Better Business Bureaus may be directed to CARU if they have a sufficient national merit.

All CARU, National Advertising Division (NAD) of the Council of Better Business Bureaus, and National Advertising Review Board decisions are published in the NAD/CARU Case Reports (issued 10 times a year) as well as in the regular press. The National Advertising Review Board is the appellate branch of the self-regulatory system and hears appeals from NAD and CARU decisions.

## STATUS OF GUIDELINES REGARDING SEXUALIZATION OF CHILDREN AND ADVERTISING TO ADOLESCENTS

Other countries have similar guidelines, yet are much stricter in their measures to protect children. For instance, self-regulatory guidelines for the European Union define a child as under 15 years of age (D. Lyle, written communication, June 2002), yet CARU's Guidelines apply to advertising addressed to children under 12 years of age. In CARU's section on Product Presentation, one Guideline states, "[p]ortrayals or encouragement of behavior inappropriate for children (eg, violence or sexuality) and presentations that could frighten or provoke anxiety in children should be avoided." The European guidelines are more direct, cautioning advertisers not to glamorize violence, present violence as an acceptable method of achieving social or interpersonal gains, or portray children in a sexually provocative manner.

Canada's self-regulatory body, Advertising Standards Canada, explicitly states that advertisements must not "appear to exploit, condone, or incite violence; nor directly encourage, or exhibit indifference to, unlawful behaviour" (2004). And the Canadian Gender Portrayal Guidelines direct advertisers to specifically avoid "inappropriate use or exploitation of sexuality of both women and men" (Advertising Standards Canada, 1993). Quebec does not allow *any* advertising to children. The process for making a complaint or appeal is clearly explained in material from Advertising Standards Canada. A detailed report on the complaints is published yearly and is available on the Web site.

In the United States, there are no guidelines on specifics regarding the sexualization of children in advertisements, no guidelines for advertising to children over 11 years of age, and no guidelines for the depiction and use of children in advertising directed toward adults. The only related material is a directive under the "Safety" section of a publication from CARU stating, "advertisements should not portray adults or children in unsafe situations, or in acts harmful to themselves or others."

### SEXUALLY EXPLICIT PHOTOS AND PROOF OF AGE

The advertising industry commonly portrays children, especially girls, who are nude, partially nude, and/or in sexually suggestive poses. Often the girls appear very young whether or not they are actually under 18 years of age. One serious consideration is that no federal law exists prohibiting the creation and publication of advertisements or other images showing nude children or adolescents as long as they are not in sexually explicit (rather than suggestive) poses.

Currently, proof of age is required for persons participating in the production of pornography (federal law) (**Table 2-1**) and for employment as a nude dancer (state laws). Similarly, the purchase of cigarettes or alcohol requires proof of age because of the illegality of use under certain ages and the deleterious effects on children's health.

Proof of age is even more important in today's environment. Girls are reaching sexual maturity earlier than in the past and are often younger than they appear (Herman-Giddens et al, 1997), and there is an increasing demand for sexualized children in the advertising, pornography, and related sex trade industries. Physical sexual maturity for US children now occurs at 15 to 16 years of age and often earlier (Sun et al, 2002). Although there is an urgent need for more research on the effects on children made the subject of pornographic and sexualized imagery, there is ample evidence of the harm of exposure to pornography to both adults and children (Dines, 1998; Itzin 1997; Wingood et al, 2001; Zillmann et al, 1994). It is likely that the effects of

| Table 2-1. Relevant Federal Statute for Pornography—18 USC 2257 |
| --- |

This statute mandates that producers of pornographic materials check age identification of all people appearing in their visual depictions and that they maintain records of that identification (and label materials according to specified regulations with information about the location of those records). The producer is required to do the following:

1. Ascertain, by examination of an identification document containing such information, the performer's name and date of birth, and require the performer to provide such other indicia of his or her identity as may be prescribed by regulations.

2. Ascertain any name, other than the performer's present and correct name, ever used by the performer including maiden name, alias, nickname, stage, or professional name.

3. Record in the records required by subsection (a) the information required by paragraphs (1) and (2) of this subsection and such other identifying information as may be prescribed by regulation.

As with nearly all laws, this statute has regulations that elaborate on the details of effectuating the code. In this case, the relevant regulations are documented in 28 CFR (Code of Federal Regulations) § 75.1 and sequence. The statute clarifies that the identification must be picture identification as defined in 28 CFR § 75.1(b): "Picture identification card shall mean a document issued by a government entity or by a private entity, such as a school or a private employer, that bears the photograph and the name of the individual identified. A picture identification card may be a passport, driver's license, work identification card, school identification card, selective service card, or identification card issued by a state."

pornography-related child sexual abuse are enhanced as compared to those of sexual abuse that do not include production of sexually explicit images, in part due to the permanence of photographs and videos as well as the unprecedented global scope of distribution. With increasing maturity, individuals used in these ways as children often exhibit anxiety, humiliation, and shame due to the knowledge that the images of them are irrevocable, uncontrollable, and may be distributed worldwide (Itzin, 1997). A source of trauma and distress may be the recognition that the permanent record of their abuse becomes entertainment for untold strangers and acquaintances and may be used to normalize viewing children as sexual targets.

Minors, especially those under 18, are less likely to be able to assess any future harm from participating in public sexual activities; therefore, proof of age is essential. Minors are simply not able to give full informed consent and are entitled to protection from the significant inherent risks. Because many documents such as driver's licenses may be fraudulently produced, it would be prudent for the laws to require birth certificates in addition to photo identification.

# RECOMMENDATIONS FOR CHANGE
## LET KIDS BE KIDS
Many groups, educational and cultural, medical and political, are investigating the impact of media on children and understanding media as a public health problem as

well as a sociological one. Because of the growing sexualization of children by the media in the United States, in 1997, the Committee on Child Abuse & Neglect of the North Carolina Pediatric Society launched a campaign against the sexual exploitation of children in advertising. The campaign, titled Let Kids Be Kids, was designed to discourage companies from using advertising that portrayed children as sexual objects. The North Carolina Pediatric Society produced brochures, videotapes, and other promotional materials that described the problem (**Figure 2-31**). These were distributed to all pediatricians across the state and were made available to others upon request. Brochure content emphasized that physicians, parents, and others interested in this issue can do the following:

— Write or call advertisers who sexually exploit children in their ads.

— Educate colleagues about the problem.

— Talk to children if they are exposed to these advertisements to address confusion such ads create.

— Discourage companies or businesses from advertising in this manner.

— Support advertisers using healthy, nonsexual, and age-appropriate themes and let them know of your support.

— Promote media literacy courses that include sexuality issues in schools.

The Let Kids Be Kids campaign targets advertisements of children wearing provocative clothing, appearing in suggestive poses, or touching private parts. It also targets ads of adult models acting sexually desirable while made to look like children. The North Carolina Pediatric Society encourages the public to support companies using healthy, nonsexual, age-appropriate advertisements. The North Carolina campaign spurred a national effort, which was supported by the American Academy of Pediatrics (AAP), which has also endorsed advertising campaigns that present youth in positive settings without relying on sexual themes.

A survey containing specific advertisements with questions regarding respondents' opinions was distributed to members of the North Carolina Pediatric Society, medical students, and medical residents. Approximately 80% of the survey respondents felt that children presented in a sexualized manner influence the general public's perception of childhood sexuality. However, more than 90% of private physicians surveyed admitted that they do not counsel families about sexualized advertising and its underlying messages.

*Figure 2-31.* This Let Kids Be Kids brochure is a way that the North Carolina Pediatric Association Society is working to protect children.

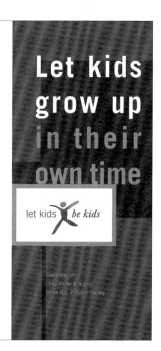

### DADS AND DAUGHTERS

Dads and Daughters (DADs), a national nonprofit membership group for fathers and daughters, conducted a write-in campaign expressing concern about the epidemic of girls' body image problems to 5 popular teen girls magazines: *Seventeen, Teen People, CosmoGIRL, Teen,* and *YM.* Only *YM* responded, agreeing to stop printing diet tips and start including larger models in its stories. DADs continues to urge all teen magazines to demand that advertisers stop glorifying unhealthy body images. The group plans to "draw positive attention to those who market successfully without undermining kids" (Kelly, 2002).

## WHAT PEDIATRICIANS CAN DO

The AAP has taken leadership in recognizing the role of mass media in child health and development, by reviewing research, advocating policy, and developing and implementing professional and public education campaigns. Its most comprehensive effort, Media Matters: A National Media Education Campaign, was launched in 1997 to assist physicians, parents, and children in recognizing the impact of media on health and providing strategies to mitigate potential problems (http://www.aap. org/advocacy/mediamatters.htm).

Programs like North Carolina's Let Kids Be Kids, organizations such as the AAP and the American Association of Child and Adolescent Psychiatrists (AACAP) and other child advocacy groups, and concerned parents and teachers are united in a public stand to protect children from harmful media. Advertising is more than just a blur of images in the pages of magazines and across the channels of the television, before the feature in the movie theater or as pop-up windows on the Internet. Author Mary Vipond states, "[a]dvertising is a form of communication and even, some would argue, of culture. Its presence in virtually all of our media is integral, not accidental. … Its influence and effect are intertwined with the influence and effect of the editorial content it surrounds and pays for … It is thus fundamental not only to the economics of our media but to their cultural impact" (1989).

Pediatricians are in a unique position to make a difference because of their proximity, and more important, commitment to the welfare of children. The question is simple: How can we as concerned individuals allow, let alone support, individuals and industries who achieve success by irresponsibly using other people's children to sell products? The answer is equally simple: Until more people demand more responsibility in advertising, we are neglecting our responsibility. While advertising is not causing society's ills nor is it even the sole factor contributing to the vulnerability of children, its influence must be studied. Reminding people by taking a definitive stand that children have a right to a positive and safe childhood, society takes a giant step forward. Yet it can seem to be an overwhelming task; voices for change can seem small and insignificant compared to the powerful and pervasive influence of the media. But there are some simple steps physicians can take now to help ensure children's safety.

The AAP and the AACAP recommend that pediatricians, child psychiatrists, and child health professionals add a simple media history as part of a health profile during routine office visits (Arehart-Treichel, 2001; Wingood, et al 2001). As part of the AAP's Media Matters program, a media history form is available, and the academy recommends that parents spend 5 minutes completing this form in addition to the usual medical history form during annual exams. If the evaluation indicates heavy media use, pediatricians can suggest healthy alternatives as well as evaluate for aggressive behavior, fears, or sleep disturbances. Brochures are available with suggestions about how to guide families toward positive uses of media, establishing a healthy "media diet" with limits and balance, and critical discussion of what they read and watch. Exploring sexual content of media preferences can help in evaluating exposure to media sexual misinformation as well as providing an opportunity for discussion of sexuality issues.

The academy has recommended providing only socially responsible, child-positive magazines, periodicals, and other media choices to patients in outpatient waiting rooms and inpatient settings. That should be expanded to include prescreening print media, videotapes, and videogames for violent content and for sexually explicit content. When evaluating print media, look at editorial content as well as advertising images and messages. Encourage and facilitate professional organizations and child advocacy groups to establish content guidelines for popular media available at all child and adolescent health care settings. Obtain child-friendly literature on developing media literacy skills and material to help educate parents on media issues that include advertising.

"[I]ntensive lobbying in Hollywood by groups such as the AAP and the Center for Population Options ... has resulted in more references to safer sex and condoms in entertainment programming and in teen magazines and music" (Brown et al, 1993). Such efforts are important and should be encouraged and expanded especially to the advertising community.

Use this successful model to develop outreach programs to increase awareness and encourage the implementation of codes of conduct within modeling agencies and professional groups of photographers (ie, the National Association of Photographers). Lobby for establishing position statements regarding the responsible portrayal of children in advertising, as well as guidelines to minimize the risk of harm to children used in the production of commercial media.

Emphasize the "profitability" as well as the "positive duty" of social responsibility within the business community. "[C]onsumers are willing to not only boycott services whose reputations are tainted by allegations of child abuse but also to pay more for services that were not provided through questionable practices. ... [A] recent study found that 78 percent of US consumers would avoid retailers known to carry products made in exploitative circumstances" (Hecht, 2001).

Encourage the AAP to form a committee to study the harm to children and adolescents used in sexual media and the desirability of working to pass legislation to raise the minimum age to 21 years old for models used in the production of sexually explicit media. Related recommendations from the AAP include advocating the following (Committee on Public Education, 2001):

— Programming supporting responsible sex

— Public service announcements encouraging abstinence

— More child-positive media, not censorship

— Media education in schools

— More research into the effect of sexual content in the media on children and adolescents.

Additional knowledge is essential about risk factors, effective deterrents to children being influenced by harmful media messages, and ways that media can be used to educate and intervene on unsafe sexual activity (Committee on Public Education, 2001). Other actions include encouraging people to do the following:

— Advocate for stricter limitations on the amount of advertising on children's television.

— Hold corporations and businesses accountable by not buying their products.

— Praise appropriate advertising and patronize responsible businesses.

— Suggest parents spend their dollars on consumer goods that do not exploit children with harmful products or advertising.

— Write offending companies letters of thoughtful concern and get other colleagues and parents to write, as well as encourage similar projects for older children and adolescents as individuals and groups.

— Write, phone, or e-mail local newspapers and radio and TV stations who run irresponsible ads.

— Encourage parents to teach media literacy and ask their children's schools to do the same; ask leaders at the neighborhood school if they have a program on media literacy that includes advertising and sexuality, if not, volunteer to serve on a committee to develop needed programs.

— Help to raise public awareness by suggesting and supporting school, civic group and church programs, and workshops on advertising, media, and sexuality.

— Support media activist groups that promote more balanced, realistic, age-appropriate, and diverse portrayals of girls and boys and men and women in advertising.

— Encourage professional associations and child advocacy organizations to develop position statements on the nonexploitive use of children in advertising and the targeting of children by advertisers.

— Build coalitions with other professional and community groups, including early childhood professions and parent-teacher organizations, education and public health departments, and state attorney generals' offices.

More important than the action as the consumer is the role of child and parent advocate. Parents are a child's first line of defense; pediatricians can use their influence to help parents raise media-resilient children with the following suggestions:

— Remind parents that advertising represents commercial speech, not free speech, and the FTC is empowered to ban advertising that is unfair or deceptive.

— Encourage parents to expect the media to take responsibility for its actions and play a role in the public health of society.

— Advise them to limit children's access and exposure to media, especially when young, and to establish good media habits early.

— Encourage them to discuss media with their children, pointing out that media are created products designed to influence and sell other products; help parents explain that advertisements entrance viewers because media-makers make it their business to do so, spending years learning techniques for influencing others.

— Reinforce that though children may protest and disagree, especially when parents critically assess popular youth culture, they will remember what was said and may not experience the images or messages in the same way again; this can keep children from feeling overwhelmed or traumatized by totally unrealistic images and highly sexualized messages and demands for appearance and behavior.

— Brainstorm ways for parents to more effectively share about media experience and impact, and establish an open and ongoing dialogue with their children.

— Support parents who may feel devalued and stigmatized for being critical of the powerfully pervasive and youth-focused popular culture.

— Encourage muting commercial breaks while viewing TV, or if not muting, pointing out marketing techniques.

Good parent-child discussions about advertising are vital. An AAP News article identified ads as the most expensive and powerful media messages, loaded with emotional material. The hundreds of thousands of commercials a child is exposed to by age 18 can condition a child to not think and shorten attention spans. "Explain and break the power of the rapid-fire images. ... Reclaim the power of your own attention from the makers of the commercials" (McCannon, 1997). The academy cites a number of ways that parents can reclaim that power and help children avoid television advertising, including exploring public TV as a viewing option, taping programs for children and editing the commercials, organizing a family video library, and avoiding program-length commercials (American Academy of Pediatrics, 1995).

Of course, the most important step is to learn more and to be able to tell the difference between what is educational, age-appropriate and developmentally appropriate, and healthy, and what is dehumanizing and exploitive. According to the AAP, "pediatricians and parents must embrace media education as the best and simplest solution to the public health risks presented by the media" (Hogan, 1999).

According to a press release from the AAP, "media are also the influence that can be most easily changed to send responsible messages to young people about sex. The policy statement recommends that broadcast media provide messages that encourage the delay of sexual intercourse and support safer, more respectful sexual behavior" (Pediatrician presents findings, 2001).

It is clear that citizens and professionals are coming together to protect children from harm caused by inappropriate portrayals in media and advertising. Expanding this global challenge, HIH Princess Takamado encouraged attendees in her welcoming speech at the opening session of the Second World Congress Against the Commercial Sexual Exploitation of Children held in December 2001 in Yokohama, Japan, by remarking, "every adult is guilty of being an accomplice if he looks the other way and allows the sexual exploitation of children to take place. ... If there were no demand, it would not be commercially viable to have a supply. This is a simple fact. If there is anyone around you that is helping to create a demand, then take courage and speak out" (The History of ECPAT, 2002).

Many children, too, know what is and is not right. An unscientific polling of a Chapel Hill, North Carolina, 3rd grade class on what the phrase "let kids be kids" means to them reveals much about this issue. "Grown-ups should help kids do the right things," says Caroline. "Kids should be able to do just kid things and not have to do grown-up things," Justin comments. "Kids shouldn't have to do things they're not ready for yet," Lauren concludes. And what does advertising tell these children? Jennifer sums up the issue perfectly: "I think that advertisers are just using kids. They just want to make more money and they think that taking pictures of kids will get them more money."

## CONCLUSION

Children Now, a child advocacy group, found that 77% of 800 kids surveyed wished there were less sexual things on TV. But according to Cobden, a director of a university school of journalism,

every year the imagery becomes louder, more aggressive, more explicit. It has to as all these mass media fight for our desensitized attention. Where will it end? One shudders to think. ... And the sexier and more violent the messages, the sexier and more violent they have to be next time to get our attention. And so it goes ... So isn't it paradoxical that our society abominates sexual crime as never before while absorbing bigger and bigger doses of sexual stimulation without protest? (1994).

The bottom line? "Society cannot claim to abhor the sexual abuse and exploitation of children ... in pornography and yet allow the portrayal of children ... as sexualized objects in the popular press and in advertising" (Elliott, 1992).

Deborah Roffman, a teacher of human sexuality and author of *Sex and Sensibility: The Thinking Parent's Guide to Talking Sense About Sex*, sums up the benefits of ending the exploitation of children in advertising:

What is going on here is nothing less than the violation of our children's most fundamental rights and needs. A sense of clear limits is not just 'nice' for children and teens, it's almost as important to them as oxygen. Limits and boundaries—those brackets we put around our children's lives to keep them safe and healthy—do for them what they are not yet able to do for themselves. A culture that screams 'There are no limits!' at every turn puts children in great peril. ... Ultimately, we'll need to create a society where our children's first and most important reference points about sexuality are families and schools, not their peers [or] the media (Roffman, 2002).

# APPENDIX 2-1: THE MARKETING MACHINE

Abercrombie & Fitch (A&F) is a national chain of retail clothing stores that has been targeting adolescents and preadolescents for more than a decade, more recently including separate stores for younger children called abercrombie. Beginning in 1997, until the withdrawal of the Christmas 2003 issue, A&F published an almost 300-page catalog 4 times a year and charged consumers $6 an issue at stores or less for annual subscriptions for this advertising vehicle. The quarterly publication, described more accurately by many as a "magalog," or magazine/catalog combination, appeared more like a lifestyle magazine and subsequently came shrink-wrapped with a warning label that it was for adult buyers 18 years and older. The warning label was added after public awareness led to organized protests and threats of legal action because this sexually explicit adult material was being purchased by middle-schoolers. Additional controversy and some media attention was generated when abercrombie children's stores sold thong underpants to girls as young as 10 years old, with messages on the underwear such as "wink, wink" and "eye candy" (Ford, 2002).

Although using sex to sell to children is not uncommon, A&F took marketing to youth to the next level of exploitation with irresponsible and hyper-sexualized advertising as well as products (such as T-shirts), and probably further lowering the threshold of what society would tolerate as acceptable for children.

Sexualized T-shirt slogans for young girls included:

— Front of shirt: PURE; back of shirt: EVIL

— Wild Honeys

— A&F Soccer shirt: We SCORE MORE

— Abercrombie Women's Water Polo shirt: WE DO IT BETTER IN THE WATER

— Front of shirt: Moon-Lite Bakery; back of shirt: We Knead It All Night

— A&F Cloud 9 Hotel, fulfilling your wildest dreams since 1892 (NOTE: "Cloud nine" is a street term for ecstasy [MDMA], an illegal and dangerous club-drug used by young people at raves [all-night dance parties].)

— "I Got Lucky at the ..." Pair-a-Dice Motel, Honey Moon Sweets, Hourly Rates Available (NOTE: Hourly hotel/motel rates are most commonly associated with prostitution.)

Sexualized T-shirt slogans for young males included:

— Want a Quickie? Quickie Car Wash, Quickie In & Out Service

— Party Animal: Individual who has trouble controlling limits ... Can be found sleeping it off on the beach

— Spring Break: Random hook-ups with several willing partners ... Stint in Mexican jail

— I schedule classes around happy hour

— Ski Fest: Spruce Mountain, "The most fun you'll have going down"

To legitimize the catalog's commercial sexual display, A&F sprinkles throughout its content miscellaneous articles, literary and music reviews, and interviews with entertainment figures including strippers, porn stars, and youth cult figures, with raunchy sex talk embedded in the text. One particularly graphic interview of a popular star in hardcore pornography included a photo of her on a bed displaying a tattoo on her buttocks. One celebrity interviewee exclaimed that having sex with a drunk female is a normal activity on campus, and that 90% of all sex would not happen without liquor. In a pseudo-advice column, a student was strongly encouraged to get a summer job stripping because this was empowering for females. Content included exhibitionism, nudity (genitals are not displayed), campus streaking, nude football, implicit couple sex in dorms and in classrooms, "threesomes," group sex, student/teacher sex, binge drinking, porno-chic, stripping, and prostitution (**Appendix Figures 2-1** and **2-2**). One photo in the issue that was eventually pulled (**Appendix Figure 2-3**) was followed by this caption titled "Group Sex":

Sex, as we know, can involve one or two, but what about even more? The ménage à trois (three-way) is not an uncommon arrangement. An orgy can involve an unlimited quantity of potential lovers. Groups can be mixed-gender or same-sex, friendly or anonymous. The risk of pregnancy and of STD transmission, including HIV, increases with each additional partner. A pleasant and supersafe alternative to this is group masturbation—sometimes called a circle jerk or Jack-and-Jill-Off. Orgies and group sex were common in the Middle Ages. Promiscuity was popular with both the peasantry and the nobility. Since divorce was forbidden by the Church, adultery was very common and socially accepted. Did you know? Both humans and porpoises have one social sex practice in common—group sex. So that's what they keep making those noises for (A&F Quarterly, Christmas, 2003).

This was shocking content to some, but provoking a strong response was the intent in order to compete with the clutter of other advertising to increasingly desensitized youth. Playing to the adolescent tasks of questioning traditional authority and institutions, A&F legitimized and glamorized high-risk behaviors while selling children logo knit tank tops and low-rise hot pants.

Regional and national citizen groups intensified protests and organized consumer boycotts. After years of ignoring complaints, in December 2003, A&F pulled the Christmas Field Guide Issue. The company failed to comment on the content of the quarterly or respond to criticism but stated that the catalogs were removed to make more room on store shelves for new products (Carr & Rozhon, 2003). A&F subsequently revealed its plan to retire the quarterly catalog without giving reasons for its decision or details for a new marketing campaign.

Apart from the changes in catalog format, the fashions themselves have an impact. The clothes have been termed "aspirational," outfits preadolescents and young teens buy to emulate "cool" college kids. Marketing and products may contribute to permission-giving beliefs for age-inappropriate behavior by exploiting teens' desire to emulate older youth. Because there is an intense need by adolescents to feel part of the sexually attractive, high-social-standing "in" peer group, A&F tries to deliver an easy answer for youngsters by promoting behavior rebellious and independent of restrictive rules or the admonitions of "old people" and "wimps." A&F sells more than logo-emblazoned T-shirts that transform kids into walking billboards; it continues to sell values and concepts of sexuality, romance, success, and normalcy.

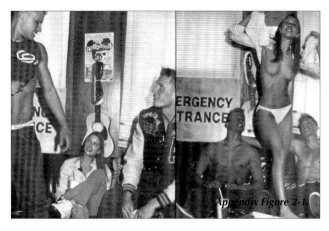

*Appendix Figure 2-1*

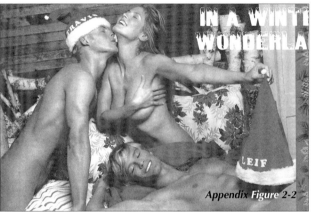

*Appendix Figure 2-2*

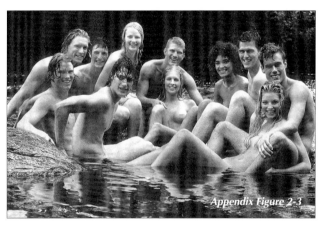

*Appendix Figure 2-3*

**Appendix Figure 2-1** *This ad implies the possibility of a threesome in a dorm room* (A&F Quarterly, *Back to School 2001*).

**Appendix Figure 2-2.** *This ad explicitly shows a group sex scene and lacks the clothes that the ad is selling* (A&F Quarterly, *Christmas 2002*).

**Appendix Figure 2-3.** *This ad depicts a group sex scene as a happy, everyday occurrence* (A&F Quarterly, *Christmas 2003*).

## References

Adatto K. Childhood: the last outpost of the soul. *See.* 1995;1(4):34-39.

Advertising Standards Canada. Canadian Code of Advertising Standards. May 2004.

Available at: http://www.adstandards.com/en/standards/adstandards.asp. Accessed September 25, 2004.

Advertising Standards Canada. Gender Portrayal Guidelines. 1993. Available at: http://www.adstandards.com/en/Standards/gender.asp. Accessed September 25, 2004.

Alan Guttmacher Institute. *Sex and America's Teenagers*. New York, NY: Alan Guttmacher Institute; 1994.

Alexander VD. The image of children in magazine advertisements from 1905 to 1990. *Communic Res.* 1994;21(6):742-765

American Academy of Pediatrics. *Media Matters*. Available at: http://www.aap.org/advocacy/mediamatters.htm. Accessed August 25, 2004.

American Academy of Pediatrics. Television and the family: guidelines for parents [brochure]. Ill: American Academy of Pediatrics; 1995.

American Psychiatric Association. *Diagnostic and Statistical Manual of Mental Disorders*. 4th ed. Washington, DC: American Psychiatric Association; 1994.

Arehart-Treichel J. Psychiatrist helps pediatricians develop antiviolence statement. *Psychiatr News.* 2001;36(24):14.

Barker C. *Cultural Studies: Theory and Practice*. London, England: Sage Publications; 2000.

Briere J, Runtz M. University males' sexual interest in children: predicting potential indices of pedophilia in a nonforensic sample. *Child Abuse Negl.* 1989;13(1):65-75.

Brown JD, Greenberg BS, Buerkel-Rothfuss NL. Mass media, sex, and sexuality. *Adolesc Med.* 1993;4(3):511-525.

Brownback hosts forum on the impact of explicit entertainment on children [press release]. Washington, DC: Sam Brownback, senator from Kansas; July 26, 2001.

Carr D, Rozhon T. Abercrombie & Fitch to end its racy magazine. *New York Times.* December 10, 2003: C1.

Carr J. Theme paper on child pornography. Paper presented at: Second World Congress on Commercial Sexual Exploitation of Children; December 17-20, 2001; Yokohama, Japan.

Children's Advertising Review Unit (CARU). Self-regulatory guidelines for children's advertising. 2003. Available at: http://www.caru.org/guidelines/index.asp. Accessed August 25, 2004.

Cobden M. Media porn onslaught affects attitudes, if not actions. In: *Healthy Relationships: A Violence-Prevention Curriculum: Gender Equality and Media Awareness*. Vol 2. Nova Scotia, Canada: Men for Change: 1994.

Committee on Communications, American Academy of Pediatrics. Children, adolescents, and advertising. *Pediatrics.* 1995;95(2):295-297.

Committee on Public Education, American Academy of Pediatrics. Sexuality, contraception, and the media. *Pediatrics.* 2001;107(1):191-194.

Davidson JO. The sex exploiter. Paper presented at: Second World Congress Against Commercial Sexual Exploitation of Children; December 17-20, 2001; Yokohama, Japan.

DeFleur M. *Understanding Mass Communication: A Liberal Arts Perspective*. Boston, Mass: Houghton Mifflin; 1998.

Dines G, Jenson R, Russo A. *Pornography: The Production and Consumption of Inequality*. New York, NY: Routledge; 1998.

Elias M. Study sizes up teen girls, magazines. *USA Today.* March 2, 1999a:1D.

Elias M. Teen mags hurt fat-fearful girls. *USA Today.* August 26, 1999b:5D.

Elliott M. Images of children in the media: soft kiddie porn. In: Itzin C. *Pornography: Women, Violence and Civil Liberties.* Oxford, England: Oxford University Press; 1992:216-221.

Estes RJ, Weiner NA. The commercial sexual exploitation of children in the US, Canada and Mexico: executive summary. Philadelphia: University of Pennsylvania; September 10, 2001. Available at: http://caster.ssw.upenn.edu/~restes/CSEC_Files/ Exec_Sum_020220.pdf. Accessed September 25, 2004.

Exton NG, Truong TC, Exton MS, et al. Neuroendocrine response to film-induced sexual arousal in men and women. *Psychoneuroendocrinology.* 2000;25:187-199.

Featherstone L. Sex, lies, and women's magazines. *Columbia J Rev.* March/April 2002.

Field AE, Cheung L, Wolf AM, Herzog DB, Gortmaker SL, Colditz GA. Exposure to mass media and weight concerns among girls. *Pediatrics.* 1999;103(3):E36.

Ford D. Abercrombie's Lolita line of thongs goes beyond bad taste. *San Francisco Chronicle.* May 26, 2002:E2.

Fox RF. *Harvesting Minds: How TV Commercials Control Kids.* Westport, Conn: Praeger Publishers; 1996.

Frontline. The merchants of cool: synopsis. 2001. Available at: http://www.pbs.org. /wgbh/pages/frontline/shows/cool/etc/synopsis.html. Accessed September 25, 2004.

Gilday K. *The Famine Within* [videotape]. Santa Monica, Calif: Direct Cinema Ltd; 1990.

Givan R. A peek at the jeans is all you need. *The News and Observer.* December 18, 1996:3E.

Grant L. Can Calvin Klein escape? *Los Angeles Times Magazine,* February 23, 1992:16.

Greenberg BS, Brown JD, Buerkel-Rothfuss NL. *Media, Sex, and the Adolescent.* Cresskill, NJ: Hampton Press; 1993.

Grossberg L, Radway J. *Controversies in Cultural Studies.* New York, NY: Routledge; 1997.

Hecht ME. The role and involvement of the private sector. Paper presented at: Second World Congress Against Commercial Sexual Exploitation; December 17-20, 2001; Yokohama, Japan.

Herman-Giddens ME, Slora EJ, Wasserman RC, et al. Secondary sexual characteristics and menses in young girls seen in office practice: a study from the Pediatric Research in Office Settings network. *Pediatrics.* 1997;99:505-512.

Herman-Giddens ME. The making of an eight-year-old woman. Presented at: Women's Health Matters Forum & Expo; January 18, 2002; Toronto, Canada.

The history of ECPAT. ECPAT International Web site. 2002. Available at: http:// www.ecpat.net/eng/Ecpat_network/history6.asp. Accessed September 25, 2004.

Hogan M. Media education offers help on children's body image problems. *AAP News.* May 1999:27.

Huston AC, Wartella E, Donnerstein E. Measuring the effects of sexual content in the media: a report to the Kaiser Family Foundation. May 1998. Available at: http:// www.kff.org/entmedia/1389-content.cfm. Accessed September 25, 2004.

Itzin C. Pornography and the organization of intra- and extrafamilial child sexual abuse: a conceptual model. In: Cantor GK, Jasinski JL. *Out of the Darkness: Contemporary Perspectives on Family Violence.* Thousand Oaks, Calif: Sage Publicatons; 1997.

Jhally S. Image-based culture: advertising and popular culture. In: Dines G, Humez J, eds. *Gender, Race, and Class in Media.* Thousand Oaks, Calif: Sage Publications; 1995.

Jhally S. Media Education Foundation brochure [package insert]. North Hampton, Mass: Media Education Foundation; 1998.

Katz J. Advertising and the construction of violent white masculinity: from Eminem to Clinique for Men. In: Dines G, Humez J, eds. *Gender, Race, and Class in Media.* 2nd ed. Thousand Oaks, Calif: Sage Publications; 2002.

Katz J. Advertising and the construction of violent white masculinity. In: Dines G, Humez J, eds. *Gender, Race, and Class in Media.* Thousand Oaks, Calif: Sage Publications; 1995.

Kellner D. Reading images critically: toward a postmodern pedagogy. In: Dines G, Humez J, eds. *Gender, Race, and Class in Media.* Thousand Oaks, Calif: Sage Publications; 1995.

Kelly J. DADs asks teen mags to take YM's step—and the next one. Dads and Daughters Web site. March 1, 2002. Available at: http://www.dadsanddaughters.org/action/teenaction.html. Accessed September 25, 2004.

Khadilkar V. Children and the media. Aarogya.com, the Wellness Site. Available at: http://www.aarogya.com/news/Story/media.asp. Accessed August 25, 2004.

Kilbourne J. *Can't Buy My Love: How Advertising Changes the Way We Think and Feel.* New York, NY: Simon & Schuster; 1999.

Kilbourne J. Beauty and the beast of advertising. In: Dines G, Humez J, eds. *Gender, Race, and Class in Media.* Thousand Oaks, Calif: Sage Publications; 1995.

Kingsley C, Mark M. *Sacred Lives: Canadian Aboriginal Children and Youth Speak Out About Sexual Exploitation.* Vancouver, Canada: Save the Children Canada; 2000.

Kuhn A. *The Power of the Image: Essays on Representation and Sexuality.* Boston, Mass: Routledge & Kegan Paul; 1985:42-43.

Lewis J. *Cultural Studies: The Basics.* Thousand Oaks, Calif: Sage Publications; 2002.

McCannon B. Fourteen ways parents can create healthy, capable learners. *AAP News.* June 1997.

The McKnight Investigators. Risk factors for the onset of eating disorders in adolescent girls: results of the McKnight longitudinal risk factor study. *Am J Psychiatry.* 2003;160(2):248-254.

Minow NN, Lamay CL. *Abandoned in the Wasteland: Children, Television and the First Amendment.* New York, NY: Hill & Wang; 1995.

O'Grady R. Moving on. *ECPAT International Newsletters.* January 1, 2002;(special issue). 18 USC § 2257.

Pediatrician presents findings that sexually explicit media has significant impact on children [press release]. Washington, DC: American Academy of Pediatrics; July 26, 2001.

Quart A. *Branded: The Buying and Selling of Teenagers.* Cambridge, Mass: Perseus Publishing; 2003.

Reisman JA. Child pornography in erotic magazines, social awareness and self-censorship. In: Zillmann D, Bryant J, Huston AC, eds. *Media, Children, and the*

*Family: Social Scientific, Psychodynamic, and Clinical Perspectives.* Hillsdale, NJ: Lawrence Erlbaum; 1994:313-325.

Rich M. Too much, too soon. Testimony to senate forum. Washington, DC; July 26, 2001.

Roberts R. Sex, violence, and advertising. *The Daily News.* July 22, 1991. Reprinted in: *Healthy Relationships: A Violence-Prevention Curriculum: Gender Equality and Media Awareness.* Vol 2. Nova Scotia, Canada: Men for Change: 1994.

Roffman D. Way too much fantasy with that dream house. *Washington Post.* December 22, 2002:B1.

Rosenbaum DE. Protecting children, tempting Pandora. *New York Times.* June 26, 2001:E1.

Rudman LA, Borgida E. The afterglow of construct accessibility: the behavioral consequences of priming men to view women as sexual objects. *J Exp Soc Psychol.* 1995; 31:493-517.

Schroeder JE, Borgerson JL. Marketing images of gender: a visual analysis. *Consumption Markets Cult.* 1998;2(2):161-201.

Spangenberg M. *Prostituted Youth in New York City: An Overview.* New York, NY: ECPAT-USA; March 2001.

Stepp LS. Nothing to wear: from the classroom to the mall, girls' fashions are long on skin, short on modesty. *Washington Post.* June 3, 2003:C1.

Steyer JP. *The Other Parent: The Inside Story of the Media's Effect On Our Children.* New York, NY: Atria Books; 2002.

Strasburger VC, Donnerstein E. Children, adolescents, and the media: issues and solutions. *Pediatrics.* 1999;103(1):129-139.

Sun SS, Schubert CM, Chumlea WC, et al. National estimates of the timing of sexual maturation and racial differences among US children. *Pediatrics.* 2002;110:911-919.

Villani S. Impact of media on children and adolescents: a 10-year review of research. *J Am Acad Child Adolesc Psychiatr.* 2001;40(4):392-401.

Vipond M. The *Mass Media in Canada.* Toronto, Canada: James Lorimer & Co; 1989.

Ward LM. Does television exposure affect emerging adults' attitudes and assumptions about sexual relationships? Correlation and experimental confirmation. *J Youth Adolesc.* 2002:31(1):1-15.

Wingood GM, DiClemente RJ, Harrington K, Davies S, Hook EW, Oh MK. Exposure to X-rated movies and adolescents' sexual and contraceptive-related attitudes and behaviors. *Pediatrics.* 2001;107:1116-1119.

Zillmann D, Bryant J, Huston AC, eds. *Media, Children, and the Family: Social Scientific, Psychodynamic, and Clinical Perspectives.* Hillsdale, NJ: Lawrence Erlbaum; 1994.

# CHILD SEXUAL EXPLOITATION FROM A GLOBAL PERSPECTIVE

Ingrid Leth, Former Senior Adviser, UNICEF*

The literature on sexual exploitation of children reflects the cultural background from which it is derived. Generally, textbooks describe the phenomenon from a Western and often urban perspective.

The purpose of this chapter is to describe the concept of sexual exploitation in different frameworks, analyze root causes and risk factors, and illuminate different aspects of sexual exploitation and abuse in a broader scope. The emphasis is on regions of the world where sexual exploitation plays a major role. The international conventions and aid organizations' efforts to combat the phenomenon will be described. The descriptions will be based on available situation analyses and research studies.

This chapter will also provide an overview of the methodology used in these studies. The studies are of variable quality, partly because the issue is sensitive. For example, brothel owners or guards may be present when children are informants, causing the conditions in which studies are carried out to be stressful. It seems highly objectionable that researchers should pretend to be customers in order to approach the children and tape the interviews without the respondents' knowledge.

Conducting reliable studies is a critical issue (Ennew et al, 1996). In fact, few studies since the First World Congress Against Commercial Sexual Exploitation, which took place in Stockholm in 1996, could be labeled reliable. Much material exists, but one problem with the nongovernmental organization (NGO) literature is that "the academic literature seems to be largely ignored or unknown" (Ennew et al, 1996). In addition, within mainstream campaign literature, certain categories become blurred. The following are among the most common sources of error:

— Prepubescent and postpubescent children are often included in the numbers given for prostituted children along with young women over age 18.

— Numbers given for Western tourist clients are confused with numbers of Western tourists as a whole, with no account given of local clients (Ennew et al, 1996).

Child sexual abuse and exploitation are universal problems, and no country can claim to be without these scourges. However, the problem is particularly widespread in Southeast Asia (eg, Thailand, the Philippines, Cambodia, Vietnam, China), southern Asia (eg, India, Nepal, Sri Lanka), and Latin America (eg, Brazil). In Africa, the problem emerges in a less visible way.

## DEFINITION OF SEXUAL EXPLOITATION

In studies and situation analyses from developing countries, *sexual exploitation* is the most commonly used term. In a background paper for the Second World Congress, O'Connell-Davidson (2001) provides a definition of *sex exploiters*. With a slight change, this definition may be used to define ***child sexual exploitation*** (CSE) as taking unfair advantage of some imbalance of power between an adult/young person

---

* The contents of this chapter do not necessarily reflect the policies or views of UNICEF.

and a child under the age of 18 in order to use her or him sexually for either profit or personal pleasure.

The term *sexual abuse* is used here to emphasize the emotional relationship between the child victim and the sex exploiter, often within the context of families.

Along with sexual abuse and commercialized sexual exploitation, this definition includes the question of consent. Children below the age of 18 can not give informed consent. The term sex exploiter may be more useful than perpetrator or sex offender, because it may encompass commercial sexual exploitation as well.

The Convention on the Rights of the Child (CRC) defines **childhood** as continuing up to age 18 years old (Office of the High Commissioner for Human Rights, 1989). This normative rule is followed in this context, even if children have to care for their families before age 18 or are married at age 10.

## THE CONCEPT OF SEXUAL EXPLOITATION FROM A GLOBAL PERSPECTIVE

In Western academic literature, the term sexual abuse is used, and there is little reference to CSE such as prostitution. This may be because in Western societies the prostitution of children is not a significant problem nor is it defined as a problem to be dealt with. Children involved in the sex trade are regarded as "bad kids" who are to blame for what happened to them (Spangenberg, 2001). Child prostitution is, thus, considered a form of sexual acting out (Hollin & Howells, 1991). This clinical approach does not include aspects of necessity and survival. Therefore, it is necessary to link this tradition to its historic background and to look at other cultures to understand this phenomenon.

In Western societies, sexual abuse and exploitation became a political issue in the 1970s largely as a consequence of the women's liberation movement. Unseen aspects of family life were brought into the open, including wife battering, child abuse, and child sexual abuse. The knowledge obtained in the past 25 years, however, can not be easily generalized beyond Western culture.

To understand the broader scope of the problem, it is necessary to include the exploitative sides of sexual abuse. We may roughly distinguish among physical injury, sexual abuse, emotional or psychological abuse, and neglect (Creighton, 2002), despite the fact that a sexually abusive act includes 2 or 3 of these aspects. From a global perspective, sexual exploitation should be added. In this context, the concept of sexual exploitation should be considered as a general term also to include both commercial and noncommercial sexual abuse. Sexual exploitation of children may occur inside and outside of families and is committed by a male or, in rare cases, a female perpetrator or sex offender (Ennew, 1986). The most common model to categorize sex offenders was developed by Groth (1979). He describes 3 types of sexual perpetrators: the regressive type, the fixated type, and the situational type. The men committing these acts by having sex with children are not considered normal but are thought to have a personality disorder.

Among the general public it is considered perverted to have sex with children, and in prisons sex exploiters are treated harshly and are placed lowest in the status hierarchy of the inmates. In Western communities, there is an outspoken condemnation of offenders because sexual exploitation is known to be harmful to children and to have long-lasting consequences. It is not only a question of a disorder but also a question of morality.

In Western countries, legislation and attitudes define childhood as a special life stage requiring nurturing, formal education, and protection up to a specific age. Children are often brought up in a world of their own and in many ways are segregated from the adult working realm.

In other societies, the distinction between children and adults is not that clear. Children are treated as adults as soon as their physical and mental development makes it possible for them to perform an adult's job and as far as they are permitted to do so by their adult caregivers. In some societies, children are viewed as small adults; they live apart from their families, they do not "play" with other children, and they are not educated as Western children are. In such cultures, children may have adult responsibilities, be involved in all kinds of child labor, and be used for sexual purposes.

In these societies, it may not be considered perverted or immoral to have sex with children. Even if sexual exploitation of children is banned, it may take place without any risk of detection due to lack of law enforcement. Sexual exploitation includes all situations where children are involved in sexual activities with an adult, ranging from fondling various parts of the body, breasts, and genitals to inter-course, oral sex, and anal sex. **Table 3-1** lists acts that may be considered sexual abuse according to the Economic and Social Commission for Asia and the Pacific (ESCAP) report (2000). This definition gives a picture of sexual abuse in the private sphere and provides the Western view of sexual abuse as mainly a 2-person relationship with a perpetrator who is attracted to the child and tries to gain access to the child through the protection of the private sphere. The advantage of this definition is the way many aspects of sexual abuse are included.

Sexual exploitation may take place in the private sphere, in institutions, or in different commercially exploitative contexts such as child prostitution, trafficking and the sale of children, and child pornography.

Commercial sexual exploitation indicates that a second party benefits from sexual activity involving a child, either by making a profit or through a quid pro quo. The more powerful person (the adult) will always take advantage of the less powerful person (the child). Being less powerful may include the physical differences but also the incapacity to anticipate the consequences or the readiness to be lured into some clandestine business.

---

**Table 3-1. Acts Considered to Be Sexual Abuse**

*Physical sexual abuse.* Touching and fondling of the sexual parts of the child's body (genitals and anus) or touching the breasts of pubescent females, or the child's touching the sexual parts of a partner's body; sexual kissing and embraces; penetration, which includes penile, digital, and object penetration of the vagina, mouth, or anus; masturbating a child or forcing the child to masturbate the perpetrator

*Verbal sexual abuse.* Sexual language that is inappropriate for the age of the child used by the perpetrator to generate sexual excitement, including making lewd comments about the child's body and making obscene phone calls

*Emotional sexual abuse.* Use of a child by a parent or adult to fill inappropriate emotional needs, thereby forcing the child to fulfill the role of a spouse

*Exhibitionism and voyeurism.* Having a child pose, undress, or perform in a sexual fashion on film or in person (exhibitionism); peeping into bathrooms or bedrooms to spy on a child (voyeurism); exposing children to adult sexual activity or pornographic movies and photographs

*Adapted from Economic and Social Commission for Asia and the Pacific.* Sexually Abused and Sexually Exploited Children and Youth in the Greater Mekong Sub-Region: A Qualitative Assessment of Their Health Needs and Available Services. *New York, NY: United Nations; 2000.*

Sexual exploitation of children may not necessarily involve any use of violence or coercion. The fact that children are easy to lure is often used as an excuse or justification of the exploitation.

The distinction between commercial and noncommercial sexual exploitation is often blurred. For instance, child pornography is clearly sexual exploitation. Much of this is based on nonprofit exchange via the Internet, although many Web sites do charge users for access. In contrast, child prostitution, as it is organized in Asia, is a clear example of commercial sexual exploitation.

In a global perspective it may be more feasible to use the term sexual exploitation and then distinguish between commercial and noncommercial sexual exploitation. There are no sharp boundaries between abuse and exploitation and there is an overlap between commercial and noncommercial sexual exploitation, clearly described by Estes & Weiner (2001) in the study, *The Commercial Sexual Exploitation of Children in the US, Canada, and Mexico.*

## THE SCOPE OF THE PROBLEM OF SEXUALLY EXPLOITED CHILDREN: SOME NUMBERS

Exact figures on the number of children who have been subjected to commercial sexual exploitation are not known. **Table 3-2** is presented only as an overview of estimates by field workers in different regions of the world, as official numbers are rarely available. The numbers are derived from different sources, using different methods. Some of them indicate children in prostitution; some refer to sexually exploited children. The reliability of these numbers is unknown and they should be interpreted with caution. The only reliable number in **Table 3-2** is the one from Indonesia because prostitutes are registered there. Of the officially registered women,

| Table 3-2. Children Subjected to Commercial Sexual Exploitation for Selected Countries | | |
|---|---|---|
| COUNTRY | ESTIMATED NUMBER OF CHILDREN | AGE RANGE |
| **Asia** | | |
| Bangladesh | 10 000-29 000* | Not known |
| Thailand | 12 000-18 000* | Not known |
| Indonesia | 40 000-70 000 (children registered as prostitutes)* | 15-18 years |
| Sri Lanka | 30 000* | Not known |
| Taiwan | 30 000-60 000* | Not known |
| China | 200 000-500 000* | Not known |
| Philippines | 100 000[†] | Not known |
| **Latin America** | | |
| Dominican Republic | 25 000* | 12-17 years |
| **Africa** | | |
| South Africa Johannesburg | 28 000 in prostitution* | Not known |
| | | *(continued)* |

**Table 3-2.** *(continued)*

| COUNTRY | ESTIMATED NUMBER OF CHILDREN | AGE RANGE |
|---|---|---|
| **Africa** | | |
| Cameroon | 15.9% of children are sexually exploited[‡] | Up to 15 years |
| **North America** | | |
| US | 244 000-325 000[§] | Up to 18 years |
| Mexico | 16 000[‖] | Up to 18 years |

*\* Data from End Child Prostitution, Child Pornography and the Trafficking of Children for Sexual Purposes (ECPAT). ECPAT International Web site. Available at: http://www.ecpat.net/eng/Ecpat_inter/ projects/monitoring/online_database/index.asp. Accessed October 7, 2003.*

*† Data from Department of Social Welfare and Development. Commercial Sexual Exploitation of Children in the Philippines: A Situation Analysis: Executive Summary. Manila, Phillipines: UNICEF; 1998.*

*‡ Data from Mbassa Menick D. Les abus sexuels en milieu scolaire au Cameroun. September 28, 2001. Available at: http://www.crin.org/docs/resources/treaties/crc.28/DMenick-Cameroon.pdf. Accessed October 7, 2003.*

*§ Data from Estes R, Weiner N. The Commercial Sexual Exploitation of Children in the US, Canada, and Mexico. September 2001. Available at: http://www.ssw.upenn.edu/~restes/CSEC.htm. Accessed August 12, 2003.*

*‖ Data from Azaola E. Stolen Childhood, Girl and Boy Victims of Sexual Exploitation in Mexico. Mexico City, Mexico: UNICEF; 2000.*

60% are presumed to be children. In a situation analysis from the Philippines there are numbers concerning children who have been reported to the authorities over a 5-year period (1991-1996) as commercial sexual exploitation of children (CSEC) cases, in total 1403 children, which constitute only 2% of the estimated CSEC incidents nationwide in 1993 (Department of Social Welfare and Development, 1998).

From a Cameroon study (Mbassa Menick, 2001) based on a population of 15-year-old school children, it was found that 21.2% of the girls and 9.6% of the boys had been sexually abused. This ratio between genders (2:1) has been found in many other studies.

The Cameroon study was a cohort study and might be a model for developing countries in order to provide information about sexual abuse legitimately. Unfortunately, the study has no information about how many children are prostituted.

# CHILDREN IN COMMERCIAL SEXUAL EXPLOITATION

Qualitative investigations of CSEC can help provide a richer picture of the problem than the severely restricted available numerical data. Such information is often presented in the form of situation analyses by official agencies or reports of NGOs from specific countries or regions. Data tend to be available from regions that have been the focus of these agencies and, as such, countries in Asia, Africa, and Eastern Europe have so far been most thoroughly investigated.

## THE FACE OF CHILD PROSTITUTION: A SITUATION ANALYSIS FROM SOUTHEAST ASIA

A study was carried out by ESCAP in 2000 in the greater Mekong subregion, which covers Cambodia, Yunnan Province (China), Lao People's Democratic Republic, Myanmar, Thailand, and Vietnam. The focus of the investigation was the health consequences of sexual abuse and sexual exploitation in children in the region. Data were collected mainly through interviews with exploited children and professionals working with these children. The study included only 110 children, which means that the group from each country was quite small.

In the Mekong subregion, prostituted children may be found in brothels, discotheques, nightclubs, massage parlors, coffee shops, and male hair salons. Children also work as "call girls." The demand for sexual services of children and youth comes from local and foreign men. Places where local men can gain access to children can be found throughout the provinces while places for foreigners are usually concentrated in large urban areas or tourist resorts. The highest incidence of female exploitation was found to occur between the ages of 11 and 15. Children are being sold to brothels for $100 to $150 (US dollars [USD]). The brothel owner obtains a higher prize when a virgin is offered to clients; once the girl loses her virginity, her value decreases.

Thailand

In Southeast Asia, prostitution is closely linked to trafficking. This is often the case in Thailand (Foundation for Women, 1988). Children are trafficked from rural areas to metropolitan cities. In many cases, a child freely agrees to follow the recruiter in order to pay off the family's debt. Recruiting takes place in remote areas, and family members are easily lured by promises that the child will get lucrative jobs in big cities like Bangkok. The syndicates are strong and if the government in Thailand succeeds in blocking a trafficking route between the Northern remote areas and Bangkok, the routes are changed to go through areas with fewer obstacles, such as Myanmar.

Philippines

An example of the historic development in the Philippines is found from a situation analysis based on multiple data collection methods and data sources, including an annotated bibliography and interviews with children, parents, government organizations (GOs), and NGOs (Department of Social Welfare and Development, 1998). It clearly illustrates how commercial sexual exploitation started to flourish due to the presence of American military bases, extended through the Vietnam War. One location, Olongapo, depended economically on the rest-and-recreation industry, and the activities were maintained and protected by the government. During the Marcos Administration (1965-1986) tourism was made a national priority, with a 6-fold increase of tourists during the late 1970s. In this period, sex tourism developed a new form, as more male and female children became victims of commercial sexual exploitation. Boys and girls from ages 9 through 16 were involved.

In the actual study, 9 out of 10 children interviewed were girls (which does not reflect the usual proportion of boys and girls in prostitution). It was found that 76% of the children lived with nonfamily members although they wished to be reunited with their families.

For boys, the situation of having been exploited by adult males seemed to be confusing. On one hand, it was shameful for them and their families and, therefore, these cases were seldom brought to court. On the other hand, the motive for staying in prostitution reportedly was that boys could not get pregnant and had nothing to lose.

When asked, the children at first claimed it was their own decision to enter the sexual exploitation trade although later they pointed out other reasons, such as peer pressure, economic factors, and problems in the family. Few mentioned abuse in the family.

Information from girls in the Philippine brothels shows that they worked an average of 6.9 hours per day, 5.6 days per week, and averaged 3 customers per day (ranging from 1-9). The income ranged from Pesos 390.35 to 1027.73 ($10-$25 USD). What they earned was spent mainly on their daily needs.

When asked about aspirations for the future, the children said that they hoped to quit the job, get a family, and complete their studies. There seemed to be more regret of not having finished school than in other developing countries. However, it is also clear that the children interviewed expressed a low degree of self-confidence.

## A South Asian Study

The life of children in a brothel has been documented in a study of a large brothel located in a red light district of Dhaka, Bangladesh (Khan & Arefeen, 1990). The researchers gained access to one particular brothel, which consisted of 27 dwelling houses with 230 rooms inhabited by 1000 to 1200 women and their children. The researchers followed 434 inhabitants.

One third of the prostituted women were affiliated with regular clients. More than two thirds of the prostitutes were between the ages of 16 and 30 and approximately 12% were below the age of 16. Most of the prostitutes had been born into prostitution. A few were pushed in from outside by extreme poverty and the lack of a male protector because of death or desertion by husbands. (One should bear in mind that female children in Bangladesh are often married at age 12 or 13.) One third of the women had children, who were born and brought up in the brothel. Both boys and girls under the age of 12 were found. However, above the age of 12 the boys had apparently moved out of the brothel and only girls were seen. Usually the girls raised in the brothel between the ages of 12 and 16 were not supposed to be inducted into prostitution, but there were several exceptions. The case studies show that some of the child prostitutes had become the breadwinners of the family starting at age 10 or 11 because the mother was too ill to earn money, and it was necessary to support a grandmother and younger siblings as well.

The children below the age of 18 were interviewed about their introduction into prostitution. Most answered that they had been "born into it." Their mothers were prostitutes and the children had lived in a brothel for their entire lives. If children came in from the outside they had either been sold to the brothel by a relative or they had fled from an abusive marriage. The children came from poor back-grounds and the girl prostitutes had only a faint hope of escaping prostitution, for example, by being married to one of their clients.

These young prostitutes were guarded by the madams of the brothel or by the mother who took care of the contact with the clients and ensured that the young girls did not have too many clients a day.

## Children Born in Brothels (Brothel Children)

Many children are born and raised in brothels, such as those in India or the Philippines. Khan & Arefeen's (1990) study also highlights the conditions of young children being brought up in brothels. The infants were reported to be in poor health, and the women reported a high infant mortality rate. However, the health of children above the age of 2 seemed to be reasonable. The mothers in this community were eager to have the children go to school, particularly their sons. The boys had to hide their identity and address, or they would be forced to leave school by their classmates' parents.

Children in brothels apparently led free lives with fewer restrictions than children outside brothels. However, the children knew very well that what took place there had to do with sexuality and its related activities, such as entertainment and various forms of addiction.

The children, like the adults, believed that prostitution was not only bad but also immoral and sinful. The social and institutional rules that condemn the brothel and treat its inmates as outcasts of society were internalized by the children and reflected in their view of the future. The girls and boys expressed a desire for jobs outside the brothel. The boys hoped to continue their studies and get jobs as government officers or policemen. The girls hoped to get decent jobs or to get married, but they said that because they were prostitutes' daughters, they were fated to become prostitutes themselves.

In several big cities in India, such as Mumbai and Calcutta, prostitution based in brothels is well organized in the same way. The girls and young women once involved in prostitution will have difficulty in ever being accepted by their families or society. Corruption is pervasive due to factors such as very low salaries for police (Friedman, 1996). The police may warn the brothel owners of impending raids so that they can hide the girls in another place. The police are deeply involved as customers and sometimes owners of brothels.

## AN EXAMPLE FROM EASTERN EUROPE

Since the decline of the Soviet Union, the economic situation in Eastern Europe has been very unstable. The rate of unemployment is high, and in this period of transition to a market economy, many people are in despair. Women and young girls are easy targets for recruiters from the Russian or Albanian mafias.

There is now organized trafficking from the former Soviet republics to Eastern Europe, the Balkans, and Italy. However, studies on these populations do not reveal how many are children below age 18 (International Organization of Migration, 2001).

Albania seems to be an ideal country for recruiters for the sex trade. It is surrounded by wealthy countries that want to receive the children, has a high prevalence of women due to immigration, is the poorest and least developed country in Europe, and has a close connection to the Italian mafia (Renton, 2001). The children often come from rural sites, are known to be docile and used to domestic violence, and, thus, are easy to control. The Albanian pimp has the reputation of being extremely ruthless. For example, 168 foreign prostitutes were killed in the year 2000 and the majority of them were Albanians and Nigerians who had been murdered by their pimps. There are estimated to be 15 000 Albanian prostitutes in Italy and 6000 in Greece, 80% of whom are children (Renton, 2001).

Often the Italian police arrest prostituted girls and deport them to Albania. Here they are rejected by their communities and blamed for what has happened to them. The girls fear going home and are often retrafficked.

Due to a shortage of men in some villages, recruiters will show up in the villages and offer marriage to young girls. (There is a tradition for marriage by the age of 16.) The recruiters will have an elderly couple pose as their parents to convince girls and their families that this is a big chance to go abroad (Renton, 2001). The brides-to-be are transported by speedboats to Italy. There seems to be a close network among the recruiters, and the young girls are threatened that their relatives will be killed if they try to escape. These threats are serious, and killings are executed; therefore, the young girls have no choice. (Note: this report, written by Daniel Renton for Save the Children, is based on focus group interviews and was carried out by researchers in different areas of Albania. Due to the clandestine nature of trafficking and its associated dangers, it is difficult to find conclusive evidence since the families and victims are afraid to talk about their experiences.)

## THE MIDDLE EAST

As described by Ennew et al, (1996), the literature on CSEC in the Middle East is dominated by legal considerations that are replacing a culture of denial. The preparatory conference for Africa and the Middle East, which took place in October 2001 in Rabat, Morocco (the author was present) leading up to the Second World Congress Against Commercial Sexual Exploitation, in some ways reflected this former denial. The issues presented concerned early marriages and female genital mutilation. However, representatives from the host country of Morocco were willing to discuss the issues in a broad perspective.

EXAMPLES FROM AFRICA

It is difficult to get information about sexual exploitation of children for commercial purposes (UNICEF West and Central Africa Regional Office, 2001). Four types of situations account for the vulnerability of children: movement and displacement of populations (eg, refugee movements, trafficking, voluntary or illegal migration), domestic labor, armed conflicts, and the phenomenon of children living or working in the street.

In many areas of Africa, there is a tradition of letting children from large families leave at an early age to stay with other relatives. Separation of children from their parents at an early age is widely accepted. Many of the countries are Muslim, and the families tend to be large; husbands are also often polygamous. Feeding all of the children in a family is, therefore, difficult. In a study from Benin (J. C. Legrand, regional advisor in UNICEF, West Africa, e-mail correspondence, September 2003), 76% of the households interviewed had at least one child away from home. The children may be domestic workers, but if they run away or are thrown out, they may become street prostitutes.

There are established trafficking routes from very poor countries in West Africa such as Mali, Benin, and Niger, There, countries are transit zones in the trafficking network. Nigeria has a reputation for being a turning point for victims of child trafficking from West Africa to Gabon. Ghana is also known as a transfer country for the departure of Togolese children to Gabon via Nigeria. From there, routes go through Mauritania, Morocco, and Spain to Italy, where a majority of child prostitutes are from West Africa. The prostitution is not as organized as it is in Asia; it is primarily street prostitution. Adult prostitutes, who may act as pimps or madams, hire the children.

Until recently, governments did not recognize the problems concerning child prostitution, and trafficking was considered part of a well-established tradition. In February 2000, a subregional consultation was held in Libreville, Gabon. For the first time, governments admitted the problems and the connection between CSE and trafficking. Some important political steps have been taken since then, such as an agreement between Cote d'Ivoire and Mali to collaborate against trafficking. (Accord De Cooperation entre la Republique du Mali et la Republique de Cote d'Ivoire contre le trafic transfontalier des enfants, 2000; UNICEF West and Central Africa Regional Office, 2001). In general, there is an increasing public awareness of the problem.

EXAMPLES FROM CENTRAL AMERICA

As a developing poor country adjacent to a large, rich country such as the United States, Mexico presents a peculiar perspective of CSE. A study at the University of Mexico (Azaola, 2000) aimed to identify the nature and causes of exploitation in 6 Mexican towns, border towns, tourist towns, and 1 metro city. The research team interviewed key informants with a professional background in dealing with children in various sex trades. There seemed to be several special traits:

— Prostituted children develop an addiction to drugs and alcohol provided by customers and prostitute themselves to acquire these substances.

— Background factors often include abuse and discord at home.

— Many children in Mexico are invited to stay in houses rented by rich Americans who, in a couple of weeks, provide the children with whatever they want and use them for pornographic and sexually abusive purposes.

— Prostitution is legal. There are 2 types of establishments: registered and nonregistered. (The latter operate clandestinely.)

— There were minors in all the nightclubs investigated in this study. The boys operate on the beaches and in the streets.

— Children in prostitution may earn a higher-than-average income. A police officer earns 1700 pesos in 2 weeks, which is what a girl in prostitution might earn in 1 night. The police may threaten the girls or beat them up to get money from them.

— Public response to these children is extremely limited, and there are no programs aimed at victims of sexual exploitation or to reduce drug abuse.

A report from Guatemala mentions the close linkages between drug addiction and prostitution/pornography, which are in particular apparent with respect to street children (Guatemalan Street Children Working in Prostitution, 2003).

# OTHER FORMS OF SEXUAL EXPLOITATION

## EARLY MARRIAGES

Early marriages have not previously been considered to be child sexual abuse or exploitation. The rationale for early marriage is economic survival and the protection of girls placed under male control. However, there seem to be good reasons to take a closer view at this phenomenon and its consequences (UNICEF, 2001).

Early marriages are still a widespread tradition in sub-Saharan Africa. Between 50% and 75% of girls between the ages of 15 and 19 are married, often as part of an exchange of goods or money, especially where virginity carries an economic prize (United Nations, Population Division, Department of Economic and Social Affairs, 2000). This most often occurs in countries such as Cameroon, Cote d'Ivoire, Lesotho, Liberia, and Mali. Many of these young brides are the second or third wives in polygamous households.

In Asia, marriage takes place shortly after puberty. Extreme examples of early marriage are in Afghanistan and Bangladesh, where 54% and 51% of girls are married between the ages of 15 and 19, respectively, compared to 9% and 5% of the boys. In Nepal, 7% of girls are married before the age of 10 (United Nations, Population Division, Department of Economic and Social Affairs, 2000).

In China, the proportion of early marriages fell during the 1970s but rose from 13% to 18% in 1987 (Demographers appeal for solution, 1991). Due to China's one-child policy, which led to the infanticide of girls, there is now a shortage of potential female spouses. As a result, there is a demand for mail-order brides. In one particular province of China, this phenomenon is increasing. These brides are often requested to be below the age of 18, and, in many cases, they become simply house slaves who also can be used for sex.

In cases of girls married before puberty, it is a normal understanding that there will be no sexual intercourse until the first menstruation. The mother-in-law should enforce this protection, but it is not always done. Cases of forced intercourse between husbands who are physically fully developed and wives younger than 10 years old have been reported. While an unmarried teenage girl may find it difficult to resist unwanted sexual advances, the married young girl may find it impossible. These young wives are very vulnerable to sexual violence.

Very few girls in developing countries have access to contraception in early marriages. In many societies, child-bearing immediately after the wedding is considered an important part of the woman's status. Mothers under the age of 15 are 5 times as likely to die in childbirth as those who are 20 to 24 years old (UNICEF, 2001).

The issue of early marriage is sensitive in many cultures, and linking it to the fact that some kinds of early marriage are unrecognized as sexual exploitation makes this issue even more critical. However, attitudes are changing in regions where this tradition is widespread.

## TEMPLE PROSTITUTION: DEVADASI

Religious prostitution is practiced in various parts of India and Nepal (Ennew et al, 1996). Devadasi cults are found mostly in southern India. The tradition reflects upper-caste temple traditions. An initiation rite during a full moon dedicates girls between ages 5 and 9 from poor, low-caste homes to the deity in the local temple. After girls are married to the deity by the tali rite, they are branded with a hot iron on both shoulders and breasts. The temple priest then employs them. Sometimes, even before their menarches, they are auctioned for their virginity; the deflowering ceremony becomes the privilege of the highest bidder, who also pays a lump sum to the family. The market value of girls falls after they attain puberty, when they are said to have no recourse other than prostitution.

### SUGAR DADDIES

An African phenomenon attached to schools is the presence of elderly men who supply teenage girls with pocket money as compensation for sexual services. They have easy access to the children at the school gates. Until recently, this has not been considered sexual exploitation.

## PSYCHOSOCIAL FACTORS WITH AN IMPACT ON THE VULNERABILITY OF CHILDREN REGARDING COMMERCIAL SEXUAL EXPLOITATION

There is no single reason that children enter prostitution. There are many contributing factors, which are summarized in **Table 3-3** and discussed below.

### POVERTY

In a global perspective, poverty is one of the main factors contributing to commercial sexual exploitation. Poverty deprives children of other options, such as going to school and receiving an education. It also makes children vulnerable to the risk of losing their families and having no protection against exploitation. According to many reports from developing countries, children are abandoned or rejected by their families, or relatives take care of the children until a good offer to sell the child is available. Despite the fact that poverty has been claimed to be a major cause for children entering the sex trade, not all poor families will sell their children. However, there is no doubt that reducing poverty would prevent many children from entering prostitution.

### POWER AND POWERLESSNESS

Another important factor is power and powerlessness. When sex is considered as personal sexual satisfaction involving use of another person and not as a mutually satisfactory encounter between 2 peer partners, the basis for exploitation is created. In societies with strong repression of women and male control of female sexuality, this

---

**Table 3-3. Psychosocial Factors Contributing to Childhood Prostitution**

— Poverty

— Power and powerlessness

— Lack of knowledge

— Child as a commodity

— Consumerism

— Macho or machismo culture

— Children sexually abused or exploited in the private sphere

— Taboos

— Lack of knowledge regarding the needs of children

— Dysfunctional families

perception will be predominant and may define the relationship between the powerful male partner and the powerless female partner. This will have an impact on women's perceptions of themselves and their acceptance of being powerless. In her book on sexual abuse of children within Indian families, Virani (2000) describes how mothers are unable to protect their children because they are socially and economically dependent on their spouses. In cases of sexual abuse within the family, divorce is not an option. The inequality between genders will facilitate and justify sexual exploitation and even be accepted by women themselves.

## Lack of Knowledge

Often parents contribute to child prostitution due to lack of knowledge about the long-term consequences of commercial sexual exploitation. Nowadays, most families know what the job in reality may include. They might hope that their children will come home safely after a couple of years, maybe even with money saved. In remote areas of Thailand, daughters send money home. According to Buddhist values, children are devoted to their parents and, therefore, they are ready to sacrifice themselves. However, it is still appropriate to regard this practice as due to a lack of knowledge, because the disastrous long-term consequences on the children's mental and physical health are not acknowledged.

## Child as a Commodity

If children are considered to be commodities, the process of selling a child is facilitated. The value of children in many countries seems to be directly related to the economic prosperity of the country. Children have rights, but even though the Convention on the Rights of the Child was adopted in 1989, it is still the tradition in many countries that children may be treated as commodities. Children belong to their families and can be sold to support the rest of the family. In many developing countries such as Bangladesh, children and youth comprise nearly one third to one half of the population. This fact may support the attitude that children are there to be used. This in particular will concern the daughters, who are considered less important than the sons in the family. This means that when daughters try to speak out, they are not heard.

Currently, a global urbanization is taking place particularly in less developed parts of the world. Many children and young people are forced to leave rural areas to find a way to survive in cities. Many recruiters are ready to pick up vulnerable youth at railway stations and bus terminals and persuade them to get jobs, and the children may find themselves sold to brothels by young men they considered to be protecting boyfriends.

## Consumerism

Consumerism is sometimes the reason children enter prostitution. Some newspapers claim that the motive for young girls or children to agree to be prostitutes is that they want products, dresses, bags, etc, that they see advertised on television. A quote from the March 8, 1984, edition of the *Bangkok Post* illustrates this attitude: "Poverty is no longer the main factor that forces parents to sell their daughters, pushing many young girls into a hellish life, and sometimes death. Rather it is out of… materialistic values, their trying to catch up with the next-door neighbors." This is also the case in Japan: "Perhaps most shockingly ahistorical, in the view of many commentators, these girls [the young prostitutes] are not members of the under-class trying to escape grinding poverty, but rather members of the middle class who want more disposable income to spend on designer goods" (Bailey, 2003). However, there is no study that clearly indicates the link between wanting luxury goods and passing the threshold into prostitution. Instead, a sort of addiction to consumerism is established after having entered prostitution. A report from World Vision gives an example of prostituted boys in Phnom Penh: "Prostitution for them was not only a means to earning a living, but part of a street lifestyle which had its own attractions" (World Vision, 1996).

## MACHO OR MACHISMO CULTURE

"Macho" or "machismo" culture is one example of the male-dominated society. According to old cultural traditions, women are supposed to be innocent and untouched before marriage. The same expectation does not exist for men, who are supposed to prove their masculinity by approaching domestic maids or going to prostitutes. These circumstances give rise to the development of another group of women who may satisfy the male need for sex. To use a separate group of women, so-called fallen women, for prostitution has been considered normal. An investigation carried out in Lima, Peru, revealed that as many as 40% of fathers said that they would like their sons to have their sexual debuts with women in prostitution (Narvesen, 1989). Twenty-five percent of a sample of teachers answered likewise. An example from the United States refers to the fact that fathers may bring their sons "to give them a good time—training on sex" (Raymond & Hughes, 2001). There has been too little attention on the demand side concerning men who frequent prostitutes. Adult prostitution is often considered sacred, something not to be dealt with, as a phenomenon segregated from prostituted children. However, it is documented that most prostitutes begin working at approximately 15 years of age (Ennew et al, 1996). Child prostitution feeds into adult prostitution. Obviously, it is difficult for children to leave prostitution.

## CHILDREN SEXUALLY ABUSED OR EXPLOITED IN THE PRIVATE SPHERE

When the issue of commercial sexual exploitation in Asia was recognized as a major problem, it seemed more convenient to consider sexual exploitation as a phenomenon due to sex tourists' demand. As mentioned earlier in this text, sexual exploitation within the private sphere and the commercialized forms constitute a continuum with no clear boundaries. In developing countries, there has been limited interest in the problem of children being sexually abused or exploited within families. Sexual abuse within families is seldom addressed by international organizations or NGOs, even if it is reported worldwide. Virani (2000) gives examples of sexual abuse within families in India. Aid organizations may have felt the taboo against passing the threshold of the family home and interfering with the family's style of rearing the children. While breastfeeding and immunization are manageable issues for the United Nations Children's Fund (UNICEF) and NGOs, family violence is considered a sensitive issue only dealt with in a few countries. Therefore, only a few studies are concerned with abuse within families. In order to truly understand the problem of sexual abuse and exploitation, that which takes place in the private sphere must also be examined.

## TABOOS

Sexual exploitation of children is a taboo. In many regions of the world, in developing and industrialized countries, it is impossible to mention the concept of sexuality, and to combine sexuality with children is even worse. This means that children have no language with which to articulate any sexual assault, or they may think that the assault is normal. Many sex exploiters do not consider that children will suffer from being sexually exploited because children are often reluctant to talk about it, thinking that they are to blame for what has happened to them. These taboos may be broken down into 2 types: taboos concerning the act of sexual exploitation and taboos about talking about it. Breaking the silence is an important message in several countries, for instance, in the Middle East.

## LACK OF KNOWLEDGE REGARDING THE NEEDS OF CHILDREN

The knowledge about children's psychosocial needs has been investigated and disseminated in the Western world. Child protection is a new issue for international organizations and NGOs, which historically have concentrated on education in safe motherhood emphasizing health aspects, such as hygienic and nutritional measures; they have not included how to fulfill the protection aspects that are important in raising children.

## DYSFUNCTIONAL FAMILIES

The risk for children to become victims of sexual exploitation seems to be greater in dysfunctional families. In the Mekong study (ESCAP, 2000) from Thailand, 69% of prostituted children had been abused by relatives, particularly by uncles and step-fathers. Seventy-seven percent had been abused by an acquaintance such as a neighbor. Only in 2 cases was the perpetrator a stranger. The study showed that most of the sexually abused children were neglected by their parents and that all of the families were reported to be dysfunctional. Substance abuse by adults was common in more than half of the families examined. This pattern is similar to what has been found in many studies from industrialized countries. The lack of social service or mandatory reporting may mean that sexual abuse will continue even if the adults in the families are aware of it. The perpetrators may be the breadwinners; in these cases, the family is often afraid of losing the income and, therefore, remains silent. Dysfunctional violent families may lead children to run away from home and place themselves in vulnerable situations.

There is a link between a history of domestic sexual abuse and commercial sexual exploitation. A study from Costa Rica (Caramunt, 1998) indicates the close connection between sexual abuse at home and the risk of entering child prostitution. In the study from the greater Mekong subregion concerning sexual abuse and exploitation (ESCAP, 2000), it was found that in Vietnam 50% of the children interviewed had been sexually abused at home before entering prostitution. Some children, particularly in the industrialized world, enter the sex trade because they are fleeing from abusive and dysfunctional families. Girls in Asia who have lost their virginity through sexual abuse see no other option than prostituting themselves. This has provided the possibility of examining the link between sexual abuse in homes and the risk of becoming a prostitute. Other studies underline the connection of sexual abuse and prostitution. Podhisita et al (1993) reported that among the prostituted girls interviewed, 0.4% had their first sexual "experience" before the age of 10, 15.2% had it between the ages of 11 and 14, and 52.2% had it between the ages of 15 and 17.

The link between sexual exploitation and the prostitution of children is generally studied without a control group. There is no knowledge about how many children are sexually abused at home, and we do not know how many are being abused without becoming prostitutes. This methodological problem is serious and should be dealt with in future studies.

## ENVIRONMENTAL FACTORS: CIRCUMSTANCES INCREASING CHILDREN'S VULNERABILITY TO SEXUAL EXPLOITATION

In addition to psychosocial factors, there may be factors in the environment—structural and cultural causes—that may contribute to the risk for a child to become sexually exploited.

### THE DEMAND FOR CHILDREN

This discussion has focused mainly on the supply side concerning the children's availability. There is, however, a demand for children caused by the widespread idea that men imperatively have sexual needs that must be gratified as soon as possible. These demands may in particular be visible among groups of men without women for extended periods of time (eg, long-distance truck drivers, sailors, soldiers). The demands may be reinforced by group pressure and the fact that they are away from home and not subject to the usual social norms.

The idea that men must have sex as soon as they experience the need seems to be a myth of masculine sexuality. In practice, however, the absence of another person to bring them to orgasm does not actually threaten their continued survival (Davidson, 2001).

A preference for children in a brothel may be a question of price. Small children are cheaper (Ennew et al, 1996). Sex with virgins is considered safe sex, and choosing young children may guarantee virginity. Many men feel that they have no risk of contracting acquired immunodeficiency syndrome (AIDS) this way. The myth of being cured by having sex with virgins is widespread, particularly in Africa.

## THE ECONOMIC IMPACT OF CHILD SEXUAL EXPLOITATION

The demand for children is a very lucrative business. It has been estimated that prostitution of children contributes $5 billion (USD) globally (United Nations, 1995). The costs spent on children in trafficking and prostitution are small compared to the large gains obtained in this sex trade. Commercial sexual exploitation contributes in some countries to the gross national product (GNP) (Lim, 1998) in a magnitude that makes it questionable whether there is a true desire to abolish this scourge or if children will continue to be sacrificed for money. An example from Albania illustrates this point (Renton, 2001). Most girls are not paid for their night's work in the streets (the most dangerous kind of prostitution), so the pimps get all of the income. Many girls are required to earn between 500 000 lira to 1 000 000 lira ($250-$500 USD). One Albanian trafficker reported that he had 3 girls in Switzerland and earned $3000 a night from his girls (Renton, 2001). Some additional circumstances that increase the risk of being sexually exploited are identified below.

## STREET CHILDREN

At the beginning of the 1990s, literature coming from Latin America was dominated by the category of street children (Rizzini, 1996). The phenomenon of street children is very visible, but this may not be a distinct group of children. Some children are expelled from their homes due to poverty, dysfunction of their families, or death of caregivers. The concept of street children covers a variety of different problems; some children are "part-time" street children and still have contact with their families. A study from the Philippines reported that 70% of a sample of 1000 street children had been exposed to sexual abuse, in most cases by a person they knew (Department of Social Welfare and Development, 1998). Street children are extremely vulnerable to violence, rape, and sexual exploitation. In particular, girls risk sexual abuse to obtain food, shelter, or dubious protection.

## CHILDREN WITH DISABILITIES

In cultures where the birth of a disabled child is considered a punishment from God, disabled children are kept away to hide the shame of the family, and these children may be sexually abused both inside and outside of the family. From Myanmar and Thailand it was reported that developmental disabilities prevented children from defending themselves from the offender (ESCAP, 2000). Blind, deaf, and mentally retarded children are particularly at risk. Since these children are not capable of adequate communication, they will be used as an occasional commodity without any risk of detection.

## ORPHANED CHILDREN

The most rampant problem concerning orphaned children is found in eastern Africa, where 12 million children are now estimated to be orphaned because of AIDS (UNICEF, 2000). Growing up without a family or a family network makes these children extremely vulnerable to exploitation. The older siblings function as caregivers and prostitute themselves in order to provide for their younger siblings. In this way, they serve as inadequate role models. These young prostitutes may already be infected with human immunodeficiency virus (HIV) in early childhood due to mother-to-child transmission. This also contributes to the rapid dissemination of AIDS. It is a catastrophe with unimaginable consequences.

## CHILDREN IN ARMED CONFLICTS

From all kinds of warfare, it is known that organized prostitution will follow and that rape and molestation may occur as side effects to armed conflicts. In the war in the Balkans (1992-1995), for example, rape was a part of combating the enemy.

In war times, there are 2 sides to sexual exploitation. First, prostitution is considered a necessity for recreation (so-called comfort women). Second, situational crimes such as rape are committed by men no longer controlled by the social context and usual norms. Sexual exploitation of children by security forces is documented in a note from the United Nations High Commissioner for Refugees (UNHCR) and Save the Children UK (2002). The level of prostitution, including the prostitution of children, increased into the present high level in Cambodia following the arrival of peacekeepers in the 1970s.

Another problem that occurs during war times is the abduction of girls by rebel armies. In Uganda, larger groups of girls have been abducted. From time to time, girls are abducted (sometimes from boarding schools) by rebel armies to serve as domestics and as mistresses. When they become pregnant, they are simply abandoned.

In situations of conflict or postconflict, norms change, the weaknesses of families become visible, and possibilities of proper protection are limited. As a consequence of armed conflict, families are displaced and may live for extended periods in refugee camps. The effects of being outside one's norms and the changed social context may result in children being left unprotected and vulnerable to sexual abuse. Many children suffer from sexual exploitation in refugee camps. It is part of the training for international staff from UNHCR and Save the Children to be aware of this fact (Actions for the Rights of Children, 2001). A neglected problem has been sexual exploitation by humanitarian agency staff, which has been investigated in Guinea, Liberia, and Sierra Leone (UNHCR and Save the Children UK, 2002). The girls were between 13 and 18 years old. In all 3 countries, agency workers from international and local NGOs as well as UN agencies were reportedly the most frequent sex exploiters. Most of the allegations involved male staff who had direct contact with the refugees. As one adolescent in Liberia expressed, "It is difficult to escape the trap of those [NGO] people; they use the food as bait to get you to [have] sex with them" (UNHCR and Save the Children UK, 2002). This is a serious problem, taking into account that the refugee camps in Guinea are over-crowded, and there is food for only two thirds of the refugee population. No wonder that although parents were aware of the exploitation, they felt that there were no other options for their family to secure a livelihood. While they did not approve of what was happening, they generally turned a blind eye.

## Indigenous Children

In the sexual abuse and exploitation of children, there is an evident and profound racist element. If the children being used for sex look foreign, they are considered more eligible because it is assumed that their culture raises them to be open to sex. The existence of early marriages in certain African and Asian cultures may support this attitude. The following examples illustrate this problem:

— In Cambodia, children trafficked from Vietnam to be prostitutes are preferred as sex partners due to the lighter color of their skin.

— It may be easier for a European middle-aged father on a business trip to think that the child is just an exotic stranger and disregard the fact that the child may be the same age as his daughter at home.

— Until recently, in Thailand, nearly 90% of the recruitment for young girls to prostitution took place from the Northern provinces, allegedly because these girls are beautiful (Narvesen, 1989). These Northern minority groups are not considered Thai people, even though their families have lived in the remote areas for more than 100 years. As non-Thai people, they do not have civil rights and do not have access to education, healthcare, or legal protection (Thailand, 2003).

— In Eastern Europe, *Roma* (a more well-known term is "gypsy"; the people themselves prefer the term Roma) children are exposed to severe discrimination including sexual abuse and prostitution (Renton, 2001).

— In Canada, a remarkable study was released in 2000 showing that aboriginal youth constituted up to 90% of the youth involved in the sex trade in some communities (Kingsley & Mark, 2000).

— With regard to prevention, awareness-raising campaigns may not have reached minority ethnic groups due to language differences or ignorance of the prevalence of sexual exploitation in minority groups.

## CHILDREN WHO WORK

When children work, they are no longer seen as children because they carry out jobs one might expect an adult to perform. In Haiti, there is a phenomenon called the *restaveks* (derived from the French words "rester avec" meaning "to stay with"). Children as young as 6 or 7 years old from poor rural areas are sent to Port au Prince to stay with a family. They call the housewife their "mother" or "aunt." They function virtually as house slaves, doing the housekeeping and looking after the children. They stay with poor families that have to work outside the house and, therefore, benefit from having a restavek. Until recently, this was considered an acceptable way of householding. Restaveks are not paid, and they do not go to school. Many of them are exposed to abuse, including that of a sexual nature. These conditions are described in Karen Kramer's 2001 documentary, "Children of the Shadows."

Domestic workers are found all over the world. In the Francophone part of Africa it is common to hire "une petite bonne," a girl whose parents have received a small loan. The child is supposed to pay off the debt for the parents. However, since the child does not attend school, she has no intellectual way of knowing when the loan is paid off and, therefore, is totally dependent on the family for whom she works. This phenomenon is well-known in many regions of Africa (Narvesen, 1989).

Many children occupied in domestic labor risk being sexually abused either by the father or the sons in the family or visiting friends of the family. In the Dhaka study (Khan & Arefeen, 1990), a 14-year-old girl interviewed in a brothel did not remember anything about her family; she had been working as a maid since the age of 7. The males in the family had severely abused her, physically and sexually. Often children will not risk bringing themselves and their families into disrepute by revealing the abuse.

## CHILDREN WHO ARE TRAFFICKED

Children who are trafficked are extremely vulnerable to any kind of violence, including sexual exploitation. They are often without protection or in a cultural setting where they may not even understand the language. Often the girls are recruited and trafficked for sexual purposes. They will be sold to a brothel when they reach their destination (Sanghera, 2000).

## SEXUAL VIOLENCE IN SCHOOLS

Human Rights Watch (2001) published a report on sexual violence against girls in South African schools. The report stated that South Africa has one of the highest rates in the world of violence against women. One in 4 young men questioned reported having had sex with a woman without her consent by the time he reached 18. From 1996 to 1998, girls aged 17 and under constituted 40% of reported rape and attempted rape victims nationally. The girls in schools are at risk of being sexually assaulted by male classmates and teachers. Teachers coerce the girls to have sex in order to get better marks or to not risk failure on examinations. This risk for girls may cause them to drop out of school.

In a recent study from Cameroon examining sexual violence (Menick, 2001), the researcher found a general prevalence rate of 15.9%, broken down by gender: boys

9.5% and girls 21.2%. The study was carried out in 10 public and private secondary schools with a sample of 1688 students aged 15 years, with a response rate of 98.7%. The girls constituted 54.2% of the sample and the boys 45.8%.

The abuse usually took place between the ages of 10 and 14 years. The characteristics of the sexual abuse were 38.7% rape and 54.6% inappropriate touching. The abuse was most likely to take place in the victim's home. The victims remained silent in 42.4% of the cases. Only 10.5% of the cases were brought to trial. Unfortunately, the breakdown of the numbers by gender is not consistently reported at every item. An interesting finding is the perpetrators' ages at the time of perpetrating: nearly 30% were between 14 and 19 years of age.

Relatives and nonrelatives were predators. Within the family, relatives such as uncles and cousins were the most frequent perpetrators. Outside the family, classmates or schoolmates constituted 29.4% and neighbors 24.9%. Teachers accounted for 7.9% and school coaches for 7.3%.

Men constituted 86.1% of the perpetrators. We may reasonably assume that the perpetrators in schools are male (classmates, teachers, and coaches). If this is the case, there is a lack of safe environments for girls in school.

This study should definitely become an item for the school curriculum and should provide support for strengthening codes of conduct for teachers and staff at schools. The study is important because we have so few studies from this part of the world (Central Africa), and it may be used to extrapolate a prevalence of sexual abuse of boys and girls; it shows that sexual abuse within families is mostly committed by uncles and cousins, while fathers are seldom reported as perpetrators (n = 1); and approximately one third of the perpetrators are very young and are often classmates of the victims.

### School Dropouts

According to the research study from the greater Mekong subregion (ESCAP, 2000), in 6 countries, children who ended up in prostitution were illiterate or had very poor education. This fact was sometimes one of the reasons for accepting prostitution—they could not see any other options, particularly if they were the eldest of the siblings and felt responsible for the rest of the family. Jobs available for girls with no education are often physically difficult, such as a sawmill worker or as a construction laborer. In these cases, the girls prefer work that seems easier to carry out and provides the option for earning a bit more money. Uneducated girls may have more difficulties understanding the consequences of such a choice.

### Children in Institutions

We know that children in institutions (such as orphanages) may be targets for physical and sexual abuse. There are people working as staff members who are especially attracted to children and seek to have close contact with them. Some institutions provide no protection against sexual abuse and maltreatment committed by other children or by staff members (Hunt, 1998).

## Health Consequences for Children Exposed to Sexual Exploitation

Only a few reports concern the health status of children who are sexually exploited or who live in prostitution. This may lead to the conclusion that the only risk is contracting AIDS or other sexually transmitted diseases (STDs). An article by Willis & Levy (2002) provides a useful overview of health consequences. Another useful study on this issue is the Mekong study (ESCAP, 2000) referred to earlier.

Although the Willis and Levy study had to be carried out in different countries in order to obtain adequate information, and although the group of sexually abused children was smaller than the group of sexually exploited children, the study provides a good qualitative analysis of health consequences related to sexual exploitation. Information was obtained through interviews with the prostituted children and with key professionals. The following physical and mental health consequences were reported:

— *Skin diseases.* In Cambodia, prostituted children were often locked up in small, dark rooms with insufficient oxygen and lack of proper sanitation, which led to skin infections.

— *Physical consequences of early pregnancy.* Lack of contraception because of ignorance or lack of power to demand the use of contraceptives may lead to early unwanted pregnancy. The risks of early pregnancy and childbirth are well known. Pregnancy-related death is the leading cause of mortality for 15- to 19-year-old girls worldwide (whether married or not). Those under age 15 are 5 times as likely to die as women in their 20s (UNICEF, 2001).

— *Susceptibility to STDs.* Young girls are much more susceptible than adult women to contract STDs, including HIV. This is caused by a young girl's more fragile tissue. Also, as mentioned above, young girls lack the power to demand safe sex or are largely ignorant of preventive measures to take against STDs. In India, the prostitution of children is considered to be a ticking bomb due to the uncontrolled and unrecognized dissemination of HIV/AIDS. When children contract STDs such as gonorrhea, syphilis, and herpes simplex virus, they are often given medicine by the owner of the brothel, or they buy medication not prescribed by medical doctors. In a study from Rwanda, 25% of girls aged 17 or younger were infected with HIV although many reported having sex only with their husbands. According to the study, the younger the age of the girl who is sexually active, the higher the incidence of HIV infection (UNICEF, 1994).

— *General poor health.* Sexually exploited girls seemed to be undernourished, complaining of general physical illnesses such as abdominal pain, headaches, body aches, fever and colds, and insomnia (possibly caused by frequent sleep deprivation).

— *Drug problems.* In Thailand, more than 90% of the prostitutes are said to be drug addicts (C. Wongburanavart, PhD, oral communication, July 1999). However, this percentage varies depending on how long they have been involved in prostitution. Over time, most of the children need to drug themselves to endure their life. (Different kinds of drugs are used, including amphetamines.) In Cambodia, none of the girls interviewed were substance abusers, while boys smoked and sniffed glue to ward off hunger.

— *Affective disorders.* Affective disorders are often difficult to observe and diagnose. Mood disturbances, self-mutilation or suicidal behavior, feelings of inferiority, self-blame, guilt, sadness, tantrums, and aggressiveness were seen. Lack of self-confidence and despair are common.

The short-term and long-term health consequences are devastating for the children involved. The information given above is based primarily on girls; unfortunately, there is no systematic information about the health of boys. This may be because boys are often very reluctant to talk about their lives. One might expect severe affective disorders among boys.

## MEASURES BEING TAKEN: RESCUE, RECOVERY, AND REINTEGRATION

Until now, there have been many interventions, but they have seldom been followed by evaluations. The First World Congress Against Commercial Sexual Exploitation of Children, which took place in Stockholm in 1996, is often considered to be the beginning of international organizations and governments acknowledging the problems already recognized by NGOs. An international agenda for action was adopted, in which the governments committed themselves to:

— Developing a national plan of action in order to combat commercial sexual exploitation.

— Identifying focal points.

— Establishing databases in each country.

The weakness of this agenda for action was the lack of follow-up mechanisms to monitor and confirm that the intentions in the Stockholm agenda were followed.

In December 2001, the Second World Congress Against Commercial Sexual Exploitation of Children took place in Yokohama, Japan, and was hosted by the Japanese government. The congress reconfirmed the Stockholm Agenda for Action.

The main progress since the First World Congress Against Commercial Sexual Exploitation has been in the legal area. International conventions and protocols have been adopted. UNICEF response has raised awareness of the problem, supported law enforcement in sensitizing the police, encouraged research, promoted advocacy, and provided legal training.

The efforts to combat trafficking with women and children have yet to show many results. This failure illuminates the complexity of trafficking and child prostitution and the need for a multisectoral approach (Sanghera, 2000).

In national areas, a large number of countries have improved their legislation, which is a step forward, but it does not necessarily result in more prosecutions. The great obstacle as described in several contexts above concerns the lack of law enforcement.

## MEASURES OF RESCUE, RECOVERY, AND REINTEGRATION IN DEVELOPING COUNTRIES

From outside there is often a focus on rescuing children who are being sexually exploited, in particular for tourists coming to countries with resorts where the sex trade with children is obvious. There are people on private initiatives who buy children out of the brothels. This can not be recommended as a proactive strategy because this will maintain prostitution as a good business and indirectly function as an acceptance of the trade.

In cities such as Phnom Penh, Cambodia and Mumbai, India, occasionally there are organized rescue actions between the trustworthy part of the police and different NGOs (UNICEF Country Office of Cambodia, oral communication, July 1999). The first step of a rescue action is to have the NGO staff members get in contact with the girls by approaching them as customers. They explain to the girls that they want to help them and have them sign a piece of paper indicating that they want to get help. This paper is required to make the police take action (ie, to raid the chosen brothel and arrest the owners, madams, and children). They are taken to the police station, but then the girls are sent to a rehabilitation home, which may be run by an NGO or by the state, supported by an international agency. In this home they receive healthcare, are offered AIDS testing, and sometimes may be offered psychosocial assessment and counseling. The most frequent procedure is to find vocational training for them so that they can become hairdressers, garment factory workers, or waitresses. Regrettably, there is seldom access to computer training or opportunities to learn more advanced skills.

In West Africa, prostituted children work in the street, and they may accept the offers for street children in general: a place to sleep, 2 levels of school classes, and vocational training in traditional handicraft wax dyeing and sewing.

There are, however, obstacles to this rescue procedure. In Asia, the shelters must be safe for children, or they risk being abducted from the shelters by their pimps and, in this way, persuaded to return to prostitution. There are no easy ways out of child prostitution, and the damage is devastatingly difficult to repair.

## RECOVERY AND INTEGRATION PROGRAMS

In most rehabilitation and recovery programs, the term *reintegration* is mentioned. Ideally, children who have been trafficked and exploited should return to their families. However, it is not such a simple thing. In Africa, children are trafficked because their families can not feed them. It could be a disaster if the child were returned. To pay for a return ticket to the country of origin or provide the necessary guidance on the journey is not an option. Often, rehabilitation at the location where the children are found is preferable.

Another obstacle is the risk of ostracism. This is a huge problem in India; these happily saved children do not have many chances outside the rehabilitation home, so they tend to stay there for years (R. Gupta, UNICEF headquarters, personal communication, February 2000).

In Asia, the children must often tell stories of success in order to be accepted in their families. This procedure may perpetuate the willingness for younger siblings or relatives to be trafficked. The girls know that their families have been dependent on the financial support they have been able to provide. Psychosocial intervention programs should focus on supporting formerly prostituted children to improve their self-esteem and develop alternative life perspectives. The children (especially young girls, who need strong role models) have to learn to stand up for their rights.

The International Organization for Migration (IOM) is an international agency that works with migrants and governments to provide humane responses to migration challenges. In addition to assisting refugees all over the world, they provide assistance to girls and women who have been trafficked for sexual purposes, particularly in Eastern Europe.

## INTERNATIONAL CONVENTIONS AND PROTOCOLS

Since the 1990s, and in particular after the First World Congress Against Commercial Sexual Exploitation of Children, several tools have been established. These include international conventions and protocols (see below) and national legislation.

The CRC was adopted in 1989 and ratified by all countries in the world except the United States of America. The CRC guides the work of UNICEF and NGOs work and provides an international framework for the protection of children against sexual abuse and sexual exploitation.

Article 19 of the CRC commits governments to protect children from all forms of physical or mental violence, including sexual abuse. Article 34 of the CRC commits governments to protect children from all forms of sexual exploitation and sexual abuse. In particular, governments are to prevent:

— The inducement or coercion of a child to engage in any unlawful sexual activity.

— The exploitative use of children in prostitution or other unlawful sexual practices or the exploitative use of children in pornographic performances and materials.

The Law on Extraterritorial Legislation enables a state to prosecute nationals and residents of the state if they are accused of exploiting children in other countries. There have been some trials according the extraterritorial legislation, but still only a limited number of countries have this kind of legislation.

The International Labour Organization (ILO) Convention No. 182 on elimination of the worst forms of child labor, which include the prostitution of children and child pornography, was adopted in 1999. Article 7 emphasizes the importance of free basic education where possible and appropriate vocational training as a preventive and reintegrating measure (ILO, 1999).

An optional protocol to the Convention on the Rights of the Child on the Sale of Children, Child Prostitution and Child Pornography was adopted in 2000. The protocol is particularly valuable in its focusing of governmental responsibilities regarding the creation of child-friendly legal proceedings.

In December 2000, a protocol was passed to prevent, suppress, and punish trafficking in persons, especially women and children, supplementing the United Nations Convention Against Transnational Organized Crime. Exploitation is defined by the protocol to include at a minimum "the exploitation of the prostitution of others or other forms of slavery, forced labor or services slavery, and practices similar to slavery" (Protocol to Prevent, Suppress and Punish Trafficking in Persons, Especially Women and Children, Supplementing the United Nations Convention Against Transnational Organized Crime, 2000). The protocol emphasizes that the consent of the child is irrelevant and that a child being trafficked is not a criminal.

In October 2001, the Council of Europe adopted the Convention Against Cyber Crime, which includes an article (Article 9) against child pornography on the Internet.

These international tools for protection of children should be integrated into all national legislation. The tools, though useful, are only one way of combating CSE.

## PREVENTIVE MEASURES: FUTURE PERSPECTIVES

Combating a problem as complex as sexual exploitation will require intervention on many different levels. In this chapter, numerous contributing factors of child exploitation and abuse have been described. As long as these factors continue to have a significant impact on the lives of children and their families, there will be a risk of sexual exploitation. It is worth noting that sexual abuse and exploitation are less frequent in countries with the following qualities:

— A tradition of education for both girls and boys

— Free access to sex education

— A high level of social control in the community

— Equality between genders

— Political and economic stability

— A high level of social and healthcare services

— Efficient legislation regarding child protection

— Efficient legislation to prosecute perpetrators

— Efficient law enforcement

— A cultural mainstream emphasizing the principles of rights of children

For the qualities listed above to be implemented in all countries, a multisectoral intervention would be needed to ensure that there would be an impact on different levels of society. Such goals would be extremely costly to attain, and any effort leading in the right direction must be applauded.

Changing well established social attitudes and eliminating social taboos is a long process. Options for prosecuting perpetrators must be strengthened, and children must be treated as victims, not criminals. The options for treating children as victims who deserve just and fair trials means respect for the rights of the child, but it may in addition help the children to regain their dignity. Unfortunately, the establishment of child-friendly legal procedures may be an ideal difficult to realize in many countries, both developing and industrialized.

Shelters should be available to these children to provide them with basic services, access to a bath, a place to sleep, and protection, in addition to relevant psycho-social assistance.

Juvenile sex offenders should be given a high priority for intervention programs. The prevalence of perpetrators in school staffs is also alarming and should be addressed properly.

International aid agencies and NGOs should consider sexual abuse taking place in families a target for further analysis and find ways of appropriate intervention for this sensitive issue, despite cultural obstacles.

## CONCLUSION

This chapter illuminates how CSE is closely knit with local culture and history although it is an official taboo. The level of denial and repression regarding many forms of sexual exploitation is overwhelming; to look at sexual exploitation of children in a global perspective may be like opening Pandora's box. Sexual exploitation constitutes a severe threat to children's physical and mental health and their chances for a better life. The measures taken to combat all forms of sexual exploitation are still in the beginning stage, so concrete results have yet to be demonstrated.

This chapter described some of the methods used in developing countries to compile data on the phenomenon in order to obtain sufficient background information for planning interventions. It should be a high priority to examine the value of cohort studies in developing countries. In addition, more accurate and detailed research studies on this phenomenon still need to be developed, as well as indicators to measure progress or steps backward.

In certain countries, the prostitution of children provides a significant contribution to the GNP, meaning that in these countries the lives of prostituted children are sacrificed to improve the economy of the country. Therefore, governments, as well as the prostituted child, may be in a situation of impossible choices. Should the world society continue to accept destroying our best investment for the future—our children?

## REFERENCES

Accord de Cooperation entre la Republique du Mali et la Republique de Cote d'Ivoire contre le Trafic Transfontalier des Enfants; 2000.

Actions for the Rights of Children. *Critical Issues: Abuse and Exploitation.* Rev ed. Stockholm, Sweden: Save the Children Sweden; 2001.

Azaola E. *Stolen Childhood, Girl and Boy Victims of Sexual Exploitation in Mexico.* Mexico City, Mexico: UNICEF; 2000.

Bailey J. Japan's teenaged prostitutes: coerced or upwardly mobile? Available at: http://www.ageofconsent.com/comments/numberfourteen.htm. Accessed August 13, 2003.

Caramunt MC. *Explotacion Sexual en Costa Rica: Analisis de la Ruta Critica de Niños, Niñas y Adolescentes Hacia la Prostitucion.* Costa Rica: UNICEF; 1998.

Creighton SJ. Recognising changes in incidence and prevalence. In: Browne KD, Hanks H, Stratton P, Hampton C, eds. *Early Prediction and Prevention of Child Abuse.* New York, NY: John Wiley and Sons; 2002.

Davidson JO. The sex exploiter. Paper presented at: Second World Congress Against Commercial Sexual Exploitation of Children; December 17-20, 2001; Yokohama, Japan.

Demographers appeal for solution to early marriage and early childbearing. *China Population Today.* 1991;8(5):3-4.

Department of Social Welfare and Development. *Commercial Sexual Exploitation of Children in the Philippines: A Situation Analysis.* Executive Summary. Manila, Philippines: UNICEF; 1998.

Economic and Social Commission for Asia and the Pacific. *Sexually Abused and Sexually Exploited Children and Youth in the Greater Mekong Sub-Region: A Qualitative Assessment of Their Health Needs and Available Services.* New York, NY: United Nations; 2000.

End Child Prostitution, Child Pornography and Trafficking of Children for Sexual Purposes (ECPAT). ECPAT International Web site. Available at: http://www.ecpat.net/eng/Ecpat_inter/projects/monitoring/online_database/index.asp. Accessed October 7, 2003.

Ennew J. *The Sexual Exploitation of Children.* Cambridge, England: Polity Press; 1986.

Ennew J, Gopal K, Heeran J, Montgomery H. *Children and Prostitution: How Can We Measure and Monitor the Commercial Sexual Exploitation of Children?* Oslo, Norway: Centre for Family Research, University of Cambridge, and Childwatch International; 1996. Available at: http://www.eldis.org/static/DOC3007.htm. Accessed October 7, 2003.

Estes RJ, Weiner NA. The commercial sexual exploitation of children in the US, Canada and Mexico. September 2001. Available at: http://www.ssw.upenn.edu/~restes/CSEC.htm. Accessed August 19, 2003.

Foundation for Women. *Report of the Kamla Project.* Bangkok, Thailand: Women's Information Centre; 1988.

Friedman RI. India's shame: sexual slavery and political corruption are leading to an AIDS catastrophe. *The Nation.* April 8, 1996:11-20.

Groth N. *Men Who Rape: The Psychology of the Offender.* New York, NY: Plenum Press; 1979.

Guatemalan street children working in prostitution. *Child Labour Today.* Available at: http://www.globalmarch.org/child_labour_today/guatemalan.php3. Accessed August 22, 2003.

Hollin CR, Howells K, eds. *Clinical Approaches to Sex Offenders and Their Victims.* New York, NY: John Wiley and Sons; 1991.

Human Rights Watch. Scared at school: sexual violence against girls in South African schools. New York, NY: Human Rights Watch; 2001. Available at:http://www.hrw.org/reports/2001/safrica. Accessed September 25, 2003.

Hunt K. *Abandoned to the State: Cruelty and Neglect in Russian Orphanages.* New York, NY: Human Rights Watch; 1998.

International Labour Organization. Convention Concerning the Prohibition and Immediate Action for the Elimination of the Worst Forms of Child Labour (ILO No. 182), 38 I.L.M. 1207. November 1999. Available at: http://www1.umn.edu/humanrts/instree/ilo182.html. Accessed August 19, 2003.

International Organization of Migration. Kosovo Anti-Trafficking Report; September 2001.

Khan ZR, Arefeen HK. *The Situation of Child Prostitutes in Bangladesh.* Dhaka, Bangladesh: Dana Publishers; 1990.

Kingsley C, Mark M. *Sacred Lives: Canadian Aboriginal Children and Youth Speak Out About Sexual Exploitation.* Vancouver: Save the Children Canada; 2000.

Lim LL, ed. *The Sex Sector: The Economic and Social Bases of Prostitution in South-east Asia.* Geneva, Switzerland: International Labour Organization; 1998.

Menick MD. Les abus sexuels en milieu scolaire au Cameroun. September 28, 2001. Available at: http://www.crin.org/docs/resources/treaties/crc.28/DMenick-Cameroon.pdf. Accessed October 7, 2003.

Narvesen O. *The Sexual Exploitation of Children in Developing Countries.* Oslo, Norway: Redd Barna; 1989.

Office of the High Commissioner for Human Rights. Convention of the Rights of the Child. Geneva; November 1989. Available at: http://www.unhchr.ch/html/menu2/6/crc/treaties/crc.htm. Accessed August 19, 2003.

Podhisita C, Pramualratana A, Kanungsukkasem U, Wawer MJ, McNamara P. Socio-cultural context of commercial sex workers in Thailand. Paper presented at: IUSSP Working Group on AIDS: Seminar on AIDS Impact and Prevention in the Developing World; December 1993; Annecy, France.

Protocol to Prevent, Suppress and Punish Trafficking in Persons, Especially Women and Children, Supplementing the United Nations Convention Against Transnational Organized Crime. December 2000. United Nations Office on Drugs and Crime Web-site. Available at: http://www.unodc.org/pdf/crime/a_res_55/res5525e.pdf. Accessed August 20, 2003.

Raymond JG, Hughes DM. Sex trafficking of women in the United States. Coalition Against Trafficking in Women. March 2001. Available at: http://www.ojp.usdoj.gov/nij/international/programs/sex_traff_us.pdf. Accessed August 22, 2003.

Renton D. *Child Trafficking in Albania.* Save the Children; March 2001. Available at: http://www.pelastakaalapset.fi/childtraffinc.pdf. Accessed September 25, 2004.

Rizzini I. Street children: an excluded generation in Latin America. *Childhood.* 1996; 3(2):215-234.

Sanghera J. *Trafficking of Women and Children in South Asia: Taking Stock and Moving Ahead.* A review of anti-trafficking initiatives in Nepal, Bangladesh and India. Commissioned by: UNICEF Regional Office of South Asia, Save the Children's Alliance South and Central Asia; March 2000.

Spangenberg M. Prostituted youth in New York City: an overview. ECPAT-USA. 2001. Available at: http://www.ecpatusa.org/pdf/cseypnc.pdf. Accessed August 21, 2003.

Thailand. Terre des Hommes Web site. Available at: http://www.tdhsea.org/Thailand.htm. Accessed August 22, 2003.

United Nations. *Sale of Children, Child Prostitution and Child Pornography.* Note by the Secretary General. September 20, 1995. A/50/456.

United Nations Children's Fund (UNICEF). *Too Old for Toys, Too Young for Motherhood.* New York, NY: United Nations; 1994.

United Nations Children's Fund (UNICEF). *The State of the World's Children.* New York, NY: United Nations; 2000.

United Nations Children's Fund (UNICEF). *Early Marriage: Child Spouses.* Florence, Italy: Innocenti Research Centre; March 7, 2001.

United Nations Children's Fund (UNICEF) West and Central Africa Regional Office. Regional Report on the Sexual Exploitation of Children in West and Central Africa. Abidjan, Cote d'Ivoire: UNICEF; October 2001. 04 BP 443.

United Nations High Commissioner for Refugees (UNHCR) and Save the Children UK. Note for Implementing and Operational Partners on Sexual Violence and Exploitation: The Experience of Refugee Children in Guinea, Liberia and Sierra Leone. Geneva, Switzerland: UNHCR; February 2002.

United Nations, Population Division, Department of Economic and Social Affairs. World marriage patterns 2000. Available at: http://www.un.org/esa/population/publications/worldmarriage/worldmarriagepatterns2000.pdf. Accessed October 7, 2003.

Virani P. *Bitter Chocolate: Child Sexual Abuse in India*. Delhi, India: Penguin; 2000.

Willis BM, Levy BS. Child prostitution: global health burden, research needs, and interventions. *Lancet*. 2002;359:1417-1422.

World Vision. Boy prostitutes in Phnom Penh. *Child Work Asia*. 1996;12(3): 20-22.

# RAPE SURVIVORS: PSYCHOSOCIAL PROBLEMS AND INVESTIGATION IN SOUTHERN ASIA

Govind Prasad Thapa, MA, BL, MPA, PhD

Child sexual exploitation has many manifestations in various parts of the world. In some countries, children are abducted from roadsides, sexually assaulted, and then sold into sexual slavery. In other countries, girls are lured into prostitution and their pimps use Internet cafes to provide clients instructions and locations. Understanding the diverse cultural circumstances that impact the investigation and prevention of child sexual exploitation is important. Southern Asia is a troublesome area in that the value of women and girls is markedly second to that of men. The level of violence, rape, and exploitation remains high, and it requires a through review as is evidenced in the following discussion.

## BACKGROUND

Rape occurs when an assailant compels a victim to submit to sexual intercourse or sexual activities by force, threat of force, threat of imminent death, serious bodily injury, extreme pain, or kidnapping (18 USC § 2241). The negative impact of rape is not isolated to the victim's life; it impacts the lives of the victim's family and the general community. In southern Asia, the joint family system is prevalent. In this type of family system, in which parents and their married children live together, the disgrace of one member is translated into the disgrace of the whole family and often the whole community.

In southern Asia women and female children suffer most. If female children are not aborted, they are often killed early in their lives or face systematic violence and crime later in their lives. Advances in science have been detrimental to female children as the illegal early detection of sex of the fetus has added more deaths. Sex determination through ultrasound results in millions of female feticides every year. In the 2001 Census of India, the number of female children was 2 million less than expected, apparently caused by abortions by parents (Shridhar, 2003).

In 2003, Child Workers in Nepal (CWIN) Concerned Center recorded 6315 incidents related to the exploitation of children, sexual exploitation of children, trafficking of children, forced prostitution of children, child labor exploitation, child death, missing children, children in armed conflict, and children in conflict with the law (**Table 4-1**).

In Pakistan, during the first 8 months of 2004, 2367 cases of physical abuse against women were reported (Madadgaar Help Line, e-mail circulation of press release, September 2004) and included 940 murders, 259 tortures, 271 mutilations, 19 stripping cases, 69 beatings, and 99 harassment in public places cases. Cases were counted in the 4 territories of Pakistan (**Figure 4-1**) and were tabulated for each month: 240 in

**Table 4-1. Child Rights Issues Recorded in Nepal (2003)**

| TYPE OF CASE | NUMBER OF CASES |
|---|---|
| Domestic violence involving children | 109 |
| Corporal punishment of children | 203 |
| Child physical abuse | 324 |
| Child sexual abuse | 137 |
| Child abandonment | 184 |
| Child abduction | 578 |
| Missing children | 948 |
| Found children | 494 |
| Child neglect | 136 |
| Child neglect because of a physical and/or mental disability | 31 |
| Orphaned children | 16 |
| Children sent for adoption | 510 |
| At-risk, migrant children | 458 |
| Child labor exploitation | 181 |
| Child trafficking | 74 |
| Children deprived of adequate facilities in childcare homes | 51 |
| Child marriages | 32 |
| Juvenile delinquency | 61 |
| Children involved in an accident | 519 (398 died) |
| Children affected by a natural disaster | 276 (124 died) |
| Children who died because of a communicable disease | 186 (3 died due to negligence) |
| Children with human immunodeficiency virus (HIV) | 41 |
| Homeless children who became sick | 84 (2 died) |
| Attempted child suicides | 52 (47 died) |
| Children directly affected by armed conflict | |
| *Child deaths* | 36 |
| *Child injuries* | 57 |
| *Child arrests* | 17 |
| Child murders | 33 |
| Infant murders | 28 |
| Child rights violations not otherwise classified | 459 |
| **TOTAL** | **6315** |

*Adapted from Child Workers in Nepal (CWIN) Concerned Center. National annual report: the state of the rights of the child–2004. Available at: http://www.cwin-nepal.org/resources/reports/roc_2004/roc_report04.htm. Accessed December 27, 2004.*

January, 250 in February, 228 in March, 213 in April, 287 in May, 413 in June, 351 in July, and 385 in August. The data pointed to the following perpetrators (Madadgaar Help Line, e-mail circulation of press release, September 2004):

— Husband (462 cases)

— Ex-husband (16 cases)

— Father (28 cases)

— In-law (250 cases)

— Uncle (17 cases)

— Son (42 cases)

— Brother (71 cases)

— Neighbor (63 cases)

— *Zameendar* or *waderas* (ie, landlord) (16 cases)

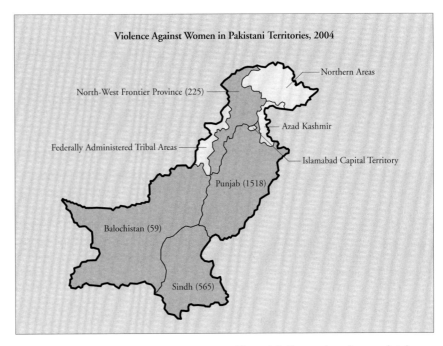

**Figure 4-1.** *The number of cases of violence against women in January through August, 2004, in the 4 territories of Pakistan.*

In southern Asia, women have become victims of crimes inside and outside of their homes. Such cases usually include harassment, torture, abuse, and murder. Dowry atrocities, child prostitution, and trafficking of women for the purpose of sexual exploitation have brought disgrace to the general population of the region.

Many children in southern Asia are abused for commercial sexual purposes every year and their lives and health are destroyed by this lifestyle. Prostituted children are raped, beaten, sodomized, emotionally abused, tortured, and killed by their pimps, brothel owners, and customers. Another significant fact, especially for law enforcement officers, is that child sexual abuse is often hidden and not discussed within the culture. In fact, these abuses are so thoroughly hidden under layers of guilt, shame, and societal pressure that the crimes often remain undetected, unreported, and unpunished. Victims sometimes accept the offenses against them as their destiny and they live with the torment for the rest of their lives.

Though this took place in Kenya rather than southern Asia, a shocking example of violence against females occurred in July 1991, at the St. Kizito mixed secondary school. Male students invaded the girls dormitory and violently raped more than 70 of them, causing 19 girls to lose their lives. The St. Kizito incident caused international outrage, especially following the headmaster's comment that the boys never meant to hurt the girls but "only wanted to rape" them (Kariuki, 2005).

Though no such large-scale incident has been reported in Nepal, the situations for the women and children of Nepal, and the attitudes of most Nepali men are identical. The following examples (in which all names have been changed) provide a glimpse of what is happening in Nepal.

## VICTIMS AND THE CRIMINAL JUSTICE SYSTEM

Throughout the world, victims' experiences with the criminal justice system vary greatly. In Nepal, helpless women and children find accessing the justice system difficult since they are typically not courageous enough to approach police officers. Even if they did so, they would become further stigmatized by their culture and community. In some instances, law enforcement officials treat victimized women and children as perpetrators of the crime, which can lead to victim apathy, distrust, and avoidance of the justice system. Consequently, offenders enjoy impunity, meaning that other people will become victims.

One case in Nepal illustrates the ignorance of judges regarding the gravity and nature of sexual assault. The district and appellate courts acquitted a rape suspect because of the absence of semen on the vaginal swab. These court decisions were inappropriate, and they were reversed by the Supreme Court of Nepal, which described the lower courts' decisions as an "inability to properly understand the nature and gravity of the crime. The suspect's animal instinct, his barbaric physical and psychological attack on a minor girl, the trauma that she has to undergo throughout her life, and the social stigma that her family has to bear are more important" (*State v Madhukar Rajbhandari*, 2001). The Supreme Court decision was exemplary and supportive of victims' rights.

When police officers are unable to uncover adequate evidence that can be used in court, sexual assault and trafficking victims can become frustrated. The legal system seems to favor hard evidence and disregards victims' willingness to be physically present in court and testify. For example, Parvati Khattri was trafficked to Mumbai, India, and sold to a brothel. *Goondas* (ie, henchmen) gang-raped her when she refused to enter into prostitution. She managed to escape from the brothel a year later and filed a complaint upon her return home. The court asked the victim to produce evidence that would prove the offenders' guilt. She did not have any evidence, only her word. During the trial, she asked, "What other big evidence can I produce other than myself as the victim? What [evidence] can I give to the government?" (What evidence can I give, 2004). Unfortunately, the impassioned pleas of sexual exploitation victims usually fall on deaf ears.

In a similar case (*State v Bir Bahadur Biswokarma*, 1991), Gita was lured, trafficked, and sold in India by Bir Bahadur, Lahure, and Kanchha. Although all 3 were involved in the crime, Gita knew only Lahure and could identify only him in court during the trial. Gita said, "I can identify only one of the accused and do not know the others." Because Gita did not recognize Bir Bahadur, he was acquitted. Innocence, ignorance, and the inability of victims to explain and prove the crime that was committed against them can result in acquittals of offenders.

Generally, people in southern Asia complain that law enforcement officials are insensitive to humanitarian issues and that they neglect human values. Psychosocial problems are ignored because of the officers' negative attitudes, lack of knowledge of victim support programs, and lack of skills to prevent revictimization. Because many law enforcement officers view the violence and crimes against women and children to be sex-related issues that are not serious matters, people generally believe that the law enforcement community considers sexual assault to be of a lower status and importance than other crimes. Additionally, law enforcement officers tend to turn a blind eye to the psychological state of mind of sexual assault victims. Others believe that these officers rarely recognize the level of skill required for work in investigations of sexual crimes. Law enforcement officers must harmonize their duties, authority, and power with humanity, which can be accomplished by sensitizing officers and the justice system to the protection of human rights.

## A Child Rape Victim

The investigation regarding the rape of Laxmi, an underprivileged 10-year-old girl, remains in progress. The preliminary investigation indicated that she had been previously abused numerous times. She could not provide specific details of her most recent ordeal; however, she was able to convey her message by signaling with her hands. According to Laxmi, a man lured her with money and then raped her. The only other evidence to corroborate her story came from the medical report, which indicated that her vagina appeared swollen and abnormal, yet her hymen remained intact, and the vaginal swab that showed the smear was negative for spermatozoa.

With little evidence, the police filed the case with the courts, leaving its fate to depend on the sympathetic attitude of the court rather than on the strength of persuasive evidence. The police officers referred her to a CWIN childcare center where she has lived for the past year. A female police counselor maintains contact with Laxmi, but her behavior remains restless, possibly indicating that her needs as a victim are not being met.

## A Repeatedly Raped Victim

Pramila, a blind girl who lived in a hostel, was repeatedly raped by her hostel warden over a period of 6 years. The warden convinced her not to tell anyone about the sexual abuse. Until Pramila left the hostel, she complied, but upon leaving to pursue higher education, she confided in her friends the details of her experience.

Pramila had last been raped in 2002. In a 2004 interview, Pramila said, "at times when capable women are not in a position to tell our worries, how could we do so? If ever we did, people would have not believed us."

In the report submitted to the National Human Rights Commission of Nepal, the fact-finding team summarized Pramila's experience summarized as follows*:

Although the investigating officers seem to be doing their level best, the team felt that investigating officers need further support to do [a] thorough investigation of the case. … As there has not been thorough investigation, the benefit of doubt [may] go to the accused [who may] be freed, in which case all the evidence available will be destroyed … and victims who revealed the atrocities will be at risk.

## A Gang Rape Victim

On December 20, 2003, a woman from the Ganeshpur village in the Bardiya district in Nepal was gang-raped in the presence of her husband by an unidentified "armed group." The rapists threatened the couple with dire consequences if they reported the crime to the police. The local people did not speak about the incident out of fear. As a result of the assault, the woman's family was uprooted and displaced after the incident. The victim continues to feel forced to remain silent because she remains afraid of retaliation by the rapist. She is reluctant to lodge a complaint for financial reasons and the inaccessibility of the criminal justice system.

# Reasons Why Rape Victims Do Not Report the Crime

Rape victims in southern Asia are unlikely to report an assault because of the physical, psychological, social, economic, and legal consequences. For example, 25-year-old Kapali of Mohammadpur village of the Bardiya district was gang-raped by Indians: "They always threaten to shoot at us; how can we report [them] to the police" (Baduwal, 2004).

In a study conducted by Deuba & Rana (2001) regarding the psychosocial impacts of violence against women and girls in Nepal, a significant number of victims cited shame, fear, and social stigma as the major reasons they remained quiet about the violence they endured. They believed that if the community knew of the crime, they and their families would feel shame. As a result, few of these victims needed to be bribed to remain silent.

A study conducted by CWIN and Save the Children—Norway, Nepal (SCNN) (2003) found that most victims were threatened or bribed by their abusers. The study confirmed many child victims did not understand what was happening to them during the abuse. Many child victims said they had remained quiet because they did not think anyone would believe them, and they thought the crime had occurred as a result of something they had done, thereby making the crime their fault.

In contrast, Soledad, a 28-year-old rape survivor, reveals the psychology of a rape survivor by suggesting the following:

---

*The information from this report was provided by Mandira Sharma, a former member of the fact-finding team on Pramila's case. The report was submitted to the National Human Rights Commission on February 3, 2004.*

Don't run away from it. Don't bury it. Don't try to produce a different reality getting all strung out on something, or eating your way through your feelings. Don't slash your wrists. Just deal with it, because it's going to keep coming back if you continue living anyway. It's painful, but you just have to keep going. It's just part of life, really (Bass & Davis, 1994).

The attitudes of law enforcement and the judicial system play a significant role in the infrequent reporting of sexual assault (**Table 4-2**). Many women realize that going to the police and testifying in court is a difficult experience for a rape victim. They are afraid that the authorities will make them feel worse about the rape rather than better. They know that the police and the courts are often like the rest of society in the way they distrust rape victims. Additionally, sometimes the lack of confidence in the law enforcement system to deliver efficient and prompt justice discourages reporting.

Additional reasons why rape victims do not report the crime include the following:

— Rape cases are difficult to prove.

— Law enforcement officers and officers of the court tend to question what rape victims say.

— Family members may discard the victims if they make the rape public.

— Witnesses in the case turn hostile against the victim.

— Victims worry they will go through the ordeal of a court case for nothing since they fear their rapists will not be convicted or will receive a light sentence.

## PHYSICAL CONDITION OF THE VICTIM AND OFFENDER

Investigators can not rule out the presence of a struggle during the commission of a rape; therefore, rape may inflict injuries to the victim's body as well as that of the rapist. As a result, the physical condition of the rapist and the victim must be examined and evaluated by medical and forensic experts. If a rape is reported, investigators are expected to ensure that detailed examinations occur to identify, photograph, and note any physical marks of evidentiary value. Some of the significant body marks that can help prove an offender's guilt include bruises, lacerations, slap marks, blunt injuries, bite marks, belt and/or strap marks, cane and/or stick marks, and burns.

---

**Table 4-2. Example Highlighting Distrust of Authorities**

In 2000, a schoolteacher repeatedly raped a 9-year-old student. A rape charge was filed in the Kathmandu courts. During the court examination, the child was cross-examined by the defense attorney while in the presence of her relatives. She was first asked, "What is rape?" The child could not answer the question. Next, the lawyer asked, "What did you feel after rape?" She meekly answered, "It was painful." Then the lawyer asked, "How did he rape?" With that, everyone present in the court objected because the question was so insulting and disgraceful. An example like this causes many people to dislike and distrust legal and law enforcement authorities.

*Thapa P. Question to a nine-year-old girl in the court: how did he rape? [in Nepali].* SpaceTime. *March 7, 2001:1.*

---

## PSYCHOLOGICAL PROBLEMS OF INCEST VICTIMS

Studies indicate that rape victims suffer from numerous psychosocial problems in addition to their identifiable physical injuries. Nepali incest victims are no different, as illustrated by this excerpt:

The respondents reported some of these feelings as being under stress most of the time (67%) and feeling scared (67%). A number of them (62%) felt guilty and blamed themselves for the … relationship and also suffered sleep disturbances (30%). The majority of them also hated themselves (53%), had frequent mood change swings (50%) and felt angry (55%). Others also expressed wanting to cry often (45%) and not wanting to talk to anybody (45%) and being upset very easily (36%). They were plagued by feelings of helplessness (40%) and did not respect themselves and even wanted to commit suicide (44%). Another large percentage (44%) felt they could never get married or even have normal emotional relationship with anybody. Thirty-five percent said that they could not do anything positive in their lives and would amount to nothing (Dueba & Rana, 2001).

Rape survivors suffer from their own hatred directed toward the offender as well as fears of social stigmatization, of being attacked by the offender again, and of the response of their parents. Unfortunately, the attitudes regarding the fears of these victims are not often realized. For example, when someone is raped, whether by a stranger or an acquaintance, most people believe that sex did occur; however, they assume the sex was consensual and that the victim must be promiscuous.

## IMMEDIATE NEEDS OF AND APPROPRIATE RESPONSES TO RAPE VICTIMS

Immediately after being raped, victims focus their attention on what has just happened. As a result, a victim's primary need is to feel safe (**Table 4-3**). Evidence is critical in rape prosecutions, so all evidence should be collected and protected. The probability of recovering evidence from the victim's body is increased if the victim does not bathe, eat, drink, urinate, or defecate prior to the medical examination. Such an examination is vital even when the rape victim feels physically unharmed by the rape.

---

**Table 4-3. Making a Victim Feel Safe**

If a person learns that someone he or she knows has just been raped, that person should

— Find out where the victim is located and if the victim is safe.

— Ask if the victim wants someone with him or her.

— Determine if there are any potential threats to the victim.

— Assure the victim of privacy and confidentiality.

— Inform the victim if the offender is under control or has been arrested.

At later stages, information about the offender should be provided to the victims. This information may include the sentence commencement date and length, the location where the sentence is being served, the date on which the offender is to be released, the date on which the offender becomes eligible for parole, and whether the offender is in custody, and if not, why.

*Adapted from Correctional Service of Canada.* Myths and Realities: How Federal Corrections Contribute to Public Safety. *2nd ed. Ottawa: Correctional Service of Canada; 2000.*

---

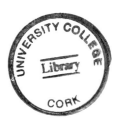

# INVESTIGATION

The investigation of crimes against women and children, particularly those involving domestic violence, trafficking, and sexual offenses, requires knowledge, skills, sensitivity, and a particular aptitude. Male and female officers should be specially trained to meet the needs of victims with professionalism and competence. The collection of facts and evidence is essential to all investigations, and investigators must pay special attention to the following:

— Collecting preliminary information and data about the case in an effort to indicate the way in which an investigation should proceed

— Showing considerable sensitivity to the victim's psychosocial problems

The investigative process begins as soon as a case is reported or, quite often in the case of trafficking (when there is no one to report the case), the process begins when a victim is released or rescued from a brothel.

## PREPARATIONS FOR AN INVESTIGATION

Since rape cases require specialized investigative skills, multidisciplinary teams specializing in sexual assault should be established in an effort to anticipate victims' needs and to be prepared for proper and effective investigation of such cases. Teams should be composed of law enforcement officers, social workers, prosecutors, medical practitioners, and counselors. An interdisciplinary effort by the team's members is essential to protect and support victims effectively.

## PHYSICAL EVIDENCE OF A RAPE

Evidence is the key factor in the investigation, prosecution, and subsequent conviction of an offender. Therefore, both types of evidence, the *mens rea* (the criminal intent) and the *actus reus* (the criminal act), must be proved in court. The most significant sources of evidence include the crime scene, as well as the bodies of the victim and the offender. A crime scene expert must visit the scene, victim, and offender to identify, locate, and handle evidence. A trained expert must bear the responsibility of collecting and caring for the evidence, which is a task that requires much patience and perseverance. The expert must have modern equipment and tools to collect, preserve, photograph, and store such evidence.

As a matter of principle, any attempt to establish facts and gather evidence calls for a survivor-centered approach. Cooperation from each member of the multidisciplinary team is essential to ensure a comprehensive compilation of material evidence, physical and psychological signs and symptoms, and social aspects of the case.

Investigators must examine all details of material evidence and/or physical signs and psychological symptoms that might connect the abuse with the suspect, indicate the way the survivor was abused or trafficked, or indicate the means by which the abuse or trafficking occurred. All forms of evidence (eg, fibers, written notes, recordings, photographs, traces of bodily fluids, head or pubic hair, skin tissue, fingerprints, shoeprints) must be collected to substantiate a survivor's testimony as well as the physical and psychological effects inflicted on the survivor by the abuser or the trafficking situation.

## INTERVIEWING VICTIMS

Reporting a sexual assault can be upsetting and emotionally draining for a victim. Similarly, the decision to investigate and prosecute a difficult rape case is a stressful experience. If the victim decides to report the assault, he or she will have to tell the story of the rape to a law enforcement officer. To ensure the report is complete, the officer must ask the victim to provide a detailed description of what the rapist said and did, and this causes the victim to relive the experience. The victim may want to have a supportive friend, relative, or counselor present when making the report. The law enforcement officer should encourage and provide such support.

An interview of a victim is a delicate matter and an art unto itself. The interviewing officer must be aware of the victim's physical and psychosocial problems as well as the victim's needs before beginning the interview. The officer should ensure that victims do not become revictimized during the course of the interview or the investigation.

Hsu Lu, a notable Taiwanese reporter, described the painful experience in the police station after she had been sexually abused:

The female officer routinely pulled out her notepad, and asked me [questions]: 'name?'; 'address?'; 'profession?' … The officer was very serious and rushed. I suddenly realized that this was an official log. At that instant, I just wanted to escape. But the door was closed. … The officer asked me about every event and detail, and I started to get a mental picture of the occurrence. I even tried to make up some rational sounding details for the memories that were utterly in pieces so that she could finish her log. … When the officer asked me, 'Did he rape you?' I violently shook my head. The officer asked again. My stomach knotted up, and I was in so much pain that I started to faint. … I then told her that my stomach hurt, and asked her if we could stop. (Su-Huan W, Ching-Li C , 2004).

Inappropriate treatment by law enforcement officers will make a victim feel miserable. By using proper interview techniques, officers can help protect a victim from reliving the tragedy. An interview with a rape victim must be conducted in a comfortable environment. Victims must feel safe and secure. Since uniforms often infuse victims with fear, thereby causing them to distance themselves from the interviewing officer, law enforcement officers should wear plain clothes instead of uniforms when conducting interviews, which should not last more than 1 hour at a time. Victims must be allowed time to relate their stories, and officers should ask open-ended questions. Since the frequent exchange of investigators often makes victims nervous, interviewers should not be changed in the middle of an interview. Having a counselor present during the interview to help the survivor cope with the trauma is recommended.

Different interviewing techniques should be used when interviewing child victims than should be with adult victims. Experts who excel at interviewing adult victims may not be as adept at interviewing young children. As a result, such officers should receive training specific to interviewing children. Tips that can be helpful when interviewing a child are to reinforce behaviors positively, give appropriate and consistent feedback, help the child verbalize his or her feelings, and reassure the child that he or she will not be blamed.

## DEALING WITH THE SUSPECT

The identification, interrogation, and prosecution of a suspect is a significant undertaking that warrants the use of special skills and processes. Understanding and identifying the starting point of the abuse process is essential to building a case. With the exception of robberies coupled with a rape, most sexual offenders assault people they know (eg, family members, friends). Deuba & Rana (2001) revealed that 73% of Nepali victims knew their rapist. In 16% of the cases, the victims identified their rapist as being a person in a position of authority over them, suggesting that the hunt for a rapist should begin with the victim's relatives, neighbors, and acquaintances, and can broadened to include friends, local officials, and persons in authority over the victim. Other suggestions for handling a suspect are the following:

— Use only lawful methods when handling a suspect.

— Control access of the suspect to the victim.

— If arrested immediately, preserve all evidence on the body and clothing.

— Take the suspect to the hospital immediately for a medical examination.

— Take photographs of bodily injuries or bruises that may be visible.

— Ensure that the suspect does not attempt to destroy or alter evidence or attempt to commit suicide.

— Never interview the suspect until all the background information and facts of the case are obtained.

— Verify all information gained from the suspect.

— Arrange for audio and video recordings of the interview.

## CONCLUSION

Violence and crime against vulnerable sections of society are considered customary and routine social evils in many countries, especially in southern Asia. These crimes are typically under-reported and poorly investigated in many parts of the world. As a result, many victims suffer silently. Quite often, the humanitarian needs of victims are neglected.

Sensitive and professional intervention and investigation are crucial. The technical phase of an investigation (ie, the application of forensic science) is equally important to establish the *actus reus* of the crime. The successful investigation and prosecution of the crime is not the only objective; victims' rights must be protected at the highest level, which requires humanization of the entire law enforcement system. The successful investigation and prosecution of sexual assault in southern Asia will depend upon a structural change of the legal system, a transformation of society's perception of rape victims, a high level of proficiency among multidisciplinary team professionals, and a multidisciplinary team's ability to work well together.

## REFERENCES

Baduwal D. *The Kathmandu Post*. January 2, 2004:4.

Bass E, Davis L. *The Courage to Heal: A Guide for Women Survivors of Child Sexual Abuse*. 3rd ed. New York, NY: HarperCollins Publishers; 1994.

Child Workers in Nepal (CWIN) Concerned Center. National annual report: the state of the rights of the child in Nepal—2004. Available at: http://www.cwin-nepal. org/resources/reports/roc_2004/roc_report04.htm. Accessed December 27, 2004.

Child Workers in Nepal (CWIN) Concerned Center, Save the Children—Norway, Nepal (SCNN). *Research Report on Silent Suffering: Child Sexual Abuse in the Kathmandu Valley, Children's Perspectives*. Kathmandu, Nepal: CWIN, SCNN; 2003.

Deuba AR, Rana PS. *A Study on the Psycho-Social Impacts of Violence Against Women and Girls with Special Focus on Rape, Incest and Polygamy*. Kathmandu, Nepal: Saathi; 2001.

18 USC § 2241.

Kariuki CW. Masculinity and adolescent male violence: the case of three schools in Kenya. Gender and Women's Studies for Africa's Transformation Web site. Available at: http://www.gwsafrica.org/knowledge/masculinities-kenya.htm. Accessed January 26, 2005.

Shridhar P. The lost girls. *Famina*. November 15, 2003; 44(22):16.

*State v Bir Bahadur Biswokarma*, Nepal Kanoon Patrika 1991, No 3/10, Verdict No 4385, 618.

*State v Madhukar Rajbhandari*, Nepal Kanoon Patrika 2001, No 10/11, Verdict No 6949, 750.

Su-Huan W, Ching-Li C. *A New Milestone in Multi-Disciplinary Criminal Case Processing: The Taiwan Experience*. Paper presented at: International Police Executive Symposium Eleventh Annual Meeting; May 14-20, 2004; Chilliwack, Canada.

What evidence can I give to the government that I was sold [in Nepali]. *Himilaya Times*. September 28, 2004:4.

Chapter 5

# The Commercial Sexual Exploitation of Children in the United States*

Richard J. Estes, DSW, ACSW
Neil Alan Weiner, PhD

## Introduction

The benefits of economic globalization, internationalization, and free trade have brought with them an unanticipated, certainly unprecedented, set of social, political, and economic problems (Bales, 1999; Estes, 1998b; Held & McGrew, 2000; Lie, 1996; UNDP, 2003; World Bank, 2003; Yoon, 1997). Among these problems is what appears to be a dramatic rise worldwide in the incidence of child exploitation (Basu, 2003; Cockburn, 2003; Cusick, 2002; ITCR, 2000; Longford, 1995; UNICEF, 2003; USDOL, 1994, 1995, 2000), including child sexual exploitation more generally (Calcetas-Santos, 1999; ECPAT International, 2001; Hughes, 1999; ITCR, 2000; IPER, 1990) and the commercial sexual exploitation of children (**Table 5-1**) more specifically (Azaola, 2001; Azaola & Estes, 2003; Barnitz, 1998; Calcetas-Santos, 1998; Ennew et al, 1996; Farley, 1998; Flowers, 1994; Hofstede, 1999; Jaffe & Rosen, 1996; Munir & Yasin, 1997; Seabrook J, 1997; UNCHR, 1994; USDOL, 1996; Williams, 1999; World Health Organization, 1996). The problems of child sexual exploitation (CSE) and the commercial sexual exploitation of children (CSEC) appear to occur more frequently in developing countries (Bales, 1999; Estes, 1995, 1996a, 1996b; Richard, 1999) and in countries characterized as "transition economies" (See United Nations Development Programme [2003] for a complete listing of officially designated "developing" and "transition economy" countries) (Caldwell et al, 1997; Estes, 1998a; Hughes, 2000; Rigi, 2003). However, the CSEC also occurs

---

**Table 5-1. Child Sexual Exploitation and Commercial Sexual Exploitation of Children**

*Child sexual exploitation* (CSE) refers to practices by which a person, usually an adult, achieves sexual gratification, financial gain, or advancement through the abuse or exploitation of a child's sexuality by abrogating that child's human right to dignity, equality, autonomy, and physical and mental well-being.

*Commercial sexual exploitation of children* (CSEC) refers to the sexual exploitation of children entirely, or at least primarily, for financial or other economic reasons. The economic exchanges involved in the CSEC may be monetary or nonmonetary (eg, food, shelter, drugs) but, in every case, involves maximum benefits to the exploiter and an abrogation of the basic rights, dignity, autonomy, and physical and mental well-being of the child involved.

---

* Funding in support of the research reported in this chapter was received from the National Institute of Justice of the US Department of Justice (Grant #1999-IJ-CX-0030), the William T. Grant Foundation, the Fund for Nonviolence, the Research Foundation of the University of Pennsylvania, and the Dean's Discretionary Fund of the School of Social Work of the University of Pennsylvania.

in economically advanced countries where the problems are largely invisible except to those directly involved in serving commercially exploited children and their families (ECPAT International, 2001; Estes, In press; Estes & Weiner, 2003; Landesman, 2004; Spangenberg, 2001; United Nations, 1995). The CSEC that occurs in "rich" countries is especially acute in those nations that serve as the destination for the hundreds of thousands of women and children that annually are known to be trafficked worldwide for sexual purposes (Hughes & Roche, 1999; Lederer, 2001; Radcliffe & MacGregor, 2003; USDOS, 2003). Child sex tourism, an especially pernicious and degrading manifestation of the CSEC, has surfaced as a major aspect of the CSEC phenomenon that is difficult to solve for rich and poor countries (De Albuquerque, 1999; ECPAT International, 2001; Klain, 1999; Pettman, 1997; Seabrook, 1997; Simmons, 1996).

## FACTORS CONTRIBUTING TO THE COMMERCIAL SEXUAL EXPLOITATION OF CHILDREN

Various personal and societal forces contribute to the CSEC. These include the following:

— Family dysfunction, including parental instability, serious mental illness, and substance abuse (Cauce et al, 2003; Ferrara, 2001; O'Brien, 1991; Paradise et al, 2001; Whitbeck & Hoyt, 1999)

— Prior history of child physical or sexual abuse or child sexual assault, including a history of child sexual abuse in the family (Boyer & Fine, 1992; Brannigan & Van Brunschot, 1997; Briere, 1988; Briere & Runz, 1988; Gelles & Wolfner, 1994; Nadon et al, 1998; Powers & Jaklitsch, 1989; Rotheram-Borus et al, 1996; Ryan et al, 2004; Seng, 1989; Silbert & Pines, 1983; Simons & Whitbeck, 1991; Stiffman, 1989; Tyler et al, 2000, 2001a,b; Whitbeck & Simons, 1990; Whitbeck et al, 1997; Widom, 1996; Widom & Kuhns, 1996)

— History of serious depression, substance abuse, and recurrent mental illnesses in the family (Cauce et al, 2000; MacLean et al, 1999; Molnar et al, 1998; Rotheram-Borus, 1993; Seto & Barbaree, 1999; Stewart et al, 2004; Whitbeck et al, 1999)

— Income poverty (Azaola, 2001; Cauce et al, 2003; Hood-Brown, 1998; Longford, 1995; MacWilliams, 2003; National Coalition for the Homeless, 1999, 2001; US Conference of Mayors, 2003)

— The promotion of the prostitution of children by parents, older siblings, and boy-friends (Faugier & Sargent, 1997; Muecke, 1992; Schloenhardt, 1999; USDOJ, 2003)

— Immaturity and poor sexual decision making on the part of extremely vulnerable (often substance-abusing) children and youth (Allen, 1980; Cates, 1989; Cates & Markley, 1992; Du Rant et al, 1998)

— Criminal and other deviant behaviors that place children at higher risk of sexual exploitation (Baron, 1997; Kaufman & Widom, 1999; Loeber & Farrington, 1998; Lucas & Hackett, 1995; McCarthy & Hagan, 1992; Whitbeck et al, 2001)

— The use of "survival sex" and prostitution by runaway and "thrownaway" children to provide for their subsistence needs (Flowers, 1994; Greene et al, 1999; McCarthy & Hagan, 1992; Yates et al, 1991)

— The presence of preexisting adult prostitution markets in communities where large numbers of street youth are concentrated (Azaola, 2001; Estes & Weiner, 2003; Farley & Kelly, 2000; Hofstede, 1999)

— The presence in local communities of large numbers of sexually unattached and transient males, including military personnel, truckers, conventioneers, and tourists (Azaola, 2001; Estes & Weiner, 2003; Moon, 1997; Sturdevant & Stolfuz, 1992)

— Sexual minority status (eg, gay, bisexual, transgender/transsexul) (Arey, 1995; Boyer, 1989; Clements-Nolle et al, 2001; Cochran et al, 2002; Diamond, 2000; Estes & Weiner, 2003; Kruks, 1991; Lock & Steiner, 1999; Nemoto et al, 1999; Tremblay, 2003)

— For some girls, attachments to "boyfriends" who, in time, reveal themselves to be pimps or traffickers (Faugier & Sargent, 1997; Hughes, 1999)

— The existence of organized criminal networks that, among other illegal activities (primarily drugs, thefts, and money laundering), engage in prostitution and the trafficking of children and women for sexual purposes (Budapest Group, 1999; Schloenhardt, 1999; United Nations, 1999; Williams, 1999; Woodiwiss, 1993)

— The trafficking of domestic children and women for sexual purposes within countries (Estes & Weiner, 2001, 2003; Spangenberg, 2001)

— The trafficking of children and women for sexual purposes across international borders (Azaola, 2001; Barnitz, 1998; Barr, 1996; ECPAT International, 2001; Lederer, 2001; Richard, 1999; Shelley, 2000; USDOS, 2003)

— For some girls, membership in gangs (Hazlehurst & Hazlehurst, 1998; Moore & Hagedorn, 2001)

## CHILD MALTREATMENT IN THE UNITED STATES

The precise number of child victims of sexual abuse, sexual assault (**Table 5-2**), and sexual exploitation in the United States is unknown; most specialists estimate such children number in the hundreds of thousands (USDOJ, 2003). For the year 2001, the Administration for Children and Youth of the US Department of Health and Human Services (USDHHS) reported that 903 000 American children had been the victims of some form of "maltreatment," ie, physical abuse (18.6%), neglect (57.2%), medical neglect (2.0%), sexual abuse (9.6%), psychological maltreatment (6.8%), and/or other forms of abuse (19.5%). These numbers do not add up to 100% because many of these children have been victims of multiple forms of abuse, and therefore, their situations are reflected under more than one category (USDHHS, 2003b).

Of the nearly 1 million cases of child maltreatment reported to federal authorities in 2001, approximately 87 000 involved children subjected to sexual abuse, or approximately 1.2 out of every 1000 of the nation's population of 73 000 000 children (USDHHS, 2003b). To these "new cases" of child sexual abuse, of course, must be added those hundreds of thousands of cases of child sexual abuse substantiated to have occurred during previous years—an unknown portion of which continued to be re-abused even after their cases came to the attention of public authorities (Gelles &

---

**Table 5-2. Child Sexual Abuse and Child Sexual Assault**

*Child sexual abuse* refers to illegal sexual activity involving persons younger than 18 years of age. Most often perpetrated by an adult, such activities include rape and molestation, pornography, and the intentional exposure of children to the sexual acts of others (Goldstein, 1999).

*Child sexual assault* refers to any sexual act directed against a person younger than 18 years of age, forcibly and/or against that person's will or not forcibly or against the person's will where the victim is incapable of giving consent because of his/her temporary or permanent mental or physical incapacity. Child sexual assault includes forcible rape, forcible sodomy, sexual assault with an object, and forcible fondling (National Incident-Based Reporting System [NIBRS] as cited in Snyder, 2000).

Wolfner, 1994; Kaufman & Widom, 1999; Simons & Whitbeck, 1991; Stewart et al, 2004; USDHHS, 2003b). Fortunately, recent trend data reported by Jones & Finkelhor (2001) suggest that the incidence of child abuse—including child sexual abuse—may be on the decline, from 1.7 out of 1000 in 1997 to 1.3 in 1999 to 1.2 in 2001 (USDHHS, 2003b). Though the reasons for the apparent decline in child abuse and child sexual abuse remain unclear, Jones & Finkelhor suggest that 2 factors likely account for the favorable trend: a real decline in the incidence of child sexual abuse and/or changes in attitudes, policies, or standards that result in fewer reports and substantiations of child sexual abuse (2001). The investigators tend to favor the first explanation, given the combination of public policy successes over the decade that have resulted in improving public awareness of the existence and seriousness of child sexual abuse; the expansion and increased effectiveness of prevention programs focused on child sexual abuse (Finkelhor & Dziuba-Leatherman, 1994); the successful incarceration of a large number of adult and juvenile pedophiles and other sexual molesters of children (Beck, 1993; Freeman-Longo, 1994); and more effective monitoring of child and adult sexual offenders living in the general community (Finn, 1997).

## THE COMMERCIAL SEXUAL EXPLOITATION OF CHILDREN IN THE UNITED STATES

No estimate in the child sexual abuse field is more contentious than that applied to the number of American children and youth who each year become victims of commercial sexual exploitation. The number of such children is believed to be "significant," but the precise numbers remain elusive primarily due to the illegal and highly secretive nature of the commercial sexual exchanges engaged in by children and their "customers," the vast majority of whom are men over the age of 30. (See Shafer [2004] for an example of the debate that surrounds the application of even modest estimates to the number of commercially sexually exploited children in a single US city.)

To the extent that data do exist, however, estimates of the annual number of CSEC cases in the United States range from as few as a couple of thousand children (Hammer et al, 2002; Sedlak et al, 2002) to several hundred thousand American children and youth who—owing to their especially vulnerable status as runaways, thrownaways, otherwise homeless, or as victims of domestic and international trafficking—are "at special risk" of becoming victims of commercial sexual exploitation (Estes & Weiner, 2001; Finkelhor et al, 1990; Goldman & Wheeler, 1986; Greene et al, 1999; Hofstede, 1999; Jaffe & Rosen, 1996; National Coalition for the Homeless, 1999, 2001; US Conference of Mayors, 2003; USDOJ, 2000, 2003). Whatever their actual numbers, the social and economic impact of CSEC on children, their families, and American society is far-reaching, long-lasting, and expensive (Estes & Weiner, 2001, 2003; Browne & Finkelhor, 1986; Franey et al, 2001; Tyler et al, 2001b; USDOJ, 2000, 2003; World Health Organization, 1996).

America's problem with the CSEC appears to be concentrated in the nation's coastal and resort cities (Estes, 2002; Estes & Weiner, 2003) as well as in those cities that border Mexico and Canada (Azaola, 2001; Azaola & Estes, 2003; Ives, 2001). However, the problem occurs in "middle America," in the nation's many smaller- and medium-sized cities and rural communities that frequently serve both as "recruiting" and "training" locales before children move (or are moved) to larger cities where higher levels of anonymity and invisibility can be achieved (Hofstede, 1999; Kral et al, 1997; Lucas & Hackett, 1995; Stiffman, 1989).

The CSEC is present in those cities where children are trafficked into the United States from developing Asia, Africa, and Latin America and from selected Eastern European and Central Asian countries that are "successor states" to the former Soviet Union (Budapest Group, 1999; Hughes, 2000; Interpol, 2003; Lederer, 2001;

Richard, 1999; USDOS, 2003). Organized crime groups appear to be heavily involved in the trafficking of such children from developing nations and transition economy countries into the United States, especially those crime groups with strong ties to Russia, the Ukraine, China, the Philippines, Thailand, and other East Asian nations (ECPAT, 2001; Richard, 1999; USDOS, 2003).

The remainder of this chapter is devoted to a discussion of the nature, extent, and severity of the CSEC phenomenon in the United States. Data come from a 3-year study focused on CSE and the CSEC in the United States, Canada, and Mexico. The chapter is divided into 3 parts: (1) a discussion of the research methods used in conducting the study; (2) a summary of the major findings obtained from the United States portion of the study; and (3) recommendations concerning ways in which the United States can strengthen its capacity for responding to the complex needs of children and families at risk of CSE and the CSEC. Trends regarding CSE and the CSEC of children in all 3 countries of the North American Free Trade Agreement (NAFTA)—United States, Canada, and Mexico—are summarized in chapter 15 in this volume.

# RESEARCH METHODS
The data reported in this chapter were collected as part of a 3-year study that began in January 1999. The study focused on CSE and the CSEC in the 3 countries of NAFTA. The organizing goals of all 3 national efforts were the same but as is useful for this chapter are the following:

— To identify the nature, extent, and underlying causes of CSE and the CSEC in the United States

— To identify those subgroups of children in the United States who are at the greatest risk of commercial sexual exploitation

— To identify those subgroups of adults—United States and foreign nationals—who initiate or otherwise promote the CSEC

— To identify other "stakeholders" and "stakeholder networks" in the United States that economically benefit from the CSEC (eg, pimps, traffickers, hotel and travel businesses)

— To identify the nature and extent of domestic and international trafficking of children in the United States for sexual purposes

— To identify the various types and levels of "functionaries" associated with the sexual trafficking of children in the United States

— To identify the contribution, if any, made by organized criminal units to the CSEC in the United States

— To assess the current capacity of the United States for acting more proactively in halting, with the goal of eliminating, national and international factors that contribute to the commercial sexual exploitation of children

## RESEARCH PARTNERS
The investigation involved a unique partnership between the following groups: leading governmental and nongovernmental organizations located in the US, Canada, and Mexico; 3 universities (1 located in each country); 2 international child advocacy organizations; the leading national child welfare organizations in the United States and Mexico; a major professional association in the United States whose practitioners deal directly with commercially sexually exploited children and their families; and for the United States, financial participation from the federal government, private foundations, and the investigators' home institutions.

The United States phase of the effort involved working partnerships with some 800 law enforcement and human service professionals in 17 American cities selected for special study. More than 200 child victims of the CSEC participated in this research as informants and partners in the project's implementation.

## PROJECT PHASING

The United States national study was implemented in the the following 13 phases:

1. Recruitment, selection, hiring, and training of the national project staff

2. Reviews of the relevant criminal justice and human service literature

3. Establishment of linkages with key governmental and nongovernmental agencies and organizations serving sexually exploited children

4. Appointment of national and regional experts in CSE to an international advisory group

5. Interviews with key decision makers in law enforcement and the human service agencies at the federal, state, and local levels

6. Implementation of city-specific focus group meetings

7. Statistical surveys of local, state, and national governmental and nongovernmental organizations serving sexually exploited children

8. Interviews with sexually exploited children

9. Interviews with traffickers of children for sexual purposes (Mexico)

10. Interviews with adult "customers" of children for sex (Canada)

11. Reviews of local, state, and federal statutes pertaining to the CSEC

12. Reviews of international agreements, declarations and covenants pertaining to the CSEC

13. Meetings with law enforcement and human service professionals to frame recommendations for strengthening the national capacity to prevent, or at least significantly reduce, the number of children who become victims of commercial sexual exploitation

(For complete details regarding all of the substeps undertaken in support of these phases, see the methodology subdirectory of the project's electronic home page: http://caster.ssw.upenn.edu/~restes/CSEC.htm.)

## COUNTRY SELECTION

The 3 countries of the NAFTA region (United States, Canada, and Mexico) were selected for inclusion in this investigation for the following 7 reasons: (1) their geographic proximity to one another; (2) the special nature of the free trade agreement in which each country participates; (3) the comparative ease with which the nationals of all 3 countries move across each nation's borders; (4) the known existence of the CSEC in all 3 countries; (5) the transnational and intraregional nature of the CSEC within and between the 3 countries; (6) the existence of formal commitments on the part of each government to work toward the elimination of the CSEC; and, as evidenced by this project, (7) a history of productive research partnerships between the region's universities and human service and law enforcement organizations.

## CITY SELECTION

Twenty-eight North American cities were selected for special study as part of the regionwide investigation: 17 in the United States, 4 in Canada, and 7 in Mexico (**Table 5-3**). Cities were selected using the following 5 criteria: (1) population size; (2) known problems with the CSEC; (3) a history of attempting to resolve problems associated with the CSEC within their communities; (4) the presence of networks of child- and youth-serving organizations with which the national research teams could partner; and, (5) for Canada and Mexico, relative proximity to the United States. Over the project's 3-year period, in-depth studies were completed as planned for all but 3 Canadian cities: Toronto, Vancouver and Windsor.

## KEY INFORMANTS FOR THE CITY, COUNTRY, AND REGIONAL STUDIES

In the United States, data were obtained from more than 1000 key informants nationwide from the following groups: sexually exploited runaway and thrownaway street children (n = 124); sexually exploited children in the care of local human service and law enforcement agencies (n = 86); representatives of federal law enforcement agencies (n = 164); representatives of state, county, and local law enforcement agencies (n = 146); representatives of public human service agencies (n = 93); representatives of local private human service agencies (n = 196); representatives of international non-governmental organizations (n = 51); and members of the project's Tri-National Research Team and International Advisory Board (n = 60). Supplementary statistical data were obtained from questionnaires completed by national and state organizations dealing with sexually exploited children and their families (n = 288).

## STATUTORY REVIEWS

Relevant national and sub-national laws, criminal statutes, and international agreements relating to the CSEC also were reviewed as part of this investigation. A summary of the major US federal laws relating to the CSEC is available in Appendix G of the electronic version of the project's major report (available at http://caster.ssw. upenn.edu/~restes/CSEC.htm). State statutes pertaining to the CSEC may be downloaded from the Web site of the National Clearinghouse on Child Abuse and Neglect (NCCANCH) (http://nccanch.acf.hhs.gov/general/statespecific/index.cfm). Electronic summaries of national laws pertaining to the CSEC in other countries may be downloaded from the Web site recently established by the Protection Project (http://www.protectionproject.org). Finally, Appendix H of the project's electronic report contains a summary of major international agreements, declarations, and covenants relating to CSE and the CSEC.

---

**Table 5-3. Cities in North America Included in the Study of the Commercial Sexual Exploitation of Children**

| UNITED STATES | CANADA | MEXICO |
|---|---|---|
| Chicago | Montreal | Acapulco |
| Dallas-Ft. Worth | Toronto | Cancun |
| Detroit | Vancouver | Ciudad Juarez |
| El Paso | Windsor | Guadalajara |
| Honolulu | | Mexico City |
| Las Vegas | | Tapachula |
| Los Angeles | | Tijuana |
| Miami | | |
| New Orleans | | |
| New York | | |
| Oakland | | |
| Philadelphia | | |
| San Antonio | | |
| San Diego | | |
| San Francisco | | |
| San Jose | | |
| Seattle | | |

# FINDINGS

The study's findings for the United States are grouped under the following 11 headings:

1. Factors that contribute to the sexual exploitation of children

2. More and less common forms of CSEC

3. Social, emotional, health, and other risks to sexually exploited children

4. Impact of sexual exploitation on children

5. Categories of sexually exploited American children

6. Profiles of child sexual exploiters in the United States

7. Pimps and child sexual exploitation

8. Organized crime and child sexual exploitation

9. Domestic and international trafficking of children for sexual purposes

10. Risk of child sexual exploitation in comparison with other social risks to which American children and youth are exposed

11. National capacity of the United States for addressing CSE and the CSEC

Electronic versions of the individual country reports can be downloaded from http://caster.ssw.upenn.edu/~restes/CSEC.htm.

## FACTORS THAT CONTRIBUTE TO THE SEXUAL EXPLOITATION OF CHILDREN

A range of factors were identified as contributing to the sexual exploitation of children in the United States. In addition to those already identified in the chapter's introductory section, they include macro/contextual factors, micro/situational factors, and individual/internal factors. **Table 5-4** identifies definitions and examples of the social forces and processes associated with each cluster of contextual factors that contribute to CSE and the CSEC in the United States.

## MORE AND LESS COMMON FORMS OF THE COMMERCIAL SEXUAL EXPLOITATION OF CHILDREN

The CSEC takes many forms, including child pornography, the prostitution of juveniles, and the domestic and international trafficking of children for sexual purposes. **Table 5-5** identifies the forms of the CSEC we encountered in the United States.

## SOCIAL, EMOTIONAL, HEALTH, AND OTHER RISKS TO SEXUALLY EXPLOITED CHILDREN

Sexually exploited children are exposed to a wide range of social, emotional, health, and other risks. These risks are varied and profound and, for many children, appear to become insurmountable trauma from which they may never fully recover (Brannigan & Van Brunschot, 1997; Briere, 1988; Cauce et al, 2003; Farley, 1998; Snyder, 2000; Stewart et al, 2004; WHO, 1996). Further, in identifying the risks (and subsequent resiliency) of children exposed to commercial sexual exploitation, we found it necessary to distinguish between the risks experienced by children living in their own homes versus risks experienced by sexually exploited children who have left home (as runaways, thrownaways, or as those who have have been forced out of their homes for other reasons, like family dysfunction, serious mental illness, substance abuse, profound poverty, or homelessness). The adaptive challenges confronting both groups of children, though shared in some respects, differ sharply especially for those children who no longer have access to their families, extended kinship systems, school, and other critical components of social life on which most American children depend.

**Table 5-4. Factors Contributing to the Commercial Sexual Exploitation of Children and Youth**

| DOMAIN | DEFINITION | CONTRIBUTING FACTORS |
|---|---|---|
| Macro/Contextual (External) | External forces and processes that exist in the larger social environment over which individuals can exercise only minimal control but which, nonetheless, exert a powerful influence on the lives of children and their families. | — Socioeconomic<br>— Societal attitudes toward children and youth<br>— Social anomie among children and youth (ie, a lack of connectedness on the part of youth with the larger society and their place within it)<br>— Poverty<br>— Child victims of crime and violence<br>— Societal responses to crimes committed against children, including sexual crimes<br>— Presence of preexisting adult prostitution "markets"<br>— Presence of groups advocating child-adult sexual relationships<br>— Sexual behavior of unattached and transient males (ie, the military, seasonal workers, truckers, motorcycle gangs, conventioneers)<br>— Community knowledge and attitudes concerning HIV/AIDS and other sexually transmitted diseases |
| Micro/Situational (External) | External forces and processes that impact children and their families directly but over which they can exert some measure of control. | — Sociobehavioral<br>  — Family dysfunction<br>  — Parental drug dependency<br>  — History of physical and/or sexual assault<br>  — Personal drug dependency<br>  — School/other social performance failures<br>  — Gang membership<br>— Active recruitment into prostitution by others<br>  — Peers<br>  — Parents or other family members (including siblings)<br>  — Local pimps<br>  — National and/or international crime organizations |
| Individual (Internal) | Psychogenic and cognitive forces that influence a child's sense of mastery over her/his own personal environment and future. | — Psychogenic<br>  — Poor self esteem<br>  — Chronic depression<br>  — External locus of control<br>— Seriously restricted future orientation |

## Risks of Sexual Exploitation and Commercial Sexual Exploitation for Children Living in Their Own Homes

Sexually exploited children living in their own homes are at substantial risk of re-exploitation over a period of many years (Boyer & Fine, 1992; Brannigan & Van Brunschot, 1997; Cauce et al, 2000; Ferrara, 2001; Goldstein, 1999; Myers et al, 2002; Nadon et al, 1998; O'Brien, 1991; Seng, 1989; Simons & Whitbeck, 1991; USDOJ, 2003). The risk of repeated sexual exploitation for these children is especially high in the following families: (1) where the exploitation has not been detected and in which no external intervention has occurred by either law enforcement or child protective authorities; (2) that move from city to city in order to avoid detection by oversight agencies or, once detected, move frequently so as to evade prosecution or supervision; and (3) characterized by high levels of domestic violence, drug use, serious mental illness, and sexual promiscuity.

**Table 5-5. Forms of the Commercial Sexual Exploitation of Children in the US, 2000**

MORE COMMON FORMS OF THE CSEC

| Form | Description |
| --- | --- |
| Sexual molestation of boys and girls by acquaintances | — 49% of all sexual assaults against children are committed by persons known either to the child or the child's family—teachers, coaches, physicians, scout leaders, and neighbors. |
| Sexual molestation of boys and girls by family members | — 47% of all sexual assaults against children are committed by members of the child's own family—father, stepfather, uncles, and older siblings. |
| Pornography | — Children are the subjects and victims of pornography.<br>— Street children frequently exchange participation in pornography for food, clothing, shelter, money, and other items of value.<br>— More than 6.5 million children with regular Internet access are exposed to unwanted sexual materials annually; more than 1.7 million of these children report considerable distress over exposure to these materials (Finkelhor et al, 2000). |
| For boys, gay sex | — At least 95% of all the commercial sex engaged in by boys is provided to adult males.<br>— Approximately half of the adult male sexual exploiters of boys are married men, many with children of their own. |
| For girls, modeling, stripping, and topless and lap dancing | — Modeling, nude dancing, lap dancing, and similar sexually provocative activities frequently are used to lure girls into prostitution.<br>— At a minimum, these activities serve as the basis for involving girls in pornography. |
| For girls, sex as a contribution to gang economy | — Approximately 25% of girls who are members of gangs perform sexual services for other gang members or to the general public.<br>— These sexual services are considered part of the girl's contribution to the gang's life as a collective to the gang's economy. |
| For girls, pimp-controlled prostitution, including street prostitution and prostitution organized through escort and massage services | — 55% of street girls engage in formal prostitution, about 75% of which is controlled by pimps.<br>— 45% of street girls engage in prostitution which, in only about 25% of situations, is controlled by pimps.<br>— Pimp-controlled juvenile prostitution is closely associated with escort and massage services; private dancing, drinking, and photographic clubs; major sporting and recreational events; major sporting and cultural events; conventions; and selected tourist destinations.<br>— Pimp-controlled juvenile prostitution exists side by side with adult prostitution, often on the same streets and along the same tracks followed by adults involved in prostitution. |
| For boys, entreprenurial pornography and prostitution | — A large percentage of boys report engaging in commercial sex for money and pleasure more often than girls.<br>— A large percentage of older boys involved in commercial sex think of themselves as "hustlers" rather than as prostitutes.<br>— Like girls, boys also exchange sex for money and other things of value to them (eg, drugs, alcohol, a place to sleep, transportation).<br>— A disproportionate number of boys involved in commercial sex, about 25% to 35%, self-identify as sexual minorities. |

*(continued)*

**Table 5-5.** *(continued)*

LESS COMMON FORMS OF THE CSEC

| Form | Description |
|---|---|
| Participation in national organized crime networks | — About 20% of children encountered in this study were trafficked nationally by organized criminal units using well established prostitution tracks. <br> — Trafficking is expensive and children are required to pay their traffickers for the services received (eg, transportation, false identity papers, a place to live, jobs). <br> — Children are trafficked into, and within, the United States by various private and public means (eg, cars, buses, vans, trucks, planes). <br> — Most trafficked children have available to them various false identity papers for use in case of arrest. <br> — The majority of nationally trafficked children use drugs and engage in drug sales. |
| Participation in international organized crime networks | — Only about 10% of the children encountered in the present study were trafficked internationally. <br> — Some children who are citizens of the United States are trafficked outside of the United States, mostly to other economically advanced countries located in Europe and Asia. <br> — Most internationally trafficked children are the citizens of developing countries located in Asia, Africa, Central and South America, and Central and Eastern Europe. <br> — International trafficking of children is highly lucrative: a single trafficked child can earn a trafficker as much as $30 000 or more in trafficking fees. <br> — International trafficking of children is highly complex and requires the involvement of a wide range of functionaries, including recruiters, trainers, purveyors of false documents, transporters, money collectors, and enforcers. |
| Servitude and indenturing | — Many children who enter the country illegally are forced into servitude by their traffickers. <br> — Child servitude includes working in sweat shops, restaurants, and hotels for virtually no wages; performing sexual services for money; panhandling or attempting to sell items of little economic value. <br> — Children in servitude frequently are required to repay their trafficking debts through commercial pornography and prostitution. <br> — In many cases, trafficked children are required to serve as "mules" in transporting illicit drugs into and/or across the US. |

All 3 of these situations place pre-pubescent boys and pre- and post-pubescent girls still living at home at the highest risk of becoming sexual targets of family members (USDOJ, 2003), including sexual assaults initiated by nonparental family relatives (32%), day care providers (22%), unmarried partners of parents (15%), foster parents (10%), legal guardians (9%), and parents (5%) (USDHHS, 2003a). Children living in their own homes are at risk of sexual exploitation from a range of unrelated adults living in the general community who are known to, and typically trusted by, the child, the child's family, or both (eg, neighbors, coaches, clergy). In the worst situations, child victims of sexual exploitation in their own homes are at risk of considerable violence, occasionally even to the point of death (Gelles & Wolfner, 1994; Gelles, 1996, 1997; Widom, 1992; USDOJ, 2003).

Risks of Sexual Exploitation and Commercial Sexual Exploitation for "Street," Homeless, and Other Children Not Living in Their Own Homes

Children living on America's streets are subject to an extraordinary range of social, emotional, physical, health, and economic risks not experienced by other groups of children. Poverty is rampant among sexually exploited homeless children, as are hunger and malnutrition (Cauce et al, 2003; Greene et al, 1999; Lucas & Hackett, 1995; National Coalition For the Homeless, 1999, 2001; US Conference of Mayors, 2003). Illnesses caused by exposure to the weather, eating rotting food from dumpsters, and sleeping in pest- and vermin-infested areas are widespread (Farrow et al, 1992; Yates et al, 1991). Sexually transmitted diseases are high among street youth (Bond et al, 1992; Clements-Nolle, 2001; Kral et al, 1997; Nemoto et al, 1999), who also regularly fall victim to violence inflicted by peers, pimps, "customers," and others (Dalla et al, 2003; Farley & Kelly, 2000; McCarthy & Hagan, 1992; Nixon et al, 2002; Scarpa, 2003; Simons, 1990; Stiffman, 1989; Tyler et al, 2001a; Whitbeck & Simons, 1990; Widom, 1992).

Street youth suffer disproportionately from serious mental illnesses, including disruptive behavior disorders, attention deficit disorders, depression, mania, schizophrenia, post-traumatic stress syndrome, suicide, and suicidal ideation (Cauce et al, 2000, 2003; Estes & Weiner, 2003; Molnar et al, 1998, 2001; Rotheram-Borus, 1993; Rotheram-Borus et al, 1996). A large percentage of street youth participate in criminal activities; much of this activity is directed at obtaining the minimal resources required to meet survival needs of the youth, including illicit drugs used to mask the psychological pain of their exploitation (USDOJ, 2003; Yates et al, 1991).

## IMPACT OF COMMERCIAL SEXUAL EXPLOITATION ON CHILDREN

No matter how children become victims of sexual exploitation, no child is able to withstand her or his molestation unharmed; all suffer long-term physical and emotional injures (Browne & Finkelhor, 1986; Ferrara, 2001; Gelles & Wolfner, 1994; Goldstein, 1999; Kaufman & Widom, 1999; Myers et al, 2002). These profound injuries remain with the majority of sexually exploited children throughout their lives and, in turn, pose complex relationship challenges for others with whom they interact, including intimate partners, their own children, friends, and various types of human service providers. The correlation is known to be especially strong between the CSEC and teen pregnancy (Boyer & Fine, 1992; Ireland & Widom, 1994; Widom, 1996; Widom & Kuhns, 1996), adult prostitution (Farley, 1998; Farley & Kelly, 2000; Widom & Kuhns, 1996), substance abuse (DuRant et al, 1998; Ireland & Widom, 1994; Kral et al, 1997), violence (Gelles & Wolfner, 1994; Nixon et al, 2002; Widom, 1992), and juvenile and adult criminal behavior (Kelley et al, 1997; Loeber & Farrington, 1998; USDOJ, 2003).

## CATEGORIES OF COMMERCIALLY SEXUALLY EXPLOITED CHILDREN IN AMERICA

Based on our field research, 14 categories of American children at risk of commercial sexual exploitation were identified in the course of this investigation (Estes & Weiner, 2001). Four of these categories are the following: (1) CSEC victims not living in their own homes (n = 4 subgroups); (2) CSEC victims living in their own homes (n = 2 subgroups); (3) other groups of CSEC victims (n = 2 subgroups); and (4) groups of domestic and foreign children involved in cross-border and international issues related to the CSEC (n = 6 subgroups). In addition to identifying the various subgroups associated with these various clusters of children at risk of the CSEC, **Table 5-6** contains working estimates of the number of potential CSEC cases in a given year associated with each cluster of children.

The estimates summarized in **Table 5-6** reflect what we believe to be the number of children in the United States "at special risk" of commercial sexual exploitation, because of their unique status as runaways, thrownaways, victims of physical or sexual

**Table 5-6. Categories of Children "At Risk" of Commercial Sexual Exploitation in the US, December, 2000\***

| Categories of Commercially Sexually Exploited Children & Youth | Operational Definitions | Number of Children Estimated "At Risk" of CSEC | Running Total[†] *Low Senerio* (75% of Estimated Cases)[‡] |
|---|---|---|---|
| **Group A: Commercially Sexually Exploited Children Not Living in Their Own Homes** | | | |
| 1. Runaways from Home | Youth under the age of 18 years who absent themselves from home or place of residence without the permission of parents or legal guardians and who, as a result of running away, are prone to becoming victims of sexual exploitation | 121 911 | 91 433 |
| 2. Runaways from Juvenile and Other Institutions | Youth under the age of 18 years who absent themselves without permission from group foster homes, juvenile detention centers, hospitals or wards for the chronically ill, mental hospitals or wards, or other types of group quarters and juvenile institutions | 6793 | 96 528 |
| 3. Thrownaway Youth | Youth under the age of 18 years who are abandoned or are forced to leave their homes by parents or guardians and are not permitted to return and who, because of their vulnerable economic status, are prone to becoming victims of sexual exploitation | 51 602 | 135 230 |
| 4. Homeless Children (Not Elsewhere Counted) | Youth not counted under runaways or thrownaways who are homeless and who, because of their social and economic status, are vulnerable to sexual exploitation | 27 972 | 156 209 |
| **Group B: Commercially Sexually Exploited Children Living in Their Own Homes** | | | |
| 5. Children Ages 10-17 Living in the General Population | Children between the ages of 10 and 17 years living in the general population who become victims of sexual exploitation | 72 621 | 210 674 |
| 6. Children Ages 10-17 Living in Public Housing | Children between the ages of 10 and 17 years living in public housing who become victims of sexual exploitation | 4447 | 214 010 |
| **Group C: Other Groups of Commercially Sexually Exploited Children** | | | |
| 7. Female Gang Members | This group includes approximately 27 000 girls between the ages of 10 and 17 years who are members of identifiable gangs, some of whom become victims of sexual exploitation as a result of their gang membership | 5400 | 218 060 |

*(continued)*

**Table 5-6. Categories of Children "At Risk" of Commercial Sexual Exploitation in the US, December, 2000\*** *(continued)*

| CATEGORIES OF COMMERCIALLY SEXUALLY EXPLOITED CHILDREN & YOUTH | OPERATIONAL DEFINITIONS | NUMBER OF CHILDREN ESTIMATED "AT RISK" OF CSEC | RUNNING TOTAL† *LOW SENERIO* (75% OF ESTIMATED CASES)‡ |
|---|---|---|---|
| **Group C: Other Groups of Commercially Sexually Exploited Children** | | | |
| 8. Transgender Street Youth | A broad category of sexually exploited youth who identify themselves as members of the opposite sex to which they were born; this includes male identifying as female, female identifying as male, and youth born with sex organs of both genders | 3000 | 220 310 |
| **Group D: The International Dimensions of the CSEC in the US: United States Children and Youth Traveling Abroad and Foreign Children Traveling to the United States for Sexual Purposes** | | | |
| 9. Foreign Children Ages 10-17 Brought into the US Legally Who Became Victims of Sexual Exploitation | Includes all children brought into the US legally as extended family members, as au pairs to private households, and to business and diplomatic communities, and who, in due course, become victims of sexual exploitation | 3000 | 222 560 |
| 10. Foreign Children Ages 10-17 Brought into the US Illegally Who Became Victims of Sexual Exploitation | Includes all children smuggled or otherwise brought into the US illegally (often in economic or sexual servitude to their smugglers/traffickers) | 8500 | 228 935 |
| 11. Unaccompanied Minors Entering the US on Their Own Who Become Victims of Sexual Exploitation | Includes all children who, on their own, enter the US and become victims of sexual exploitation | 2500 | 230 810 |
| 12. Non-Immigrant Canadian and Mexican Children Ages 10-17 Crossing into the US for Sexual Purposes | Includes all Canadian and Mexican youth who enter the US on a more or less casual basis and who, while in the US, engage in sexually exploitative activities | 2500 | 232 685 |
| 13. US Youth Ages 13-17 Living Within Driving Distance to a Mexican or Canadian City | Includes American youth living in cities and towns in close proximity to Mexico or Canada who cross into these countries in pursuit of sex | 14 329 | 243 431 |
| 14. Non-Immigrant US Youth Ages 13-17 Trafficked from the US to Other Countries for Sexual Purposes | Includes youth between the ages of 13 and 17 years who travel outside the US to provide sexual services to the nationals of other countries | 1000 | 244 181 |

*\* The methodology used to construct these estimates is described in at the end of part V in Estes & Weiner (2001).*

*† A cumulative total of the number of estimated number of children at special risk of commercial sexual exploitation in that row plus the number of estimated cases in all preceding rows.*

*‡ The "low scenario" adjusts the total number of children estimated to be a special risk of commercial sexual exploitation by 25% in order to minimize the likelihood of duplicate counting of the same children in one or more categories, ie, the same child being counted as a runaway and a thrownaway.*

abuse, users of illegal drugs and other substances, members of sexual minority groups, illegally trafficked children, and children who cross international borders in search of cheap drugs and sex, among others.

Owing to the illegal and highly secretive nature of the CSEC, the numbers reported in **Table 5-6** do not reflect an actual "head count" of the number of confirmed cases of commercial sexual exploitation associated with each risk group of children. Even so, the estimates achieved the following: identified groups of children in American society who are judged to be at the highest risk of commercial sexual exploitation; identified groups of children not previously associated with the CSEC (including American children who cross international borders in search of cheap drugs and sex, unaccompanied minors, nonimmigrant Canadian and Mexican youth, children trafficked domestically and internationally for sexual purposes, sexual minority youth, youth affiliated with gangs, and others); and suggested a plausible range within which the actual number of child victims of commercial sexual exploitation likely fall.

At the time of completing work on the investigation, a new study called the *National Incidence Studies of Missing, Abducted, Runaway, and Thrownaway Children-2* (NISMART-2) was completed (Hammer et al, 2002; Sedlak et al, 2002). Inasmuch as 60% of the children we estimate to be at risk of commercial sexual exploitation fall within the runaway and thrownaway categories (Rows 1, 2, 3 and 4 of **Table 5-6**), the findings from this updated national incidence study of runaway and thrownaway children likely will impact future estimates of the number of children judged to be at special risk of commercial sexual exploitation (eg, children away from home for extended time periods and living in unsafe or unsupervised living conditions). Preliminary discussions with investigators associated with NISMART-2, for example, suggested that the number of runaway and thrownaway children may have declined by as much as 30% to 40% between 1988 and 2000, a finding that would be consistent with more favorable trends reported for children in situations of sexual risk (Jones & Finkelhor, 2001).

### PROFILES OF CHILD SEXUAL EXPLOITERS IN THE UNITED STATES

The investigation succeeded in identifying discrete groups of persons who regularly exploit children for sexual purposes. While the "membership" of these groups consists primarily of men not all child sexual exploiters are men. As reported in **Figure 5-1**, a portion of the sex crimes committed against children are perpetrated by women, couples, and even other juveniles—including other commercially sexually exploited youth (De Albuquerque, 1999; NCCANCH, 2003; Righthand & Welch, 2001; Simmons, 1996; Snyder, 2000; USDHHS, 2003a; USDOJ, 2003).

Similar to the conceptual decision made in identifying child victims of commercial sexual exploitation, the investigators found it useful to distinguish between perpetrators of sex crimes involving children living in their own homes and sex crimes perpetrated against street and other children not living in their own homes. Sex crimes committed against children in their own homes typically are classified as child sexual abuse or child sexual assault and only rarely include a "commercial" nexus. Rather, sexual assaults inflicted on children living in their own homes tend to be opportunistic in nature and involve primarily perpetrators who are known to the child, the child's family (eg, neighbors, friends, clergy), or both (USDHHS, 2003a).

*Figure 5-1.* Type of child maltreatment and gender of offender, including male only, female only, and male and female couples Data Source: USDHHS (1998) as cited in *OJJDP*, 2000: 46.

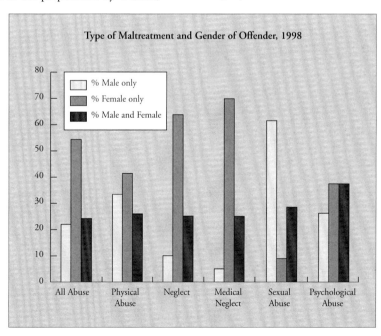

Sex crimes committed against street and other children not living in their own homes, however, are nearly always economic or commercial in nature in that children require, or are forced, to exchange sex for money or something else of commercial value. The perpetrators of these crimes are rarely known to the child or the child's family personally and, typically, such perpetrators tend to perceive their child victims as a temporary "means" to the satisfaction of some personal need (eg, sexual satisfaction, control, power). Such perpetrators rarely develop long-lasting relationships with their child victims; many may express "affection" and other "fuzzy feelings," but only as a means for persuading the child or children to "cooperate" with the sexual initiatives.

While the faces of the children victimized by each form of sexual exploitation may differ somewhat, the underlying sociocultural dynamics responsible for all forms of child sexual abuse remain constant—in almost every situation the exploitation is initiated by a more powerful offender, usually an adult, who seeks to exert his or her will over the child in order to secure some sexual, economic, or other benefit of value to the offender (Lanning, 1992; Myers et al, 2002; Tyler & Cauce, 2002). In situations involving the commercial sexual exploitation of children, the rights and human dignity of child victims are compromised further given the maturational disparities and unequal power relationship that exists between child victims and that majority of their "customers" who are adults. In every case, the CSEC operates to the sexual benefit of the "customer" and at a loss of dignity and well-being for the child.

## Sexual Exploiters of Children Living in Their Own Homes

There are more than 300 000 cases of alleged child sexual abuse reported to the National Center for Child Abuse and Neglect each year. Of these, some 105 000 (approximately 1:3) cases are confirmed to be *substantiated* (includes cases in which the allegation of maltreatment or the risk of maltreatment was supported or founded [USDOJ, 2000]) or *indicated* (includes cases in which the allegation of maltreatment or the risk of maltreatment could not be substantiated, but there was reason to suspect the child was maltreated or at risk of maltreatment [USDOJ, 2000]). The majority of these cases involved sexual crimes inflicted on children 12 years of age or younger and nearly all (84%) occur in the privacy, and hence secrecy, of the child's own home (USDOJ, 2000).

Further, data reported by the USDHHS confirm that 96% of all cases of sexual abuse of children living in their own homes are perpetrated by persons known either to the child or to the child's family (49%) or by members of the child's own family (47%). Contrary to widely held beliefs, only a small number of confirmed cases of sexual abuse are perpetrated against children by strangers (4%).

Reflected in the child maltreatment data summarized in **Figure 5-1** is that perpetrators of child sexual abuse include men, women, couples, and juveniles. *Males only* were the offenders in 62% of all confirmed cases of child sexual abuse whereas *males and females acting together* were the offenders in 29% of the cases. *Women only* were the offenders in fewer than 10% of all confirmed cases of child sexual abuse.

Patterns of child sexual assault are similar to those reported to child sexual abuse. As reported by the Federal Bureau of Investigation (FBI) in its National Incident-Based Reporting System (**Figures 5-2** and **5-3**), persons over the age of 18 were responsible for more confirmed cases of child sexual assault (57%) than persons younger than 18 years. Beginning at perpetrator age 18, however, sexual assaults of very young children living in their own homes is more likely to be committed by a member of the child's own family (58%).

The above findings are especially important given the strong relationship that this investigation and other studies have confirmed to exist between child sexual abuse, child sexual assault, and the subsequent involvement of children in the CSEC (Boyer & Fine, 1992; Brannigan & Van Brunschot, 1997; Kaufman & Widom, 1999; Nadon et al, 1998; Prentky et al, 1997; Righthand & Welch, 2001; Seng, 1989; Simons & Whitbeck, 1991).

## Sexual Exploiters of Children Not Living in Their Own Homes

In addition to the sexual abuse of children living in their own homes, the study of the NAFTA countries confirmed that tens of thousands of American children living outside of their homes fall victim to sexual exploitation each year. The majority of these children live on the streets or sleep in emergency shelters, cheap motels, "squats" (ie, abandoned and usually seriously deteriorated houses occupied without the permission of the owner), cars, vans, and in some cases trash dumpsters.

Based on interviews with children and focus group meetings with law enforcement and human service professionals, the investigators were able to identify 6 discrete categories of sexual exploiters of children not living in their own homes: (1) pedophiles (adults with sexual desires and arousal fantasies that often culminate in sexual acts with pre-pubescent and adolescent children of the same or opposite sex); (2) "transient males," including members of the military, truck drivers, seasonal workers, conventioneers, and sex tourists; (3) "opportunistic" exploiters, (persons who will sexually abuse whoever is available for sex including children); (4) pimps; (5) traffickers; and (6) other juveniles.

The precise number of predators associated with each category of child sexual exploiters could not be determined by this investigation; with certainty, though, their demographic characteristics and psychosexual histories are quite varied (Davidson, 1996; Faugier & Sargent, 1997; Hughes, 1999; Lanning, 1992). Considered together, sexual predators are young and old, well educated and not, and are equally as likely to come from middle America as well as from the nation's coastal cities.

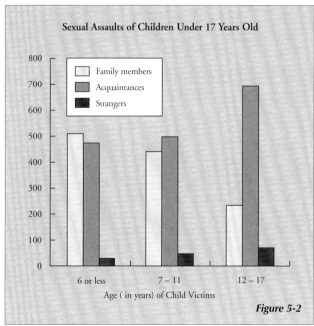

Figure 5-2

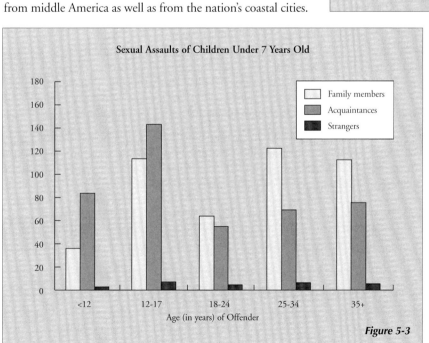

Figure 5-3

*Figure 5-2.* Sexual assaults of youth by victim age and relationship of offender per 1000 typical incidents within each age group, 1991-1996. Data Source: FBI National Incident-Based Reporting System (NIBRS) as cited in *OJJDP, 2000: 29.*

*Figure 5-3.* Sexual assaults of youth younger than 7 by age and relationship of offender. Data Source: FBI National Incident-based Reporting System (NIBRS) as cited in *OJJDP, 2000: 29.*

ed by one of 3 criteria: (1) the ages of the children involved—children older than 12 years of age are preferred except in cases involving electronic pornography; (2) the nationality of these children—domestic children are easier to move around than foreign children who may or not speak the language or understand the cultures of the sexual "customers" for whom these children are intended; and (3) the profit potential associated with the recruitment, selection, training, and movement of children as they are compelled to engage in commercial sexual services. Our experience suggests that organized criminal units, in general, and with the sole exception of child pornography, tend to avoid involving themselves to any great extent in the commercial sexual exploitation of children 10 years of age and younger, not out of any false sense of morality but because such young children are "too difficult" or "too hot" to handle. Further, the CSEC typically constitutes only one element provided by organized criminal units to their "clients." A much larger "portfolio" of illegal services they provide includes drugs, adult prostitution, sexual trafficking, sometimes counterfeiting, and almost always money laundering. See **Table 5-5** for examples drawn from the public media of the highly diversified nature of most national and international criminal networks that, among other illegal activities, engage in the CSEC.

## DOMESTIC AND INTERNATIONAL TRAFFICKING OF CHILDREN FOR SEXUAL PURPOSES

The investigation in the United States encountered many children who were being trafficked into and across the country for sexual purposes (**Table 5-6**, Group D). These children included citizens of the United States who are trafficked as part of regional and national sex crime rings; a limited number of foreign children who, along with adult women, are trafficked into the United States from other world regions (USDOS, 2003).

### Regions and Countries of Origin of Sexually Exploited Trafficked Foreign Children in the United States

**Table 5-7** identifies the regions and countries of origin of foreign children the investigators encountered who had been trafficked for sexual purposes into the United States. **Table 5-7** also identifies the focus group cities in which these children were encountered, but like trafficked adults, these children are moved quickly from one city to the next to avoid detection.

### Adult Traffickers of Children for Sexual Purposes

Many adults benefit financially from national and international trafficking of children for sexual purposes. Groups of such persons include amateur traffickers; small groups of organized criminals; and multilayered trafficking networks that are organized both nationally and internationally (Graycar, 1999; Lederer, 2001; Richard, 1999; Schloenhardt, 1999; USDOS, 2003; Yoon, 1997).

In addition to these 3 broad groups of trafficking "organizers" and promoters, a large network of trafficking "functionaries" were identified in this investigation. As initially conceptualized by Schloenhardt (1999) and Graycar (1999), trafficking functionaries include arrangers/investors; recruiters; transporters; corrupt (ie, "bribable") public officials; informers; "guides" and crew members; enforcers; supporting personnel and specialists; debt collectors; and money movers. **Table 5-8** summarizes the major "responsibilities" assigned to each type and level of trafficking functionary and illustrates the application of these roles via stories that have appeared in the public media.

## RISK OF CHILD SEXUAL EXPLOITATION IN COMPARISON WITH OTHER SOCIAL RISKS TO WHICH AMERICAN CHILDREN AND YOUTH ARE EXPOSED

**Figure 5-4** places the risk of child sexual exploitation, including the online sexual victimization of children (Finkelhor et al, 2000), in the context of other major social risks to which American youth are exposed (eg, truancy, pregnancy, drug use, violence, homicide). The number of incidents associated with each type of risk are standardized at the rate of cases per 100 000 age-specific population.

The summary data contained in **Figure 5-4** present a convincing and disturbing picture of the large numbers of American children and youth who, each year, are at risk of becoming victims of commercial sexual exploitation.

### NATIONAL CAPACITY OF THE UNITED STATES FOR ADDRESSING CHILD SEXUAL EXPLOITATION

Another goal of the project was to assess the adequacy of the existing network of law enforcement and human service systems for responding to the needs of sexually exploited children and their families. Below are the patterns that emerged from analysis of the data collected through surveys of governmental organizations (hereafter "GOs") and nongovernmental organizations (hereafter "NGOs") serving sexually exploited children and their families.

— Sizable numbers of GOs and NGOs are coming face to face with CSE and the CSEC.

— "Official" GO reports of the nature and extent of the CSEC in the United States, in our judgment, seriously underestimate the number and types of such children in the American population.

— Substantial gaps exist in the conceptual reach and range of services provided to commercially sexually exploited children by GOs and NGOs.

— The magnitude of the policy and service gaps that characterize GOs and NGOs serving CSEC is serious and reduces the nation's ability in responding effectively to combat the root causes of CSE and the CSEC.

The following policy, administrative, and service issues are judged to be the most problematic with respect to the capacity of the nation's GOs in responding effectively to the needs of commercially sexually exploited children (and their families):

— Strategic intelligence concerning the nature, extent, and dynamics of the CSEC in the United States at the present time is lacking at almost all levels of public life, including in those organizations charged with the responsibility of preventing, or at least reducing, the risks of child commercial sexual exploitation.

— The vast majority of GOs lack an adequate understanding of the complex nature, causes, and dynamics of commercial child sexual exploitation at all levels of social organization.

— Most GOs lack clear policies and procedures for dealing with cases of the CSEC that come to their attention.

— The vast majority of GOs are severely understaffed and underresourced in being able to respond adequately to the complex service needs represented by children and families struggling with commercial sexual exploitation.

— To the extent they are available at all, the CSEC-focused services of most GOs are largely uncoordinated and fragmented.

— Comparatively few GOs work cooperatively with NGOs at any level of political organization in identifying child victims of sexual exploitation or the adults who perpetrate these crimes against children.

— In addition to severe fiscal and personnel shortages, nearly all GOs continue to lack adequate electronic and other surveillance systems for tracking adults and juveniles convicted of commercial and noncommercial sex crimes against children.

**Table 5-7. Regions and Countries of Origin Commercially Sexually Exploited and Trafficked Foreign Children in the US, 2000**

| World Region | Country of Origin | Focus Group Cities in Which Children Were Found |
|---|---|---|
| **Asia-Oceania** | Australia | Honolulu, New Orleans |
| | Burma | Chicago, New York |
| | Cambodia | Honolulu, New Orleans, San Francisco, Seattle |
| | Hong Kong | Honolulu, New York, Seattle |
| | India | Berkeley, Chicago, New York, San Jose |
| | Japan | Honolulu |
| | Korea | Detroit, Honolulu, New York, San Francisco |
| | Laos | Honolulu, Los Angeles |
| | China | Chicago, Detroit, Honolulu, Los Angeles, New York, Seattle |
| | Philippines | Honolulu, Los Angeles, Miami, New York, Philadelphia, San Diego, Seattle |
| | Sri Lanka | Chicago, Los Angeles |
| | Taiwan | Honolulu, New York, San Francisco |
| | Vietnam | Chicago, Honolulu, New Orleans, New York |
| **Africa** | Benin | Seattle |
| | Burkina Faso | Seattle |
| | Cameroon | New York, Seattle |
| | Eritrea | New York, Seattle |
| | Ethiopia | New York, Seattle |
| | Ghana | New York, Seattle |
| | Nigeria | Seattle |
| | Somalia | Chicago |
| | Sudan | Chicago |
| **Central and South America** | Belize | San Diego |
| | Colombia | Chicago, El Paso, San Diego |
| | Costa Rica | El Paso, San Diego |
| | El Salvador | Chicago, El Paso |
| | Guatemala | Chicago, El Paso, New York |
| | Honduras | Chicago, El Paso, Miami |
| | Nicaragua | Chicago, El Paso, Los Angeles, San Diego |
| **Caribbean** | Dominican Republic | Fort Lauderdale, Homestead (Fla), Miami, New York |
| | Haiti | Fort Lauderdale, Homestead (Fla), Miami, New York |
| | Jamaica | Miami, New York |
| **North America** | Canada | Chicago, Honolulu, Las Vegas, Los Angeles, Miami, New Orleans, New York, Seattle |
| | Mexico | Chicago, Detroit, Honolulu, Los Angeles, Miami, New York, Philadelphia, San Antonio, San Diego, San Francisco, Seattle |
| **Eastern Europe** | Bosnia | Chicago, New York |
| | Belarus | Chicago, Seattle |
| | Czech Republic | Honolulu, New York |
| | Hungary | Los Angeles (via Mexico), New York |
| | Poland | Chicago, Honolulu, New York |
| | Russia | Chicago, Honolulu, Los Angeles (via Mexico), New York, Seattle |
| | Ukraine | Baltimore, Los Angeles (via Mexico), New York, Seattle |

NGOs serving commercially sexually exploited children and their families confront yet another set of service challenges. The following are assessed to be the most serious issues confronting the effectiveness of CSEC-focused NGOs:

— The activities of the nation's CSEC-focused NGOs are largely uncoordinated and fragmented.

— The lack of coordination between and among NGOs severely restricts their ability to intervene effectively in dealing with occurrences of the CSEC other than at the local level.

— Sharp ideological disagreements exist between often competing NGOs concerning the magnitude of child sexual exploitation in the United States and the appropriate courses of action that should be taken to address the situation.

— Sharp ideological divisions exist between competing NGOs advocating positions on behalf of adult women and men victimized by prostitution versus those seeking to extricate children from commercial sexual exploitation. Some organizations would like to merge the issues confronting the 2 age populations into a common agenda for action (eg, dealing with male privilege, reorganizing the human service and justice systems dealing with youth), whereas others wish to keep the agenda for commercially sexually exploited youth separate from issues affecting adults.

— Nearly all CSEC-focused NGOs are small and severely underfunded. Most compete with one another for the very limited programmatic resources that are available.

— Though certain exceptions were found, in the main, sexually exploited boys, sexual minorities, difficult-to-handle street youth, and street youth with serious mental illnesses are seriously underrepresented in the service populations of most NGOs seeking to serve sexually exploited children and youth.

*Figure 5-4. Risk of CSE in groups with other social risks.*

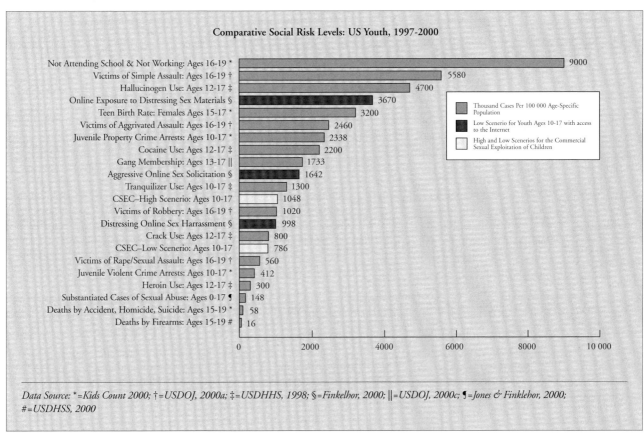

**Table 5-8. Trafficking "Functionaries" Associated with the Commercial Sexual Exploitation of Children in the US, 2000**

| CATEGORIES | OPERATIONAL DEFINITIONS | EXAMPLES FROM THE PUBLIC MEDIA OF TRAFFICKING "FUNCTIONARIES" IN THE US |
|---|---|---|
| **Arrangers/ Investors** | Persons who invest money in the trafficking operation and oversee the whole criminal organization and its activities. These persons are rarely, if ever, known to the lower levels of employees and to the migrants being trafficked. An organizational pyramid structure insulates the arrangers, who stand back and are not easily connected with the commission of specific criminal offenses. | — Yu Zheng and Sheng Deng, Chinese nationals, were ultimately sentenced to 2 years in federal prison for their involvement in smuggling 12 Chinese nationals into the US. The aliens had been confined inside sealed steel shipping containers and were required to pay the smugglers as much as $60 000 each. (See Human smugglers try new tactic. *MSNBC News.* February 8, 2004. Available at: http://www.msnbc.com/news/354350.asp. Accessed August 17, 2004.)<br>— Thirteen people were charged when a Chinese gang, the Snakeheads, forced women to repay trafficking "contracts" worth $30 000 to $40 000 each by working as prostitutes. Some brothels in which these women worked grossed an average of $1.5 million over a 2.5 year period. (See Booth W. 13 charged in gang importing prostitutes. *Washington Post.* August 21, 1999:A03) |
| **Recruiters** | Persons who work as middlemen between the arranger and the customers of the criminal enterprise. Recruiters are responsible for finding and mobilizing potential migrants and collecting their payments. The recruiters that work in the country of departure are usually not informed about the precise trafficking passage. They get paid for casual jobs only and not on a permanent basis. Investigations show that in many cases, the recruiters come from the same region as the migrants and frequently are members of the same culture and are well respected people within the local community. | — A man smuggled a 14-year-old Mexican female into the US through Texas to Orlando under the pretext of working in the hotel industry. In fact, she was raped by 1 of "the many bosses" responsible for the operation, beaten, and forced into prostitution. (See testimony of "Rosa," a trafficking survivor, before the *US Foreign Relations Committee.* April 4, 2000.)<br>— The CIA found modern US slaves, some as young as 9 years old. The report describes case after case of foreign women and children who answered advertisements for jobs in the US as au pairs, sales clerks, secretaries, or waitresses but found, once they arrived, that the jobs did not exist. (See CIA finds modern US slavery. *Philadelphia Inquirer.* April 3, 2000:A06) |
| **Transporters** | Persons in charge of assisting the migrants in leaving the country of origin by any means (land, air, sea). Transporters in the destination country bring undocumented immigrants from an airport, seaport, or coast to the big cities. The transport providers and operators have to be technically sophisticated to change their operations in reaction to law enforcement and coastal surveillance activities. Transporters usually do not get inside | — Dominican immigration officials uncovered a child trafficking ring that operated at the Santa Domingo airport which, in many cases, used pregnant women as "covers" to transport Dominican children into the US and Puerto Rico. Ring operators collected between $10 000 and $12 000 for each child they managed to slip illegally into the US. (See Pregnant women used in scheme to transport children. *Agencia EFE S.A.* June 25, 2000.)<br>— A Thai boy got involved in a fight against sex trafficking because at age 2, he was brought into the US along with a man and a woman, the latter destined to be a sex slave somewhere in America. The boy was a human decoy, designed to make them look like a family on holiday. (See Rosin H. Thai boy caught up in fight against sex trafficking. *Washington Post.* May 15, 2000:A.02) |

*(continued)*

**Table 5-8.** *(continued)*

| Categories | Operational Definitions | Examples From the Public Media of Trafficking "Functionaries" in the US |
|---|---|---|
| | information on the criminal organizations and structures. They stay in touch with the organization through intermediaries who contact them casually. | |
| **Corrupt Public Officials, ie, "Bribable" Protectors** | Traffickers have to pay government officials to obtain travel documents for their customers. Law enforcement authorities in many transit countries have been found to accept bribes to enable migrants to enter and exit countries illegally. The corruptees individually or collectively protect the criminal organization through assault of their position, status, privileges, and other violations of the law. | — Senior Chinese government officials were believed responsible for bribing authorities in Guatemala to get Mexican visas to use for human trafficking. Immigrants paid up to $50 000 for the documents and transport to North America. (See Mitrovica A. Smuggling network extensive, officials say China's reach 'way beyond.' *The Globe and Mail.* May 5, 2000.) |
| **Informers** | For trafficking operations, it is necessary to have systems of information-gathering on border surveillance, immigration and transit procedures and regulations, asylum systems, and law enforcement activities. The accumulated knowledge is used to the best advantage of the criminal organization. In some cases, it was found that information-gathering resided in a core group of informers who managed the information flow and had access to well-organized and centralized communications systems through sophisticated technology. | — Officials in Guatemala were bribed by Chinese government officials to send Mexican visas through "middlemen" in Canada in a complex human trafficking ring. Five Canadians were charged, one who was under investigation by the USDOJ. (See Mitrovica A. Smuggling network extensive, officials say China's reach 'way beyond.' *The Globe and Mail.* May 5, 2000.) |
| **Guides and Crew Members** | Guides are responsible for moving illegal migrants from one transit point to the other or by helping the migrants to enter another country by sea or air. Crew members are people employed by the traffickers to charter trafficking vessels and accompany migrants throughout the illegal passages. | — Dominican immigration officials uncovered a child trafficking ring that operated at the Santa Domingo airport which, in many cases, used pregnant women as "covers" to transport Dominican children into the US and Puerto Rico. Pregnant women traveled with the children, their travel and destination fares paid. (See Pregnant women used in scheme to transport children. *Agencia EFE S.A.* June 25, 2000.)<br>— A Thai boy got involved in a fight against sex trafficking because at age 2, he was brought into the US along with a man and a woman, the latter destined to be a sex slave somewhere in America. The boy was a human decoy, designed to make them look like a family on holiday. (See Rosin H. Thai boy caught up in fight against sex trafficking. *Washington Post.* May 15, 2000:A02) |

*(continued)*

**Table 5-8. Trafficking "Functionaries" Associated with the Commercial Sexual Exploitation of Children in the US, 2000**
*(continued)*

| CATEGORIES | OPERATIONAL DEFINITIONS | EXAMPLES FROM THE PUBLIC MEDIA OF TRAFFICKING "FUNCTIONARIES" IN THE US |
|---|---|---|
| **Enforcers** | Often themselves illegal migrants, enforcers are primarily responsible for policing staff and migrants and for maintaining order, often involving the use of violence. | — Unless they were accompanied by guards, the women owned by a gang that imported women as prostitutes, were not even allowed to run errands. (See Booth W. 13 charged in gang importing prostitutes. *Washington Post.* August 21, 1999:A03)<br>— To pay off her ticket and arrange for her visa, a woman trafficked from Thailand to the US was expected to have sex with more than 300 men. She was held captive behind the locked doors of a Chinatown brothel where she was known by a number rather than her name. Bars covered the window and buzzer-operated gates controlled the doors. (See Goldberg C. Sex slavery, Thailand to New York. *New York Times.* September 11, 1995:B1, B2.) |
| **Supporting Personnel and Specialists** | These persons consist mostly of local people in transit points who provide accommodation and other assistance to illegal migrants. Traffickers also depend on skilled individuals who provide specialized products and services to the criminal organization. These individuals are usually paid for casual duties only and do not share a continuing commitment to the group. Children interviewed provided a long list of types of support personnel they encountered in the course of being trafficked including taxi drivers; operators of "safe houses," including family homes; persons who prepared false or stolen documents; "coyotes" who crossed into the US with the children at strategic border points; persons who provided children with housing and, sometimes, jobs as domestics or in restaurants or bars; and persons who introduced the children to their buyers persons who bought the children or owned their contract | *See the following stories, illustrative of the depth, complexity, and violence associated with these drug and human trafficking networks:*<br>— Thompson CW. 7,898 from 39 nations held in anti-smuggling raids. *Washington Post.* June 28, 2001:A02<br>— Alvord V. Drug bloodshed threatens to flow over border. *USA Today.* March 15, 2000:29A ff.<br>— McCarthy T. Coming to America: the long, harsh odyssey of a Chinese illegal smuggled from Fujian province to New Jersey. *Time.* May 1, 2000.<br>— Shannon E, Padgett T. Valley of death: how arrogance and violence breed a massive drug-war slaughter. *Time.* December 13, 1999. |
| **Debt Collectors** | Persons based in the destination country who are responsible for collecting the trafficking fees. | — Thirteen people were charged when a Chinese gang, the Snakeheads, forced women to repay trafficking "contracts" worth $30 000 to $40 000 each by working as prostitutes. Some brothels in which these women worked grossed an average of $1.5 million over a 2.5-year period. (See Booth W. 13 charged in gang importing prostitutes. Washington Post. August 21, 1999:A03) |
| **Money Movers** | Persons who are experts at laundering the proceeds of crime, disguising their origin through a string of transactions or investing them in legitimate businesses. | |

# CONCLUSION

The findings summarized in this chapter offer a sobering picture of the nature, extent, and seriousness of the commercial sexual exploitation of children in contemporary America. When considered together with the high, even if currently declining, rates of child sexual abuse and child sexual assault, the CSEC affects substantial numbers of American children and families. In addition to large numbers of child victims, the CSEC also involves large numbers of adults, including pedophiles; "transient" and/or sexually unattached males; married men with families and children of their own; "opportunistic" exploiters; pimps; traffickers; and other juveniles. Several of these groups have not been associated with the CSEC in other studies. International traffickers in children for commercial sexual purposes also play a major role in the CSEC, as do local and national sex crime rings.

Until now, the CSEC has been the most neglected in the field of child abuse in the United States. Based on the findings presented in this chapter, as well as the recommendations for action summarized in the volume's last chapter, nothing short of a comprehensive approach to combating the CSEC will succeed in ending this horrific form of child abuse.

# REFERENCES

Adams M. *Hustlers, Escorts and Porn Stars: An Insiders Guide to Male Prostitution in America.* Las Vegas, Nev: Insiders Guide; 1999.

Allen DM. Young male prostitutes: a psychosocial study. *Arch Sex Behav.* 1980;9: 399-426.

Arey D. Gay males and sexual abuse. In: Fontes LA, ed. *Sexual Abuse in Nine North American Cultures: Treatment and Prevention.* Thousand Oaks, Calif: Sage Publications; 1995:200-235.

Azaola E. *Stolen Childhood. Girl and Boy Victims of Sexual Exploitation in Mexico.* Mexico City, Mexico: UNICEF; 2001.

Azaola E, Estes RJ, eds. *La Infancia Como Mercancia Sexual: México, Canada, Estados Unidos [The Commercial Sexual Exploitation of Children in México, Canada, and the United States].* Mexico City, Mexico: Siglo Veintiuno Editores; 2003.

Bales K. *Disposable People: New Slavery in the Global Economy.* Berkeley: University of California Press; 1999.

Barnitz LS. *Commercial Sexual Exploitation of Children: Youth Involved in Prostitution, Pornography, and Sex Trafficking.* Washington, DC: Youth Advocate Program International; 1998.

Baron SW. Risky lifestyles and the link between offending and victimization. *Stud Crime Crime Prev.* 1997;6:53-71.

Barr CW. *Child Sex Trade: Battling a Scourge.* Boston, Mass: Christian Science Publishing; 1996.

Basu K. The economics of child labor. *Sci Am.* October 2003;289:84-91.

Beck AJ. *Survey of State Prison Inmates, 1991.* Washington, DC: US Dept of Justice, Office of Justice Programs, Bureau of Justice Statistics; 1993.

Bond LS, Mazin R, Jiminez MV. Street youth and AIDS. *AIDS Educ Prev.* Fall 1992 (suppl):14-23.

Boyer D. Male prostitution and homosexual identity. *J Homosex.* 1989;17:151-184.

Boyer D, Fine D. Sexual abuse as a factor in adolescent pregnancy and child maltreatment. *Fam Plann Perspect.* 1992;24:4-11,19.

Brannigan A, Van Brunschot EG. Youthful prostitution and child sexual trauma. *Int J Law Psychiatry.* 1997;20:337-354.

Briere J. The long-term clinical correlates of childhood sexual victimization. *Ann NY Acad Sci.* 1988;528:327-334.

Briere J, Runtz M. Symptomatology associated with childhood sexual victimization in a non-clinical adult sample. *Child Abuse Negl.* 1988;12:51-59.

Browne A, Finkelhor D. Impact of sexual abuse: a review of the research. *Psychol Bull.* 1986;99:66-77.

Budapest Group. *The Relationship Between Organized Crime and Trafficking in Aliens.* Austria: International Centre for Migration Policy Development; 1999.

Calcetas-Santos O. *Report of the Special Rapporteur on the Sale of Children, Child Prostitution and Child Pornography.* Sales No E/CN.4/1999/71. New York, NY: United Nations; 1999.

Calcetas-Santos O. *Report of the Special Rapporteur on the Sale of Children, Child Prostitution and Child Pornography on the Issue of Commercial Sexual Exploitation of Children to Mexico.* Sales No E/CN.4/1998/101/Add.2. New York, NY: United Nations; 1998.

Caldwell G, Galster S, Steinsor N. *Crime & Servitude: An Exposé of the Traffic in Women for Prostitution From the Newly Independent States.* Moscow, Russia: Global Survival Network; 1997.

Cates JA. Adolescent male prostitution by choice. *Child Adolesc Social Work J.* 1989; 6:151-156.

Cates JA, Markley J. Demographic, clinical, and personality variables associated with male prostitution by choice. *Adolescence.* 1992;27:695-706.

Cauce AM, Paradise M, Ginzler JA, et al. The characteristics and mental health of homeless adolescents: age and gender differences. *J Emotional Behav Disord.* 2000;8: 230-239.

Cauce AM, Stewart A, Rodriguez MD, Cochran B, Ginzler J. Overcoming the odds? Adolescent development in the context of urban poverty. In: Luthar SS, ed. *Resilience and Vulnerability: Adaptation in the Context of Childhood Adversities.* New York & London: Cambridge University Press; 2003.

Clements-Nolle K, Marx R, Guzman R, Katz M. HIV prevalence, risk behaviors, health care use, and mental health status of transgender persons: implications for public health intervention. *Am J Public Health.* 2001;91:915-921.

Cockburn A. 21st century slaves. *Natl Geogr Mag.* September 2003;204:2-20.

Cochran BN, et al. Challenges faced by homeless sexual minorities: comparison of gay, lesbian, bisexual, and transgender homeless adolescents with their heterosexual counterparts. *Am J Public Health.* 2002;92:773-777.

Cusick L. Youth prostitution: a literature review. *Child Abuse Rev.* 2002;11:230-251.

Dalla RL, Xia Y, Kennedy H. "You just give them what they want and pray they don't kill you." *Violence Against Women.* 2003;9:1367-1394.

Davidson JO. The sex exploiter. Paper presented at: World Congress Against Commercial Sexual Exploitation of Children; August 28, 1996; Stockholm, Sweden.

De Albuquerque K. Sex, beach boys, and female tourists in the Caribbean. In: Dank B, Refinetti R, eds. *Sex Work and Sex Workers: Sexuality & Culture.* Vol. 1. New Brunswick, NJ: Transaction Publishers; 1999.

Diamond LM. Sexual identity, attractions, and behavior among young sexual-minority women over a 2-year period. *Dev Psychol.* 2000;36:241-250.

DuRant RH, Krowchuk DP, Sinal SH, et al. Victimization, use of violence, and drug use at school among male adolescents who engage in same sex sexual behavior. *J Pediatr.* 1998;133:113-118.

ECPAT International. *Five Years After Stockholm: 2000-2001.* Bangkok, Thailand: ECPAT International; 2001.

Ennew J, Gopal K, Heeran J, Montgomery H. *Children and Prostitution: How Can We Measure and Monitor the Commercial Sexual Exploitation of Children? Literature Review and Annotated Bibliography.* New York, NY: UNICEF; 1996.

Estes RJ. *At the Crossroads: Development Dilemmas of the New Century.* Dordrecht, Netherlands: Kluwer Academic Publishers. In press.

Estes RJ. The silent emergency: the commercial sexual exploitation of children in the US, Canada and Mexico. In: Walker NE, ed. *Prostituted Teens: More Than A Runaway Problem.* Briefing Report No. 2002-2. Lansing: Michigan State University, Institute for Children, Youth and Families; 2002:15-22.

Estes RJ. Social development trends in Africa: the need for a new development paradigm. *Soc Dev Issues.* 1995;17:18-47.

Estes RJ. Social development trends in Asia, 1970-1994: the challenges of a new century. *Soc Indic Res.* 1996a;37:119-148.

Estes RJ. Social development trends in Latin America, 1970-1994: in the shadows of the 21st century. *Soc Dev Issues.* 1996b;18:25-52.

Estes RJ. Social development trends in the successor states to the former Soviet Union: the search for a new paradigm. In: Kempe RH, ed. *Challenges of Transformation and Transition From Centrally Planned to Market Economies.* UNCRD Research Report Series No. 26. Nagoya, Japan: United Nations Centre for Regional Development. 1998a: 13-30.

Estes RJ. Trends in world social development, 1970-1995: development prospects for a new century. *J Dev Soc.* 1998b;14:11-39.

Estes RJ, Weiner NA. *The commercial sexual exploitation of children in the US, Canada and Mexico.* September 2001. Available at: http://caster.ssw.upenn.edu/~restes/CSEC.htm. Accessed August 17, 2004.

Estes RJ, Weiner NA. La explotación sexual comercial de niños en Estados Unidos. In: Azaola E, Estes RJ, eds. *La Infancia Como Mercancia Sexual: México, Canada, Estados Unidos [The Commercial Sexual Exploitation of Children in Mexico, Canada and the United States].* Mexico City, Mexico: Siglo Veintiuno Editores; 2003:44-90.

Farley M. Prostitution in five countries: violence and post-traumatic stress disorder. *Fem Psychol.* 1998;8:405-426.

Farley M, Kelly V. Prostitution: a critical review of the medical and social science literature. *Women Crim Justice.* 2000;11:29-64.

Farrow JA, Deisher RW, Brown R, Kulig JW, Kipke MD. Health and health needs of homeless and runaway youth: a position paper of the Society for Adolescent Medicine. *J Adolesc Med.* 1992;13:717-726.

Faugier J, Sargent M. Boyfriends, "pimps," and clients. In: Scambler G, Scambler A, eds. *Rethinking Prostitution: Purchasing Sex in the 1990s.* London, England: Routledge; 1997.

Ferrara FF. *Childhood Sexual Abuse: Development Effects Across the Life Span.* Pacific Grove, Calif: Brooks/Cole; 2001.

Finkelhor D, Dziuba-Leatherman J. Children as victims of violence: a national survey. *Pediatrics.* 1994;94:413-420.

Finkelhor D, Hotaling G, Sedlak A. *Missing, Abducted, Runaway, and Thrownaway Children in America (NISMART)—First Report: Numbers and Characteristics, National Incidence Studies.* Washington, DC: US Dept of Justice, Office of Juvenile Justice and Delinquency Prevention; 1990.

Finkelhor D, Mitchell KJ, Wolak J. *On-line Victimization: A Report on the Nation's Youth.* Alexandria, VA: National Center for Missing & Exploited Children; 2000.

Finn P. *Sex Offender Community Notification.* Washington, DC: US Dept of Justice, Office of Justice Programs, National Institute of Justice; 1997.

Flowers RB. *Victimization and Exploitation of Women and Children: A Study of Physical, Mental and Sexual Maltreatment in the US.* Jefferson, NC: McFarland & Co; 1994.

Franey K, Geffner R, Falconer R, eds. *The Cost of Child Maltreatment: Who Pays? We All Do.* San Diego, Calif: Family Violence & Sexual Assault Institute; 2001.

Freeman-Longo RE. *Nationwide Survey of Juvenile and Adult Sex Offender Treatment Programs and Models.* Orwell, Vt: The Safer Society; 1994.

Gelles RJ. *The Book of David: How Preserving Families Can Cost Children's Lives.* New York, NY: Basic Books; 1996.

Gelles RJ. *Intimate Violence in Families.* 3rd ed. Newbury Park, Calif: Sage Publications; 1997.

Gelles RJ, Wolfner GD. Sexual offending and victimization: a life course perspective. In: Rossi AS, ed. *Sexuality Across the Life Course.* Chicago, Ill: The University of Chicago Press; 1994.

Goldman R, Wheeler V. *Silent Shame: The Sexual Abuse of Children and Youth.* Danville, Ill: The Interstate; 1986.

Goldstein SL. *The Sexual Exploitation of Children: A Practical Guide to Assessment, Investigation, and Intervention.* 2nd ed. Boca Raton, Fla: CRC Press; 1999.

Graycar A. Trafficking in human beings. Paper presented at: International Conference on Migration, Culture, and Crime; July 7, 1999; Israel.

Greene JM, Ennett ST, Ringwalt CL. Prevalence and correlates of survival sex among runaway and homeless youth. *Am J Public Health.* 1999;89:1406-1409.

Hammer H, Finkelhor D, Sedlak AJ. *Runaway/Thrownaway Children: National Estimates and Characteristics.* Washington, DC: US Dept of Justice, Office of Justice Programs, Office of Juvenile Justice and Delinquency Prevention; October 2002. NCJ 196469.

Hazlehurst K, Hazlehurst C, eds. *Gangs and Youth Subcultures: International Explorations.* New Brunswick, NJ: Transaction Publishers; 1998.

Held D, McGrew A, eds. *The Global Transformations Reader.* Cambridge, UK: Polity Press; 2000.

Hofstede A. The Hofstede Committee report: juvenile prostitution in Minnesota. 1999. Available at: http://www.ag.state.mn.us/consumer/PDF/hofstede.pdf. Accessed September 16, 2004.

Hood-Brown M. Trading for a place: poor women and prostitution. *J Poverty.* 1998; 2:13-33.

Hughes D. *Pimps and Predators on the Internet: Globalizing the Sexual Exploitation of Women and Children.* Kingston, RI: Coalition Against Trafficking in Women; 1999.

Hughes D, Roche C, eds. *Making the Harm Visible: Global Sexual Exploitation of Women and Girls.* Kingston, RI: Coalition Against Trafficking in Women; 1999.

Hughes DM. The "Natasha" trade: the transnational shadow market of trafficking in women. *J Int Aff.* 2000;53:625-652.

International Tribunal for Children's Rights (ITCR). *International Dimensions of the Sexual Exploitation of Children.* Montreal, Canada: International Bureau for Children's Rights; 2000.

International Criminal Police Organization (Interpol). *International Crime Statistics, 2003.* St. Cloud, France: Interpol; 2003.

Institute of Psychological and Educational Research. *Child Exploitation and Abuse: A Global Phenomenon: A Report of the First Asian Conference on Child Sexual Exploitation and Abuse.* Calcutta: Sree Saraswaty Press; 1990.

Ireland T, Widom CS. Childhood victimization and risk for alcohol and drug arrests. *Int J Addict.* 1994;2:235-274.

Ives N. *Final Report From the North American Regional Consultation on the Commercial Sexual Exploitation of Children.* Philadelphia: University of Pennsylvania School of Social Work; 2001.

Jaffe M, Rosen S, eds. *Forced Labor: The Prostitution of Children.* Upland, Pa: Diane Publishing Co; 1996.

Jones L, Finkelhor D. The decline in child sexual abuse cases. *OJJDP Bulletin.* Washington, DC: US Dept of Justice, Office of Justice Programs, Office of Juvenile Justice and Delinquency Prevention; January 2001:1-12. NCJ 184741.

Kaufman JG, Widom CS. Childhood victimization, running away, and delinquency. *J Res Crime Delinq.* 1999;36:347-370.

Kelley B, Thornberry T, Smith C. In the wake of child maltreatment. Washington, DC: US Dept of Justice, Office of Justice Programs, Office of Juvenile Justice and Delinquency Prevention; August 1997:1-16.

Klain EJ. *Prostitution of Children and Child-Sex Tourism: An Analysis of Domestic and International Responses.* Arlington, Va: National Center for Missing and Exploited Children; 1999.

Kral A, Molnar BE, Booth RE, Watters JK. Prevalence of sexual risk behavior and substance use among runaway and homeless adolescents in San Francisco, Denver and New York City. *Int J STD AIDS.* 1997;8:109-117.

Kruks G. Gay and lesbian homeless/street youth: special issues and concerns. *J Adolesc Health.* 1991;12:515-518.

Landesman P. Sex Slaves on main street: the girls next door. *New York Times Magazine.* January 25, 2004; section 6:30-39, 66-67,72,75.

Lanning KV. *Child Molesters: A Behavioral Analysis for Law Enforcement Officers Investigating Cases of Child Sexual Exploitation.* 3rd ed. Arlington, Va: National Center for Missing and Exploited Children; 1992.

Lederer L. *Human Rights Report on Trafficking of Women and Children.* Baltimore, Md: Johns Hopkins University, The Paul H. Nitze School of Advanced International Studies; 2001.

Lie J. Globalization and its discontents. *Contemp Sociol.* 1996;25:585-587.

Lock J, Steiner H. Gay, lesbian, and bisexual youth risks for emotional, physical, and social problems: results from a community-based survey. *J Am Acad Child Adolesc Psychiatry.* 1999;38:297-304.

Loeber R, Farrington D, eds. *Serious and Violent Juvenile Offenders: Risk Factors and Successful Interventions.* Thousand Oaks CA: Sage Publications; 1998.

Longford M. Family poverty and the exploitation of child labor. *Law Policy.* 1995;17: 471-482.

Lucas BM, Hackett L. *Street Youth: On Their Own in Indianapolis.* Indianapolis, Ind: Health Foundation of Greater Indianapolis; 1995.

MacLean MG, Paradise MJ, Cauce AM. Substance use and psychological adjustment in homeless adolescents: a test of three models. *Am J Community Psychol.* 1999;27: 405-427.

MacWilliams B. Forced into prostitution. *Chron High Educ.* October 2003:A34-A36.

McCarthy B, Hagan J. Surviving on the street: the experiences of homeless youth. *J Adolesc Res.* 1992;7:412-430.

Molnar BE, Buka SL, Kessler RC. Child sexual abuse and subsequent psychopathology: results from the National Comorbidity Survey. *Am J Public Health.* 2001;91: 753-760.

Molnar BE, Shade SB, Kral AH, Booth RE, Watters JK. Suicidal behavior and sexual/physical abuse among street youth. *Child Abuse Negl.* 1998;22:213-222.

Moon K. *Sex Among Allies: Military Prostitution in US-Korean Relations.* New York, NY: Columbia University Press; 1997.

Moore J, Hagedorn J. *Female Gangs: A Focus on Research.* Washington, DC: US Dept of Justice, Office of Justice Programs, Office of Juvenile Justice and Delinquency Prevention; March 2001: 1-12. NCJ 185234.

Muecke MA. Mother sold food, daughter sells her body: the cultural continuity of prostitution. *Soc Sci Med.* 1992;35:891-901.

Munir AB, Yasin S. Commercial sexual exploitation (of children). *Child Abuse Rev.* 1997;6:147-153.

Myers JEB, Berliner L, Briere J, Hendrix CT, Jenny C, Reid TA, eds. *The APSAC Handbook on Child Maltreatment.* 2nd ed. Thousand Oaks, Calif: Sage Publications; 2002.

Nadon SM, Koverola C, Schludermann EH. Antecedents to prostitution: childhood victimization. *J Interpers Violence.* 1998;13:206-221.

National Center on Child Abuse and Neglect. *Child Maltreatment, 2001.* Washington, DC: Administration for Children and Families of the US Dept of Health and Human Services; 2003.

National Coalition for the Homeless (NCH). *Homeless Families With Children, NCH Fact Sheet #7.* Washington, DC: NCH; 2001.

National Coalition for the Homeless (NCH). *Homeless Youth, NCH Fact Sheet #11.* Washington, DC: NCH; 1999.

Nemoto T, Luke D, Mamo L, Ching A, Patria J. HIV risk behaviors among male-to-female transgenders in comparison with homosexual or bisexual males and heterosexual females. *AIDS Care.* 1999;11:297-312.

Nixon K, Tutty L, Downe P, Gorkoff K, Ursel J. The everyday occurrence: violence in the lives of girls exploited through prostitution. *Violence Against Women.* 2002;8: 1016-1043.

O'Brien M. Taking sibling incest seriously. In: Patton MQ, ed. *Family Sexual Abuse: Frontline Research and Evaluation.* Newbury Park, Calif: Sage Publications; 1991.

Paradise M, Cauce AM, Ginzler J, Wert S, Wruck K, Brooker M. The role of relationships in developmental trajectories of homeless and runaway youth. In: Sarason BR, Duck S, eds. *Personal Relationships: Implications For Clinical and Community Psychology.* New York, NY: John Wiley & Sons; 2001: 159-179.

Pettman JJ. Body politics: international sex tourism. *Third World Q.* 1997;18:93-108.

Powers JL, Jaklitsch BW. *Understanding Survivors of Abuse: Stories of Homeless and Runaway Adolescents.* Lexington, Mass: Lexington Books; 1989.

Prentky RA, Knight RA, Lee AF. *Child Sexual Molestation: Research Issues.* Washington, DC: National Institute of Justice; 1997.

Radcliffe L, MacGregor K. Preying on children: the number of kids trafficked into virtual slavery in Europe is on the rise. *Newsweek.* November 17, 2003:26-27.

Richard AO. *International Trafficking in Women to the US: A Contemporary Manifestation of Slavery and Organized Crime.* Washington, DC: US State Dept Bureau of Intelligence and Research; 1999.

Righthand S, Welch C. *Juveniles Who Have Sexually Offended: A Review of the Professional Literature.* Washington, DC: US Dept of Justice, Office of Juvenile Justice and Delinquency Prevention; 2001.

Rigi J. The conditions of post-Soviet dispossessed youth and work in Almaty, Kazakhstan. *Crit Anthropol.* 2003:23:35-49.

Rotheram-Borus MJ. Suicidal behavior and risk factors among runaway youth. *Am J Psychiatry.* 1993;150:103-107.

Rotheram-Borus MJ, Mahler KA, Koopman C, Langabeer K. Sexual abuse history and associated multiple risk behavior in adolescent runaways. *Am J Orthopsychiatry.* 1996;66:390-400.

Ryan KD, Kilmer RP, Cauce AM, Watanabe H, Hoyt DR. Psychological consequences of child maltreatment in homeless adolescents: untangling the unique effects of maltreatment and family environment. *Child Abuse Negl.* 2004;24:333-352.

Scarpa A. Community violence exposure in young adults. *Trauma Violence Abuse.* 2003;4:210-217.

Schloenhardt A. The business of migration: organized crime and illegal migration in Australia and the Asia-Pacific region. Paper presented at: University of Adelaide Law School; May, 1999; Adelaide, Australia.

Seabrook J. *North-South Relations: The Sex Industry.* Penang, Malaysia:Third World Network Features; 1997.

Sedlak AJ, Finkelhor D, Hammer H, Schultz DJ. National estimates of missing children: an overview. *OJJDP NISMART Bulletin Series.* Washington, DC: US Dept of Justice, Office of Justice Programs, Office of Juvenile Justice and Delinquency Prevention; October, 2002. NCJ 196465.

Seng MJ. Child sexual abuse and adolescent prostitution: a comparative analysis. *Adolescence.* 1989;24:665-675.

Seto MC, Barbaree HE. Psychopathology, treatment behavior, and sex offender recidivism. *J Interpers Violence.* 1999;14:1235-1248.

Shafer J. Doubting Landesman: I'm not the only one questioning the *Times Magazine's* sex-slave story. *Slate.* January 27, 2004. Available at: http://slate.msn.com/id/2094502. Accessed August 17, 2004:5.

Shelley L. *Trafficking in Women and Children: Trafficking and Organized Crime.* Paper presented to: staff of the Protection Project; October 4, 2000; Washington DC.

Silbert MH, Pines AM. Early sexual exploitation as an influence in prostitution. *Soc Work.* 1983;8:285-289.

Simmons MJ. *Hookers, Hustlers, and Round-Trip Vacationers: The Gender Dynamics of Sex and Romance Tourism.* Paper presented at: Society for the Study of Social Problems; August 1996; New York, NY.

Simons RL. Life on the streets: the victimization of runaway and homeless adolescents. *Youth Soc.* 1990;22:108-125.

Simons RL, Whitbeck LB. Sexual abuse as a precursor to prostitution and victimization among adolescent and adult homeless women. *J Fam Issues.* 1991;12:361-379.

Snyder HN. *Sexual Assault of Young Children as Reported to Law Enforcement: Victim, Incident, and Offender Characteristics—A Statistical Report Using Data from the National Incident-Based Reporting System.* Washington, DC: US Dept of Justice, Office of Justice Programs; 2000.

Spangenberg M. *Prostituted Youth in New York City: An Overview.* New York, NY: ECPAT-USA; March 2001.

Sterry D. *Chicken: Self Portrait of a Young Man For Rent.* New York, NY: Regan Books; 2002.

Stewart AJ, Steiman M, Cauce AM, Cochran BN, Whitbeck LB, Hoyt DR. Victimization and post-traumatic stress disorder among homeless adolescents. *Child Adolesc Soc Work J.* 2004;21:325-331.

Stiffman AR. Physical and sexual abuse in runaway youths. *Child Abuse Negl.* 1989; 13:417-426.

Sturdevant SP, Stoltfuz B. *Let the Good Times Roll: Prostitution and the US Military in Asia.* New York, NY: The New Press; 1992.

Tremblay P. Interacciones sociales entre pedofilos Canadienses. In: Azaola E, Estes RJ eds. *La Infancia Como Mercancia Sexual: México, Canada, Estados Unidos [The Commercial Sexual Exploitation of Children in Mexico, Canada, and the United States].* Mexico City, Mexico: Siglo Veintiuno Editores; 2003:91-139.

Tyler KA, Cauce AM. Perpetrators of early physical and sexual abuse among homeless and runaway adolescents. *Child Abuse Negl.* 2002;26:1261-1274.

Tyler KA, Hoyt DR, Whitbeck LB. The effects of a high-risk environment on the sexual victimization of homeless and runaway youth. *Violence Vict.* 2001a;16:441-455.

Tyler KA, Hoyt DR, Whitbeck LB. The effects of early sexual abuse on later sexual victimization among female homeless and runaway youth. *J Interpers Violence.* 2000; 15:235-250.

Tyler KA, Hoyt DR, Whitbeck LB, Cauce AM. The impact of childhood sexual abuse on later sexual victimization among runaway youth. *J Res Adolesc.* 2001b;11:151-176.

United Nations. *World Situation With Regard to International Traffic in Minors.* Costa Rica: UN Latin American Institute for the Prevention of Crime and the Treatment of Offenders; 1995.

United Nations. *Global Programme Against Trafficking in Human Beings: An Outline for Action.* Vienna, Austria: United Nations; 1999.

United Nations Children's Fund. *The State of the World's Children, 2003.* New York, NY: Oxford University Press; 2003.

United Nations Commission on Human Rights (UNCHR). *Rights of the Child: Sale of Children, Child Prostitution, and Child Pornography.* New York, NY: UN General Assembly, January 14, 1994. Document E/CN.4/1994/84.

United Nations Development Programme (UNDP). *Human Development Report, 2003: Millennium Development Goals—A Compact Among Nations to End Poverty.* New York, NY: Oxford University Press; 2003.

US Conference of Mayors. *Hunger and Homelessness Report, 2003: A 25-City Survey.* Washington, DC: US Conference of Mayors; 2003.

US Department of Health and Human Services (USDHHS). Perpetrators of child maltreatment, 1997-2001. Washington DC: USDHHS, Administration for Children & Families; 2003a. Available at: http://www.acf.hhs.gov/programs/cb/publications/cm01/chapterfour.htm. Accessed March 15, 2004.

US Department of Health and Human Services (USDHHS). Victims of child maltreatment, 1997-2001. Washington, DC: USDHHS, Administration for Children & Families; 2003b. Available at: http://www.acf.hhs.gov/programs/cb/publications/cm01/chapterthree.htm. Accessed March 15, 2004.

US Department of Justice (USDOJ). *Juvenile Offenders and Victims: 1999 National Report.* Washington, DC: US Dept of Justice, Office of Juvenile Justice and Delinquency Prevention; 2000.

US Department of Justice (USDOJ). *Juvenile Offenders and Victims: 2002 National Report.* Washington, DC: US Dept of Justice, Office of Juvenile Justice and Delinquency Prevention; 2003.

US Department of Labor (USDOL). *The Use of Child Labor in US Manufactured and Mined Imports.* Washington, DC: US Government Printing Office; 1994.

US Department of Labor (USDOL). *The Use of Child Labor in US Agricultural Imports and Forced and Bonded Child Labor.* Washington, DC: US Government Printing Office; 1995.

US Department of Labor (USDOL). *Forced labor: The Prostitution of Children.* Washington, DC: US Government Printing Office; 1996.

US Department of Labor (USDOL). *By the Sweat and Toil of Children (Volume VI): An Economic Consideration of Child Labor.* Washington, DC: US Government Printing Office; 2000.

US Department of State (USDOS). Trafficking in persons report. Washington, DC: US Dept of State; July 2003.

Whitbeck LB, Hoyt DR. *Nowhere to Grow: Homeless and Runaway Adolescents and Their Families.* New York, NY: Aldine de Gruyter; 1999.

Whitbeck LB, Hoyt DR, Ackerly KA. Abuse family backgrounds and later victimization among runaway and homeless adolescents. *J Res Adolesc.* 1997;7:375-392.

Whitbeck LB, Hoyt DR, Yoder KA. A risk-amplification model of victimization and depressive symptoms among runaway and homeless adolescents. *Am J Community Psychol.* 1999;27:273-296.

Whitbeck LB, Hoyt DR, Yoder K, Cauce A, Paradise M. Deviant behavior and victimization among homeless and runaway adolescents. *J Interpers Violence.* 2001; 16:1175-1204.

Whitbeck LB, Simons RL. Life on the streets: the victimization of runaway and homeless adolescents. *Youth Soc.* 1990;22:108-125.

Widom CS. *The Cycle of Violence.* Washington, DC: National Institute of Justice; 1992.

Widom CS. *The Cycle of Violence Revisited, Research Preview (of the NIJ).* Washington, DC: National Institute of Justice; 1996.

Widom CS, Kuhns JB. Childhood victimization and subsequent risk for promiscuity, prostitution, and teenage pregnancy: a prospective study. *Am J Public Health.* 1996; 86:1607-1612.

Williams P, ed. *Illegal Immigration and Commercial Sex: The New Slave Trade.* London, England: Frank Cass Publishers; 1999.

Woodiwiss M. Crime's global reach. In: Woodiwiss M, ed. *Global Crime Connections.* Toronto, Canada: University of Toronto Press; 1993.

World Bank. *World Development Report, 2003: Sustainable Development in a Dynamic World.* New York, NY: Oxford University Press; 2003.

World Health Organization (WHO). *Commercial Sexual Exploitation of Children: The Health and Psychological Dimensions.* Stockholm, Switzerland: CSEC World Congress; 1996.

Yates GL, MacKenzie RG, Pennbridge J, Swofford A. A risk profile comparison of homeless youth involved in prostitution and homeless youth not involved. J Adolesc Health. 1991;12:545-548.

Yoon Y. *International Sexual Slavery.* Washington, DC: CG Issue Overviews; 1997.

# Chapter 6

# WHAT IT IS LIKE TO BE "SERVED" IN THE "SYSTEM": A SURVIVOR'S PERSPECTIVE*

Aaron Kipnis, PhD

The editors of this book have asked me to write about my personal and professional experiences with the child welfare and juvenile justice "system." As a professor of psychology, author, and practicing psychologist today, I enjoy a rich life. But that was not always the case. From ages 4 to 23, I was largely a ward of the state.

Like the parents of many children at risk for abuse and neglect, mine were teenagers at my birth. They divorced when I was 3 years old. My mother, Dorothy, won custody. She only had a high school education and no job training. Unfortunately for my mother and I, she was a flaming alcoholic. Although my father regularly sent child support, she was not able to cope with the economic or emotional burdens of single motherhood. She put me into foster care the year following their divorce as the government drafted my father, Kip, and sent him off to the Korean War.

From ages 4 to 9, I lived in numerous foster homes. Being given over to the care of strangers so early in life caused me to feel I had little worth. I took the abandonment personally. The confusing disorientation of a life lived with strangers and the irrational childhood belief that "it must be my fault" set the stage for an angry young male identity to flourish in the years that followed. The majority of children who wind up in the system today experience some similar sense of early abandonment from one or both parents and often by society as well.

## FOSTER UNCARE

Coming mostly from young family systems that fail to thrive, more than half a million American children will be in government-run foster care homes this year. Although the foster care system was designed to provide temporary care for abused, abandoned, and neglected children, once committed, many, like myself, remain in state custody for years. In that girls are highly favored over boys for adoption, boys tend to remain in the system longer. One in 5 foster boys spends more than 5 years in foster care. Many are simply warehoused in understaffed environments until they are 18 (Courtney, 1998).

Foster care does not ensure the rescue of children from abuse. In one facility, when I was 9, I was forced to chop firewood all day and repeatedly slapped if I failed to work. I was stripped of my clothing and humiliated by a male staff member when I tried to run away. Even more severe abuse is widespread in many foster care arenas.

Los Angeles County has more than half of California's foster kids—about 73 000 (one in 70 children)—the highest rate in the nation. In 1997, a Los Angeles grand

---

* This chapter is mostly excerpted from Kipnis A. Angry Young Men: How Parents, Teachers, and Counselors can Help "Bad Boys" Become Good Men. San Francisco, Calif: Jossey-Bass Publishers; 1999. This material is used by permission of John Wiley & Sons, Inc.

jury looked into the foster care system and found that, in many foster homes, food was bad, clothing was in short supply, and children were physically abused by their caretakers. Inappropriate mixing of children of different ages also subjected younger children to sexual, emotional, and physical abuse by older ones. Many foster children, especially boys, were being given drugs several times a day to control their "depression and rage." Some were as young as 3 (Craig & Derek, 1997; Weber, 1998).

Further investigations found that *all* the small boys in some foster group homes were sedated. Many foster children were given behavior modification drugs inappropriate for their age, size, and mental condition; the doses of psychiatric drugs exceeded the upper end of recommended adult usage and were combined in dangerous mixtures of drugs, so-called cocktails (Pasco, 1998). Unexplained deaths were attributed to the abuse of these medications as well as drug-induced psychosis, abnormal heart activity, uncontrollable tremors, liver damage, learning disabilities, loss of bowel control, and other problems. Some mental health professionals defend the use of drugs to control children's behavior, saying they can be used safely if they are correctly monitored; however, such monitoring is rare in most foster care facilities. Also, most foster kids come into their next placement with little or no medical history accompanying them.

The abuses in the foster care system of Los Angeles are not unique. What is unusual is that child advocates had the courage and resolve to encourage the convening of a grand jury to investigate this underworld of the child welfare system. Many American cities appear to suffer worse abuses, but I included Los Angeles here because it is the largest in the nation and also the system in which I grew up. Many of these reports ring true to me from my own experience and those of my dozens of foster sisters and brothers along the way.

Most public foster care agencies are financially discouraged from seeking adoptive homes for their wards because government subsidies are based on the number of children in foster care per day. There is no financial incentive to move children into adoption, where care that is in their better interests and our society's can be provided. Foster care organizations, with staff and facilities to maintain, are instead financially rewarded for warehousing kids.

Consequently, abandoned and neglected children, as veritable commodities, are often cycled through a series of foster homes, group homes, and other institutions as they age. Every one of my foster homes was in a different community, with a different school and a new set of siblings and caretakers. Many of the children I have worked with have been in a dozen different foster homes, some more than that.

Abusive, neglectful, and abandoning parents dominate the early lives of most foster children. Such parents are followed by an ever-changing parade of strangers: child protection workers, welfare officials, lawyers, court investigators, judges, psychiatrists, police officers, surrogate parents, foster siblings, social workers, counselors, and teachers. Each new foster home has its own particular rules and regulations. It is confusing for foster children, who get tumbled around in these whirlwinds of inconsistency, to learn the behavioral guidelines in any given situation or how to please the new adults around them.

These children are innocent. They are victims of abuse, not criminals—yet. Every effort should be made to get all abandoned children into a normalized family setting. I remember taking walks in the evening and peering into windows, from the sidewalk, where families were sitting down for dinner. My palpable longing for a real home was extraordinary.

Unintentionally, the well-meaning public servants that administer our child welfare system lead thousands of boys to the iron gates of our criminal justice system instead of to the pleasures of productive lives. Most of these children go through a bewildering and demoralizing process of disorientation from which, in both my personal and professional experience, it is hard to recover. This sort of background is a virulent medium for the incubation of conduct-disordered and antisocial behavior. As adults, foster children are highly overrepresented among the unemployed, homeless, addicted, violent crime victims, and prisoners (Roman & Phyllis, 1995).

## HOME AGAIN

Periodically, my mother moved in with various men and made abortive attempts to bring me out of foster care into their households. I liked most of the guys. But the affairs never lasted long. There were hysterical departures in the middle of the night and subsequent returns to foster homes.

When I was 10, Dorothy married a "nice Jewish boy" from her hometown. He turned out to be an unstable person and inveterate gambler. I fainted at their wedding. It was as though I had some premonition that he would bring only suffering into my life. Dorothy got me out of foster care, however, and tried her best to provide a stable home. But by the time I was 11, I began to rebel. My new stepfather, "Zombie," as everyone called him, proved to be hostile and violent.

Mom was always a little uneven herself. When I was 2, I fell out of a laundry sink full of bath water, where she had left me alone, and cracked my skull on a steam radiator. It left 2 parallel scars that are still engraved on the back of my head. When I was 4, I mysteriously fell out of the back seat of her speeding car and tumbled down the middle of the freeway. When the police confronted her later, she told them she just did not notice I was gone until she arrived at her destination, miles away.

Dorothy often left me in the back seat of her car, which had a broken emergency brake. Once it rolled downhill into the middle of heavy traffic. Her boyfriend ran out and rescued me. Another time, I accidentally hit the gearshift, and the car rolled away into the side of a building. She often shared these stories with others as amusing anecdotes of my childhood. And I would laugh along with her as she retold the tragicomic stories that defined our relationship.

As a child, I loved my mother. She was vivacious, beautiful, and witty. However, she made me pretty nervous. Once, in a drunken rage, she swung my thick leather Davy Crockett belt, hitting me in the face with the heavy, solid, brass buckle end. The belt hook embedded just below my eye, which still droops a little to this day. After that, it was difficult for me to trust her judgment.

One night, Dorothy slapped me hard for some reason, long forgotten. I slipped out my bedroom window in the middle of the night and ran away. A nurse found me in the morning, sleeping in the doorway of a hospital. Mother's handprint was still vividly etched on my face. I was surprised that the obviously concerned hospital staff returned me to her care. I had a fantasy that they would take me away to a better place where little boys were safe. I was soon to learn that there were no such magical lands for boys at risk for abuse.

## ABUSED BOYS

In later years, as I counseled "incorrigible" boys in treatment centers, I came to believe that a primary inculcator of their "bad" behavior was their experience of neglect, physical violence, and emotional or sexual abuse in the home. Boys often express distress more physically than girls do. As some child therapists say, "boys act out, girls act in." Though some boys may act out because of neurological or mental illness, domestic abuse is a major factor that turns active, inquisitive, and sensitive boys into angry young men.

Abused children, or those who merely witness domestic abuse, are highly overrepresented among those suffering academic, emotional, and economic failure (Burton et al, 1994). Many experience early difficulty in school. They drink more, abuse more drugs, and suffer more juvenile arrests at earlier ages than nonabused boys (Cooley-Quille et al, 1995). Abused boys are 3 times as likely to become aggressive and violent, and, thus, are the majority of felons serving long prison sentences and men on death row (Gilligan, 1996; Smith & Thornberry, 1995).

Girls represent the majority of sexually abused children. However, the majority of children who are murdered, seriously injured, physically abused, or medically neglected are boys. Boys with special needs or disabilities, in particular, are overrepresented in all abuse categories, comprising two thirds of abused children with disabilities (Sobse et al, 1997). Protection of boys from domestic violence should be a priority of our social programs. But for the most part, in my clinical experience over the years, violence against males is rarely a leading concern.

One of the many factors accounting for this is that boys are far less likely than girls to tell anyone about abuse. A 1998 survey of 7000 children found that 48% of boys, as compared to 29% of girls, said they would never tell anyone if they were abused. Over 3 times as many girls as boys said they would, at the least, confide in a friend who might, in turn, tell a concerned adult (Louis Harris and Associates, 1998).

It is egodystonic—not in accord with their self-image and traditional gender identity—for boys to complain about pain. Until I was a middle-aged adult in therapy, I never told anyone, except my wife, about my own abuse. As a boy, it never occurred to me that abuse was not the normal experience of childhood. Tragically, in our culture, the problem of child abuse has worsened considerably since I was a boy.

To remedy this lacuna in psychological treatment theory and training, clinicians, educators, and other helping professionals may need education that better sensitizes them to the often silent suffering of boys. To speak of males as victims, however, rubs against the dominant cultural grain. To get needed male sensitivity training on the agenda of our mental health and educational institutions, our culture must confront its apathy toward the often hidden vulnerability and pain of angry young men.

Reports of child abuse in the United States have steadily risen over recent decades (Sedlak & Broadhurst, 1996). In the latter half of the 1990s, reports of child abuse and neglect doubled. Over a million children suffer moderate injuries each year, about 160 000 are severely injured, and over 1000 children die from parental abuse or neglect. At the end of the 20th century, reports of abuse and neglect exceeded 3 million, up fourfold in 2 decades. Physical abuse now affects 1 in 50 American children (US Dept of Health & Human Services [USDHHS], 1993).

Nearly 80% of perpetrators are parents; an additional 10% are other relatives. The average age of an abused child is 7. The average age of the abuser is 31; 58% of the time, the abuser or neglecter of a boy is female. As a precursor to future incarceration, neglect may be as damaging to boys as physical abuse (Smith & Thornberry, 1995). Therefore, in our analysis of the role of childhood trauma in the etiology of angry young male behavior, we can not dismiss neglect as a lesser evil.

Children who live with both biological parents have the lowest reported rates of maltreatment (Blankenhorn, 1995). Divorced fathers with custody show slightly higher rates, and children living with single mothers, particularly those with a nonbiological male in their home, suffer the highest abuse rates by far (Margolin, 1992). Why do single fathers show lower rates of abuse and neglect of boys than single mothers? The generally better economic welfare of single fathers may partially account for this, since child poverty is highly correlated with abuse (US Bureau of the Census, 1998). Children from families with annual incomes of less than $15 000 report maltreatment almost 7 times more frequently than children from higher income families. Single mothers with young children living below the poverty line, together with alcoholic and drug-addicted parents of both sexes, have the greatest statistical risk of abusing or neglecting boys (Horn, 1998). My own teenaged parents met all of the above criteria.

## PROTECTING BOYS

Even though I went to school on several occasions with black eyes from my stepfather's beatings, no one ever questioned me. I believe this was true because many adults still unconsciously uphold these toughen-up-the-boys codes, which are deeply embedded in our cultural psyche. This code is also reflected by the professional literature, which publishes significantly more research about abused females than abused males even though males represent the majority of victims of violence.

Advocates for women and girls have displayed great courage and commitment in bringing long-overlooked, critically important issues to our social and political discourse. I hope, thanks to those efforts, that it will not take our culture as long to become sensitized to boys' specific needs. We can model women's effective leadership by maintaining a warm, positive, fiercely protective, nurturing, male-responsive environment for boys wherever they are.

## RUNAWAY TO JAIL: FIRST OFFENSE

One night, in my 11th year, I ran away from my mother's home again, this time to escape my stepfather's violence. He said it was "all my fault" that he had so many problems with my mother. I thought I could simply fix things for them both by leaving. But that just made him angrier. With Zombie on my tail like a hound after a rabbit, I tore through the neighborhood and climbed over a 12-foot fence surrounding the Budweiser brewery. I hid in some bushes most of the night. Plant security guards discovered me the next morning, sleeping in a parked car. Though my face was obviously bruised, the police charged me with "incorrigibility" and took me to juvenile hall. Click.

On the morning after my first despairing night in juvenile hall, foreshadowing hundreds of nights to come in locked cells, a guard brought me out to the day room where about 100 boys sat on wooden benches in front of a black-and-white TV. The majority of the boys were Latino, with a number of African Americans, Caucasians, and few Asians. I later learned from the chaplain that I was the only Jewish boy there.

The "barber" shaved my head bald. A trustee issued me the uniform that every inmate wore, a white T-shirt and worn-out jeans. In exchange for a purloined cigarette or match, he would give out better quality clothing that fit. But I had no contraband, so he doled out misfit seconds from the bottom of the pile to me. Despite our differing backgrounds, our uniformly shorn appearance sent a message to me that we boys were all part of the same outlaw tribe. I was startled when I saw myself in the mirror for the first time. My new countenance was grimly reminiscent of the pictures of other European Jews interned during the previous decade's Holocaust.

One of the boys there was a 13-year-old named Peter. He was overweight, had blotchy skin, and wore thick glasses. I thought he was rather funny looking. But after a few weeks we became friendly. Peter was originally from Louisiana and spoke with a curious lilt. His family moved to California, which, in those days, still had a number of small farms. After a neighbor caught him having sex with a ewe inside his barn, he was arrested for sodomy.

Peter was an expert "hambone" player who would entertain us with rapid rhythmic slaps against his thighs and chest. But this unusual behavior, plus his odd appearance, speech, and the nature of his crime, made him subject to ridicule in this hard-edged, urban juvenile detention center. Jails are extremely conservative places. Their behavioral protocols tend to be rigid and narrow. Like the Jewish "Kapos" who turned against their own in concentration camps, those who have suffered society's intolerance can become equally hostile toward others' deviations from the norm.

Other boys taunted and hit Peter. One night, after I had been there for a while, a gang of older boys raped him in the shower. The rest of us continued showering, acting as if nothing unusual was happening. None of us wanted to be known as the one who attracted the guards' attention and, thus, risk suffering a similar fate at the hands of the same gang.

There was a toilet at one end of the day room in full view of the guards and everyone else in the room. The extreme lack of privacy made defecating difficult for me. But eventually, if you have to go, you have to go. The next day, I noticed Peter had been sitting on the toilet in the day room for a long time. He looked pale, which was understandable considering what he had been through the night before. Suddenly, he pitched over and landed hard on the floor with a sickening thud. Blood streamed down his legs and began pooling on the floor.

Apparently, while sitting there in plain view, Peter reached beneath his groin and sliced his testicles with a razor blade. He then just sat there on the toilet, bleeding in front of the guards and all us boys. Many of the boys thought it was hysterically funny. I was horrified. Unconscious, he was taken to the hospital. The next day the authorities released me, on probation, to my mother's home. I never did find out if he lived or died from his suicide attempt. But the immutable fact that juvenile hall was an extremely dangerous and degrading place for children became indelibly stamped on my soul.

The punitive atmosphere of juvenile hall had its desired deterrent effect on me. I was highly motivated to avoid future incarcerations. Despite my loathing of jail, however, I was to spend several years of my coming adolescence behind bars and my entire youth and young adulthood as a ward of the state under the critical eye of probation and parole officials. Deterrence simply does not work for most angry young men. But, as discussed later in this chapter, many sorts of interventions do help abused boys to recover.

## TODAY, MY SON, YOU ARE A MAN

After my return from spending several months in "Juvi," my mother never hit me again. But more severe beatings from Zombie replaced her sporadic outbursts. For a time, I suffered his abuse as the price of my freedom. But one day, I reached my limit.

Early one Saturday morning, Zombie attacked me for failing to get out of bed to mow the lawn. He came into my room yelling at me. When I sleepily told him to "bug off," he jumped on the bed and began slugging me in the face. My experiences in juvenile hall, however, had toughened me up. I had also learned how to stick up for myself in the street fights that often occurred in our working-class neighborhood. I learned that even the older boys, who went after my lunch money as I cut through alleyways on the 3-mile walk to school, would leave me alone when I started fighting back. For the first time, I was undaunted by his rage.

That morning, yanked straight from sleep into a violent assault, I suddenly reached a boiling point. Having grown stronger and more confident about my fighting ability, I hit back, swift and hard. Zombie was stunned. He instantly became frenzied. His face turned red. He began bellowing and punching me in earnest. I weighed about 100 pounds and he weighed over 200, so clearly I had no chance of winning the fight. But I did not care. I felt he had to learn that, from now on, there would be a price to pay for hitting me.

A running battle ensued. We tumbled out of the bedroom into the living room where my mother tried to break it up, screaming and swinging a hammer at us. To this day, I do not know whether she was aiming the hammer at her husband or me. I was not so sure at the time either, so I broke free and ran out the door with Zombie in hot pursuit.

I ran into the garage. Like many boys, I kept a variety of special things in a secret hollow among the storage boxes: a raven's wing, my marble collection, fishing lures, some firecrackers, pages from a *Playboy*, and a hunting knife my father gave me. Zombie chased me around the pool table (a prize Dorothy won on a game show) screaming, "I'm going to kill you, you little punk!" When he picked up a pool cue and swung it at me, I believed he meant it. I plunged into my secret space and grabbed the knife. Brandishing it, I cried, "Go ahead, take your best shot, Zombie. But if you miss I'm going to stick this knife in your fat belly." Standing there with blood streaming down my face, I was suddenly perfectly calm.

I had no shred of doubt in my mind that I was ready and able to kill him. He must have seen it in my eyes somehow. A resolute look can communicate a great deal, man to man. He put the pool cue down and backed away. It was the one and only time in my life that I was completely prepared and resolved to kill another human being—coldly.

The experience of repeated abuse alone can drive boys into sociopathic behavior. Had I killed Zombie, however, my life would have been destroyed as well. I would have spent the rest of my youth incarcerated. Few survive that experience with their souls intact.

I was lucky that he backed off. Having caused a grown man to back down from a violent attack, I felt a new sense of power. I had proved my "manhood" to my stepfather. To assault me now he knew that he would risk the same consequences he could incur for hitting another adult male—a man.

# DON'T MESS WITH ME!

For many bad boys, violence toward an abusive "caretaking" adult paves their road toward long-term incarceration. Sadly, by the time they commit a violent crime, little is available to most boys but more abuse from the criminal justice system. One study indicates that over 60% of all murders by teenaged boys are against adult men or family members who were abusing them (Dawson & Langan, 1994). In a cycle of violence that affects generations, boys who were abused by their mothers as children are more likely to abuse their spouses as adults. Women abused by their spouses are, in turn, more at risk for abusing their boys, thus completing a grotesque circuit of family violence.

Even though crime rates dropped from the mid-1990s to 2001, violence toward children remained at epidemic levels in America. Over the last decade, our adolescent male homicide rate averaged 50 times that of Japan's and 12 times that of most other industrialized societies (Centers for Disease Control and Prevention, 1997; Krug et al, 1998; World Health Organization, 1995). Boys who present a hard-edged, violent posture to the world around them are not necessarily looking for trouble. Many angry young men develop a menacing demeanor as an unconscious defense designed to keep the violence in their world at bay. Often, it is merely a sociopathic facade covering an inner experience of pro-found anxiety.

The rest of the short time I lived in my mother's home, I marked my boundaries through hostile looks, through a "ready-for-action" walk/posture, and by remaining continually armed. Dorothy took the hunting knife away one day when I was out of my room, so I stole her butcher knife from the kitchen and hid it inside my box spring mattress. Every night I took it out, put it under my pillow, and slept with my fingers wrapped around the handle. For weeks, she complained about the loss of her favorite knife.

During the day, I kept a switchblade hidden in the lining of my jacket. I had bought the knife from a Mexican boy at school. Zombie knew I was armed with a knife; moreover, that I was resolved to use it. He never hit me again. The resolution I made—never again to suffer abuse by others, regardless of the cost—helped keep me alive during the incarcerations I faced in the years ahead. Now, as an adult, I find myself equally resolved to help protect other children from abuse.

## DISCIPLINING BOYS OR BREAKING THEIR SPIRITS?

There were a number of reasons I failed in the 2 dozen or so schools I attended prior to dropping out. Like many boys, I was restless in the classroom. I was bored and distracted. I interrupted the teacher and acted out, goofing around with other kids. I was a wise guy, the one who asked tough questions or responded to queries with a sarcastic retort. I was a dreamer who wrote poetry and short stories, often not paying attention in class.

Consequently, teachers often sent me to detention or "social adjustment" classes. Though I did not show it, I usually felt ashamed for being singled out and punished. If I was tardy, talkative, or missed detention, I was sent to the vice principal's office for punishment. That, however, only made me feel more rebellious and defiant.

In the seventh grade, I received over 100 welt-raising swats from the vice principal's hickory paddle, delivered with the full force of his athletic strength. After receiving the hundredth swat, boys got the privilege of signing his paddle. While other kids were out playing ball after school, I was in social adjustment, meeting other boys who had signed the paddle. They became my first gang, "The 100s."

Social adjustment consisted of writing 500 "I will not _____" affirmations. We also received more swats for infractions such as breaking room silence or failing to complete the assignments on time. Insidiously, the assignments were often impossible to finish in the time allotted.

The posture the social adjustment "teacher" made us assume was to bend over, grasp our ankles, and then raise our heads so we looked straight ahead. Then, wham! A good swat could knock a boy halfway across the room. Florid bruises remained for days thereafter. When swats came daily, the hematomas overlapped one another.

During these "classes," I became friends with Denny Slayter, the class clown, Chuck Mendez, a tough Chicano who "ruled" the schoolyard, and other bad boys. In the bathroom one day, the 3 of us showed off the vivid palette of colors on our behinds and upper thighs as though they were merit badges or other hard-won symbols of achievement. We began to wear triple pairs of underwear to soften the blows. But that did not make much difference.

Eventually, our pain thresholds increased. This only incensed the social adjustment teacher. As a measure of our manhood, we prided ourselves on not showing any reaction when hit and derided one another if we failed in our stoic display. Sometimes, despite our resolve, tears leaked out. It was good training for turning restless and mischievous boys into cynical, angry, and violent young men. After detention, we were so wound up, we sometimes took vengeance on the community. Vandalism and fights with other boys after school were frequent after these sessions.

One day, our gym teacher broke Andy Lipinsky's tailbone with his paddle. After that and the ensuing lawsuit, they stopped swatting kids at my school. Years later, the state legislature made corporal punishment illegal in California.

In his book *Beating the Devil Out of Them*, Murray Straus notes, "It is virtually certain that part of the link between corporal punishment and crime occurs because 'bad' children [who] are hit go on to have a higher rate of criminal activity than other children" (Straus & Donnelly, 1994). Despite the evidence, the institutionalized practice of disciplining boys with paddles, belts, rulers, and other implements widely persists in school and at home (National Center for Education Statistics [NCES], 1997). In the half of our states that still permit it, boys still receive 2 to 3 million applications of corporal punishment a year. The majority occur in Southern states, where, coincidentally, higher incidences of gun violence occur at school. In fact, states in which teachers are allowed to hit children have the most student violence and higher murder rates overall.

Thousands of boys punished at school require medical attention. But this is one of many arenas in which authorities apply different standards of protection for boys. Although corporal punishment may effect short-term changes in bad boys' behavior, it ultimately does more to fuel young male anger and aggression than assuage it.

Combat sports, such as football, also proliferate in school. Annually, over 300 000 high school boys are injured, 14 000 are hospitalized—many with permanent disabilities such as paralysis—and several are killed playing football. Sports with the highest injury rates are largely reserved for boys (Kipnis, 1991). Annually, 4 million visits to emergency rooms result from high school sports (Mayo Clinic, 1998). The promise of full-paid college scholarships, gargantuan professional sports contracts, the adoration of cheerleaders, and praise from older men all tell boys that a willingness to enact violence, suffer injury, and endure pain is the formula for success.

## VIOLENCE 101

Today, many of us ask why boys seem more prone to violence and acting out than previous generations. I believe the socially tolerated abuse of boys and young men, in many arenas, is one cause of unarticulated, young male rage. Our schools have come to tolerate a social ecology of punishment, neglect, and even outright abuse of some boys. Highly publicized school shootings have desensitized many teachers to more common forms of violence and made them less likely to report it or intervene in other ways (Yi, 1998).

As numerous surveys of domestic violence bear out, violence against males is often substantially underreported (Gelles & Loseke, 1993; Straus et al, 1988). Boys tend to believe that complaining about injuries from assault is not manly, whereas most girls are encouraged to ask for help. Many boys also fear that informing will subject them to retaliatory assaults. Statistics on school safety are, therefore, deceptive when it comes to boys. In 1995, almost half of all boys surveyed in grades 9 through 12 reported involvement in a physical fight during the previous year (Sickmund et al, 1997). Yet official school statistics cite a rate closer to only 10%, in itself an unacceptably high incidence of victimization (Friedfel, 1998).

Although I was involved in numerous school fights, several of which drew blood, authorities were never called in response to a single incident. I never received a single session of counseling to help me extricate myself from the violence at or near school, where most fights occurred. In a strange quirk of male culture, I instead became friends with several of the boys who fought with me.

After battling Denny Slayter on the basketball court one afternoon, we wiped the blood off one another with paper towels in the school bathroom, laughed about the whole thing, and were fast friends thereafter. During the time (ages 12 to 14) that my identity was transforming from wimp to wild boy, I never felt there was a single adult I could go to at school for help or guidance. After I refused to back down when Chuck Mendez, who ruled the schoolyard, challenged me on the football field, he invited me to join his gang. The idea of inclusion and protection by a group, any group, sounded good. I joined.

Today, some school safety guidelines list behaviors typical of half the adolescent boys in school as predictive of students most at risk for violent outbreaks. Because bad boys are referred to programs in which the staff usually has the lowest level of training, poorest tools, and most dilapidated facilities, our highest risk students tend to become the least well cared for. In particular, most boys lack a strong male presence in the classroom. Increased father involvement and minority male teacher recruitment can go a long way to improving opportunities for at-risk boys to succeed in school (Addison, 1998).

The predominant response of schools today, however, is zero tolerance toward any acting out behavior from boys (NCES, 1997). Consequently, increasing numbers of boys are being forced out of the educational system and what protections from abuse it could afford those children at risk if more effort was put into creative student-retention programs (Cantelon & LeBoeuf, 1997).

## SENTENCED TO THE STREETS

In addition to boys being sentenced to the streets by escalating expulsions, suspensions, dropouts, and school failures (Sickmund et al, 1997), between 5 and 15 million children of working parents are home alone after school. More than half of all juvenile crime occurs between 2:00 and 8:00 PM (Morton-Young, 1995). During the few years I lived in the homes of my working parents, I hung out at the railroad tracks or drainage basins with other wild boys after school. There was nowhere else to go except home, alone.

Not only homeless children populate the streets. Many live in homes that are essentially crash pads with family members only marginally involved in their lives. Unsupervised children swell the ranks of kids on the street. There, male loiterers are much more subject to suspicion and arrest than females. Boys near the street generate significantly more police contacts for noncriminal activity than do more socially integrated boys. They are much more likely to be arrested and incarcerated for the same crimes that divert more affluent and sheltered youth into mental health treatment. Boys who are "hangin' with the homies" know they are targeted more than other citizens. Their first experience with police is often a negative encounter. This can make them cynical about justice. Inequity, in any arena, tends to breed contempt for the law.

Most of the street kids I knew during my homeless years lived in fear of the police. Many of us suffered abuse in police custody. Few would approach police if victimized by crime ourselves. We legitimately feared that we were more likely to be arrested than assisted. A Hollywood vice officer raped a homeless girlfriend of mine, Angela, in his police car the night of her 16th birthday. Many years later a police commission finally held several officers at that Hollywood substation accountable for their sexual abuse of homeless kids and prostitutes over the years.

## LIFE ON THE STREETS

When not in locked juvenile institutions, I spent most of my adolescence living in or near street life. I was usually broke. Survival took up a good portion of each day. I regularly looked for work but was repeatedly refused because of my age, few skills, and the lack of an address or phone number. Also, using only public bathrooms for hygiene, I could not stay impeccably clean. I imagine my appearance got somewhat scruffy over time. The hungrier I got the more I fantasized about stealing as an immediate way to get food or money. Like most low-level offenders, I was not particularly violent, but I wanted to survive. So, I started committing petty thefts.

Armed with a coat hanger, I would walk the streets of the Hollywood Hills late at night. Many cars were unlocked. Others I would open with the hanger, sticking it down between the window and the doorframe to catch the locks. Rifling cars produced a steady stream of spare change, an occasional item I could sell on the street, and often a place to sleep.

Though I always tried to wake before dawn, I preferred sleeping in underground garages where I could hear people approaching in the morning if I overslept. The few times someone discovered me, I bolted and ran, hopping fences and working my way through the tangles of poison oak, manzanita, honeysuckle, and sage that filled the rugged canyons below. I always got away quickly and was never caught. But for many years, I was haunted by exhausting dreams about endlessly running away from pursuers. Generally, however, all these petty thefts were insufficient to even provide me with steady meals.

# SURVIVAL SEX: THE PROSTITUTION SOLUTION

I never wanted to get involved with prostitution. I simply drifted into it as I got more desperate. Hustling gay men proved to be the only steady income I could produce as a homeless 15-year-old. I "turned" my first "trick" at 4:00 AM in a Hollywood hotel. A man bought me drinks in a bar till 2:00 AM, fed me steak at an all-night diner, and then took me to his room. He was a dumpy, pasty white guy with a wife and kids in the suburbs. So were many of the others along the way.

One day, I met a guy, Gary, on the Sunset Strip who took me to a large abandoned house in the hills. There, about 10 gay men were squatting. They had turned the gas on at the street and were cooking a pot of stew over a gas log in the fireplace. The only furniture consisted of some mattresses lying around and a stained, threadbare couch rescued from some alleyway. I shared their meal. Gary let me sleep on the couch.

Because "you dance with whom you came," I "belonged" to Gary. The other guys left me alone. But there was a high-strung guy, Patrick (Patty), who kept asking for sex when Gary was not around. Patty was a jerk and had nothing to offer. So, I just kept putting him off. After all, sex was my only coinage at the time. I tried to spend it only for survival.

After a week or so Patty got agitated about being refused. Then he got aggressive. I fought him off, giving him a black eye. A few nights later I was at the After Hours club, where I often hung out and danced. During a break, I went out to the alley to cool off. A couple of dealers, who regularly sold drugs at the club, suddenly attacked me. Patty had told everyone that I was a police informant, doubly dangerous because I was a minor. The first part was not true. Though today at times I work professionally with law enforcement, at that stage of life I had nothing but contempt for the police. But I was banned from the club and the house, exiled to the street again.

A man who worked for Bank of America picked me up and took me to his apartment late that night. After being coerced into having sex with him, I became so distressed that I tried to slash my wrists with a razor blade in his bathroom. This was my third suicide attempt, having unsuccessfully overdosed with pills twice in recent years. I was unable to cut myself deeply. I remember feeling like a coward. The bank teller discovered me bleeding in his bathtub; even those superficial cuts made quite a mess. He was furious. It was about 3:00 AM. He taped up my wrists, made me get dressed, put me in the car, drove me back to Hollywood, and pushed me out of the door. I spent the rest of the night sitting in a 24-hour diner drinking coffee.

## ON THE ROAD

Broken, bruised, depressed, and no longer feeling safe in Hollywood, I hitchhiked out of town the next morning. I caught rides up Highway 101 along the California coast, generally heading for San Francisco. A couple picked me up in Big Sur, took me in, fed me, tended my cuts, and shared their infinite supply of excellent pot. He was a burly, heavily bearded sculptor. His willowy, long-haired wife grew herbs, vegetables, and marijuana in a large organic garden. This was the first of many times in my life that I was blessed by unconditional compassion emanating from countercultural strangers. I worked around the house and garden for a few days, gained strength, and moved on.

A week of bumming my way up the coast brought me to San Francisco's Tenderloin district. After a few homeless days, 2 Hell's Angels offered me a place to crash. I moved into their single, $20-a-week room in a hotel near Turk and Eddy Streets. Betty, a teenaged runaway from Indiana, was also there. We slept in shifts, generally using the room at different times than the bikers.

Betty was also hustling for survival. We walked the streets and worked the clubs from about 10:00 PM until 2:00 or 3:00 in the morning. Sometimes we would hang out together. But just like Hollywood, the straight and gay trolling grounds were on different streets, so we mostly had to go it alone. Then, unless we were spending the night with a trick, we would come home and crash. We often held one another in the bed for comfort.

The 2 bikers were running a scam that kept them on the street from 3:00 AM until dawn. They had a key that opened parking meters. They would raid them in the small hours, coming back to the hotel room in the late morning to wrap coins after their breakfast. I would get up then, hit the streets, and come back sometimes to sleep in the afternoon when the bikers were usually out.

I do not know why they let me live there. I found, as I made my way along the underground corridors of our culture, that outlaws were often unexpectedly kind. While the churches and synagogues barred their doors at night and my middle-class relatives just did not care, it was usually the poor, the outcasts, the freaks, and the downtrodden who offered me a hand. They asked for little. More often than not, they asked for nothing in return.

My first night in San Francisco I slept in the bushes above the Union Street parking garage. It was a cold night. A raggedy alcoholic bundled up in the same hedge told me, "Hey, this is no place for a kid." He gave me a musty blanket he had bundled under his head for a pillow and dug into his pocket for 50 cents. He told me to buy a bowl of soup in the diner across the street so as not to go to sleep hungry. That was probably all the money he had. The blanket was half his personal property. Like Blanche in *A Streetcar Named Desire*, I survived primarily because of the kindness of strangers. The generosity of this bum in the bushes touched me deeply. In my current good fortune, the memory of him ensures that I consider those with less.

The bikers got busted one night. Cops came in the middle of the night. Betty and I were in the bed. They searched the place and hauled away coin wrappers as evidence. They asked us if we knew anything about an extra parking meter key. We said no, we just used the room to sleep when the guys were not there—the truth. The cops left us there. Why they did not haul us in, I will never know. Betty took off for unknown parts the next day. I never saw her again.

## MAKING THE SCENE

I could not afford the next week's rent on the room, so I moved in with 2 gay men down the hall, Jackie and Johnny. They taught me tricks of the street-hustling trade. It seemed like a good deal at the time. In addition to $10 or $20 in my pocket, sometimes a decent meal or a bath in a comfortable hotel also came along. Ten bucks equaled 20 chili dogs or a week's rent-share for my Tenderloin fire-trap. It was not until years later, when a friend's sister told me she made $500 a night hooking, that I realized my innocence was so cheaply sold. In a strange twist of "equity pay," boys do not command nearly as much for their bodies as girls. One day, as winter began to cool the streets, Jackie went off to Mexico. I hopped a Greyhound bus with Johnny and went back to Los Angeles in search of warmer nights.

I stayed away from the After Hours club. Patty had ruined my reputation there. But Johnny introduced me to new haunts in the arts and theater district of West Hollywood. The 8727 was an underground gay club on Melrose Avenue. Outside, nothing advertised its presence but the address. Inside, the flame of Hollywood gay culture burned with bright intensity.

We hustled a little but mostly just hung out. Night after night I reveled in the scene. Actors came in after the theaters closed. Intellectuals lit up the night with articulate debate. Drag queens preened occasionally, adding a campy hilarity to the night. And there was a steady stream of food, drugs, and lodging. The occasional payment of sex assured the older men who paid for it all that I was a player.

I spent nights drinking bottomless cups of coffee, chain-smoking cigarettes inside and marijuana outside, dropping bennies (benzedrine) like M&Ms, and talking with everyone about anything and everything. The richness, tempo, and depth I missed in school were abundant in the coffeehouses. I learned about art, music, poetry, literature, dance, cinema, sex, radical politics, and the engaging psychology of those living outside society's norms.

Like a vampire, I left before the full sun of first light, lest it somehow return me to the demon hells of depression stored behind the manic mask I wore in those nocturnal parades. The amphetamine-drenched nights heightened the mystical quality of dawn as I often walked to the boulevard for breakfast awash in beauty.

Abandoned as I was by straight culture, gay men kept me alive. But they also took their toll. Some tricks abused me, cheated me, gave me disorienting drugs, pressured me, or threatened me. I often felt afraid of things getting out of control. On 2 occasions, "gay bashers" (men who beat homosexuals for sport) assaulted me.

Ironically, I never regarded myself as gay. Men have never sexually attracted me. Many adolescent male hustlers self-identify as heterosexuals. But since few women seek male prostitutes, street boys, gay or straight, work the gay clientele. In Los Angeles today, just as in my time 35 years ago, women and girls still work the straight crowd on Sunset while boys walk the streets of Selma or Santa Monica, a few blocks south. The whole bizarre milieu intrigued me in some perverse way. It has taken a lifetime, however, to recover from the shame and sexual confusion resulting from some of these experiences as a teen prostitute.

## THE TOLERATED SEXUAL ABUSE OF BOYS

During my street years, I met numerous kids selling sex for food, lodging, or drug habits frequently incurred to medicate the pain they felt as discards. It was not until I began working intensively with male clients, however, that I began to understand these experiences as sexual abuse.

Most people would immediately regard a homeless, teenaged girl prostitute as a victim of predatory adults. But I never thought about my life that way, in part because no one else ever framed it in that light. Like many victims of child sexual abuse who blame themselves, for years I felt that any deviance in my experience must have been my own. Although it is essential for people in recovery to take responsibility for their actions, it is also important for abuse survivors to understand the impact that predatory sex can have on their psyches. For most men and boys, however, this topic is so taboo and shameful that they rarely find forums supporting forthright discussions about the impact of uncomfortable, early sexual experiences.

Today, there is a serious drought of compassion for males. Cynicism abounds. I have conducted seminars in a number of mental health institutions with blatant double standards of care for young men. However, at least one third of all child sexual abuse, perpetrated by women and men, is against boys. Yet many sex abuse treatment programs still predominately focus on female victims and male abusers.

In California, legislators did not even make the statutory rape of boys illegal until 1993. Yet various studies and the stories many young men tell me indicate that sexual abuse creates as many psychological problems for boys as girls. When working with male clients, I am still surprised at how often sexual abuse emerges from their personal histories. Few, however, report that anyone previously showed much concern about it.

Today, thousands of children continue to walk the nation's streets with little support from social services. When they become bad boys and they attract the interest of the criminal justice system, then most of these children get significant attention. For many of them, by the time they get into juvenile justice, it is too late. What does it say about our society that we cavalierly abandon thousands of children to prostitution, drug addiction, AIDS, and the violence that accompanies life on the streets?

# WHY ARE SO MANY CHILDREN HOMELESS?

More than any other issue, poverty is the key element pushing increasing numbers of children onto the streets. With welfare reform, as more mothers' benefits shrink below the capacity to maintain a home, more women and children of both sexes are put at risk. Boys and young men, however, still comprise the majority of the homeless.

In *The Grapes of Wrath*, John Steinbeck wrote that during the Great Depression, "It was obvious to all but the most dense that vast and uncontrollable economic forces were responsible for the millions thrown into poverty" (Steinbeck, 1939). But today, as most policy makers enjoy wealth and privilege, the injuries of class do not seem so obvious. Though Americans enjoy one of the highest levels of affluence in the world, an equally extreme moral and spiritual poverty seems to sanction the disenfranchisement of millions of citizens. Disenfranchisement, like shunning practiced in early America, excludes those deemed offensive to societal norms through incarceration, narrowed economic and educational opportunity, and revocation of rights normally accommodated enfranchised citizens.

The National Law Center on Homelessness and Poverty estimates that about 760 000 Americans are homeless on any given night. One to 2 million experience homelessness sometime during the year. About 13 million American adults today were homeless at some point in their lives, so I am not alone in my experience. But I do not take much comfort in the company. It is getting worse. More than half report that their homelessness occurred in the last decade (Shinn & Weitzman, 1996). Homelessness is expected to keep expanding at 10% to 30% a year, and the death rate for homeless people also keeps growing.

Children under the age of 18 account for roughly 25% of the urban homeless (Waxman & Trupin, 1997). Single men—40% of whom served in the armed forces—constitute 47% of the homeless (Marin, 1991; National Coalition for the Homeless [NCH], 1997-1998). High rates of addiction plague the homeless, particularly young men, 20% to 25% of whom also suffer severe, persistent mental illness (Greene et al, 1995). Every night about 150 000 youth live homeless nationwide. One out of 4 reports a history of abuse and neglect at the homes they left. More than half report that their parents told them to leave or just did not care what they did. One in 5 homeless youth has attempted suicide. For gay youth, the attempted suicide rate leaps to an astounding 65% (Gibson, 1989). Overall, adolescent boys have the highest "successful" suicide rate in the nation—4 to 5 times that of girls the same age (USDHHS, 1993). In 1999 about 3% of homeless persons under age 25 were HIV-positive. For homeless young men alone, the rate leaps (Wendell et al, 1992). By some estimates, 1 in 10 male prostitutes is infected.

Many youth become homeless because of family poverty. In our affluent nation, over 20% of American children live in poverty. Our "war on poverty" parallels our similar "success" in Vietnam and the "war on drugs." American youth in the mid-1990s were 50% more likely to be poor as in the mid-1970s (May, 1995).

Forty percent of the homeless were once foster children, a history that also correlates with becoming homeless at an earlier age and remaining so for a longer time. Eighteen months after discharge from placements, 1 in 4 former foster kids reports having been beaten, seriously hurt, or incarcerated; a third have not completed high school; and half are unemployed (Roman & Phyllis, 1995). Many young men are also discharged from jails and prisons without any housing or employment waiting.

When abused and neglected boys fall through the safety net of the community and crash onto the streets, the next step for many is a juvenile institution of some kind. Ninety-five percent of prisoners are male. Incarceration frequently severs boys' few threads of continuity with jobs, housing, social support systems, and family. As a result of insufficient shelter beds for youth in general and admission policies often biased against boys over the age of 10, few are housed in emergency shelters. Youth shelters, when available, however, are not merely interim safe housing. They also frequently function as sites for drop-in crisis counseling, legal aid, and health services for street kids. Without safe and simple access to these services, these children needlessly suffer.

According to the National Coalition for the Homeless (1997-1998)

[h]omeless adolescents often suffer from severe anxiety and depression, poor health and nutrition, and low self-esteem. Furthermore, homeless youth face difficulties attending school because of legal guardianship requirements, residency requirements, proper records, and lack of transportation. As a result, homeless youth face severe challenges in obtaining an education and supporting themselves emotionally and financially.

Throughout my childhood and adolescence, as I bounced among family, friends, foster care, the streets, and institutions, I never lived in the same place for one year. The cumulative effect of this chaos gradually instilled a belief that nothing was stable, the world was unsafe, everything was subject to change, all relationships were conditional, and no one could really be trusted.

Perhaps, because I longed to create some illusion of normalcy in an otherwise bizarre life, I made one abortive attempt to attend Hollywood High when I was 16 years old. I enjoyed being around regular teenagers, but just maintaining my life took most of my energy. No school programs helped students living independently. After a few weeks, I dropped out again.

## BACK TO THE STREET

My second homeless period started after I turned 17, and the California Youth Authority released me as an emancipated minor. I rented a cheap apartment in the same part of Hollywood I had worked as a prostitute 2 years earlier. About 6 months later, however, I lost my job as a county clerk and started washing dishes at a trendy French restaurant on the Sunset Strip.

I was stunned by the quantity of food wealthy diners left on their plates. This was my first ongoing encounter with affluent adults, or, at least, their leftovers. Steaks that skinny women hardly touched, half-finished lobster tails, mounds of salad, whole baked potatoes, and piles of vegetables filled the plates sent back to me for cleaning.

I lined my coat pockets with plastic and stuffed them nightly with leftovers. That fed me during off-work hours as well as my unemployed roommate and other kids I knew living on the fringes of Hollywood. I was appalled that the restaurant wasted so much expensive food. I realized then that wealthy people lived in an entirely different universe of privilege.

One of my most visceral memories from the street years is one of persistent hunger. I would go into fast-food restaurants and finish food left on tables, glean garbage cans, and retrieve discarded sand sharks from fishermen at the Venice pier. Shark stew was pretty good. Even a small shark, combined with vegetables plucked from a supermarket dumpster, would feed a lot of kids.

I had a whimsical moment, years later, while visiting my publisher's home near Beverly Hills, following the release of my first book in 1991. Earlier that day, a limousine provided by a television talk show had driven me around town. As I relaxed, sipping Perrier and listening to jazz in the air-conditioned embrace of the limo's plush interior, I felt strangely amused as we passed through the same streets where I once struggled.

In my mind, I waved to that skinny boy on the streets and told him to take heart, that the wheel of life kept turning and many delightful surprises were ahead. He just had to persevere and keep hope alive. That evening, my publisher told me he had occupied his exquisite home for over 30 years. I realized that he had once been on my

Wednesday night trash-picking route. But not wishing to spoil an enchanting dinner with a sordid tale, I just kept this story to myself, as with most of these memoirs, until now.

## CAGED

Although my early experiences of fragmentation created paranoid tendencies in my thinking, they also led me on a spiritual quest for enduring values. As circumstances worsened, I began to look within for places of refuge. My first transcendental experience occurred in a solitary confinement cell in the subbasement of the Cook County Juvenile Detention Center.

This happened a few months after I had been shipped to Chicago to live with relatives. The home was violent and I ran away with my girlfriend, 15-year-old Sandy. We had just enough money for a ticket to St. Louis. So, that is where we went. We slept in a derelict building, on a tattered mattress amidst a debrislittered floor. We huddled together for warmth as the first snow of the season fell on the street outside the broken windows of our new home. But we were happy.

We panhandled and performed petty thefts to survive. Sandy charged a man who approached us on the street for the gifts she gave me free. I felt ashamed that we were so broke. But we were basically starving, so I was grateful for the money. After a week on the streets, the police picked us up for loitering. We had destroyed all of our identification. But an interstate, all-points police bulletin was out on Sandy. With a few phone calls, the police figured out that we were those runaways from Chicago.

The police charged me with violating the Mann Act (interstate kidnapping) and statutory rape. But since I was a minor, and because Sandy convinced her parents that she was a willing conspirator, the authorities dropped those charges. They just held me for being a runaway. I remained in the St. Louis Detention Center for about a week. The guards gave me a thin mattress on the floor in a cell with 4 young men, who filled the double bunk beds on either side. They began taunting me. The oldest one said that as soon as the lights were out they were going to take turns "fucking me in the ass" while I "sucked their cocks." Each one of them was larger than me.

Being raped by a cage full of urban psychopaths was not an experience I was looking forward to. I acted unfazed, making whatever attempts I thought might garner their good will. I made them see me more as a brother gangster than "fresh white meat." I made some progress during the day, to the point where their behavior became less hostile and belittling. Toward the end of the evening, one man was almost apologetic about their plans. He explained that they had all been in youth prison for several years, were just being held there for a hearing the next day, and they had needs. "You'd understand if you been in the Missouri pen like us," he said.

I felt a foreboding despair but silently resolved to fight. I figured that at best I would be raped and, at worst, badly beaten, maybe killed. Miraculously, I was spared those fates. Thousands of other boys are not so lucky. Just before lights-out, our cell door suddenly opened. Three deputies charged in. They made all 5 of us strip. Then they conducted an exhaustive search of the cell and our clothing. They found a few cigarettes and matches hidden in personal items belonging to the other men.

Possession of contraband is a serious offense in the netherworld of juvenile justice. The breaking of institutional rules can send a boy to solitary confinement or add to his incarceration time, without any due process hearing. A thread of hope glimmered in the impending doom. I said, "That's mine," hoping, like Br'er Rabbit longing for the briar patch, that they would punish me with solitary confinement. No such luck.

The guards knew the cigarettes belonged to the other men. But I insisted, "They belong to me." The others did not deny it. The guards left in disgust. The other prisoners were grateful that I, now a "stand-up guy," took the rap. They left me alone that night. The next day, they went to court, were loaded into a bus, and were sent back to youth prison. A week later, St. Louis police shipped me, in handcuffs on an airplane, to the Chicago Juvenile Detention Center.

## CHICAGO BLUES

Sandy went home. Her parents reconciled whatever issues they had with her. I spent the next 4 months in Juvi. Beatings by guards for slight infractions were frequent. They hit us hard with the flat of their hands in ways that hurt but did not leave significant bruises or break bones. I contracted severe bronchitis. It went untreated. Forced every day to run in circles in the gymnasium, I would sometimes collapse with a racking cough. The guards told me to continue running or I would be sent to solitary confinement—the ultimate punishment in jail.

Nights were terrifying. The dormitories housed about 100 boys each, sleeping in cots side by side and head to toe. In the deep of night, various predatory activities occurred. Some boys were raped. Others boys received "blanket parties," during which a group would beat a boy under a blanket so he could not identify his attackers. Some of the older gang boys slept with tightly folded blankets on their chests, held in place by T-shirts or towels, as armor to protect them from being stabbed.

One night, I awoke to some boys setting fire to a heap of toilet paper they had piled on my bed. I had no idea why. I did not even know them. They fled as I let loose a bloodcurdling scream that erupted from some previously untapped depth within. After that, I slept on the floor under my bed. For years afterward, a part of my psyche remained vigilant in the night.

When I was in my early 20s, my first wife, Satri, would sometimes rouse me early for work. I would often break out of sleep with a scream and fists flailing. Fortunately, I never hurt her. But she was badly shaken the first few times it happened. After the first occurrence, she learned to wake me from a distance. It took me about 20 years to grow out of this posttraumatic stress response. And to this day, like gunslingers in the Old West, I pick the restaurant seat with my back to the wall and my gaze toward approaching people. But the more extreme responses have waned as I keep reminding myself that, today, I live in a safe and loving environment.

One day, as I was sitting in the Juvi's day room, watching TV with a few hundred young hoodlums, I accidentally poked the guy in front of me with my foot. He stood up, all 6 feet of him. His pumped-up jailhouse muscles rippled across his torso. He punched me so hard in the nose that I flew into the benches behind me. A melee ensued. Guards hauled me off to solitary confinement to serve a month in the "hole" for fighting.

## LIFE IN THE HOLE

The windowless cell was in the basement of the cold, damp concrete tomb in which Chicago housed its discarded youth. I could almost touch both walls simultaneously by outstretching my hands. The cell was slightly longer than the steel cot bolted to the floor. A stainless steel, lidless toilet was alongside the foot of the bed.

Three times a day a guard opened a slot at the bottom of the solid steel door. He slid a paper plate of food and a paper cup of Kool-Aid through the door. A cardboard spoon accompanied the meager meals. That flimsy spoon seemed ironic to me at the time. They did not want to give me an implement with which to hurt myself, since suicide attempts are rampant in solitary. Yet they created an environment of sensory deprivation that was psychologically the most brutal experience of my life.

There was no light in the room. A naked light bulb further down the dimly lit corridor bleakly illuminated the room through a small, thick, Plexiglas observation port in the cell door. If I looked out at just the right angle, I could see a clock on the wall under the light. So, by keeping track of meals and checking the clock I could figure out whether it was day or night. I do not know why that felt so important, but I did not want to lose psychological connection to daylight. I found the perpetual twilight of my cell unnerving.

The lack of any reading material or any other distraction was tortuous. For days, an agony of loneliness and boredom, intense as intractable physical pain, filled my every waking moment. The only relief was frequent masturbation and the meals that I ate as slowly and methodically as possible, prolonging every mediocre bite. I ate the canned corn a kernel at a time and rolled the two slices of white bread into little dough balls that I could chew on throughout the day.

One day, a few weeks into my confinement, I felt I could not bear another single hour. I began carving on my arm with the edge of a plastic comb that I sharpened on the concrete floor. The pain helped distract me. My cough worsened. When it racked my body, my nose kept spewing blood. Since there was no towel I used my T-shirt to staunch it. I could have used toilet paper but did not want to run out of my limited supply. That had already happened when, to amuse myself, I used up the last roll by braiding it into paper twine that I then wove into little funny animals. When it ran out, a week passed until I received a new roll.

Laundry, however, was exchanged once a week through the same slot in the door that the food and toilet paper came through. I sent the bloodstained T-shirts through the door like messages in a bottle. I hoped they would land on some distant shore where someone cared about a teenager with declining health locked in a basement.

Someone finally determined that I genuinely needed medical care. All my senses were heightened as I was taken, in handcuffs, to Chicago General Hospital. Outside it was 14° below zero. Though sunlight blinded my unaccustomed eyes, the glittering crystals formed by breath in the winter air delighted me. Everything looked beautiful. After months inside, every aspect of the outer world was novel. The simplest icicle overwhelmed me as an exquisite wonder.

The doctor determined that the blow to my nose had caused a deviated septum. When I sneezed or coughed hard, broken cartilage kept opening blood vessels. They cauterized the inside of my nose, gave me antibiotics for the bronchitis, a shot for anemia, and topical treatment for the now infected, self-inflicted wound on my arm. I remember the doctor telling me that I was lucky I had not contracted pneumonia in my weakened state. He told me to stay warm, rest, and drink plenty of liquids.

The guard took my comb away when he returned me to my cold, damp, solitary cell with its bare metal cot and one thin blanket. The bleak contrast to the sensory richness of the trip to the hospital made my solitary confinement all the more unbearable. I instinctively knew I had to find a new way of coping with sensory deprivation or go insane.

Set into the wall was a round, stainless steel button that flushed the toilet when depressed. When staring at it I noticed that if I fixed my gaze unblinkingly, the surrounding visual field would begin to fade. After a while, the entire cell would disappear into a gray haze until, eventually, only the silver button remained. Then the button itself would disappear as patterns of light, colors, and other visual effects swam into my vision. Hours would pass this way as I sat watching whatever was playing on my mental TV.

Like Alice through the looking glass, I stumbled into another world. Or perhaps, as do countless prisoners in isolation, I had a psychotic break. Either way, I learned from this self-taught meditation that no matter how inescapable the agony a soul feels in the underworld, some avenue of escape may still yet lead us from the blinding terrors of the maze. A few years later, I learned that meditation could be more than simply an escape from pain. It proved to also be a path toward healing, renewal, and a spiritual life. Most prisoners, however, find little respite from the torture they experience behind bars. The mere thought of prisoners spending years in solitary confinement today, regardless of their crimes, is like a steel knife scraping on the slate of my psyche. Despite sanctions from Amnesty International for violations of human rights, protracted solitary confinement is still practiced by the American juvenile institutions (United Nations, 1988).

## PRISONERS OF OUR IMAGINATION

Many believe that the need to keep expanding juvenile institutions is inevitable. But prisons, juvenile or otherwise, are not an indelible fact of life. Our culture invented penitentiaries. Our evolving society has modernized many other archaic institutions to meet the needs of a changing world. The time is overdue for the leaders of a new era also to revise our juvenile justice system, much of which is still guided by 19th-century beliefs. The crumbling cell I first occupied in the Los Angeles Juvenile Hall had been built in 1903.

## CHANGES IN THE SYSTEM

Parenting classes, mentoring programs, home visits by health professionals, and anger and stress management for parents can all help prevent child maltreatment. The high incidence of child abuse and neglect by female caretakers points to a need for our social programs to teach anger management to women as assiduously as they do men suspected of domestic violence or child abuse. This can be done in a blame-free approach that is sympathetic to the specific stresses that women face, especially when there is turmoil in their homes. In 1998, Congress allotted over a billion dollars to protect women from violence. This official attention was hard-won and a long time coming for women. But because children do not vote and boys, in particular, have few organized or effective advocates today, no such largess has yet come forth for their protection.

The following measures would help to reduce the incidence of child abuse in America:

— Provide better support for impoverished parents in achieving economic self-suffi-ciency and education, understanding that economic stress alone can contribute to their higher incidences of abuse and neglect of children.

— When any violence occurs in a home, assure that parents and caretakers of either sex are mandated to anger management programs and drug and alcohol treat-ment programs where applicable.

— Dedicate more public resources to protecting foster children, knowing they do not have the political power to lobby on their own behalf.

— Support male-involvement programs to assist fathers in developing the emo-tional, technical, and financial capacity to be more positively involved with their children's lives.

— Initiate aggressive adoption campaigns, including economic incentives and professional support networks, for all America's children currently abandoned to institutions.

— Require high schools and marriage license grantors to provide all teenagers and newlyweds with parenting instruction.

— Require all divorcing couples with children to attend joint child-care planning before granting a divorce.

— Implore teachers, doctors, coaches, counselors, clergy, parents, and neighbors to speak directly to children who appear abused or to contact authorities. Whenever safe to do so, talk to adults who are abusing their children in public.

— Abolish the notion that any adult should be allowed to strike any child, any-where, for any reason.

Foster children need special attention to give them the same chances for a productive life afforded those from intact families. Many of these children are abandoned by parents whose lifestyles caused their children to be born with fetal alcohol syndrome, narcotic addictions, or AIDS. To ensure that these children get the extra help they need and deserve, governments could begin to eliminate obstacles to the adoption of abused children.

To help turn the growing tide of disenfranchised youth in our culture, more concerned citizens need to offer safe homes for children at risk for abuse and neglect from their caretakers. For this to happen fully, however, society would have to change many of its attitudes, particularly toward boys who represent the vast majority of unwanted and institutionalized children, contributing to the public agency child welfare budget of some $12 billion a year.

Another change that can help foster children is to reduce social workers' caseloads to levels that ensure they can, at the least, visit kids once a month to check on their welfare. Also, community-oriented social work, in which, as with community policing, the staff are familiar with the residents and resources of one specific area, can help provide more consistent and stable foster care environments. With community care, even if a placement fails, a child can be placed in a new home nearby where he can enjoy continuing contact with known teachers, clergy, counselors, and friends instead of being ripped up by the roots every time he is transferred. And these community resources, as a stable part of the child's extended family, can back up foster parents. Wherever possible, foster parents who work intimately with noncustodial, biological relatives can also expand the continuity and range of support in children's lives.

Carefully coordinated efforts in which one committed advocate stays with a foster child's case all the way from home removal to either family reunification or adoption would help enormously. Consistent, integrated care of wards and vigorous management of the foster care system could go a long way toward providing security for children.

Homeless children and young men benefit most from programs that meet immediate needs first and then help them address other aspects of their lives. Programs that minimize demands for strict adherence to normative behavior models and offer a range of support services are consistently the most successful in helping homeless children regain stability (Greenblatt & Robertson, 1993). Educational outreach, job training and living wage employment, transitional living programs, counseling, affordable housing and healthcare, all specifically designed for and directed toward homeless children, are sorely needed (Cwayna, 1993; Robertson, 1996). Today, more programs for homeless youth are coming on line. A former graduate student of mine runs just such a program in my old neighborhood. Male prostitutes and gay, lesbian, transgender, and homeless youth come from all over the city to attend this public school. There, sensitive adults warmly accept them as they are, while providing as many services as possible to aid them in their education, safety, mental and physical health, and their interactions with the broader culture.

The child welfare system could make a greater effort to prevent children from ending up on the street, if for no other reason than to save us taxpayers money on the inevitable social costs that follow homeless children throughout their lives. The documented costs of increased hospitalization rates, mental health services, welfare dependency, substance abuse, violence, AIDS and other diseases, crime, and incarceration for this population far exceed the investment needed to create zero tolerance toward child homelessness.

The following measures would help to reduce the incidence of homeless children:

— Provide shelters for all homeless youth with the educational, medical, and vocational support needed to help them stay off the streets.

— Challenge the biases that bar homeless boys and young men admittance to many shelters.

— Train social workers how to reach out to homeless young men on the streets where they live.

— Ensure that all youth leaving foster care, juvenile institutions, or jails have the resources needed to transition from institutional to independent living.

— Implement primary prevention, treatment, and diversion programs, wherever possible, to keep children in the community in the first place.

— Support mentoring programs that can connect children at risk with caring, capable, and responsible adults.

— Increase entry-level employment opportunities for youth in jobs with upward mobility and a living wage.

Some costs are involved to improve child welfare. But the investment in protecting boys is considerably less than the resources needed to contain the criminal behavior of angry young men who, as a result of child abuse, may not properly develop into mature adults. A year of imprisonment costs $30 000 to $36 000 per boy, roughly the same amount as tuition for one year at Harvard. Troubled youth need facilities designed for rehabilitation and restoration of a sense of human worth, an institution somewhere between a university and a prison (Baum & Bedrick, 1994). Recovering bad boys need opportunities to give back to their community instead of returning from abusive lockups with a desire for revenge against a culture that subjected them to rape and torture. Numerous learning and behavioral studies demonstrate that punishment is the least effective means for creating lasting change in people. Positive reinforcement for new behaviors and education produce the most significant results (Clark, 1991). Broken homes, poverty, neglect, abuse, parental substance abuse, and criminality all contribute, as they did for me, to children becoming abandoned to the wasteland of the juvenile justice system.

The bulk of public money, however, continues to go toward punitive restraint, a practice that has little or no efficacy in reducing violence. Many fear that humanistic treatment of young offenders reads as "soft on crime" or encourages lawlessness. Politicians pander to voters' fears, urging more police and prisons, as though this will magically solve the deep-rooted economic and social problems that cause most violent crimes.

When we create opportunities for alienated youth to come into positive contact with public safety officials, however, it can go a long way to bridge the divide between angry young men and the law. Police officers who demonstrate that they regard young men as a part of the community they "protect and serve" can win their respect. After all, boys on the street have the highest victimization rates of all citizens.

In community law enforcement, cops walk the street and live in the same neighborhoods they patrol. They get to know the people there. They may know the kids by name and where they live. Positive community policing can go a long way to forging strong alliances with at-risk youth while better ensuring public safety at the same time. Midnight basketball games, often sponsored by police organizations, are successful in creating a context where bad boys and police officers can begin to forge positive and productive relationships with one another. When a pilot program in Arizona kept basketball courts open until 2:00 AM, juvenile crime dropped about 50%. The cost of the program was 60 cents per boy (Chaiken, 1996).

A graduate student of mine runs summer workshops where police officers and gang members act in Shakespearean plays together. They become a community of creative artists, and, at least for a few months, largely transcend their antagonistic roles. Most bad boys are hungry for positive attention, especially from older males with strength and power. Police officers fit that bill. These sorts of activities are as legitimate a form of crime prevention as enforcement. Some boys, unconsciously, act out just so some strong man will show up in their lives, even in a negative role. Bad boys often respond well when any powerful adult shows a genuine interest in their welfare. Many long to come in from the cold.

Recommendations for rehabilitation programs include the following (Miller, 1998):

— Move youthful offenders out of remote, isolated institutions into secured environments near populations that can provide educational and social services, community volunteer programs, and regular interactions with family members.

— Reduce caseloads of probation officers so they can provide intensive supervision and integrated support services for youth returning to the community.

— Establish citizen oversight of locked institutions—similar to police review boards—to assure zero tolerance toward the abuse and neglect of boys behind bars.

— End solitary confinement and corporal punishment in all juvenile institutions.

— Provide rights for juvenile mental patients against involuntary commitment and medication equal to those granted adults.

— Increase public awareness about how expanded criminalizing and pathologizing of young male behavior is skyrocketing the rates of hospitalizations and incarcerations.

— Provide substance abuse treatment, therapy, education, parenting education, and literacy and vocational training in all locked juvenile facilities to help break generational cycles of poverty and violence.

— Enact zero tolerance toward rape, sexual slavery, and forced prostitution commonly perpetrated on youth in prisons.

— Create more voluntary community treatment centers, staffed with professionals trained to help youth at risk, that can stand between troubled boys and locked institutions.

— Once the centers are established, eliminate juvenile jails and prisons except for the minority of incarcerated youth who are a proven threat to public safety.

Today, I am a taxpayer instead of a burden on the state. I am one of the few lucky ones who got an opportunity to get an education. That made all the difference. Education is a far less costly and a significantly more effective rehabilitative tool than incarceration. Knowing that, there is much we can do. First we must change our attitudes about the intrinsic worth of youth on the margins and their capacity to exhibit real and significant change, once given a genuine chance to do so.

# REFERENCES

Addison L. Fathers joining ranks of school volunteers. *Los Angeles Times.* June 21, 1998:A3.

Baum N, Bedrick B. *Trading Books for Bars: The Lopsided Funding Battle Between Prisons and Universities.* San Francisco, Calif: Center on Juvenile and Criminal Justice; 1994.

Blankenhorn D. *Fatherless America.* New York, NY: Basic Books; 1995.

Burton DF, Bwanausi C, Johnson J, Moore L. The relationship between traumatic exposure, family dysfunction, and post-traumatic stress symptoms in male juvenile offenders. *J Trauma Stress.* 1994;7:83-93.

Cantelon S, LeBoeuf D. *Keeping Young People in School: Community Programs That Work*. Washington, DC: US Dept of Justice, Office of Justice Programs, Office of Juvenile Justice and Delinquency Prevention; 1997.

Centers for Disease Control and Prevention. Recommended framework for presenting injury mortality data. *MMWR Recomm Rep*. 1997;46(RR-14):1-30.

Chaiken M. *Youth Afterschool Programs and the Role of Law Enforcement* [videotape]. Washington, DC: National Institute of Justice; 1996.

Clark CH. *Analysis of Return Rates of the Inmate College Program Participants: Follow-up Study of a Sample of Offenders Who Earned High School Equivalency Diplomas While Incarcerated*. New York, NY: State Dept of Correctional Services; 1991.

Cooley-Quille M, Turner S, Beidel D. The emotional impact of children's exposure to community violence: a preliminary study. *J Am Acad Child Adolesc Psychiatry*. 1995; 34:1362-1368.

Courtney M. *Foster Facts*. Madison: Irving Piliavin School of Social Work, University of Wisconsin; 1998.

Craig C, Derek H. *The State of the Children: An Examination of Government-Run Foster Care*. Washington, DC: Institute for Children, National Center for Policy Analysis; 1997.

Cwayna K. *Knowing Where the Fountains Are: Stories and Stark Realities of Homeless Youth*. Minneapolis, Minn: Fairview/Deaconess Press; 1993.

Dawson JM, Langan PA. *Murder in Families*. Washington, DC: Bureau of Justice Statistics; 1994.

Friedfel S. *Research on Improving School Safety: The Role of Technology and Reduced Class Size*. National School Board Association Survey. Washington, DC: National Center for Education Statistics; 1998.

Gelles RJ, Loseke DR, eds. *Current Controversies on Family Violence*. Thousand Oaks, Calif: Sage Publications; 1993.

Gibson P. *Gay Male and Lesbian Youth Suicide: Report of the Secretary's Task Force on Youth Suicide*. Washington, DC: US Dept of Health and Human Services; 1989.

Gilligan J. *Violence: Our Deadly Epidemic and Its Causes*. New York, NY: Putnam; 1996.

Greenblatt M, Robertson MJ. Lifestyles, adaptive strategies, and sexual behaviors of homeless adolescents. *Hosp Community Psychiatry*. 1993;44:1177-1180.

Greene J, Ringwalt CL, Kelly JE, Iachan R, Cohen Z. *Youth With Runaway, Throwaway, and Homeless Experiences: Prevalence, Drug Use, and Other At-Risk Behaviors*. Washington, DC: US Dept of Health and Human Services, National Clearinghouse on Children, Youth, and Families; 1995.

Horn WF. *Father Facts*. 3rd ed. Gaithersburg, Md: National Fatherhood Initiative; 1998.

Kipnis A. *Knights Without Armor: A Practical Guide for Men*. Los Angeles, Calif: Jeremy P Tarcher Inc; New York, NY: Putnam and Sons; 1991.

Krug EG, Powell KE, Dahlberg LL. Firearm-related deaths in the United States and 35 other high- and upper-middle-income countries. *Int J Epidemiol*. 1998;27(2): 214-221.

Louis Harris and Associates. Poll for the Commonwealth Fund. *Washington Post*. March 31, 1998;Health section:5.

Margolin L. Child abuse by mothers' boyfriends: why the overrepresentation? *Child Abuse Negl*. 1992;16(4):545-546.

Marin P. Why are the homeless mainly single men? *The Nation.* July 8, 1991:46-51.

May R. *Income and Poverty Trends.* Washington, DC: Center on Budget and Policy Priorities; 1995:22-23.

Mayo Clinic. A parent's guide to prevention of sports injuries. Available at: http://www.mayoclinic.com. Accessed August 28, 1998.

Miller J. *Last One Over the Wall.* 2nd ed. Columbus: Ohio State University Press; 1998.

Morton-Young T. *After-School and Parent Education Programs for At-Risk Youth and Their Families: Guide to Organizing and Operating a Community-Based Center for Basic Educational Skills Reinforcement, Homework Assistance, Cultural Enrichment, and a Parent Involvement Focus.* Springfield, Ill: Charles C. Thomas Publisher; 1995.

National Center for Education Statistics (NCES). *The Condition of Education.* Washington, DC: Dept of Education; 1997.

National Coalition for the Homeless (NCH). Fact Sheets # 3, 6, & 11. May 1997-January 1998. Available at: http://www.nationalhomeless.org. Accessed August 11, 2003.

Pasco JO. Orange County unveils children services plan. *Los Angeles Times.* September 3, 1998:A1, 24.

Robertson M. *Homeless Youth on Their Own.* Berkeley, Calif: Alcohol Research Group; 1996.

Roman NP, Phyllis BW. *Web of Failure: The Relationship Between Foster Care and Homelessness.* Washington, DC: National Alliance to End Homelessness; 1995.

Sedlak AJ, Broadhurst DD. *The Third National Incidence Study of Child Abuse and Neglect: Final Report.* Washington, DC: US Dept of Health and Human Services; 1996.

Shinn M, Weitzman B. Homeless families are different. In: Baumohl J, ed. *Homelessness in America.* Washington, DC: National Coalition for the Homeless; 1996:109-122.

Sickmund M, Snyder HN, Poe-Yamagata E. *Juvenile Offenders and Victims: 1997 & 1996 Updates on Violence.* Washington, DC: Office of Juvenile Justice and Delinquency Prevention; 1997.

Smith C, Thornberry TP. The relationship between childhood maltreatment and adolescent involvement in delinquency. *Criminology.* 1995;33:451-479.

Sobsey D, Randall W, Parrila RK. Gender differences in abused children with and without disabilities. *Child Abuse Negl.* 1997;21(8):707-720.

Steinbeck J. *The Grapes of Wrath.* New York, NY: The Viking Press; 1939.

Straus MA, Donnelly DA. *Beating the Devil out of Them: Corporal Punishment in American Families.* New York, NY: Lexington Books; 1994:112-113.

Straus MA, Gelles RJ, Steinmetz SK. *Behind Closed Doors: Violence in the American Family.* London, England: Sage Publications; 1988.

United Nations. *Special Rapporteur on Torture.* New York, NY: UN Document E/CN; 1988.

US Bureau of the Census. *Money Income in the United States: 1997. Current Population Reports, P60-200.* Washington, DC: US Government Printing Office; 1998.

US Department of Health and Human Services (USDHHS). Child maltreatment 1999: reports from the states to the National Child Abuse and Neglect Data System.

Available at: http://www.acf.hhs.gov/programs/cb/publications/cm99/index.htm. Accessed September 22, 2004

US Department of Health and Human Services (USDHHS). *Survey on Child Health.* Washington, DC: National Center for Health Statistics; 1993.

Waxman L, Trupin R. *A Status Report on Hunger and Homelessness in America's Cities.*

Washington, DC: US Conference of Mayors; 1997. Weber T. Caretakers routinely drug foster children. *Los Angeles Times.* May 17, 1998:1, 30-32.

Wendell DA, Onorato IM, McCray E, Allen DM, Sweeney PA. Youth at risk: sex, drugs, and human immunodeficiency virus. *Am J Dis Child.* 1992;146(1):76-81.

World Health Organization (WHO). *World Health Statistics Annual 1993: Causes of Death by Sex and Age.* Geneva, Switzerland: WHO; 1995.

Yi D. A closer look at campus fights. *Los Angeles Times.* May 4, 1998:B1.

# Adult Survivors of the Child Sexual Exploitation Industry: Psychological Profiles

Mary Anne Layden, PhD
Linnea W. Smith, MD

Children who are victims of child prostitution and child pornography become adults, but what kinds of adult lives do they lead? In this chapter, we will examine the adult consequences for the survivors of the child sexual exploitation (CSE) industry. Children suffer not only immediate consequences but as adults they also suffer long-term consequences. Looking at the adult outcomes of these childhood catastrophes, we can unpack and unscramble the beliefs the children learned and what they learned about coping with these events. We can see what skills they did not learn and how all of these factors have affected their adult functioning. Some victims never make it to adulthood; some victims become adults whose functioning is minimal. Others suffer the damage and show the signs but then work to rise above it and move from being victims to being survivors. These are stories about their journey toward healing.

## The Victims

### Claire

When Claire walks down the street, she looks at each man she passes, and mentally she asks, "Have you seen them?" She is referring to the pictures taken of her uncle having sex with her when she was a child. Her uncle had stacks and stacks of pornographic magazines with kids in them. He would show her the pictures and then ask her to replicate what the kids were doing. Sometimes he would show her pictures of adults in pornographic magazines and tell her how proud he would be if she could do those things. She felt physically and visually invaded by him. She would argue with him, but he said he would hurt her family if she did not do what he asked and finally she would give up. He would call his friend in to take the photographs and Claire would mentally leave her body.

Now as an adult when she walks down the street, she feels invaded and vulnerable all over again. She feels ashamed and bad all over again. She feels her hatred and mistrust of men all over again. She relives the agony each day. She is like a combat veteran who still thinks he is being shot at when he hears a car backfire. The trauma of her experience in child pornography does not end for her just because she is an adult. The images are a record of her abuse, and the images are still available. They are out on the market. They are traded on the Internet. They show up in pedophile magazines. The incestuous abuses by her uncle and the abuses by the child pornographer who took the photos were followed by the abuses by all of the pedophiles who have looked at the images since then. She feels completely helpless and believes that there is nothing she can do to end the cycle. She is constantly waiting for someone to find the pictures and confront her. She thinks that it might ruin the life she has built for herself now. Her whole life could be upended in an instant.

Her thoughts when she sees women and children are very different. She thinks women and children can see her "badness." She thinks that her defectiveness and her brokenness show through. She describes it like a stain on the wall that shows through even after it has been covered with new paint. She thinks she is different from other people and there is nowhere to hide. Her pain is close to the surface.

Whenever she is in a relationship and thinks the other person cares for her, she thinks that she has fooled them. She thinks that they do not know her "real self"; her real self is dirty. She thinks the others are stupid or pretending to care about her or just about to stop caring about her. She has no idea how other people make their relationships last so long. She has no idea how they behave or talk to each other. She assumes that her relationships end because of her core of badness and that it has nothing to do with how she behaves in intimate interactions. She gets clingy in relationships when she thinks the other person is about to leave the relationship. When that does not work, she reverses her strategy and starts to distance herself from others and stays aloof.

## GLORIA

Gloria has a different history from Claire, but in some ways their stories are similar. Gloria's history includes being raped by her father when she was 8 years old. Her mother had just moved out and her father got drunk. He kept his soft-core pornographic magazines in the living room on the TV stand. After her mother left, he would get drunk once or twice a week, look at the magazines, and rape her. Her father said that Gloria dressed "slutty" and that is why he raped her. Gloria silently tried to challenge the idea that it was her fault, but the child in her believed that what adults said was true. The rapes continued until she was 13, when she ran away. She took money out of her father's wallet and bought a bus ticket. Her destination was anywhere but where she had come from. She could afford a ticket to a large city about 100 miles from her home, so that is where she went. Once she arrived, she had no idea what she would do. That's when she met Fran. Fran gave Gloria a place to stay, food, and advice. It felt like she was being cared for at a moment in her life when she was the most alone and scared. Fran had a plan; Gloria could earn some money by being sexual with some of Fran's friends. The first night it was just manual masturbation and oral sex. By the third night it was intercourse. The next week she was walking the streets looking for men to have sex with. Gloria was still 4 months shy of her 14th birthday.

Gloria is now 36. She feels the same shame and badness felt by Claire. She feels the same defectiveness, vulnerability, and powerlessness felt by Claire, although she covers it with a tough exterior. She often uses her voice and face to send daggers of contempt at people. She uses it to protect herself. Sometimes she threatens to physically hurt other people. She has the same mistrust and hatred for men that is felt by Claire, but Gloria also hates women and even sometimes children. She has missed out on how to show compassion and care to others.

## JANE

Both Gloria and Claire remember what happened to them. In contrast, Jane does not remember everything that happened. Jane's family was large, with 9 children. Her parents were so dysfunctional that they would not have been able to take care of even one child effectively. Jane was the oldest so she got the message that she was in charge of taking care of her younger siblings. Later Jane would get the message that she was in charge of taking care of her parents as well. Jane remembers some of the physical abuse. If she was bad, she would have her head held under water or be locked in a closet for many hours. She also remembers some of the sexual abuse; she recalls being taken by her aunt and uncle to their house so that they could take some pictures. Although she does not remember the pictures being taken, she does remember later getting her younger sisters to pose sexually (eg, spread their legs or turn around and bend over) and pretending to photograph them. She can not remember where she had learned such poses, but she remembers feeling very shameful doing it. Jane thinks that the pictures that were taken of her and the pictures she pretended to take of her sisters were her fault.

Jane is now 28. She spent 10 years taking drugs to numb the pain. She spent years unemployed. Her anxiety was debilitating, and she could not speak in front of groups. She started to work part-time and worked for a while with abused children. The children's problems triggered strong emotional reactions in Jane, so she switched to working with the elderly and that was somewhat better. She has the same beliefs as Claire and Gloria. She believes she is bad and powerless and that others can not be trusted. She tries to control things so that she will not get hurt. The idea of relaxation feels foreign and more than a little scary to her.

## Joyce

Finally, there is Joyce. Her stage name is Sabrina. She says she was not sexually abused as a child. At least that is what she said when she started therapy. She said she knew at 6 years old that she would be a stripper and a pornography model. It did not seem strange to her that she knew about strippers and pornography models at 6 years of age. She remembers sitting on her grandfather's lap when she was 4 or 5 or 6; he would show her pornographic magazines. He would show her Playboy and tell her she was just as pretty as the models were. Later he would show her pornographic movies and have her watch with him. He once smuggled her into a strip club so she could see the strippers. Her mother was a stripper, and her grandfather wanted Joyce to see her mother strip. He took pictures of Joyce doing the same moves she had seen her mother do. This all seemed normal to Joyce. She thought none of this was child sexual abuse. Sex was how you got attention. Everyone she knew was involved with the sexual exploitation industry, so she felt that it must be normal. She came into treatment because she was concerned that her drinking and drug use had gotten out of control. When she would try to stop drinking, the manager at the strip club would insist that she accept drinks from the customers. Joyce did not feel that she was using alcohol to cover up pain. She also knew that if she tried to cut down on the drugs she used, she would feel so bad that she "had to use."

Joyce said that all of her relationships were short-term, and that troubled her. She had little insight as to why the men she picked never seemed to develop and sustain a relationship with her. She said that her self-esteem was fine. It had been "improved" years before with artificial breasts. She figured with these assets that she should be having a fine career and attracting many men. However, stripping was not turning out financially as she had expected, and the pornographic magazines and videos did not pan out. She had started to engage in prostitution to supplement her stripper earnings, although she denied that what she was doing was prostitution. She said she just had intercourse for money in the VIP room of the strip club but that she "wasn't a prostitute."

When Joyce entered treatment, she had no idea what she would do if she did not work in the sexual exploitation industry. She had never considered what she liked to do, what her talents were, or how to interact with others except through the sexual economy. Both her relationships and her work life showed the effects of the damage.

# Childhood Trauma

The lives of Claire, Gloria, Jane, and Joyce exemplify the lives of many others. These victims came into treatment as adults as the walking wounded. By the time they enter therapy, their childhood traumas are 10, 20, or even 30 years old. Sometimes their experiences with the sexual exploitation industry are part of their child-hood pasts; sometimes such experiences have spilled over into their adult present. Sometimes the therapist is the first person they have told about the trauma. Some of them do not even think of it as trauma when they first begin therapy. At the time of the original trauma there may have been physical damage. There may have been torn vaginal tissue or bruises, or there may have been physical restraint, but now all evidence has disappeared. There may have been hurtful people populating their lives. Many of the original hurtful people are gone now as well. These all may have been elements of the original trauma, but since these elements no longer exist, how does past trauma impact their present life? The effects of trauma on adult survivors of CSE comprises 3 elements: the beliefs the child learned at the time, the behaviors they developed to cope with those beliefs, and the life skills that they did not learn. As adults, they often think and behave like they did as children. They learned the lessons well. They are burned in, seared in, by the fire of the emotion that was present at the time. Their minds and hearts and souls were branded with the meanings of these events. They have tried to construct an adult life with wounds and missing pieces, and it shows.

## TRAUMA BELIEFS

The trauma beliefs are the child's perception and interpretation of the trauma. These may be the conclusions that the child drew about herself or others. The beliefs that are focused on herself tend to revolve around 2 areas: lovability and power. The beliefs about others often involve issues of trust. These beliefs are summarized in **Table 7-1** and are discussed below. The child learns to rationalize their experiences with these beliefs, which then persist into adulthood.

---

**Table 7-1. Beliefs of Childhood Sexual Industry Victims**

BELIEFS ABOUT THEMSELVES: LOVABILITY

— I'm dirty, disgusting, bad, and morally corrupt.
— I'm to blame for what happened to me. I caused it.
— I must have liked what happened to me. If I liked any part of it, it means I liked all of it.
— Sex is the only thing about me that is valuable. Sex is the only currency.
— In order to get others to pay attention to me, I have to use sex. I'm so broken I can't trust my feelings. Others say I like things that I don't think I like.
— If I can get people to have sex with me or to want to have sex with me, it means I am lovable and worthwhile. Sex is lovability.

BELIEFS ABOUT THEMSELVES: POWER

— I'm weak and vulnerable.
— There is nothing I can do to make my situation better.
— I have no right or I am unable to tell others that I don't want to have sex with them, and they wouldn't stop even if I did. I can't protect my boundaries or stop or limit the visual or physical invasion.
— If I get people to have sex with me or to want to have sex with me, it means I am powerful. Sex is power.

BELIEFS ABOUT OTHERS: TRUST

— Other people will use me, abuse me, take advantage of me, and then leave me.
— People you think you can trust or who are the most intimate with you hurt you the most.
— Other people will find out what happened to me and judge me or hurt me because of it.
— Don't expect sex, love, and long-term commitment to be connected. People will never love me, and they will always leave. Take sex as a substitute.
— Others only want sex from me and they want to hurt me. Sex and violence are connected.

## Beliefs About Themselves: Lovability

Self-esteem is the core of the human psyche. The need for self-esteem seems to be hard-wired into the human species. People want to think well of themselves; they want to believe they are lovable and worthwhile. They want to be accepted as they are. This desire drives and propels people. Those who do not possess self-esteem will be in pain, and they will strive to increase it. Self-esteem is to the psyche as air is to the body. If the body does not have enough air, nothing else will matter at that moment, and the body will strive with focus and intensity and do whatever is necessary to obtain it. The desire for self-esteem seems to be just as psychologically important. The drive for self-esteem in those who do not have it is similarly intense, focused, and hard-wired.

However, while the desire for self-esteem is hard-wired, the content of self-esteem must be learned. Each family, each subculture, and each culture send messages about what is valuable and needed to achieve self-esteem. The content messages indicate what one needs to do, be, own, or have in order to experience self-esteem. For example, some families, cultures, and subcultures believe money is a path to self-esteem. The ones who have the most money are the ones who can think well of themselves; often, members of these groups think they are better than others. In some families, cultures, and subcultures, job status or productivity is the criteria. If one works a lot, works well, and/or works at a prestigious job, then he or she is high on the self-esteem continuum. Some measures of self-esteem tend to be gender-related. If a woman is beautiful, large-breasted, and slender, she may have self-esteem. These beliefs also tell us what we must do if we do not have self-esteem. If money is the measure of self-worth and we have none, then we must attain money. If we still do not think that we are worthy, then we must attempt to attain even more money.

The tutoring of these messages may be subtle or blatant. In some families, the socialization is spoken clearly, directly, and repeatedly and may include criticism if one does not measure up. "Why don't you get a better job that makes more money? Others make more money than you do. What is wrong with you that you can't get ahead financially?" "That's great that you got a job! How much does it pay?" "Don't major in that area in school. You can't make much money doing that." All of these messages send some version of the same message. "I will think well of you, and you may think well of yourself, if you make money. I think well of others who make money, and they should think well of themselves. I don't respect those who don't make money, and they should not respect themselves."

If a child has been sent a message by her family and/or society that she is not good enough, these messages about how to increase self-esteem may get activated, and the child may use these messages to direct her efforts. Often school, friends, church, and the media support or challenge these messages. When there is a great deal of commonality in the messages from a number of different sources and little challenge from competing sources, the lessons are deeply learned. If the family messages are the same as the subculture, the larger culture, the school, and the media, these messages may be seen as truisms.

In addition, the child or adult will often seek out sources that support the messages that were originally learned from other places. She will seek out friends and media messages that support what she has been taught elsewhere. These feel familiar. Contradictory messages may seem not just unfamiliar but strange, bizarre, silly, and/or misguided. The child or adult may judge others who disagree with her as odd or stupid. Having rejected other sources that disagree, she feels affirmed. This can either strengthen self-esteem if the child or adult feels that she is meeting the criteria for self-esteem or strengthen a desire for self-esteem if she feels that the criteria are not being met. For example, if money is the issue, the adult may bask in her financial success or spend energy and time striving for more money.

This pattern is diverted if the child or adult thinks she will never meet the criteria for self-esteem. If this conclusion is reached early in childhood, it may develop into an unconditional belief. "I'm completely, totally, and irreversibly worthless and broken. I'm bad and unlovable and therefore permanently lacking in self-esteem." This situation is devastating. Rather than striving to win the game, the child or adult believes that she is unable to do so. She may try to develop cover-up strategies to keep other people from being aware of her worthlessness or publicly try to deny feelings of inadequacy. The child or adult can develop counter-self-esteem strategies. These counter-strategies may support antagonistic values. For example, if others think that money is what gives one self-esteem, then the child or adult will think that poverty is what gives one self-esteem.

The child who has been victimized by the sexual exploitation industry is like any other child and wants to think that she is lovable, worthwhile, and deserving of self-respect. This ingrained desire for self-esteem does not seem to be diminished by the abuse. When a child does not feel worthwhile, she wants to figure out the rules for raising self-esteem. However, the messages that are being sent to the child are ones that are the opposite of what she needs to receive. The child leaves the traumatic childhood experience thinking that she is not lovable. "My only worth to others is in sexually servicing them and meeting their sexual needs. My needs are unimportant. I can only get love and attention through sex."

One frequent belief of sexually abused children is self-blame. "I must have caused this" is often thought. Sometimes the perpetrator directly tutors this belief. "Look what you make me do" is common perpetrator talk. The perpetrator often uses denial to deal with his or her own reactions to his or her own behavior. This denial of responsibility by the perpetrator encourages the child to feel responsible. If a child thinks she caused her abuse, her self-esteem can be damaged. "What kind of person causes this kind of terrible event? Since I caused it I must now be disgusting, broken, defective, or degraded by the experience." So by causing the event or by experiencing the event, she feels that she is or has become worthless.

Some perpetrators tell victims that they liked the abuse. The child may think, "What kind of person would like this experience? I must be disgusting." It may also confuse the child. She may think, "I don't think I like this, but I am told that I do." A child can conclude that she does not know her own feelings and can not trust her own re-actions. She may decide that she does not like this but that she should, so something is wrong with her reaction. Often the perpetrator shows the child pornographic im-agery to convince her that this kind of behavior is pleasurable. The child believes that she can not trust her own reactions because she is being told to enjoy something that seems so painful. The children in the pornography seem to be enjoying the expe-rience, making the abused child think she is different. So the raped, molested, pros-tituted, or pornographically photographed child may leave the experience thinking, "I caused it. I liked it. I can't trust my reactions. I'm degraded, dirty, and worthless. Sex is the only thing I'm good for and the only way to get attention."

The adult survivor may still believe some or all of these things. The consequences in the adult life are devastating. They can affect self-esteem, relationships with others, or work. If an adult thinks, "I'm bad," she may be prone to depression. There may be periods when she finds it hard to function because of depression. She may not be able to get daily tasks done. If the adult has a job, her work performance may suffer. Even getting out of bed or taking a shower may seem hard. She may have trouble sleeping and may eat too much or too little. Emotions may be constantly low and mixed with crying spells. Social interactions may be avoided. Things that used to give the adult pleasure have stopped making her feel good, so they are avoided. All of these symp-toms of depression are maintained and exacerbated by the badness belief.

This belief may progress in the adult to self-injurious behaviors. She may cut herself, burn herself, or punch herself in the stomach with her fist. Sometimes the physical pain caused by these behaviors can temporarily distract the adult from the psychological pain of thinking about her own badness.

The adult might develop an eating disorder supported by this badness belief. If she is taught that she can increase self-esteem by having others think she is attractive, she may do anything to gain that reaction. The adult may starve herself to control eating. She may vomit, take laxatives, or exercise for hours daily to control weight.

A sense of worthlessness adversely affects her relationships as well. She feels most comfortable with others who agree with her self-assessment. She will gravitate toward relationships and behaviors that feel familiar. This leads to relationships that are abusive, degrading, and based upon sex as a commodity. They all feel like "home." Such a woman may be willing to tolerate fake intimacy because real intimacy is unfamiliar. In her early experiences, others did not care enough about her to protect her, get to know her, support her growth, or teach her to make decisions that enhance her life. Relationships that include support and stability make her feel strange and uncomfortable.

Some of these women seem to get involved only with men who are antisocial, and some of them have pimp-like relationships with all men. Often, a woman will chose a man who uses her either emotionally or psychologically. Usually these men control the woman by offering acceptance and love and then withdrawing it. They tell the woman that she is to blame and has done something wrong. This "look what you made me do" stance feels familiar from childhood. She is primed to believe that and to work harder to get the acceptance back. The men she is with may rape her or expect to have sex whenever they want. They may watch pornographic movies and then demand that the woman do whatever is seen in the movie. The woman often does not think she can say no to sex even if it involves violence or other activities that she finds painful or distasteful. She may think that she does not have the right to refuse sex just because she does not want to have sex right now. She may feel that she has to go along with requests that she look a certain way, dress a certain way, or wear her hair a certain way. He may demand that she maintain her body in a way that pleases him sexually. He may also believe that he is entitled to have sex with other women and that she should not object. Her home life may in many ways symbolically resemble a strip club or a brothel. The men have beliefs that this is all normal, and they have often been involved in the sex industry in some aspect as "customer" or "boss," which lends support to their beliefs. These permission-giving beliefs held by the men make them feel justified in how they treat women, and the women have also been tutored by the sexual exploitation industry to share the same permission-giving beliefs. This all feels like a repeat of childhood and is familiar to the exploited woman.

Some men may batter a woman and say that she caused the beating. They may use threats of violence against the woman, her children, or even her pets to keep her in line. They may break her things or be violent to others to let her know what they are capable of doing. If a woman leaves such a man, he may stalk her or harass her by phone or in person. He may come to her job or approach her coworkers or her boss to try to cause problems for her. He acts like (and she may also think that) she is his property. All of this feels like versions of the woman's childhood.

These factors increase risk for involvement with the adult sexual exploitation industry. Such a woman has men in her life who have the permission-giving beliefs that are spawned by the sexual exploitation industry, including pornography and prostitution. The woman is used to abusive, battering, pimp-like men who use her to meet their own needs. She feels degraded, and she is drawn to others who agree. The woman believes that her worth is attached to sexual attractiveness and availability and that an increase in self-esteem can come from increased sexual attention.

## Beliefs About Themselves: Power

Children need to feel competent and safe. They need to know that they can get what is important to them. When children live in a benign environment, they expect that adults, usually parents, will protect them. They think that parents will provide for them and if they have a need, it will be met. Their sense of safety and protection comes from living in this loving, nurturing, and providing environment.

As they get older they need to know that they can provide for themselves. They need to think they are powerful and competent and that through their own actions they can get what they need and make themselves safe. When their competence is tested, they need to think that they can do well in areas that are important. Self-esteem is connected not only to being lovable but also to being competent and powerful. Most parents send messages to kids about which areas of life are important in order to succeed. These areas could be academics, sports, or moral behavior. The society, the culture, the subculture, the school, the media, and the church can echo or negate these messages. Children's self-esteem is affected by knowing what the important areas of life are and trying to shine in those areas. If they fail in these areas, they feel powerless and incompetent.

Children who have been abused also have strong beliefs about their safety, power, and competence. In the area of safety, the abuse sends a strong message that the world is not a safe place. If the abuse happens in the home, the place that was supposed to be the safest is not safe at all. Sometimes the abuse happens because the child ran away from a home situation that was not safe.

All of this leaves children feeling powerless. They think, "I should have been able to stop the abuse. So I must be powerless and therefore worthless." "I should have been able to take care of myself or control the situation when I was on the street." They often forget the threats, force, coercion, or blackmail that is used to get them to participate. They also forget that they are children and perpetrators are adults. Sometimes children begin to think of themselves as mature and powerful before the abuse takes place. So when the abuse starts, they think they should do something about it. They do not remember that children have significantly fewer resources than do adults. They do not have knowledge of the world as a resource. They do not have money and multiple ways to earn money. Often they do not have a car or may not be old enough to even get a driver's license. Sometimes children, rather than think of themselves as victims, start to think of their exploitation as a failure to protect themselves.

Given these factors, what can children do to feel powerful, competent, and safe? What are the messages from the family, the subculture, the culture, and the media that tell children what they can do to think well of themselves in terms of competence and power? Often sexual abuse victims come from families or experiences in which sexuality is the currency of power. "I am powerful if I attract sexual attention and sexual partners. I can feel powerful if I control this experience." "I can get money through sex and no other way, and money is power. So sex is the only power." "I can only feel powerful if I run away from my perpetrators."

The results are children who are primed to run away to feel powerful and safe; children who are primed to use sex as power and self-esteem. These are children who have few resources to care for themselves, which puts them at great risk to fall into prostitution and child pornography. If this happens, it will reinforce all the messages that were learned in the abuse that predated it. The prostitution and pornography will solidify the belief that worthiness is achieved through sex. These experiences also repeat the message that other people's needs are primary. The CSE industries are replicas of child sexual abuse. They have the same dynamics and are supporting and spreading the same messages—sex equals power equals self-esteem.

For adults who were abused by the CSE industry, their sense of power and competence often mirrors the child's. Some work in the adult sexual exploitation industry and say they feel powerful. For them, getting paid money to be sexually exploited feels more powerful than having the experience for free. For some women, controlling certain aspects, such as the hours they work at the strip club or the number of customers they have sex with that night, seems more powerful than when they were children and had no other choices. In reality, they are reenacting their childhood abuse.

Even those who do not work in the adult sexual exploitation industry often try to control things to feel powerful. They may control other people, their households, their food, or their work. Any of these can add to the sense that the world is under control. If they control their food intake, they feel more in control in general. If they still feel out of control, then they may try to monitor their food intake even more. Their eating disorders are supported by the beliefs in their badness and powerlessness, which may be why eating disorders such as anorexia and bulimia appear so frequently in these women. Some control their emotions as a way to feel powerful. Emotions are messy and, therefore, they can not afford to have any. They seem determined not to let anything affect them.

All of these forms of power and control are, in reality, pseudo power and control. These are not totally free decisions. They do not reflect the true desires and wishes of the individual. They do not really make the world safer and less chaotic. Many of them have harmful consequences; individuals who are truly free to decide do not pick outcomes that cause self-harm. Lesser forms of exploitation are still exploitation.

## Beliefs About Others: Trust

Children are also trying to learn about other people in the world. Can others be expected to help you or hurt you? Parents are the gold standard. These are the people that we can trust the most. Children naturally expect that no one can be trusted more than their parents. If the parents are abusive, then that sets the standard. If parents can not be trusted, then no one can be trusted.

Trust of others is often extremely difficult for adults who were victims of the CSE industry. They have been emotionally and sexually exploited as children. If the parents were involved in their abuse, it is especially devastating. If there were many people involved, that encourages generalization. Their experience tells them that no one can be trusted. These adults often think of abuse from others as the norm.

They may become distrustful of all others or distrust only those in a certain category, for example, men, authority figures, or people who "pretend" to care about them. They may think, "All men are the same" or "Caring behavior is just a strategy that people use to get you to do what they want." If these beliefs are applied broadly rather than specifically, the expectation is that everyone will abuse you, manipulate you, exploit you, and then probably leave you. No relationship feels safe or dependable.

This expectation of abuse leads them to accept abuse from others and think it is normal. Thinking that everyone will hurt them encourages lingering in abusive relationships. Expecting abuse reduces the shock when it happens. They may not think that abusive relationships must end or that abusive relationships can be replaced with nonabusive ones.

Some of the mistrust is directed at sexual relationships. Their mistrust is shown in their beliefs about the nature of male sexuality. They may think that male sexuality is innately narcissistic, predatory, and out of control. They may expect that sex, violence, and pain are connected. They may think that men always want sex, only want sex, or want and take sex from others even if others are hurt by it. Sexual abuse is expected and tolerated. If they are raped, they often do not report it to the police. ("Rape is just part of life, and the police won't help anyway.") Some women hate the men with whom they are involved.

Personal sexual relationships tend to be difficult because of the issue of trusting others. Some women may expect that men will abandon them if they withhold sex on any occasion. They may be vulnerable and anxious when they expose themselves physically to men. They may also feel vulnerable if they allow themselves uninhibited sexual feelings with partners. Some decide to be sexually promiscuous in an attempt not to be sexually or emotionally attached to anyone in particular.

Some of the mistrust is directed at emotional intimacy. Abused women may feel uncomfortable sharing intimate reactions with their partners. They may hide information, believing it will be used against them, misunderstood, or ridiculed. They may be concerned about asking for help. Support of any sort is unexpected. Intimate relationships are difficult to maintain or deepen when paths to intimacy are avoided.

Sometimes the mistrust is directed at other women or children. They may feel competitive and think that all women will try to take from them what they have. They may not ask women for help or expect they will get help if they do ask. They may expect that other women will harshly judge them. Children, even their own, are sometimes seen as a threat. Some decide not to have children; some are abusive or harsh to their children. In very few cases, they sexually abuse their own children. Some women involve their own children in the CSE industry.

Some women who work in the adult sexual exploitation industry have hate-filled or violent thoughts while they are working. Strippers may be thinking that the customers are repulsive while they are behaving as if they find them attractive and desirable. They may smile at their customers while at the same time having a running commentary going through their heads that includes extremely disparaging thoughts about men. Prostitutes may have thoughts that include insults about the customers while they are engaging in sex. This mismatch between their thoughts and their behaviors is in many ways similar to the childhood abuse in which there was a mismatch between what they wanted, what they were feeling, and what they were doing. In the adult sexual exploitation industry they are meeting other people's sexual needs at the expense of their own psychological health, which is also similar to the childhood abuse. This intensifies their distrust and sense of abuse.

## COPING BEHAVIORS

The trauma for abused or exploited adults is not just what they learned to believe but also what they learned to do to cope with childhood events and beliefs. When they were children, they tried to cope with these awful events as best they could. These traumas are the kinds of events that often can not be coped with even with adult resources, and children have even fewer resources. Children do not have the power to make adults stop doing what they are doing. Children do not have a car and a driver's license so they can leave. They do not have the money to buy a lock to put on the door or to set up a new household or the work skills to get a job and support themselves. Sometimes no adults other than the perpetrators know what is happening to the children. Most children would not know whom to tell even if they decided to tell someone. This leaves them with very few coping skills.

The beliefs children have about themselves and others will also affect their coping behaviors. If children believe that they are bad and worthless, they will try to find ways to deal with it or try to hide that information from others. They might try to be people-pleasing to make up for their presumed badness or to avoid people so their badness will not be revealed. If children believe that others can not be trusted, they may use aggression to handle the situation. If children believe they are powerless, they may use dependency and clinging to cope. They will try to manage the situations so that the events are shorter, less frequent, or less painful. They will often hold on to strategies that work only slightly or part of the time. In fact, that may be the best outcome that can be obtained. Coping strategies employed by children are summarized in **Table 7-2**.

Adult survivors of CSE employ the same childhood coping strategies, even when the situations and the people may be very different from those that were present in their childhood. If as adults they still believe they are bad, they may be people-pleasing to cope. They may go along with requests that they dislike. They may make their own needs secondary to everyone else's. They may think that they do not have a right to have their needs met. They may do anything a man asks them to do sexually, do any favor a friend asks them to do, or give in to any request by their children.

Some believe so totally in their own badness that self-harming becomes a coping strategy. The self-harming may be very direct; they might hit, cut, or burn themselves. It could also be more indirect; they might overspend, drive recklessly, have unprotected sex, or eat in a self-abusive manner. These self-harming strategies can distract from the pain momentarily but often lead to an increase in pain due to the consequences or the self-criticism that follows.

Dependency is used to cope with the belief about powerlessness. These victims cling to others who will help and manage their lives for them. They may become enmeshed with others, especially males. They may take on their friends' activities and opinions as they merge their own personalities with those of the men in their lives. Using this strategy, it is very hard for them to maintain their own personalities. Others who feel powerless may become underfunctioning and passive. They may not go to work, get a job, or do anything at home. Some may cling to relationships. This strategy often chases people away rather than binds them.

| Table 7-2. Coping Strategies of Childhood Sexual Exploitation Industry Victims | |
|---|---|
| — People-pleasing | — Avoidance |
| — Self-harming | — Distancing |
| — Dependency | — Overfunctioning |
| — Enmeshment | — Denial |
| — Underfunctioning | — Dissociating |
| — Passivity | — Sex |
| — Clinging | — Aggression |
| — Self-medicating with drugs and/or alcohol | |

If others can not be trusted, these women may cope using aggressive or hostile strategies. They may be quick to anger or quick to strike back. Some may even use preemptive strikes against others who they assume will soon try to hurt them. ("Since others are surely trying to hurt me, then I should hurt them first.") They can be raging with others and angry all the time. Often the angry ones will try to cause problems for others and feel justified. They may treat others unfairly and feel that this action evens out the scales somewhat or is justified by what others would have done to them given the chance. Some may steal, lie, or become physically abusive.

If aggression does not work, they may try avoidance or distancing. They could physically stay away from people by living alone or having few friends, or they may interact with people but psychologically stay at a distance. They may not share personal information or develop close ties.

Some strategies are supported by more than one belief. Overfunctioning may be used for multiple reasons. They think that if they are bad, perhaps they can make up for it by doing more than their share. If the world is full of powerful abusers, then maybe if everything is controlled it will be all right. If they do everything perfectly, then no one can criticize them and nothing will fall apart.

Denial, self-medicating, and dissociating are all caused by multiple factors. Denial makes what is true unbelievable and what is untrue believed. ("I really liked being a child prostitute; I really liked posing for child pornography.") Denial requires a lot of physical and psychological energy. Those who use it have to work mightily to keep it intact. Self-medicating can be used to deal with the pain that comes from beliefs about badness, powerlessness, or mistrust. Drugs and alcohol anesthetize the pain. Self-medicating mixed with denial means that the beliefs do not have to be confronted and changed because they are not even acknowledged. If these strategies fail, they may use dissociation, which is a more extreme form of coping. People who dissociate are not psychologically in their bodies. Mentally they shut down and leave. In the most serious versions, they may lose track of time and not remember what has happened for a period of time or not know how they got where they are.

Adults who work in the adult sexual exploitation industry may use any or all of these coping strategies. They may believe they are bad and deserve to be degraded, that they are powerless and have no other options, or that no one can be trusted, so that working in an industry based on abuse by others may seem run-of-the-mill. The adult sex industry supports and exacerbates these beliefs; the pain level is often very high. They may use denial to justify the work. Denial is often mixed in with permission-giving beliefs such as "Prostitution is normal" or "All men use pornography, so it is normal." Often the customers of the sexual exploitation industry have the same permission-giving beliefs. The customers use these beliefs to justify what they are doing.

The sexual exploitation industry workers may try to bolster their denial by pointing to the money made or the things they can buy or do with the money. Their denial may have to be applied to these statements as well. Often they do not really make as much money as they claim or do not have all the material possessions in their current life as they say they do. Often they are expecting to get things that never seem to materialize. Spending can be used like a drug to dull the pain. They often say that they are saving for a good purpose such as going to college, but usually they do not follow through.

In some cases the denial is a response to their helplessness. ("I'm really powerful now because I make them pay for it this time." "I'm powerful because they want me sexually, and I control how much they get.")

The main coping skill tends to be sex. It is the universal strategy. Sex is a way to get attention, love, self-esteem, money, and protection. The sex act gets disconnected from the sex drives of abused women. For some, the sex drive seems irrelevant or scary; often other drives are mistaken for the sex drive. The thing these women call the "sex drive" could be the urge to be held, the desire to feel safe, the need to defuse someone else's anger, the need for money for food and drugs, the need to feel in control and powerful, or the desire to act out anger toward men. All of these factors could be part of the decision to have sex. For any problem, the answer for these women is sex. The sex drive seems important only if wanting to have sex is an integral part in the decision to have sex. For many of these women, the desire for sex is not part of that decision.

All of these strategies and many more are used to cope with the beliefs that children learned in the trauma and are still believed as adults. The belief that they are bad and powerless and that others can not be trusted spawned coping behaviors that are still used by abused or exploited adults. These behaviors do not work well to make life rich and satisfying, but often the victims think there are no other choices.

## MISSING LIFE SKILLS
The lack of other choices comes from what abused children did not learn to do when

they were growing up. They should have been learning an array of life skills that would help them successfully negotiate the adult world. Children are in "life school." It is a school that trains them to deal with the coming job of adult life. Children need an array of skills that will help them cope (**Table 7-3**). They need communication skills so that they can communicate directly and effectively. They need problem-solving skills and decision-making skills so that they can handle difficult situations and increase positive outcomes. They need intimacy skills, boundary protection skills, trust-judgment skills, and parenting skills to help in relationships. They need self-soothing skills and affect modulation skills so that they are not at the mercy of their emotions. Life is much more difficult if one does not have these skills.

| Table 7-3. Missing Life Skills of Childhood Sexual Exploitation Industry Victims | |
| --- | --- |
| — Intimacy skills | — Decision-making skills |
| — Trust-judgment skills | — Communication skills |
| — Boundary protection skills | — Self-soothing skills |
| — Parenting skills | — Affect modulation skills |
| — Problem-solving skills | — Employment skills |

Typically children begin their education in these skills by watching their parents. For victims of the sexual exploitation industry, this is often impossible. Often the parents were abusers or were so woefully inadequate that they could not stop the abusers. Neither the parents nor the abusers could teach the children the life skills they needed because the adult often did not have these skills. Many times, the skills that these children do learn to use to negotiate the world are maladaptive and learned from perpetrators.

Individuals who would manipulate and lie to a child perpetrated the abuse that they experienced. So children learn that manipulation and dishonesty are common tactics in relationships and that exploitation of others for selfish needs is central to relationships. These children do not learn that honesty, sharing, and mutual care-taking are part of relationships.

As adults, these survivors often lack intimacy skills. The very nature of their childhood experience makes it difficult for them to learn how to interact in healthy ways with others. The lack of intimacy skills causes a number of problems. Adults may still see dishonesty, manipulation, exploitation, and narcissism as normal parts of intimate relationships. They will pick partners who do the same things and will tolerate it when they do. Adults may even behave in the same way toward their partners.

These children learn that no one can be trusted, so they do not learn to judge levels of trustworthiness. Adults may still believe that and are still lacking this skill. This forces adults to interact with people whom they do not trust and to be wary of people who are more trustworthy. People who are only 10% trustworthy are lumped in with those who are 80% trustworthy and are treated the same. Men who are antisocial, drug-addicted, and child-abusing may be trusted to the same degree as men who do not call them the day they say they will. A stranger they meet in a bar who might steal their money might be just as likely to be invited to their home as a relative who teased them as a child.

Intimate revelations in a relationship are typically a gradual process. Without intimacy skills it is hard to know what is appropriate to tell and when. Some victims will tell any stranger the most intimate details of their life; others will not tell even minor intimacies to those who are the closest to them.

Adult survivors may have difficulty protecting their boundaries. They may not know how and when they can limit others' physical and emotional access to them. They may think that they have to have sex with anyone who wants to have sex with them. They may think that they have to answer any question that is put to them. Often they will answer questions that are intrusions on their privacy because they do not know that they can say, "That's none of your business."

Parenting can be a relationship skill that is particularly problematic. Most people's parenting style is similar to their own parents' style. No matter what we promise ourselves when we are children, much of what we do as parents is automatic and is programmed from what was done to us. This is usually effective, but not when parents were abusive or the childhood was fraught with abuse from other adults. For children who were involved in the sexual exploitation industry, their adult model of parenting will reflect that. They may be physically, emotionally, or sexually abusive. They may even get their own children involved in the industry. They sometimes introduce their children to prostitution, stripping, or pimping. They may overtly or covertly pass on their own beliefs, coping skills, and missing life skills to their children.

When difficult situations arise, the adult survivors may have few problem-solving skills to help them cope. They may use sex to "solve" work problems, relationship problems, financial problems, or emotional upsets. The sex might be with partners, coworkers, bosses, or strangers. If this leads to other problems, they have difficulty seeing that the "sexual solution" was implicated in the problematic outcome. Decision-making skills are compromised, and sex may be used again in the future to "solve" the problem. Relationships may be broken, jobs may be lost, diseases may be contracted, and arrests may occur, but they do not stop using sex as a solution. From their point of view, there may be no other choice because they did not learn any other skills. Not knowing how to choose and develop healthy relationships, they often get stuck with others who are willing to also believe that sex is the solution to all problems. Marriages are hard to maintain, and friendships are limited.

The lack of communication skills exacerbates all the other problems. As children they may have experienced "no-talk" rules to keep the secret about what was going on. They may have learned to communicate indirectly, never saying exactly what they meant to the person who needed to hear it. As an adult these missing life skills are devastating. Healthy communication skills are the foundation of good relationships. Effective conflict resolution depends upon communication. Appropriate boundaries and intimacy can not be maintained without communication. Assertiveness is critical when there is a tendency to let abusers into their lives.

When there are emotional upsets, as there will be inevitably, it is important to know how to soothe emotions in healthy ways. Self-medicating with drugs and alcohol may reduce stressful emotions in the short term but produce significant problems later. Unfortunately, drugs and alcohol are often the only self-soothers that the victims know. They might never think to take a walk, talk to a friend, exercise, listen to music, say a prayer, or breathe deeply. In addition, they may not know how to modulate their emotions when what they want to do is experience it but just not at such a high level. Their self-talk may take each emotional reaction and raise it to an extreme level, and they may have no idea what to do when that happens. Emotional overreaction can cause others to avoid them and bosses to fire them; it also develops for them a reputation of being a "loose cannon."

Work is also compromised by the missing employment skills. There are few legitimate jobs that follow the rules embedded in the sex industry. Basic work skills are missing, and a work ethic and good employment behaviors are often missing as well. How to talk and act and the expectation of how to be treated are strange territory. Some who try to make the transition make mistakes of dressing and acting in sexually provocative ways on the job. They may get negative or mixed messages in return for that behavior. Given all that is missing, it should not be surprising how many CSE industry victims manage their relationships with difficulty and underfunction on their jobs. The adult sexual exploitation industry is a natural destination. Few healthy life skills are utilized. Quite the contrary, healthy thinking and behaving may work against entering and staying in the industry.

PSYCHIATRIC OUTCOMES

These beliefs about themselves and others combined with the dysfunctional coping skills and the missing life skills leave exploited children at risk for numerous and serious adult psychiatric problems. The list in **Table 7-4** is a partial list of disorders that show the effect of these problems. A complete list might be exhaustive, because exploited children might be at risk for almost all psychiatric problems. Treatment is not readily available for those who continue to work in the industry; the most typical outcome may be increasingly serious problems with little to mitigate the damage and even less chance of any spontaneous recovery. The stories that follow show the outcomes that may occur if help is available.

# FROM VICTIM TO SURVIVOR OF THE CHILD SEXUAL EXPLOITATION INDUSTRY

Child sexual abuse, the CSE industry, and the adult sexual exploitation industry are part and parcel of the same phenomenon. They are inextricably linked. The cognitions that support them and are produced by them are similar. The damage that is produced by child sexual abuse positions children to be abused in the CSE industry, which positions adults to be abused in the adult sexual exploitation industry. Denial and permission-giving beliefs in children or adults do not mitigate the damage.

The adult lives of women with this kind of history are often an extension of their childhood histories. The cognitions that were produced in childhood are still there, and now they may be more firmly entrenched. They may have found adult manifestations. The denial and the permission-giving beliefs may have been elaborated with adult rationales. However, the dynamics are the same and they are long-lasting. If as adults they tell about the childhood prostitution and pornography experiences for the first time, the pain is so raw that the events seem as if they happened last week. These experiences produce outcomes that do not seem to spontaneously remit. Patients often criticize themselves for that fact. ("It was so long ago. I should be over it by now.") However, the beliefs that they developed at the time of the trauma are still present and are still producing damage. The strategies that they developed at the time of the trauma are still being used to cope. The missing life skills may still be missing. They are still being drawn to what is familiar and are repeating versions of what they first knew. If they work in the adult sexual exploitation industry, they repeat the sexual abuse, and the customers play the role of the perpetrators. These women work in the sex industry because it feels like home.

---

**Table 7-4. Adult Psychological Disorders of Childhood Sexual Exploitation Industry Victims**

| | |
|---|---|
| — Depression | — Substance abuse disorders |
| — Generalized anxiety disorder | — Avoidant personality disorder |
| — Panic disorder | — Dependent personality disorder |
| — Posttraumatic stress disorder | — Borderline personality disorder |
| — Eating disorders | |

---

# SURVIVORS

Let us return to the stories of Claire, Gloria, Jane, and Joyce. In these lives we can see the adult consequences of child prostitution and child pornography.

## CLAIRE

Claire's beliefs about herself that she learned in her early sexual trauma are still present in her adult life. She believes that sex is something people use to hurt other people. When she has sex, she has flashbacks to the childhood abuse. She dissociates to get through it. She wants to be in an intimate relationship and craves the connection, but she thinks that everyone can see her badness and that she is different from the "normal people." She sometimes accuses unsuspecting dates of dating her only because they saw her in child pornography. She has shocked several dates with that accusation. Any relationship that progresses beyond the initial dating phase brings on anxiety for Claire. She feels fraudulent and fears she will be exposed at any moment. She often starts to act aggressively and then switches to dependency and neediness even when neither of these strategies makes sense to her. She is like a wounded animal that has a leg caught in a trap. When someone approaches, she fluffs up her fur and makes growling noises to try and scare them away. If they start to leave, she whimpers to get them to come back. She has never had a relationship that has lasted more than 3 months, although she often "recycles" old boyfriends.

For Claire, the idea that one can say "no" to sex is alien. It never occurred to her that she could tell a man who wanted sex with her that she did not want to have sex with him. She was so startled by the concept when raised in therapy that she asked for specific language that one might use to turn down a man for sex. She wrote the sentence down and said she would spend some time thinking about it. She came back for the next session and discussed it again. She realized that she was subtly sending the wrong signals to men. She never sent any signals to men that she did not want to have sex, and she never set up any boundaries. She would act pleased if a man made sexual innuendo remarks to her even if she did not want to have sex with him. She would invite men over to her apartment and invite them to sit on her bed with her to watch TV when she did not want to have sex with them. The whole concept that she could decide if she wanted to have sex based upon her own sexual desire was alien to her since her childhood led her to believe sex was about other people's needs. On one date, she managed to show some indication that she did not want to have sex. The man picked her up and started to carry her upstairs to the bedroom anyway. She managed to say no again. He finally set her down. After he left she realized that she could have been raped. She was frightened of this man, but when he asked her out again, she said yes. It did not occur to her that she could refuse.

Sexually inappropriate behavior on the part of others is not recognized as such by Claire. When she was a student, she told her brother she was taking a class in sexual studies and was writing a paper on masturbation. Her brother told her father, and her father called Claire. He wanted to know details about the paper and asked Claire if she was masturbating while she was talking to him on the phone. Claire brought up this experience in therapy. She felt uneasy about it but was not sure that she had a right to feel uneasy. She had no sense of what constituted appropriate sexual and privacy boundaries. Even if she knew she felt uneasy, she could not give herself permission to act on that uneasiness. Finally, even if she gave herself permission to act on that uneasiness, she had no skills to do so.

Claire's early sexual experiences and her consequent beliefs also affect her work life. She is often underemployed despite her significant intelligence. She gets upset at work when her mistrust of men is activated. Her bosses are often men, and she finds it hard to think that they might have a benign intent for anything they do. She also enters sexual relationships with male authority figures, including 2 bosses. On one job she got sexually involved with the supervisor who was in charge of ensuring that sexual relationships did not occur between supervisors and employees. She does not see this in any way as contradictory or problematic. She became involved sexually with bosses whom she did not like or with whom she did not want to be sexual. It just seems as if all relationships are based on sex from Claire's point of view. These work relationships end as badly as her personal relationships. Sometimes supervisors threaten her when they decide to end relationships and are concerned that she might cause a problem on the job. In one situation, a supervisor generated a false excuse to fire her.

Her self-esteem is almost defined by her sexuality. She sees her lovability and her competence as sexually based. Even after a number of bad experiences, she feels deeply drawn to men who find her sexually attractive. It feels like this is her only validation. She spends enormous amounts of time, money, and psychological energy in making herself sexually appealing. Everything has to look just right. Hair, clothes, and nails are hugely important. She reads fashion magazines that support that perspective.

She feels powerless without sex and powerless over her sexual behavior. Sex is the only power she has, and if she feels helpless, she reverts to increasing her sexual activity.

## GLORIA

Gloria has given up prostitution, but she still shows signs of the belief system. She lives with a man whom she fears will hurt her physically. He has hit her in the past and even though he says he will not do it again, she does not completely believe him. She lives with him because he has money and will pay all the household bills and she can take her current salary and spend it at her own discretion. She sees this as a completely equitable plan. She has a deep hatred for men, including her father, and she feels this is payback. She works in a legitimate business now but trusts no one. Women are out to get her; men are incompetent and evil. When she talks about the prostitution that started when she was a child and went on until she was well into her 20s, she says the customers taught her about life. She believes she learned skills and other lessons from them. The contradictory reaction to the experience does not seem to register with her. One minute she says the sexual exploitation industry was like going to college, and the next minute she is overcome with rage at everyone who used her. She never sees sex as an intimate act.

Her sense of lovability is often secondary in importance to the issue of power. She wants to make changes in her work life but is concerned about her competence. She realizes that her education was shortchanged. This limits her prospects. Her lack of self-esteem limits her even more. She mistrusts the talents she does have. When she performs well in skilled areas, she seems proud, but it is hard for her to generalize her talent to have expectations about her performance in other areas. The self-esteem boost seems always to be temporary. The self-image she constructed of herself early on seems to be permanent.

In childhood, no one helped Gloria, and now she continues to believe that no one will ever help her. For example, she found it hard to ask for small accommodations at work so that she could take a course. It was also hard for her to ask her life partner if she could skip making dinner one evening a week so she could take the course.

She is missing the life skills of direct communication and trust judgment. Since she does not really trust anyone, she puts everyone in the same category. There are flare-ups with the therapist if the therapist starts the session late. The therapist is assumed to be just as untrustworthy as Fran, the woman who introduced her to prostitution. If the therapist does not return a phone call as soon as expected, the therapist has shown her untrustworthiness again. This inability to recognize trustworthy situations has caused many problems in Gloria's life. Sometimes she involves herself with people she should not and at other times she will not involve herself with people who are consistently supportive. She shrugs it off with, "What's the difference?"

## JANE

Jane does not remember all of what happened to her as a child. She showed signs of sexual abuse by acting out scenes from child pornography with her siblings but does not remember where she learned to do it. She recalled going to a relative's house to be photographed. She later found sexual pictures of her younger brother taken by the same relatives. This was enough evidence to strongly suspect that she was sexually abused in a similar way.

Jane's most prominent self-beliefs concern her helplessness. She feels constantly under threat. Being alone in the house frightens her, as does doing a yoga pose in which she lays on the floor face down, talking in front of groups, getting a job, and speaking up when someone is hurting someone less powerful. Her anxiety was so bad early in her life that she spent years in a drugged and drunken haze. Drugs and alcohol were her main coping strategy.

As Jane struggled to find her way, she got jobs in which she had to protect abused children. This took a psychological toll on her as she struggled not to be overly involved with the kids. This kind of job is difficult for anyone, but for Jane it was excruciating. The childhood message that she was powerless to resist harm confilcts with her adult responsibility to ensure that harm does not befall others. She works tirelessly to try to live up to all of it.

As an adult she follows a similar pattern. She is responsible for everything. She needs to prepare perfect meals after having done perfect shopping. She needs to eat in a perfect way, and it is important to control her food intake. She does not let herself eat "bad foods," but then she will binge on bad foods and criticize herself harshly for being out of control. Jane believes that anything that is not powerfully controlled will spin into damage. Her husband shares these beliefs and expects Jane to do all the household work and to do it perfectly. He is often critical of her if she does not. Her husband mades all of these demands despite being ineffective in his own job. This pattern seems to replicate Jane's childhood. Jane's father was ineffective and expected Jane to take on the responsibilities.

Jane's siblings, who are now all adults, seem to carry with them the belief that Jane is in charge and will fix everything. When her adult siblings act out and get arrested or end up in a hospital, they call Jane instead of their spouses. One brother is active in the adult sexual exploitation industry. This has caused all manner of problems that Jane is expected to fix. When her brother has problems with his marriage because he secretively mortgaged the house to pay for sexual exploitation industry activity, Jane is the one who was approached for a solution. When another brother is arrested for sexually abusing his daughter, Jane is expected to pick up the pieces and save the day. Overfunctioning, responsibility, and control are her coping strategies. In many ways she thinks that if she can fix everyone's problems, it will not only prove that she is worthwhile and lovable but will also keep her safe from the abusers. None of this happens. She never feels worthy, and she never feels powerful and safe.

## JOYCE

Joyce was sexually abused, although she denied it at the beginning of therapy. Showing pornographic magazines to a 4-year-old child is sexual abuse, as is showing her pornographic movies, taking her to a strip club, and photographing her in sexual positions. When a patient denies childhood sexual abuse, one reason may be that it was so normalized that she did not think of it as abuse. Some patients think that only forced intercourse is child sexual abuse. One patient told her therapist that even intercourse was not abuse because the perpetrator did not have a weapon.

One area of dysfunction for Joyce is in the connection of sex and love in relationships. She does not see sex as an intimate act but as a commodity. She thinks of her artificial breasts as a sexual commodity that should attract men and then they should want to have sex with her and that should lead to a relationship. She is confused when it does not. As she says, she has paid "the relationship price" and she has "nice goods," but the relationships do not seem to last. She has never considered what kind of men she attracts with her attitude; that if a man wants her for her artificial breasts that he might not want her for her core personality. She has never considered that the men she is attracted to resemble abusers of her childhood. She has never considered what kind of men she would meet who would be involved with the sexual exploitation industry. Sex as a commodity gets disconnected from intimacy and as such does not function as part of the glue that holds relationships together. When it is a commodity, and it wears out or we tire of it, then we get a new commodity. We buy up to a newer and better model. The commodity belief has obsolescence built into it and as such functions to weaken the bonds of a relationship. The men she picks believe this, and the whole system feels familiar to Joyce.

Joyce continued to work at the strip club even when it did not financially reward her the way she had hoped. She mostly hated the customers and hated the managers as well. When she was stripping she would either "deliberately" dissociate or she would have a running monologue of invectives against the men who watched her. She said she learned to smile while mentally spewing this hate speech against men. Sometimes she said it made her feel powerful to take the money from the men she hated so much. She felt that fooling them into thinking she found them attractive made them pathetic and put her in charge.

Joyce learned to ignore the atmosphere in the strip club. She initially denied it was bad. She gave the line that it was "upscale" because she wore a sequined dress. She denied that on her first occasion of stripping she felt scared. She said she felt fine right away. Only later did she say that she had thrown up in fright the first night. She denied that anyone "messed" with her at the club. Later she admitted that she was punched and grabbed and called horrific names. Denial was the coping skill that she used the most.

# RESEARCH

These clinical observations are supported by a number of research findings. Much of the research is indirect in this area. There is not a great deal of research specifically on the adult survivors of child pornography. There is more research about prostituted children and adult prostitutes. Finally, there is a considerable amount of research on adult survivors of childhood sexual abuse.

## CHILDHOOD SEXUAL ABUSE

The negative psychological consequences of childhood sexual abuse have been examined by a number of writers. Cheasty et al (1998) found that 37% of depressed interviewees versus 23% of nondepressed interviewees had been sexually abused before they were 16 years old. Higher frequencies of depression, posttraumatic stress disorder (PTSD), alcohol and drug dependency, phobia, suicidal behavior, anxiety, general impairment in psychological adjustment, borderline personality disorder, generalized anxiety disorder, panic disorder, and eating disorders have been found in childhood sexual abuse survivors (Bryer et al, 1987; Burnam et al, 1988; Cheasty et al, 1998; Felitti, 1991; Fergusson et al, 1996; Gorcey et al, 1986; Kendler et al, 2000; MacMillan et al, 2001; McCauley et al, 1997; Mullen et al, 1993; Neumann et al, 1996; Pribor & Dinwiddie, 1992; Stein et al, 1988; Vize & Cooper, 1995; Weiss et al, 1999).

Research has also found that the more severe or frequent the abuse, the more likely are these outcomes (Briere & Runtz, 1988; Cheasty et al, 1998; Mullen et al, 1993; Walker et al, 1992). For example, depression is more likely if the abuse involved intercourse or if the abuse was repeated than if the abuse was a single episode that did not involve intercourse (Bifulco et al, 1991; Fergusson et al, 1996). In addition, patients indicate that they believe their childhood sexual abuse had a negative impact on their lives (Cheasty et al, 1998). Childhood sexual abuse tends to produce more negative consequences than adult sexual assault (Burnam et al, 1988).

Childhood sexual abuse also produces many negative social consequences, including increased incidence of teenage marriage, divorce, separation, and lower socioeconomic status (Bagley & Ramsey, 1985; Bifulco et al, 1991; Mullen et al, 1988).

## CHILD AND ADULT PROSTITUTION

Research indicates that there is a connection between childhood sexual abuse and prostitution. Seng (1989) reported that 28% to 65% of prostituted teenagers had been sexually abused; 57% of prostituted adults indicated that they had been sexually assaulted when they were children (Farley & Barkan, 1998). James & Meyerding (1977) found that 33.8% of prostitutes indicated that they had no further contact with their first sexual partner as compared to 14% of nonprostitutes. Prostitutes are also likely to be victims of incest, to experience physical force during their first intercourse, to be raped, and to have experienced multiple rapes (James & Meyerding, 1977).

The adult lives of prostitutes tend to be difficult. Farley & Barkan (1998) found that prostitutes are likely to experience a number of negative outcomes, including violence (82%), rape (68%), and homelessness (84%). Prostitution tends to reduce the likelihood of marriage. One study found that only 6% of prostitutes were married and living with their spouses as compared to 41% in the control group (O'Sullivan et al, 1996). Another study found that 10% of prostitutes were married (Silbert & Pines, 1983).

Prostitutes also suffer from psychological problems. A study by Ross et al (1990) found prostitutes suffer from depression (60%), substance abuse (80%), borderline personality disorder (11%), and dissociative identity disorder (5%). Farley & Barkan (1998) found that prostitutes suffered from PTSD (68%), drug abuse (75%), and alcohol abuse (27%) and were suicidal (5%). Is it any wonder that 88% of prostitutes want to leave prostitution (Farley & Barkan, 1998)?

# WHERE ARE THEY NOW?

Let us return to the stories of Claire, Gloria, Jane, and Joyce. Change is slow, but they do continue to make progress. They are beginning to understand the extent and nature of the damage caused to them by CSE. They are trying to heal, change beliefs, develop new coping skills, and add missing life skills. They seem determined not to give up. Sometimes their resolve may waver, and they do not believe that they will ever be able to erase the damage, but all of them see themselves as survivors. They view recovery as learning to speak a second language. They may learn the new language well, but they will always speak with an accent.

## CLAIRE

Claire decided to spend a period of 3 months with no sexual activity. She was able to do it over one summer and said it felt like a relief. It seemed to remove a burden from her shoulders not to be sexual with everyone who wanted to have sex with her. She is now trying to start relationships more slowly and to think before each date about whether she wants to have sex with this man on this date. She does not always maintain her resolve, but she is always willing to discuss it and to try again to decide. She is using her own sexual drive, attraction to the man, and safety in her decision to be sexual. These still seem like strange components to her, but they are becoming more familiar. Claire has decided to attend graduate school and is hoping to become a lawyer.

## GLORIA

Gloria is becoming more assertive in her relationships. She is asking for her needs to be met. She is making it clear that violence and aggression will not be tolerated. She is pursuing a career that she enjoys and for which she has a talent. She has softened her hardened exterior a little; she spends some time with female friends and has gotten a puppy.

## JANE

Jane has improved her relationship with her husband. She is talking to him directly and clearly about sexual needs, likes, and dislikes. Household responsibilities are more evenly shared, and she no longer feels compelled to do everything perfectly. She is more casual about food preparation and what she allows herself to eat. She is less anxious at home and at work. She feels less responsible for everything at work. She has distanced herself from her siblings and their expectations that she will always rescue them. She takes no drugs or alcohol and has reduced her use of antianxiety medication. She does more things for pleasure and is working on feeling that she deserves to do so.

## JOYCE

Joyce is still struggling, but she is also making progress. She left her job in the sexual exploitation industry and took a job as a receptionist. It was difficult initially not to interact with her boss in a sexually provocative manner. Her dress and her demeanor encouraged him to be flirtatious. That balance is still tenuous but is being maintained. She has signed up for some college courses, though whenever things get rough, she is strongly tempted to go back to stripping. She is dating a man who does not know she was a prostitute or a stripper. He likes to go out to dinner and talk to her. She finds this strange and is not sure what "his agenda is." She is trying to let normal dating behavior become more familiar so it will not feel so alien. She is thinking about having her artificial breasts removed.

## CONCLUSION

The prostitution of children and child pornography seem to produce all of the same negative adult outcomes as child sexual abuse, but these outcomes seem expanded in intensity, duration, and frequency. In addition, there seem to be additional negative outcomes that are particular to this kind of abuse, such as the fear that the pictures will resurface or that the prostitution history will be exposed. These added problems increase the fear, shame, and hypervigilance that already exist and add a sense of identity fraud that that is not always seen in victims of childhood sexual abuse.

The damage produced by CSE increases if the victim enters the adult sexual exploitation industry. This ongoing reenactment keeps the damage at a high level through this rewounding.

The damage can be characterized to include damage to core beliefs, particularly, "I am unlovable," "Sexual activity is my only value and the only way to get attention and self-esteem," "I am helpless and powerless," and "Other people are all manipulators and exploiters." The damage is also seen in the dysfunctional coping strategies that are developed to deal with these beliefs. Behaviors such as self-medicating with drugs and alcohol or dissociating tend to be used with tremendous costs. The missing life skills make alternatives in short supply. All of this leads to a tremendous array of psychological disorders such as depression, PTSD, and borderline personality disorder; social problems such as divorce; and employment problems.

The lives described in this chapter are just a narrow sample of the lives that we could have chosen to describe. We chose stories that did not have the worst damage and stories in which there was help to move from victim to survivor. These stories are closer to the best-case scenario than the typical scenario. We suspect that many, if not most, of the victims of the CSE industry have stories that are worse than these, and the resources for help are fewer.

In addition, we have limited our stories to those of females. This is not to deny that there are male victims. There are, and they exist in significant numbers. However, it has been our experience that fewer males end up in treatment. Males seem to have more negative attitudes about treatment and asking for help. Male victims of CSE also tend to get less support from the general culture. The male myth is that males like and want any kind of sexual experiences they can get. So the culture often sends a diminishing message about the pain experienced by male victims. Sometimes the people in their personal lives send that same message. Male victims often feel shame and pain about their experience and then feel more shame and pain because of these feelings. It has been our experience that males are more likely not to tell anyone what happened and to never to ask for help.

Lives can be improved, but damage of this sort is difficult to erase. The only way to truly deal with the devastation produced by the CSE industry is to prevent it. This means educating the public about the problem; helping parents and adults to protect children; reducing the permission-giving beliefs that are spread by pornography, stripping, and prostitution, which become excuses for the behaviors in the perpetrators; and strengthening the laws to discourage those who would persist in damaging children. We owe the children nothing less.

# REFERENCES

Bagley C, Ramsey R. Sexual abuse in childhood: psychosocial outcomes and implications for social work practice. *J Soc Work Hum Sex*. 1985;4:33-48.

Bifulco A, Brown GW, Adler Z. Early sexual abuse and clinical depression in adult life. *Br J Psychiatry*. 1991;159:115-122.

Briere J, Runtz M. Symptomatology associated with childhood sexual victimization in a nonclinical adult sample. *Child Abuse Negl*. 1988;12:51-59.

Bryer JB, Nelson BA, Miller JB, Krol PA. Childhood sexual and physical abuse as factors in adult psychiatric illness. *Am J Psychiatry*. 1987;144:1426-1430.

Burnam MA, Stein JA, Golding JM, et al. Sexual assault and mental disorders in a community population. *J Consult Clin Psychol*. 1988;56:443-450.

Cheasty M, Clare AW, Collins C. Relation between sexual abuse in childhood and adult depression: case-control study. *BMJ*. 1998;6:198-201.

Farley M, Barkan H. Prostitution, violence, and posttraumatic stress disorder. *Women Health*. 1998;27:37-49.

Felitti VJ. Long-term medical consequences of incest, rape and molestation. *South Med J*. 1991;84:328-331.

Fergusson, DM, Horwood LJ, Lynskey MT. Childhood sexual abuse and psychiatric disorder in young adulthood: II. Psychiatric outcomes of childhood sexual abuse. *Am Acad Child Adolesc Psychiatry*. 1996;35:1365-1374.

Gorcey M, Santiago JM, McCall-Perez F. Psychological consequences for women sexually abused in childhood. *Soc Psychiatry*. 1986;21:129-133.

James J, Meyerding J. Early sexual experience and prostitution. *Am J Psychiatry*. 1977; 134:1381-1385.

Kendler KS, Bulik CM, Silberg J, Hettema JM, Myers J, Prescott CA. Childhood sexual abuse and adult psychiatric and substance use disorders in women: an epidemiological and cotwin control analysis. *Arch Gen Psychiatry*. 2000;57:953-959.

MacMillan HL, Fleming JE, Streiner DL, et al. Childhood abuse and lifetime psychopathology in a community sample. *Am J Psychiatry*. 2001;158:1878-1883.

McCauley J, Kern DE, Kolodner, K, et al. Clinical characteristic of women with a history of childhood abuse: unhealed wounds. *JAMA*. 1997;277:1362-1368.

Mullen PE, Martin JL, Anderson JC, Romans SE, Herbison GP. Childhood sexual abuse and mental health in adult life. *Br J Psychiatry*. 1993;163:721-732.

Mullen PE, Romans-Clarkson SE, Walton VA, Herbison GP. Impact of sexual and physical abuse on women's mental health. *Lancet*. 1988;1:841-845.

Neumann DA, Houskamp BM, Pollack VE, Briere J. The long-term sequelae of childhood sexual abuse in women: a meta-analytic review. *Child Maltreat*. 1996;1:6-16.

O'Sullivan DM, Zuckerman M, Kraft M. The personality of prostitutes. *Pers Individ Dif*. 1996;21:445-448.

Pribor EF, Dinwiddie SH. Psychiatric correlates of incest in childhood. *Am J Psychiatry*. 1992;149:52-56.

Ross CA, Anderson G, Heber S, Norton GR. Dissociation and abuse among multiple-personality patients, prostitutes, and exotic dancers. *Hosp Community Psychiatry*. 1990; 41:328-330.

Seng MJ. Child sexual abuse and adolescent prostitution: a comparison analysis. *Adolescence*. 1989;24:665-675.

Stein JA, Golding JM, Siegel JM, Burnam MA, Sorenson SB. Long-term psychological sequelae of child sexual abuse. In: Wyatt GE, Powell GJ, eds. *Lasting Effects of Child Sexual Abuse*. Newbury Park, Calif: Sage Publications; 1988:135-154.

Vize CM, Cooper PJ. Sexual abuse in patients with eating disorders, patients with depression and normal controls: a comparative study. *Br J Psychiatry*. 1995;167:80-85.

Walker EA, Katon WJ, Hansom J, et al. Medical and psychiatric symptoms in women with childhood sexual abuse. *Psychosom Med*. 1992;54:658-664.

Weiss EL, Longhurst JG, Mazure CM. Childhood sexual abuse as a risk factor for depression in women: psychological and neurobiological correlates. *Am J Psychiatry*. 1999;156:816-828.

# EXPERIENTIAL YOUTH PERSPECTIVES: CANADA

Nadine Grant, Save the Children Canada

Save the Children Canada works overseas and in Canada to bring immediate and lasting improvements to children's lives worldwide through the realization of their rights. This nonpolitical, nonreligious organization is committed to long-term development at the grassroots level through partnership with local communities, government bodies, and international organizations.

Save the Children Canada has been working for more than 80 years to protect children from neglect, cruelty, and exploitation. Save the Children Canada is a member of the International Save the Children Alliance. With 30 member organizations and operational programs in more than 120 countries, the alliance is the world's largest global movement for children.

## LANGUAGE AND RESPECT

To begin, it is important to address the terminology. "Sexual exploitation trade" is sort of an oxymoron. It is irresponsible and unjust for us to assume that the word "trade" can be used in conjunction with "sexual exploitation." Sexually exploited youth should not be grouped under the terms *sex trade, sex industry*, or *sex work* because these terms imply that there is a choice; when children and youth are involved in this industry, it may seem like a choice, but conditioning and society play a huge role in how this type of child maltreatment is viewed.

Second, sensitivity must be used regarding topics of sexual exploitation. In the Declaration and Agenda for Action, it was declared that the term *child prostitute* is no longer acceptable when working with or referring to sexually exploited youth. In this text, "prostituted children/youth" is used so that the noun becomes the youth. This reinforces the concept that these youths are not offenders, but are under someone else's control. In the interests of children and youth plagued by this popular form of sexual abuse, it is important to ensure that the proper language is used.

This chapter is written by 3 young persons who slipped into commercial sexual exploitation. As youth with experiential knowledge of exploitation, they have been involved in the nonprofit sector and have worked tirelessly as advocates for youth who are being commercially sexually exploited across Canada. The firsthand victim impact of child maltreatment is often excluded from published educational resources for professionals. We are fortunate to have contributors who survived a very dangerous form of abuse, sexual exploitation, and who are willing to share their experiences so that we may learn.

The stories of Monica, Justin, and Chris are combined and presented under the following 3 sections:

1. How did you enter commercial sexual exploitation?

2. What kept you in commercial sexual exploitation?

3. How did you exit commercial sexual exploitation?

# How Did You Enter Commercial Sexual Exploitation?

## Monica

Shortly after turning 19 and while attending college, I called an escort agency in the telephone yellow pages out of curiosity and because of financial desperation. Money was tight, and I had little, if any, financial support from my family. The initial phone call was awkward as I did not know what to expect. I asked about what the job entailed and was rather naïve to expect that escorts were just escorts. Betty, the independent owner of the legal establishment, asked me a few questions. She was curious about my looks, my age, and my interest in calling. Although I did not know how to respond, I answered her questions, as a young adult should, with professionalism. She explained that if I were interested in working for her company, I would be required to have a criminal record check and pay a $115 licensing fee. From what I recall, she was careful about her choice of words with me over the phone and was far more interested in meeting me in person. Within a couple of hours, we had discreetly met to discuss what the job entailed. While I did have some concerns about my safety and the fear of being charged for soliciting, I was advised that the owner worked closely with the police and that safety would not be a concern. It took a couple of days, and then I was registered with the licensed escort agency.

Betty explained the job description of an escort through phone conversations. She did not provide the explicit details of being an escort—this I would have to learn on my own.

Being an escort means offering sexual services at the cost of $180 per 1-hour "call." Twenty dollars of the $180 would go to the driver who would pick me up at my home, stay at the hotel or apartment where the call would take place, and then drive me home after the call. The remaining money would be for me. Although I realized that I would be offering sexual services for money, I was in desperate need of money and did not read too much further into it.

Betty informed me of a suggested dress code and the equipment I would need for calls. I bought lubricant, condoms (nonlubricated, lubricated, and ribbed), thigh-high leggings, and lacy lingerie. She emphasized the importance of looking sexy, professional, and presentable.

Betty showed me the rented apartment from which most of the girls "worked." It was a fully furnished apartment with a queen-size bed, living room, kitchen, and bathroom. This apartment was used on an appointment basis and was paid for by the hour. Clients would pay an extra charge for the use of this apartment in addition to the escort agency fee. Betty explained the routine of taking a call. I was allowed to set my own hours, work on call from my home, and was to be addressed only by my working name, "Monica." She said I would be successful in this business due to my mixed Aboriginal and European ancestry and being only 19.

Betty explained what I had to say to each client and emphasized the importance of receiving the money first before offering any of my so-called services. Professionalism was important to her. As time went by, I began to learn more about her, her background, and why she got involved in such a business in the first place. She spent many years in the Canadian Armed Forces and maintained a private life. She had a strong business sense and always treated me with professionalism.

Her role was to solicit me over the phone and profit from my service. Clients would call, ask for new girls, and inquire about their looks and age. She often portrayed me as a young Asian/Hawaiian girl with tan skin and big brown eyes.

In retrospect, it is hard for me to explain what I was thinking when I got myself into this business. It all seemed to happen so fast. I told my roommate (who should or could have been diagnosed as a nymphomaniac; she always had men in and out of our apartment) what I had decided to do. Her opinion had little weight on my decision of becoming an escort as her own promiscuous activity was given for free. I reasoned that I would at least be paid for my sexual services.

Within a few days of having my criminal record check done, the phone began to ring. My first call was at the apartment, and this was the first time that I met my driver. I was nervous and did not know what to expect. Betty explained the procedure of being at the apartment, greeting the client, exchanging the money, making small talk, and getting down to business. My first client was an old man. Money justified the reason why I had put on my charm and gradually seduced this old guy. I was extremely timid and shy, unlike the outgoing, outspoken person that I normally am. I felt more than uncomfortable undressing and lying half-naked beside this man who appeared to want only comfort, sex, of course, and to be caressed and have someone to talk to and ease the loneliness. Doing the deed was a challenge as he was old and sexual attraction or arousal was nowhere to be found on my part. After he left, I cleaned the apartment, changed the linens, and emptied the ashtray, leaving no trace of my presence. When I got home I felt degraded and like a tramp, but pushed whatever negative thoughts aside and enjoyed the hard-earned money I had made from 1 hour's work.

I did not have many boundaries when I first started as an escort and was quite naïve to say the least. I was always safe with my clients and was strict about condoms for fear of getting an STD or becoming pregnant. However, I did not quite have the street smarts and assertiveness in regards to what I would and would not do. There was no job description for this, and my boundaries had to be learned along the way.

It did not take long before my phone was ringing off the hook and I was in demand at all hours of the day. Meanwhile, I was attending school half-heartedly, realizing school was not meant for me at that time. I was partying more frequently with the extra cash that I was earning and eventually moved out of my apartment as my roommate was driving me crazy. I moved in with a friend that I had made in school and informed her of my job. I did not want to have to make up stories for my whereabouts and felt she should know for safety purposes. Hiding my new job from friends and family was a whole other story. I told them I had a cleaning job on an on-call basis, which explained the cut-off jeans and big bag I carried that held my sexy clothes, nylons, condoms, etc.

It did not take long for me to get caught up in the money. I was living a double life. Taking calls with other girls and working until the wee hours of the morning and at the same time deceiving my friends and family by playing the role of girlfriend and niece. My family was so proud of me because I was attending college and on my way to a successful career. What few people knew was that my other life that consisted of running off to the homes and hotels of strangers who were lonely and in need of company. Never did I feel unsafe or fearful of violence. Never was I offered drugs and only on one occasion was I offered alcohol. My crutch rather was to smoke, and boy, did I smoke, mostly out of nervousness; there was the occasional complaint that I was a chain smoker. Everyone has his or her vice.

## Justin

I guess I was 12 the first time that I was sexually exploited. My biological mother gave me up for adoption when I was 2 years old. When my adoption was rescinded, Social Services was unsure what to do with me, so they placed me back to live with my biological mother. Being 12 and idealistic, I had pushed to move back in with my blood relatives, hoping that I would finally fit in somewhere.

My mother was fostering a serious heroin addiction, and the support I was receiving from youth workers and the like was nil. In a few short weeks, I, too, started down the road of serious drug use. I was in my bedroom, and my mother knocked on the door; she came in and there was a man with her, in his 40s with dark hair and looking strung out. She did not say anything and then just left. The man was still in my room, standing by the door. It's sort of funny; I kind of knew what was going on and I needed little introduction. I had been sexually abused before and understood my role. The only difference this time was that I was receiving "compensation" for the acts. In my mother's world, she was teaching me survival skills. I had full knowledge in the short time that I lived with her of the "comings and goings" of sex work and at the time thought that my body was my only commodity.

When I was 13, I decided that instead of feeding money to my mother's addiction, I would strike out on my own and leave home. In the gay community to which I was introduced, there were many older men willing to "help out" a young guy new to the big scene. What I mean by this, of course, is that there would be an exchange of sex acts for shelter, introductions to other older men, food, clothes, and pretty much anything else they wanted. These men are labeled "sugar daddies."

### CHRIS

My life began in the 1970s. I was born in Canada, daughter to an Asian mother and a South American father. Ever since birth, my life has been tumultuous. At the time of my birth, my mother was young and in love and my father was every stereotype of a South American you could possibly imagine. So, I was brought into the world amongst anger, violence, betrayal, and heartache. My childhood was far from a happy one. Even to this day I can not recall most of my life before age 8, and I know that there is a good reason for that.

I was physically and mentally abused, neglected, and, at times, tortured as a child. I was unusually quiet and antisocial and did not do well in school. There was a period that I never saw "my mother" for days. I would wake up and breakfast, lunch, and dinner were made for the day. The key to the house was always tied to my lunchbox. I had been taking care of myself in many ways since the age of 6. My mother had many rules, and if I broke a rule, a beating with a water-soaked bamboo cane was my punishment. On the other hand, my father was a shattered man and, depending on the alcohol, drug, or day, I would get a beating. If I was lucky, what was nearby and accessible would be something relatively harmless; if not, a jelly slipper could deliver quite the blow. Sometimes for no reason, he would push me down the stairs or burn me with a cigarette. That was my life then.

It was during this period of my life that I created "Chris." Chris was someone no one knew about; she was my alter ego, my secret. With Chris I learned to deal better with my daily life. Chris allowed me to have a secret personal space to be myself away from everyone else, and no one could ever touch her emotionally or physically. Being able to come and go as Chris gave me power, and it trained me to take on the sex trade in the future. Dissociation had become an art form for me over the years, and it was perfected by the time I entered the sex trade at 21.

Eventually, I left Canada with my mother and went to her homeland. It was a culture shock for me and, try as I might, I never fit in. I was always different from the rest of the Asians there, and the language did not come easy in the beginning. Eventually, I could speak fluently, but I could not read or write the language.

While in this country I had to adapt to many differences. Child abuse was a part of life, and children were to be seen, not heard. One day while my mother was out, my uncle molested me. The memory was so painful that I repressed it for many years and it did not resurface till I was 16. To this day I can not remember how old I was or if it happened more than once, but I knew one thing—it did not matter. In this country, my uncle was the only boy in the family and could do no wrong; I was a half-breed daughter of a divorced woman, and I was a shame to the family anyway.

Being a teenager was awkward for me. I was fatter, darker, and definitely had bigger boobs then anyone else. This brought me nothing but trouble. Every so often some guy would grab my breasts. At school or at home, my boobs were the focus of ridicule. My grandmother was always asking me if someone had touched me yet, if I was engaged, if I had sex, or if I was pregnant. Her comments were always something about sex. If I wore a tank top, my uncle would say out loud to my mother that I was going to sell my flesh *(prostitute)*. My aunt was referring to my boobs as watermelons and telling me I would grow up to be a *whore*. Everywhere I went I was a *slut*, a *whore, worthless, useless,* and *stupid*. Eventually, I accepted these words as reality, and every day I wanted to die.

By then I was a full-grown tomboy. This did not sit well anywhere in an Asian country. I fought like a boy, talked like a boy, swore like a boy, and even walked like a boy. I did it because boys got everything they wanted and I never got anything I wanted. I rebelled, and what better way to piss off the world than to be exactly like I shouldn't—a nongirl girl. Then I flunked out of school and had no choice but to go to secretarial school.

So one day, my mother gave me a plane ticket to go back to Canada, and I was packing the next week. Decisions around me were never discussed with me, but I was thankful to get out of the horrid family and life there.

I think my mother realized that Asia did not suit a girl like me as I was "too friendly" with bus drivers and teachers. Even then, I was a virgin and all this sex talk confused me.

So, I returned to Canada when I was 16, with 3 suitcases and a rice cooker. Although my mother arranged for me to live with friends of friends, when I got off the plane, I felt completely and utterly alone with no family and no friends, like an immigrant. My mother did not have much money, and I immediately had to get a job. I got a job that month selling "dim sum" for $5 an hour. When I tried to enroll in high school, my credits from Asia did not count and I was back in Grade 10/11, although I had finished Grade 12.

At first I was not even allowed to enroll because I had no legal guardian in Canada. When I enrolled, they tried to make me take English as a second language (ESL). I was working and going to school and living with strangers. I had to make money to buy my food, cook, clean, and do homework all by myself, I never really had any time to adjust, and it was around this time that I was diagnosed with depression. I did not understand a lot of things, but mental illness was something I really could not understand. The shame—I could not even tell my mother because she would just tell me to get over it. I thought if I made up my mind, I could.

For the next 2½ years I was put in a group home, admitted into the psych ward more than 50 times, restrained more than 20 times, taken in by cops more than 10 times, and given enough pills to knock a horse dead. From chlorpromazine to Ativan, from imipramine to Haldol, from Kemadrin to Fluanxol, from lithium to Epival, to name a few. One pill for behavior, one to calm me down, one for the cutting, one for the panic attacks, one to help me sleep, one to help the side effects, one for seizures, one to stabilize moods, and the list went on.

When I began taking the pills, I was depressed and suicidal. By this time, with the pills, I was hallucinating, delusional, catatonic at times, bulimic, slicing and burning myself, and having uncontrollable body tics. This was attributed to the fact that some of my pills had side effects "that cause Parkinson's-like symptoms." One day, I had smoked a joint with some guys, and I went catatonic. (That is when you can not move your body but are fully aware of what is happening.) For a long time afterward, I wondered if they had spiked the joint so that they could rape me, but then, I do not really know. Those were my pill days; I did not ever know what was what. I can not remember most things from that time, and I could not control my mind or body.

I was already promiscuous at the time and was on phone chat lines finding men to sleep with. I dated one of these men; he bought me food, took me out, and gave me tokens. I was 20 and he was 31; he was controlling and insensitive. I felt hostage to his presents, so I dumped him, and I was back to eating soya sauce and rice.

One day on the chat line, an older man offered me money. I thought it was a lucrative sum and so I took up the offer. It basically covered my rent for the month, and that was fine by me. This "date" was into the rough trade, and I complied with his wishes, since I thought the customer is always right. After an hour of degradation, physical assault, and unmentionable activities that left me bleeding, I got paid. I did not feel anything; the only thing that crossed my mind was that I did grow up to be a *whore*, and I learned after that to take cash up front. I told some of my friends I would only do it for 6 months till I made enough money to move out of the "hole in the ground." Six years later, I was still in the business.

## WHAT KEPT YOU IN COMMERCIAL SEXUAL EXPLOITATION?

### MONICA

When I look back to the lifestyle that I was living, the financial freedom I had while working as an escort allowed me to seize the opportunity. If I wanted to go to a concert, I simply went, not concerned about how much it would cost, as I would earn the money in a night's work. I gradually began partying more frequently and parallel to this neglected my studies. I had no inclination to read, study, or write papers. It is no wonder I failed so miserably while I lived my double life. Perhaps I was addicted to the lifestyle, the fast and easy money and the freedom to buy the luxury items my schoolmates and friends were shoplifting. With the hard-earned money I was making, I was able to buy the gifts for my family and friends that I could not previously afford. Having a generous character and little means due to the lack of financial support from family, I was living a generous and carefree life.

It did not take long for me to establish my own clientele, or regulars, as we call them. They were seen as sugar daddies; men with the awkward introverted persona who possessed what appeared to be an endless amount of cash to throw around. One in particular was fond of me and liked the company of me overnight. I would be required to pay the first and last hour to the agency along with the driver, and the remainder would come to me. I would see him on a monthly basis at the cost of $1000 a night. He would buy me sweet gifts, order me room service, massage and spoil me for the night. In turn and to my relief, one session of sex was often enough for him and many of my clients.

I can not help thinking that it was a confusing and senseless time for me. I was living a risky lifestyle and one of which I was ashamed. I frequently took calls at fancy and elegant hotels as well as "divey" ones, discreetly whisking through hotel lobbies in my sexy but presentable clothing only to leave an hour or two later, paranoid that they would equate my short visit to their establishments and realize that I was a working girl. I also feared the day that I would encounter someone that I knew and that they would make the connection to my work or that I would have a client that I knew on a personal basis. To my relief this never happened. I also had great difficulty with younger, handsome clients, as I feared that I would run into them at a bar, restaurant, or somewhere in the city that I lived. I often questioned why some of these handsome, seemingly nice guys would need to use my service in the first place. Many of my clients were construction workers, businessmen, and old guys, and some were not so attractive. Some liked my company early in the morning, others right before lunch; however, most liked me in the late evening. It was challenging to pretend to family and friends that I was working and continuously having to make up lies as to my whereabouts. Furthermore, it was a challenge to mask my interest in sex at the convenience of my clients, although I found myself consumed with the lifestyle and the money. I was living on the edge, young and invincible, resilient and secretive.

## JUSTIN

At the time I felt like I was in a position of power and that these men needed me to compensate for their feelings of loneliness, inadequacy, or other shortcomings. It is clear to me now that I was not the one in control and that I was being sexually abused under the guise of prostitution and glamorization of the sex industry.

I had basically "taken control" of my identity as a male hustler, and as with any repressed minority, started to "own" my abuse. I was unsure of the acceptance that my peers would have toward this particular activity and found that as I entered junior high school, those supports and social circles started to exclude me. I was no longer seen as a person but as a problem child or wild child. For me, all of this was about survival, and I soon had to let go of my need for acceptance and my need to please others. This was a huge turning point for me; instead of making social contacts and friends and support through school, I ended up only facing off and befriending other hustlers (most of whom were adults) and not really focusing on my development. I felt like an outcast and began to get emotionally unattached to anything that was not bathed in sex, money, or drugs. These were all things that I thought I could control, so when I engaged in those activities, I felt powerful. When I got a taste of power, it was more addictive than any drug.

When I would take drugs, it started small, like the occasional joint, then moved on to cocaine, Ecstasy (E), heroin, crystal meth, Special K, and just about anything else that would be able to boost my confidence, confuse my feelings, or ultimately just shut them off.

The nightclubs that I went to were more than happy to house me. At 15, I learned that I could pretty much "be the party" wherever I went, and in a roundabout way this was the family I craved and the acceptance that I desperately needed. I would go to these clubs and after-hours parties where there were an abundance of older men (some of whom were clients) and a lot of drugs because people started to catch on to the fact that I would do almost anything when I was high, which made it easier for them to take advantage of me. I was the "life of the party," and when you are a child, you do not realize that these people would not blink if you were hauled out of a dumpster the next morning. This was something I began to tune into later when friends my own age would be raped at these parties or in some cases overdose and be left outside to die. Not wanting to be the "party pooper" and also watching my investments in the sex trade, I did not want to be ostracized, so I could sustain my habits and lifestyles, so for the most part I stopped making friends in the trade. When someone was killed or OD'd I could blame them and say, "They should have known better" or "Why would they get into a car with 3 guys?".

The West Coast was supposed to be the new start that I was looking for, but as they say, your problems will follow you. I did not really make much of an attempt to change my life around. I think that it was because all my support systems were no longer there, and I self-inflicted a life of solitude in the trade.

When I was 19, I briefly left the sex trade for an extremely abusive relationship, which to me has almost everything to do with my final exit. My partner at this stage had basically conned a young guy into supporting him while he slept around. He was violent, but I felt that I needed him, when what I was craving was abuse. When I finally left the trade, I had to deal with that addiction to pain.

When that relationship ended, I had no financial resources and had to make the connection to the sex trade again. I achieved this very easily since there were ads in every local rag for "masseurs" or "Get paid today—adult movies"; the list goes on.

After a few of these auditions, I was given my own Internet show twice a week for 2 hours. Later I "acted" in more of these "films." I came to be dependent on a high income quickly and did not realize that the drugs were costing me the money that I was abusing my body to make, and in return the drugs were passing me the courage, abandon, and recklessness I needed to carry these things out in the first place. I became seriously addicted to crack once more, but this time I was losing weight, starving myself, and homeless, so I was looking worn; gigs became scarce.

So, once again doing what I knew best, I took to the streets, roaming, waking up in Calgary, then Winnipeg, the next day in jail. It was always an adventure, and I guess looking at it that way contributed to the whole thing, too.

## CHRIS

Because I was not thin, blonde, or exceptionally beautiful, I relied on "extras" to pay the bills. Extras were anything from kissing to the rough trade. I was Asian with big boobs so that worked as well. I made up personas with their own history and personalities, and it was an easy business for me in the beginning. My family equipped me with the social skills needed for the trade, Asia equipped me with the ability to accept the business and its clientele, and my self-esteem, or lack of it, took care of the rest. I used to joke to myself: self-esteem—what's that?

So, in the long run I learned to fight, bluff, and control situations with force; otherwise, force could be used against you. I learned about pressure points, using everything as a weapon, and how to manipulate police officers. The business makes you feel like your back is against the wall at all times and you have to watch what's coming or else. I remember telling this girlfriend of mine that they only see us as interactive blow-up dolls. After a while, you forget that what you do for a living is *not* who you are; it all just gets muddled up.

The money got more and more of a hold on me; it wasn't enough to pull a date or two a week anymore. Slowly I was pulling 10, then 15, and when weeks got slow, I would curse and lie awake at night thinking it was me, that I had finally sold myself too much and no one wanted me anymore. By the end of year 3, I was on escort schedule 24/7 until my boss got busted in 1999. No other agency would hire me, so I took to the streets. If there was a time the business did break me, it was then.

Random violence, bottles, rocks, and eggs thrown at me, every second person passing by telling me their thoughts of me, police harassment, and people taking pictures while driving by. I was hard, tough, and mean on the streets. I was always in a bad mood and I had to drink, smoke weed, or take E to make up for being out there after work every day. I robbed girls, I robbed dates, and I kicked in car doors. I can not remember why I did not just quit; I do not remember thinking it was an option. Several times I tried to get a real job, and several times someone would out me, and then the stares, the innuendos, the bullshit would begin.

I would be the best employee they had, but the minute there was a mention of me being a *prostitute*, suddenly money was missing, rumors were flying, and I could not do right by them to save my life. Inevitably, I would go back to work full time; I thought that if I were miserable, why not make more money being so? I was lost; I did not know why I went in the business, and I did not know that I wanted out or that I could get out. Then I got another square job that was 15 feet from my usual corner, but abusive customers and too many *hooker* jokes pushed me back in. To top it all, I had been couch surfing for 4 years and felt completely like a deer caught in headlights.

In 1999, I had been in an abusive relationship. A broken finger and 15 punches to the head had gotten me charged, and I had to drop out of university, so in short, my life fell apart and it was back to the business full time. I spent New Year's Eve, 2000, working at my square job on a 15-hour shift and then getting off work at 5 in the morning to being utterly and completely homeless with a broken finger. In 2000, I was working with my freshly-out-of-jail boss again and making money; this time, I managed to save some as I went. With about $13 000 saved up, I took a 4-month hiatus from the business, got my own apartment, and furnished it. I was then offered a job and worked full time by the beginning of 2001 and worked part time at night. I felt like I never knew when I would have to fall back on the "game."

In the back of my head, I did not know if I could keep this job or if it was going to work out, so I stayed in both businesses. I was working Thursdays to Saturdays on the street and working 9 to 5 Mondays to Fridays. I felt torn and confused. Some clients would ask what I did besides the business. If I told them I worked full time, they would laugh; if I told them I was in university, they would laugh. Guys in cars yelling nasty words, women in cars telling me what I was, police never coming to help even when my life was threatened—it just felt like it never, ever got better. Then one night, a car with a dog, a woman, and a man drove by. As they drove by, the woman clicked her camera and a flash went off.

I started to cry out in the open. My girlfriend kept on telling me not to let people see that they got to me and I just cried and yelled. I wanted them to see me cry. I wanted people to understand I had feelings, and I wanted them to feel my wrath. How dare someone who has no relation to me come in my life and bring stuff up. The flash brought back memories that I did not want to deal with at this time, and all the while my girlfriend said it was gonna be okay. That annoyed me because it was never okay. How complacent we had become to the bullshit people gave us; we just took it, and every day we would lie to ourselves and say it would be okay.

I told her about my uncle taking pictures of me as a child while I was sleeping and while I was showering, and she was quiet. I just knew deep down inside that as long as I worked in this business, people would not care about me and my feelings. I would never be someone to them; I would represent *something* to them but never a person. I was just street trash to them, low-level scum who fed off their tax dollars. How I wished I could tell the whole square world that I had managed to infiltrate the system, and I was even one of them. I wondered how they would see me then, as one of them.

I thought to myself, What do these people know about me? Did they know that I am capable of being in a university? Did they know that I did not do any drugs besides pot? Did they even care that I actually did pay taxes? I asked myself if it would have been different if I had called from my day job. I knew the truth was that as long as I was working on the streets, other people would see me for what I do and care never for who I am.

# How Did You Exit Commercial Sexual Exploitation?

## Monica

Eventually my life as an escort began to catch up to me. The glamour was replaced with shame and further entrenched my self-esteem. I found myself looking in the mirror, crying after calls, screaming at myself and accusing myself of being slutty, trampy, gross, and degrading. I could no longer justify my acts. I questioned whether or not I did in fact perhaps like the sex. Seducing complete strangers, pretending to enjoy their company and conversation, smoking up a storm, and meanwhile leading a normal life. To further complicate things, while I was an escort I had a few relationships with guys that I went to school with. Varsity boys, good, wholesome, athletic, smart guys sweet on me, were assuming nothing but complete loyalty and faithfulness on my part. Sexually, my body, the job, and my relationships began to take a toll on my mental and spiritual state. On more than one occasion, I felt like I was having a nervous breakdown from being overwhelmed by the darkness of my character.

I was forced to look back into my childhood and ask myself why I willingly agreed to be involved in such a business. My memories of child sexual abuse began to surface more often than I appreciated; that chapter in my life was supposed to be closed. The memories were pushed so far from my mind that I thought they were gone forever. It was not until I began working as an escort that I began to put all of the pieces together. I recalled how the pedophile sexually abused me when I was 10. Over the course of 3 months, he treated me like an adult, seduced me like I was an adult, forced his heavy body on top of me in the wee hours of the night like an adult, and perversely placed his semen in my mouth when he thought I was sleeping. The memories haunted my sex life, especially when I took calls. I felt numb to my actions as well as that of my clients. Oral sex made me dry heave, and no matter how hard I faked it, I always wanted to get sick.

The lingering issue of the innocence I lost as a child was surfacing in my life, and I did not know how to cope with it all. I had oppressed all of the feelings I could not identify when I was young. Was it the fact that I did not have a father in my life? Was I seeking a replacement figure in my life, someone that cared or pretended to care for a moment? Or perhaps it was the *various* men in and out of my mother's life? Was it the poverty I lived in and the envy of my peers who *seemed* to have everything? Was it simply that I was just fucked up and did not *value* myself? Did I know what valuing myself meant? Nobody taught me any of these things. Respect for yourself. Valuing what life had in fact offered me. Health, resilience, and a warrior spirit. I was forced to come to terms with some of these questions when I had a nervous breakdown in the fourth month that I was an escort.

I had been out drinking with some friends and could not look at myself in the mirror. Ashamed and disgusted with myself, drunk and hysterical, I swallowed a bottle of Extra Strength Tylenol. I had been on the phone with my aunt, whom I am very close with; I explained what I had been doing and how I did not want to live. I was fed up with the endless challenges I was forced to face in my young life. She tried to comfort me, telling me how special I was and that the family cared for me. I was too stubborn to listen and hoped for nothing more than to die. Taking 75 pills is a weak attempt to commit suicide, as so many people pointed out, but it was, as my counselor put it, "a cry for help." I have always been quite expressive with my feelings and found living such a deceitful, isolating life challenging, which explains why I called my aunt at 2 o'clock in the morning, revealing my shameful secrets. She immediately called the police, who arrived only minutes after I got off the phone with my aunt. Just as they arrived, the Tylenol had begun taking its course. I felt ill and wanted to vomit, but I could not imagine doing so all over a police car. When I arrived at the hospital, they quickly began asking questions—why and how many? I could not answer those questions but explained while having a tube down my throat that the purpose behind taking the pills was in fact to die! I was angry that I was being punished for my actions; however, their rebuttal was that I was the one who took the pills. I was forced to talk to psychologists about my actions and behavior. I was encouraged to answer the question *why*. I was hospitalized for 4 days and isolated in my thoughts.

Although my friends and family supported me, there was still always that awkward silence of *why?* Why would I do such a thing when my life appeared to be going so well? I was always told that my family was so proud of me because I was beautiful, smart, and special. What I have come to realize over the course of the last couple of years through counseling and talking about it, is this: Children of abuse and dysfunction are forced to grow up, beyond their years, denied the carefree childhood that we are supposed to experience. My life experiences taught me how to detect the shadiness in people's character, how not to trust or get really close to anyone, and how to mask whatever I was feeling or thinking. I have come to the conclusion that the many challenges and trials I have faced in my life have taught me, in an informal way, to mask what I was feeling or thinking. My life has been an endless game of survival, sporting whatever mask that was required of me. I was the lover, mistress, girlfriend, escort, call girl one minute, and the successful student, daughter, granddaughter, niece, and friend the next. When things were bad at home, I learned how to occupy my time and avoid home until it was safe. My external strengths have been noticed as people make such statements as, "Oh, you are so strong, you should be so proud of yourself." I can say with confidence I have overcome some of these obstacles and have faced the many demons in my closet. The reality for me is one that I must face and cope with the past in order to move on. My life as an escort still haunts me, and there have been moments when money has been tight and I have considered calling Betty to list me for the night to take the occasional call. However, those thoughts have not crossed my mind for some time as I rethink what that life entailed.

The realization that nothing in fact is free in this world and that children who are abused and exploited are in fact robbed of something money can not buy— innocence and the right to be protected—has guided my voice as an advocate for children and youth. Some chapters have been closed in my life and are not meant to be reopened; however, the importance of including this piece for this resource is to provide an example of just how complicated this subculture truly is and the long-lasting effects it has on one's life. Unfortunately, this is why finding a solution for the violation of children's rights and social problems is so challenging to address due to the number of factors that contribute to the sexual exploitation of children and youth. Currently, I am an advocate for sexually exploited children and youth and a leader in my community for the rights of Aboriginal children and youth. To make sense of the abuse I endured as a child, I have had to search deep within myself and have been rewarded with the gift of a strong voice. A voice that has been heard, as I am the product of sexual exploitation, as are so many children and youth around the world. But I choose to make sense of the abuse and not let it consume me and my future. As an elder once said at a National Aboriginal Conference, "We must support the champions in our community that give voice to the issues that affect us."

## JUSTIN

I had one last major experience that influenced me, a 23-year-old hustler, to finally leave the trade. I was living with a great friend of mine who was older, but I cared about him. He had become sick with pneumonia and was hospitalized, so I ended up with his wallet and drained all of his accounts, then skipped town. Eventually he tracked me down and told me if I paid him back I could live back with him; I considered this to be my only stable home to this day. I paid my debts to him and others; then I was on the road to exiting, a clear way out.

I came back to the West Coast from the prairies, and I was exhausted and strung out. I detoxed at home for 2 weeks or so. Later, my financial aid worker (social worker) requested I take a preemployment program to finish high school and get a job.

I still remember the first day that I walked into that school. I was going back to school; it was like I was 16 again, and that's how I acted. It took awhile for me to calm down; when I did, I somehow attained my general equivalency diploma, first aid certification, computer/office skills, and general behavior in the work place. I was so proud.

That was when I applied for a job with a nonprofit agency as a participant in a test pilot program looking at youth exiting the streets. The outcome was to exit the trade and produce a resource/exiting guide for youth who are sexually exploited. This program was successful for me and allowed me to acquire the skills and knowledge of the issue to continue the fight against exploitation on my own. After this project ended, I was immediately put onto another project called Street Fest. It was a street festival that reached over 300 street-involved youth in a West Coast city to help them gain knowledge of local services through art, music, spoken word, and dance. I was again extremely proud of my work. (For a full discussion of this program, see chapter 40, Exiting Route: A Peer Support Model for Exiting and Healing Programs.)

Without delay, I was renewed once more, this time to put on a photography exhibit for sexually exploited youth, where they would take, develop, and show their world through their eyes. It was also a smash success. I have always believed that when you take a bad action/habit or situation away, you have to replace it with something else.

For me all of this work has been a healing process. Through my work, I have benefited in ways that were unforeseeable to me 3 years ago. I have been to Europe and to conferences, and finally people are allowing me the respect, and sometimes tolerance, that I have craved for years. Now I am taking a sort of break from exploitation and the issue of abuse to find out who I am. I have changed a great deal, and I acknowledge the roles of friends, government, and social supports. I hope through my experience, you gain what is needed to stop the commercial sexual exploitation of children and youth.

### CHRIS

I have had many friends who, upon quitting the business, make no mention ever again of being in the business. There has been an unspoken black mark on them, and they knew if anyone else knew it would be used against them. I have felt how a person's opinion of me changes when they find out—the looks, the whispers, and the pats on the head. I can feel their biases oozing out of them, and yet they claim to me to be unbiased. When I have done a good job, I hear the patronizing tone of voice.

I know that some think I can not make it on my own. I think some people think I do not understand how the world works, and they constantly tell me what is standard in their world. I do not want to live anyone else's life; I do not want to live by rules I did not make, but a lot of people take that as a level of my already low intelligence. Even the way I speak; oftentimes I have heard the comment, "Oh, but you don't like reading anyway." The truth is, I love reading. All my life it has been my one and only best friend. I like to read but maybe not books others would consider.

A lot of people believe that when I talk about my life I want sympathy and pity or that I need to be held and told it will all be okay. I do not need that; what I need is space to define my own journey, respect that I am an individual, and faith that I can become great at who I am. Over the years, I have felt smothered by my experiences, and not because I went through them but because I am not supposed to talk about them, and because I have to be constantly defined by them. "You did well considering"—I do not usually hear that phrase used with others, but with me, it is "considering," not just a job well done. Not to mention the excuses why my life story is not good dinner conversation, the reasons range from it not being appropriate to people do not want to hear stuff like that to it makes people uncomfortable.

No one ever listened to me when I said I was not crazy, when I said I did not need pills, when I said being in care was not good for me and in the end *prostitution* was a better experience because it allowed me to be independent and be exactly who I needed to be at the time. Unfortunately, I underestimated the pull it would have in the long run and how quickly it could spiral out of hand. But in the end, I was worse off before it in many ways than I was after; I learned not to compromise, to fight back and to say "no" when I wanted to. Before I entered the business, I let people do whatever they wanted with me.

The business has its shadows over me. People will judge me for it, and people will make assumptions about me because of it. My strength of character will always be weakened by my conceived loose morals. My life has made me who I am today, and when I look back, I would not change a damn thing about it. All I ask from others is do not bind me by rules I did not make, do not shame me for the experiences I have had to grow from, and do not judge me as black or white. I am a full spectrum of color, and if you can see past those labels, then you would know that.

The last year and a half of the business had become unpleasant. Friendships, living arrangements, dates, and just life in general had become negative. So, after saving a lot of money, I moved into a moderately priced apartment alone and was taking time off from the trade (from November to January) and figured that I would return when my money ran out. Then a really cool job opportunity that was totally up my alley came up in January, and I decided to take the job and "work" on the weekends, in case everything did not work out. At this time the trade took a turn for the worse with bad dates, terrible bosses, and not a lot of money. Nine months into the job I had the confidence to try and square up, so I looked for a part-time job to keep me occupied.

But mostly it was getting lucky at the right time with the right job. This job was not a dead-end, monotonous cashier, check-cashing, or customer service job. It was a job that did not have verbal abuse as part of the description. It was a job that had responsibilities, and most of all, it was a job that challenged me intellectually and satisfied my thirst for knowledge. Somehow, I suddenly figured out this was my ticket out and that maybe there was a life for me beyond the sex trade, but I was always careful to not say to myself I was out of the business forever. I had said that on several occasions and always had to bite myself for it. But somehow, somewhere, I hoped that the seventh time would be the last. I am still hoping. I guess you never know what can happen, and I would not rule out my return if my housing depended on it. On several previous occasions, I returned only because of being outed at previous employments and basically being harassed out of a job, but if not, I would have toughed it out.

# TOP 20 GUIDELINES FOR PROFESSIONALS DEALING WITH EXPLOITED YOUTH

1. Listen.

2. Make decisions with the person.

3. Always be very clear about where you are and what you have to do.

4. Respect the person.

5. Do not make any assumptions.

6. Remember that some people like to choose their own path. Your function is to help increase their options and help them prepare for their future.

7. Always have faith in the person.

8. Think outside of the box when necessary.

9. Always be realistic about your own capacities.

10. Do not force your values or morals on someone else.

11. Remember to treat youth professionally and not personally.

12. Practice objective—not subjective—thinking with sexually exploited youth.

13. Proactive versus reactive; if a young person is in need of assistance, set aside biases and condemnation and replace them with support and alternatives.

14. If working with this population of young people is too hard and you find youself desensitized, imagine living the life so many young people have to live to suvive.

15. Broken promises prevent young people from seeking help. Be clear as to what exactly you can offer as a professional.

16. Treat sexually exploited youth as if they are your own children. Protect them, do not oppress them.

17. Continually educate yourself on the complexities of this issue. In this way, you are better equipped to help sexually exploited youth exit and heal.

18. Youth often feel as if they are treated with condescending attitudes. Your role is that of support and assistance. In time, your efforts will pay off.

19. Encourage youth and provide opportunity whenever possible to help them believe that they are something more than nothing, valued and loved, not worthless and forgotten.

20. Take time for yourself and remember that there is power in one. You may be the light in a sexually exploited youth's life.

Always remember that the sex trade is not about sexuality, morals, or values. The sex trade is about power and control, not sex or one's perception of sex. People involved in the trade are just people, like everyone else.

# Understanding the Impact of Pornography on Adults and Children

Bruce Watson, LLB, CA
Shyla R. Lefever, PhD

Today, pornography is often discussed primarily as a legal issue as if no other factors are involved. Most adults intuitively sense that children and pornography are not an appropriate combination, but such concerns are often not discussed because of First Amendment issues. This legal prism is doubly unfortunate because (a) by historical standards, the reach of the First Amendment is unusually broad on this issue today, and (b) the term *legal* does not mean *harmless*; tobacco, after all, is legal.

This chapter addresses the underlying issue of whether pornography—regardless of its legal standing—is wise, healthy, or consequence free, particularly when it involves children. The evidence shows that any combination of children and pornography is inherently harmful, whether adults are viewing child pornography or children are viewing adult pornography.

Pornography is routinely described as the earliest and most consistent commercial success on the Internet. Part of this success comes from using free samples to attract customers. Unfortunately, these samples are often accessible by anyone, including children. A study in the summer of 2000 found that 1 in 4 youths between the ages of 10 and 17 years old had experienced an unwanted encounter with online pornography in the previous 12 months (Finkelhor et al, 2000).

## The Nature of Pornographic Material

Assessing the influence of pornography requires an understanding of the types of images involved. However, lack of knowledge about the material available today, particularly on the Internet, inhibits meaningful discussion.

Some people are simply unaware of the extent to which pornography has changed in recent decades. Pornography no longer consists solely of coyly posed centerfolds (eg, those in early *Playboy* magazines), which seem almost nostalgic now compared with current offerings. Other people are aware that pornography has changed but are understandably uncomfortable discussing issues related to hard-core pornography (eg, close-up images of clearly visible, vaginal penetration) and the industry's "truly incredible emphasis on anal sex" (Amis, 2001). The explicit images found too easily on the Internet, such as those involving "facials" (ie, ejaculating on another person's face), "water sports" (ie, urinating on another person), bestiality, bondage, and torture are difficult to discuss frankly and honestly. Even high-profile pornographer Larry Flynt, publisher of *Hustler* magazine, observed that "there's an awful lot of material on the Internet that children should not have access to. There's material that even I, in my wildest imagination, would not consider publishing" (Beggy & Carney, 1998).

It is important to be realistic about the nature of the material available today. Pre-serving artistic works such as the nude statue *Venus de Milo* or ensuring the availability of scientific facts such as acquired immunodeficiency syndrome (AIDS) information are legitimate concerns. However, such artistic or scientific works have nothing in common with today's commercial pornography and are mere distractions from the real concerns.

# THE INFLUENCE OF PORNOGRAPHY

It is sometimes considered fashionable to classify sexual activities as just another human function, such as eating or sleeping. Such an attitude makes pornography seem fairly ordinary and routine. However, experience suggests that ignoring the complexities of human sexuality (ie, its emotional, spiritual, and intellectual dimensions as well as its physical aspects) rarely leads to happiness and fulfillment.

Likewise, before dismissing pornography's caricature of human sexuality as harmless fun, it is worthwhile to consider the various indicators of its influence. Indeed, a glance at a *Playboy* magazine does not turn a man into a rapist, but evidence suggests that pornographic messages have a strong, negative influence capable of affecting attitudes and thus behavior. Pornographic images promote the same attitudes toward women that lead to sexual harassment and destroy relationships. They promote attitudes toward sexuality that breed promiscuity and irresponsible sexual behaviors that lead to the spread of sexually transmitted diseases (STDs). Pornographic images clearly model self-gratification at the expense of others. Unlike tobacco, these images do not come with a Surgeon General's warning.

## PORNOGRAPHY AS ADVERTISING

To believe that viewing pornography has no effect on values, attitudes, and behaviors, a person would need to believe that exposure to media, including image-driven media, has no impact on individuals. Advertising professionals know that images do have an effect. Communication experts note that effective advertisements appeal to human emotion—not human reason (Postman, 1994):

TV commercials do not use propositions to persuade; they use visual images … and only rarely … verifiable assertions. Therefore, commercials are not susceptible to logical analysis [and] are not refutable. … It is not facts that are offered to the consumers but idols, to which both adults and children can attach themselves with equal devotion and without the burden of logic or verification.

Which types of "idols" are offered by pornography's highly visual images? With some consistency, pornographic images advertise a particular brand of human sexuality, just as Marlboro cigarettes are associated with a particular type of person, the brawny, rugged Marlboro Man. Scholars note that human sexuality in pornography is never more than physical and is usually fairly one-sided.

— "Depictions of other basic aspects of human sexuality—such as communication between sexual partners, expressions of affection or emotion (except fear and lust) … and concerns about … the consequences of sexual activities—are minimized" (Brosius et al, 1993).

— "[Women are depicted as] malleable, obsessed with sex, and willing to engage in any sexual act with any sexual partner" (Diamond, 1985).

— "The characteristic portrayal of women in pornography [is] as socially non-discriminating, as hysterically euphoric in response to just about any sexual or pseudosexual stimulation, and as eager to accommodate seemingly any and every sexual request" (Zillman & Bryant, 1984).

Of course, such messages would be irrelevant if advertising had no effects on its audience. However, the willingness of profit-oriented companies to spend or invest staggering amounts of money is proof of the influence of advertising. In 1997, America's top 10 advertisers spent a total of $5.2 billion encouraging consumers to part with their money (Ciabattari, 1998). Though people like to believe they are immune to advertisers' messages, the numbers tell a different story—advertising works.

SEXUALLY ORIENTED BUSINESSES

The curiously toxic nature of pornographic images is illustrated by the consistently negative impact that sex businesses have on their surrounding vicinities. The impact of sexually oriented businesses (SOBs) on the areas in which they are located has been demonstrated by numerous land-use studies. In fact, American courts are so convinced that these businesses are harmful, they allow restrictive zoning of SOBs.

The so-called "secondary harmful effects" of SOBs are distinct from the primary harmful effects on the pornography customer, which can not be used as a constitutional basis for zoning ordinances. Secondary harmful effects in neighborhoods with SOBs include a significant increase in property and sexual crimes (including voyeurism, exhibitionism, and assault) and an overall decrease in property values (National Law Center for Children and Families, 1997). For example, reported rapes dropped dramatically in Oklahoma City from 1984 to 1989, the years in which the city closed 150 of 163 sexually oriented businesses.*

In the words of one *Newsweek* columnist, "[o]ne doesn't need a moral micrometer to gauge the fact that the sex industry turned Times Square into a slum" (Will, 1996). Former New York City Mayor Giuliani launched a plan to clean up the city and largely drove the sex industry out of Times Square: "Times Square sex shops [were] replaced by skyscrapers and family-friendly businesses" (Giuliani shows leaders, 2001). According to the vice president of the Times Square Business Improvement District, "[t]he neighborhood is a lot safer. It is a heck of a lot cleaner" (Rutledge, 1998). It is easy to assume that the secondary harmful effects of SOBs reflect something inherently harmful in the material being sold.

EMPIRICAL RESEARCH

Empirical research on pornography is similar to research on most topics, yet the findings are sometimes argued to be inconclusive when conflicting results arise from different studies. This view is promoted strongly by lawyers defending pornographers, who demand a degree of certainty impossible to attain in any social science research. Setting the hurdle impossibly high (ie, by requiring irrefutable proof) is the same device the tobacco companies used for decades to evade admitting the link between smoking and cancer. A basic tenet of the philosophy of science is that scientists do not prove; instead, they fail to disprove. In other words, strong theories exist that are based on repeated tests. Little or nothing can be *conclusively* proven, so the best that can be hoped for is strong evidence and theories that have not yet been disproved. Social science studies rarely have unanimous findings—the rule of random variability dictates that 5 of every 100 studies will contradict the other 95—so it is reasonable to assess the preponderance of the evidence.

The most compelling academic evidence in any social science context comes from reviewing numerous research studies and detecting patterns. Such work can take the form of ***review studies***, which compare the results of numerous original research studies, and ***meta-analyses***, which aggregate the results of original research studies meeting stringent comparability criteria. Examples of review studies and meta-analyses are the following:

— A 1994 review study based on 81 original peer-reviewed research studies on pornography and aggression (35 of which involved aggressive stimuli and 46 of which involved nonaggressive stimuli) concluded that "the empirical research on the effects of aggressive pornography shows, with fairly impressive consistency, that exposure to these materials has a negative effect on attitudes toward women

---

* See the February 22, 1991 letter from Hon. Robert Macy, District Attorney, Oklahoma County, and the March 2, 1990 letter from Ray Pasutti, Uniform Crime Reporting Program supervisor, Oklahoma Bureau of Investigation, to George Harper, leader of an Oklahoma citizen's group. Available from the National Center for Children and Families.

and the perceived likelihood to rape." The study noted that 70% of the 46 non-aggressive studies reported clear evidence of negative effects of exposure (Lyons et al, 1994).

— A 1989 review of a series of studies of "common" pornography found that it leads to insensitivity toward victims of sexual violence, trivialization of rape as a criminal offense, trivialization of sexual child abuse as a criminal offense, an increased belief that lack of sexual activity leads to health risks, and increased acceptance of premarital and extramarital sex. The study noted that "habitual male consumers of common pornography appear to be at greater risk of becoming sexually callous" about female sexuality and related concerns (Zillman, 1989).

— A 1995 meta-analysis of the results of 24 original experimental studies found that "violence within the pornography is not necessary to increase the acceptance of rape myths" (ie, the myth that women secretly desire to be raped). The authors of the study noted that the link between acceptance of rape myths and exposure to pornography stems from a simple premise, "that most pornography commodifies sex, that women become objects used for male pleasure, and that as objects of desire, they are to be acted on." The authors noted that such attitudinal changes are of concern because "several recent meta-analyses demonstrate a high correlation (approximately $r=.80$) between attitude and behavior" (Allen et al, 1995b).

— A 1995 meta-analysis of 33 pornography studies found that "violent content, although possibly magnifying the impact of the pornography, is unnecessary to producing aggressive behavior" (Allen et al, 1995a).

None of these studies suggests that the majority of those who use pornography, particularly pornography consisting of nonviolent images, will commit rape. However, it is important to recognize that when images consistently dehumanize people, as pornography frequently does, the effect on the viewer's attitudes is never positive. The sexually callous attitudes often fostered by exposure to even nonviolent pornography have real-world consequences (Saunders & Naus, 1993; Weaver, 1994). This fact is particularly disturbing in light of research indicating that some people, particularly college-age men, use pornography to teach themselves about sexual behavior (Duncan, 1990; Duncan & Donnelly, 1991; Duncan & Nicholson, 1991).

The foregoing research was conducted largely in controlled, laboratory circumstances, to measure cause and effect without extraneous variables. Another type of research looks at the "laboratory of life" to measure actual experience though with less ability to neutralize extraneous variables. This type of research can prove ***correlation*** (that certain things happen together) without necessarily proving ***causation*** (that one thing caused the other). For this reason, correlational studies must be used with caution, but they are not without value. For example, in some areas where laboratory research is ethically constrained (eg, studies of fatal accidents involving drinking and driving), almost all the evidence is based on correlational studies.

A number of studies have found "strong evidence of a very robust, direct relationship between the circulation rates of sex magazines and rape rates," even after controlling for other variables. Such studies—when taken in conjunction with the controlled laboratory research already discussed—are a valid part of the assessment process.

## EXPERIENCE OF CLINICAL PSYCHOLOGISTS
For years, clinical psychologists treating sexually related addictions have expressed concerns about pornography because of its impact on their patients. For example, in a study by Carnes (1991) of 932 sex addicts, 90% of the men and 77% of the women indicated that pornography played a significant role in their addiction. Carnes later noted, "[m]ost of my patients are CEOs or doctors or attorneys or priests. We have corporate America's leadership marching through here" (Morris, 1999).

As described by Cline (1994), the following is a commonly used classification scheme describing 4 stages through which patients progress after their initial exposure to pornography (Cline, 1994):

1. *Addiction.* Having the desire and need to keep seeking out more pornographic images.

2. *Escalation.* Having the need for more explicit, extreme, and deviant images to obtain the same sexual effect.

3. *Desensitization.* Considering material that was once viewed as shocking or taboo as acceptable or commonplace.

4. *Acting out.* Performing the behaviors viewed, including exhibitionism; sadism, masochism, or both; rape; or sex with children.

Though not all men are equally vulnerable to habitual pornography use, Cline concluded that for some men, pornography "is the gateway drug to sexual addiction" (1994). The evolution of the entire pornography market in the last 2 decades has progressed through the second and third stages experienced by Cline's patients.

The body's biological responses contribute to the power of pornography. The release of the adrenal hormone epinephrine is triggered by any emotional stimulus, including pornography. Epinephrine encourages memorization of what is seen as it "rewards" the body with surges of feelings. Memories are subsequently locked into the brain, which explains the reason people can remember pornographic images seen years before (Cline, 1994). Chemicals called *opioids* are released by nerve endings in response to pleasure and reinforce the body's desire to repeat the process causing the release. Thus, the biological response to pornography rewards the person for viewing the image and reinforces the messages presented. Because these messages often include antisocial attitudes about women, relationships, and behavior, this can be a particularly toxic situation if pornographic images are a child's first exposure to sexuality, and no other point of reference exists.

## DAMAGE TO CHILDREN

Sexuality is among the secret topics adults traditionally refrain from discussing with children until the children are mature enough to understand it. When prematurely exposed to adult sexuality, children are thrust into a world they are in no way prepared to handle.

Adult sexuality is not about simple nudity. Children can be exposed to nude statues such as Michelangelo's *David* or the *Venus de Milo* without an impact to their innocence; 2-year-olds can look at themselves unclothed and see the same thing—a nude body. Adult sexuality involves context and is prepared for incrementally. For example, seeing a loving kiss between parents is quite different from seeing sexual intercourse, and seeing elements of sexuality associated with a loving relationship between parents is quite different from seeing strangers demonstrate poses from the *Kamasutra*.

Children advance through 4 to 5 stages of cognitive development fairly predictably (Atkinson et al, 1987). As Dr. Benjamin Spock posited,

[a]ccording to Piaget (and to almost every scientist that has followed him), children do not simply get smarter as they grow. They actually think in different ways.

What drives the development of thinking is the child's inborn urge to understand the world of people, things, and ideas. At each stage, the child creates theories about the way the world works (2004).

The ramifications of being exposed to concepts too advanced for their developmental stage can have serious, far-reaching effects. Williams (1998) explains

[w]hen a child experiences reality beyond their readiness, they have no means of processing the material intellectually or emotionally. At that time, they will bury the experience in their unconscious, where it will lurk in the shadows, haunting them, possibly for the rest of their lives.

As children progress through the cognitive stages, they develop morally. "Most research supports the view that cognitive development is necessary but not sufficient for advances in moral understanding" (Fogel & Melson, 1987). If children have a traumatic experience that is beyond their understanding, it can hinder their mental and moral development. A case can be made that any deliberate, premature exposure of children to adult sexuality is sexual exploitation.

In contrast, some people suggest that unfettered access to all material, including Internet pornography, helps children develop critical thinking skills. Unfortunately, talking with children about what they have seen or might see does not mitigate the effects of media. Studies indicate that mediation from a variety of perspectives (eg, factual, evaluative) to mitigate the effects of television violence on young children is largely ineffective (Dorr et al, 1980; Nathanson, 2004; Watkins et al, 1988). Studies indicate that among adolescents "there is often a distinction between what is known (on a rational level) and what is desired (on an emotional level)" (Austin & Nach-Ferguson, 1995). In addition, "even adolescents who conclude that television images are unrealistic are susceptible. … Simply put, appeals to rational argument may not be effective" (Nathanson & Botta, 2003). Furthermore, adolescents may believe that the media are a more trustworthy source for determining what is necessary for peer approval (Strasburger, 1995). Clearly it is unrealistic to hope that allowing adolescents access to inappropriate media, whether it is violent, is sexual, or encourages undesirable behavior, and then educating them about the material will somehow make them wiser or more sophisticated.

For one obvious reason, no empirical studies demonstrate that exposing children to adult pornography is harmful—no ethical researcher would conduct experimental studies of pornography's effects on children. The ethical principles of the American Psychological Association (APA) state that "the fundamental requirements are that participants have made *a fully informed and competent decision* to participate and that they emerge from their research experiment unharmed—or, at least, that the risks are minimal, *understood by the participants*, and accepted as reasonable" [emphasis added] (1982). Clearly, no child could give such informed consent. In addition, even researchers not bound by the APA ethics code are monitored by institutional review boards that assess research designs to ensure minimal potential harm exists for participants. No researcher can ensure that sexually explicit material will do little or no harm to children, so studies of children and pornography do not exist.

# CHILD PORNOGRAPHY

At its essence, child pornography is a photographic record of child sexual abuse. Though it might seem obvious that child pornography is harmful, some argue for its legalization on the grounds that although child sexual abuse itself is harmful, the resulting pictures are not the perpetrators of abuse. This is an unfortunately naïve view of the purpose and uses of child pornography. In the abstract, child pornography and pedophilia could be considered separate phenomena. However, as with all forms of pornography, the purpose of child pornography is sexual arousal: Who other than pedophiles are aroused by sexually explicit pictures of children?

Child pornography is used to lower the natural, innate resistance of children to performing sexual acts, thus functioning as a primer for child sexual abuse (Schetky & Green, 1988). By showing resistant children photographs of other children engaged in sexual activities, pedophiles can convince their potential victims, who naturally trust adults and seek their approval, that sexual acts are normal activities children will or should enjoy (Densen-Gerber & Hutchinson, 1979).

Concomitantly, child pornography is used as a type of instruction manual to teach children behaviors that are completely foreign to them. Though children are naturally curious about sexuality, they are only prepared for incremental portions of additional knowledge about sexuality; for example, understanding that a baby can come from Mommy's tummy is quite different from understanding how to perform sexual intercourse.

Pornographic images of an actual child can not be created without sexually exploiting and molesting the child. However, it is the uses of child pornography discussed in the previous paragraph that make "synthetic" child pornography equally dangerous. Synthetic pornography involves computer-generated images, such as those that combine a child's face with an adult's body (or vice versa) or combine different children so the images are not of one specific child. Because children (and often adults) can not distinguish between "real" and "synthetic" images, computer-generated images are just as effective as true pictures for luring children into sexual activities.

Pedophiles often refer to their abuse of children in terms of "love"; for example, one network of pedophiles promoting the elimination of "age of consent" laws is called the North American Man/Boy Love Association (NAMBLA). Its behavior toward children is anything but loving. Pedophiles use child pornography for their own sexual arousal and gratification, and collections of child pornography are often central components of pedophiliac psychology, social orientation, and behavior (Rush, 1981). Children are blackmailed into silence by photographs of themselves engaged in sexual activities arranged by the pedophile. The photographs serve as a permanent record of their experience, the memory of which they can never fully escape.

As with other types of pornography, a significant problem associated with pedophiliac attraction is the process of desensitization and escalation. An increasing level of explicitness or dehumanization may be needed to achieve the same initial thrill. Pictures of nude children cease to be sufficient, creating a child pornography market that suits various types of pedophiles. Photos exist that include children being forced into sexual contact, being sexually tortured, or worse (Burke et al, 2000).

Illegal magazines with such titles as *Lust for Children* and *How to Deflower Your Daughter* (Densen-Gerber & Hutchinson, 1979) were driven so far underground by law enforcement officials in the late 1980s that they became nearly extinct. However, with the advent of the Internet, child pornography exploded (Nordland & Bartholet, 2001). The anonymity provided by Internet interaction, combined with instant access to people of like deviancies, provides an easy method for the exchange of photographs, videos, and audiotapes of child exploitation. In 1998, the discovery of an international child pornography ring called the Wonderland Club provided a clear example of the way pedophiles use the Internet, with more than 100 000 images being traded among 100 suspects in 14 countries (Grunwald, 1998). Law enforcement officials began arresting participants sooner than ideal because later evidence revealed that new images were being created for exchange at the time of the arrests.

Child pornography and pedophiliac activity are particularly dangerous to children online. Children use the Internet from home, school, the library, and other familiar, traditionally safe locations—locations where they can be unexpectedly confronted with unsafe material. Children's combination of innocence and innate sense of security makes them vulnerable to the intrinsic dangers of child pornography and pedophilia and to becoming new victims.

## CONCLUSION

Can the harm caused by pornography be established with the certainty of a geometry proof? No, because this level of certainty does not apply to behavioral research. The correct scientific question is, has the harm that can be caused by pornography been *disproved*?

Evidence demonstrates that pornographic material is not just a source of harmless fun. Pornography does not portray real-life human sexuality; it is a dehumanizing, synthetic version of sex that eliminates love, honor, dignity, true intimacy, and commitment. The image of sexuality offered by pornography is one devoid of relationships, responsibility, or consequences—a largely fraudulent picture. Pornographic movies never portray a girlfriend getting pregnant at the age of 16, a young man getting AIDS, or a man's marriage crumbling because of his infidelity.

The research demonstrates that these fraudulent messages are internalized and affect attitudes and behavior. Countless studies show that the basic messages of pornography (eg, that a woman's purpose is to satisfy a man sexually, women have no value, women's desires and needs are irrelevant) breed sexual callousness and worse.

The attitudes promoted by pornography lead to sexual harassment, failed relationships, promiscuity at a young age, and the spread of STDs. Unless a person believes that attitudes and behaviors are unrelated, it should not be surprising that a correlation between pornography usage and sexually abusive behaviors has been found. Considering the damage pornography does to adults, it is foolish to suggest that it is not a real danger to children.

People protect themselves and their communities using their values as a guide. Treating every human being with respect, equality, and dignity is a value people should embrace, as a society and as individuals. Pornography replaces respect, equality, and dignity with a candy-coated message of hate. Rather than passively believing that the First Amendment can silence those who oppose pornography, society should recognize that it actually enables the community to speak out against pornography by discussing it honestly.

# REFERENCES

Allen M, D'Alessio D, Brezgel K. A meta-analysis summarizing the effects of pornography, II. *Hum Commun Res.* 1995a;22:258-283.

Allen M, Emmers T, Gebhardt L, Giery MA. Exposure to pornography and acceptance of rape myths. *J Comm.* 1995b;45(1):5-26.

American Psychological Association. *Ethical Principles in the Conduct of Research with Human Participants.* Washington, DC: American Psychological Association; 1982.

Amis M. A rough trade. *Guardian Observer.* March 17, 2001. Available at: http://www.guardian.co.uk/weekend/story/0,3605,458078,00.html. Accessed August 27, 2004.

Atkinson RL, Atkinson RC, Smith EE, Hilgard E, eds. *Introduction to Psychology.* San Diego, Calif: Harcourt Brace Jovanovich; 1987.

Austin EW, Nach-Ferguson B. Sources and influences of young school-age children's general and brand-specific knowledge about alcohol. *Health Commun.* 1995;7:1-20.

Beggy C, Carney B. Friends of Abbie to gather at Avalon. *Boston Globe.* November 20, 1998.

Brosius HB, Weaver JB, Staab JF. Exploring the social and sexual "reality" of contemporary pornography. *J Sex Res.* 1993;30:161-170.

Burke J, Gentleman A, Willan P. British link to 'snuff' videos. *Guardian Observer.* October 1, 2000. Available at: http://observer.guardian.co.uk/uk_news/story/0,6903,375883,00.html. Accessed August 27, 2004.

Carnes P. *Don't Call It Love: Recovery from Sexual Addictions.* New York, NY: Bantam; 1991.

Ciabattari J. Who spends the most on ads? *Parade Magazine.* August 16, 1998.

Cline VB. *Pornography's Effects on Adults and Children*. New York, NY: Morality In Media; 1994.

Densen-Gerber J, Hutchinson S. Sexual and commercial exploitation of children: legislative response and treatment challenge. *Child Abuse Negl*. 1979;3:61-66.

Diamond S. Pornography: image and reality. In: Burstyn V, ed. *Women Against Censorship*. Vancouver, Canada: Douglas & McIntyre; 1985.

Dorr A, Graves SB, Phelps E. Television literacy for young children. *J Commun*. 1980;30(3):71-83.

Duncan D. Pornography as a source of sex information for university students. *Psychol Rep*. 1990;66:442.

Duncan D, Donnelly J. Pornography as a source of sex information for students at Northeastern University. *Psychol Rep*. 1991;78:782.

Duncan D, Nicholson T. Pornography as a source of sex information at Southeastern University. *Psychol Rep*. 1991;68:802.

Finkelhor D, Mitchell KJ, Wolak J. *Online Victimization: A Report on the Nation's Youth*. Alexandria, Va: National Center for Missing & Exploited Children; 2000.

Fogel A, Melson GF, eds. *Child Development: Individual, Family, and Society*. St Paul, Minn: West Publishing; 1987:418.

Grunwald M. Global Internet child porn ring uncovered. *The Washington Post*. September 3, 1998:A1.

Giuliani shows leaders how to lead [editorial]. *Peoria Journal Star*. December 29, 2001:A04.

Lyons JS, Anderson RL, Larsen D. A systematic review of the effects of aggressive and nonaggressive pornography. In: Zillman D, Bryant J, Huston AC, eds. *Media, Children & the Family: Social Scientific, Psychodynamic, and Clinical Perspectives*. Hillsdale, NJ: Lawrence Erlbaum Associates; 1994:271-312.

Morris B. Addicted to sex: corporate America's dirty secret. *Fortune*. May 15, 1999; 139:66-82.

Nathanson AI. Factual and evaluative approaches to modifying children's responses to violent television. *J Commun*. 2004;54:321-336.

Nathanson AI, Botta RA. Shaping the effects of television on adolescents' body image disturbance: the role of parental mediation. *Commun Res*. 2003;30(3):304-331.

National Law Center for Children and Families. *National Law Center Summary of "SOB land use" Studies: Crime Impact Studies by Municipal and State Governments on Harmful Secondary Effects of Sexually Oriented Businesses*. Fairfax, Va: National Law Center for Children and Families; 1997.

Nordland R, Bartholet J. The web's dark secret. *Newsweek*. March 19, 2001:44-51.

Postman N. *The Disappearance of Childhood*. New York, NY: Vintage Books; 1994: 107-108.

Rush F. *The Best Kept Secret (Sexual Abuse of Children)*. New York, NY: McGraw-Hill; 1981.

Rutledge M. New York proves zoning can chase out sex shops. *Cincinnati Post*. April 2, 1998:1A.

Saunders RM, Naus PJ. The impact of social content and audience factors on responses to sexually explicit videos. *J Sex Educ Ther*. 1993;19:117-131.

Schetky DH, Green AH. *Child Sexual Abuse: A Handbook for Health Care and Legal Professionals.* New York, NY: Brunner/Mazel; 1988.

Spock B. Stages in cognitive development. Dr. Spock Web site. Available at: http://www.drspock.com/article/0,1510,4986,00.html?r=related. Accessed November 11, 2004.

Strasburger VC. *Adolescents and the Media: Medical and Psychological Impact.* Thousand Oaks, Calif: Sage Publications; 1995.

Watkins LT, Sprafkin J, Gadow KD, Sadetsky I. Effects of a critical viewing skills curriculum on elementary school children's knowledge and attitudes about television. *J Educ Res.* 1988;81:165-170.

Weaver JB. Pornography and sexual callousness: the perceptual and behavioral consequences of exposure to pornography. In: Zillman D, Bryant J, Huston AC, eds. *Media, Children, and the Family: Social Scientific, Psychodynamic, and Clinical Perspectives.* Hillsdale, NJ: Lawrence Erlbaum Associates; 1994:215-228.

Will GF. Big stick conservatism. *Newsweek.* November 11, 1996:96.

Williams L. Letter. *Enough Is Enough Newsletter.* December 1998:6.

Zillman D. Effects of prolonged consumption of pornography. In: Zillman D, Bryant J, eds. *Pornography: Research Advances and Policy Considerations.* Hillsdale, NJ: Lawrence Erlbaum Associates; 1989:127-157.

Zillman D, Bryant J. Effects of massive exposure to pornography. In: Malamuth NM, Donnerstein E, eds. *Pornography and Sexual Aggression.* Orlando, Fla: Academic Press; 1984:115-138.

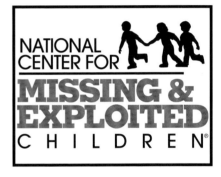

Chapter

## 10

# RESOURCES OF THE EXPLOITED CHILD UNIT AT THE NATIONAL CENTER FOR MISSING & EXPLOITED CHILDREN®

Kathy A. Free, MA
Michelle K. Collins, MA

## THE CREATION OF THE NATIONAL CENTER FOR MISSING & EXPLOITED CHILDREN®

In 1981, 6-year-old Adam Walsh was abducted from a shopping mall in Florida. His desperate parents, John and Revé Walsh, came to Washington, DC, seeking help to recover their child. They were frustrated by the lack of a coordinated response to their child's case. The Walshes turned their anger into action and went to Congress to mandate the creation of an agency to assist in missing children's cases. In 1984, John and Revé Walsh co-founded the private, nonprofit National Center for Missing & Exploited Children (NCMEC) (**Figure 10-1**). The NCMEC serves as a central clearinghouse in providing assistance to parents, children, law enforcement, other professionals, schools, and the community in recovering missing children and raising public awareness about ways to help prevent child abduction and child sexual victimization. The NCMEC has worked on more than 89 500 cases of missing and exploited children, helped recover more than 73 000 children, and raised its recovery rate from 60% in the 1980s to more than 95% today due to the increased use of technology to disseminate information regarding missing children. The NCMEC has received national and international recognition as the resource for missing and exploited children.

**Figure 10-1.** Logo of the National Center for Missing & Exploited Children (NCMEC). Reprinted with permission from the NCMEC.

## THE GROWTH OF SEXUAL EXPLOITATION ON THE INTERNET

The Internet has created an exciting world of information and communication for anyone with access to online services. While this new world offers unparalleled opportunities for children and adults to learn, some risks and dangers exist, especially for children. This may include access to illegal content on the Web or receiving inappropriate or unsolicited e-mail or chat messages. In addition, individuals who prey on children often use computer technology to seek unsupervised access to, and contact with, children. Due to perceived anonymity on the Internet, a sexual predator may approach multiple children online to begin "grooming" the child for a sexual encounter offline. The nature of the Internet allows these individuals to create numerous profiles online, which a child is unable to verify. In addition, new technologies and free online services with little authentication of users allow individuals to target children or trade illegal material with little risk.

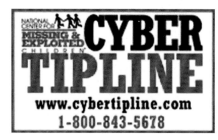

***Figure 10-2.** Logo of the NCMEC's CyberTipline. Reprinted with permission from the NCMEC.*

# THE EXPLOITED CHILD UNIT

After several high-profile cases in the mid-1990s involving children meeting adults online and being lured offline for sexual activity, the US Congress mandated the creation of the Exploited Child Unit (ECU) within the NCMEC to better safeguard children from sexual exploitation. In 1996, the ECU opened its doors to serve as a resource center for the public, parents, law enforcement, and others on the issues of the sexual exploitation of children. The 3 main services provided by the ECU are:

— *CyberTipline.* The CyberTipline (**Figure 10-2**) is an online mechanism for the public to report incidents of child sexual exploitation (CSE). Staff members at the NCMEC process these reports and disseminate the leads to federal, state, local, and international law enforcement agencies for further investigation.

— *Child Victim Identification Project* (CVIP). The ECU has become a leading resource on the identification of children depicted in child pornography images. The ECU has developed several resources to assist law enforcement and prosecutors in cases involving child pornography.

— *Exploited Child Unit Technical Assistance Services.* Based on their knowledge and experience in handling CSE cases, ECU staff members provide assistance to federal, state, local, and international law enforcement agencies with their investigations.

## THE CYBERTIPLINE: THE PUBLIC'S RESOURCE FOR PROTECTING CHILDREN

On March 9, 1998, key public and private sector leaders joined with the NCMEC to launch the CyberTipline. The CyberTipline was created for individuals to report incidents of CSE (NCMEC, 2003) including the following:

— *Possession, manufacturing, and distribution of child pornography.* Child pornography has been defined under federal statute as a visual depiction of a minor (child younger than 18) engaged in sexually explicit conduct (18 USC § 2256).

— *Online enticement of children for sexual acts.* This refers to the use of the Internet to entice, invite,or persuade a child to meet for sexual actions or to help arrange such a meeting (18 USC § 2425).

— *Child prostitution.* **Prostitution** is generally defined as performing, offering, or agreeing to perform a sexual act for any money, property, token, object, article, or anything of value (18 USC § 2423a; 18 USC § 2431).

— *Child sex tourism.* Under federal law, a US citizen can not travel abroad to engage in sexual activity with any child under the age of 18 (18 USC § 2423b).

— *Extrafamilial child sexual molestation.* This category includes sexual abuse of a child by someone other than a family member.

— *Sending unsolicited obscene material to a child.* Criminal law states that knowingly attempting to send or transfer obscene material to another individual   who has not attained the age of 16 years is illegal (18 USCA § 1470).

As of July 2003, more than 135 000 leads have been reported to the CyberTipline, with the number increasing each year (**Figure 10-3**). It must be pointed out that the ECU handles Internet and non-Internet related cases. However, most of the reports received on the CyberTipline have some connection to the Internet. Approximately 90% of the reports received on the CyberTipline are categorized as child pornography or online enticement of children for sexual acts.

### How Does the CyberTipline Work?

When an incident occurs, the reporting person accesses the CyberTipline online at www.cybertipline.com or via telephone at 1-800-843-5678. The NCMEC has worked with law enforcement to develop a reporting form that captures relevant information needed to begin an investigation. The reporting person is asked to provide information on the incident, suspect, and child victim.

Staff members in the NCMEC's communication center (which operates 24 hours a day, 7 days a week) review and prioritize each lead by assessing the immediate danger to the child. With approximately 1000 reports a week, this triage is critical for the ECU because it provides a starting point for staff members. ECU staff members analyze each CyberTipline report and "add value" to the lead for law enforcement. That analysis may include visiting a reported Web site to review posted content and determine its legality under federal law, contacting the reporting person to gather additional information regarding the incident, and conducting searches using various Internet tools. The report is then disseminated to the appropriate law enforcement agency for further investigation. (eg, Federal Bureau of Investigations [FBI], Internet Crimes Aginst Children [ICAC] task force) **Figure 10-4** shows the architecture of the CyberTipline (US General Accounting Office [US GAO], 2002).

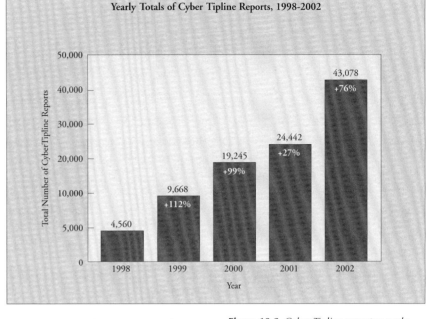

**Figure 10-3.** *Cyber Tipline reports: yearly totals, 1998-2002. Percentages indicate the percentage increase from the previous year. Reprinted with permission from the NCMEC.*

*Mandated Reporting From Internet Service Providers*
Recognizing that the battle against the proliferation of child pornography could not be won solely through the public's vigilance, Congress passed legislation in 1999 mandating that electronic communication service providers report any instances of child pornography to law enforcement through the NCMEC's CyberTipline (42 USCA § 13032):

Whoever, while engaged in providing an electronic communication service or a remote computing service to the public, through a facility or means of interstate or foreign commerce, obtains knowledge of facts or circumstances from which a violation of section 2251, 2251A, 2252, 2252A, or 2260 of Title 18, involving child pornography (as defined in section 2256 of that title), is apparent, shall, as soon as reasonably possible, make a report of such facts or circumstances to the CyberTipline at the National Center for Missing & Exploited Children, which shall forward that report to a law enforcement agency or agencies designated by the Attorney General.

To comply with this additional mandate, the NCMEC created a separate online mechanism for providers to report incidents of child pornography. The new site was launched in February 2001. Currently, the NCMEC has more than 110 providers registered to report to the CyberTipline. Reports from providers comprise approximately 50% of the total number of reports received on a weekly basis.

CHILD VICTIM IDENTIFICATION PROJECT
Each year, the volume of child pornography images circulating on the Internet increases rapidly. The faces of the children being sexually victimized stare emptily at the camera lens. The exact moment when the children are most exposed and vulnerable is permanently recorded. Child pornography images act as a tool to ensure that the victimization of the children will never truly end. With the advent of the Internet, these images featuring children being physically and emotionally assaulted will continue to be viewed by Internet users all over the world. Questions beg to be answered: Who are the children seen in these images? Have their offenders been brought to justice? Have the children received therapeutic assistance to aid in the recovery from their molestation?

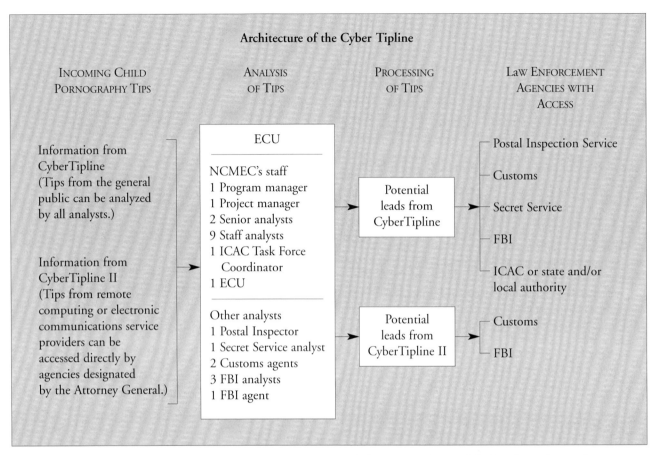

**Architecture of the Cyber Tipline**

| INCOMING CHILD PORNOGRAPHY TIPS | ANALYSIS OF TIPS | PROCESSING OF TIPS | LAW ENFORCEMENT AGENCIES WITH ACCESS |
|---|---|---|---|

Information from CyberTipline (Tips from the general public can be analyzed by all analysts.)

Information from CyberTipline II (Tips from remote computing or electronic communications service providers can be accessed directly by agencies designated by the Attorney General.)

**ECU**

NCMEC's staff
1 Program manager
1 Project manager
2 Senior analysts
9 Staff analysts
1 ICAC Task Force Coordinator
1 ECU

Other analysts
1 Postal Inspector
1 Secret Service analyst
2 Customs agents
3 FBI analysts
1 FBI agent

Potential leads from CyberTipline

Potential leads from CyberTipline II

Postal Inspection Service

Customs

Secret Service

FBI

ICAC or state and/or local authority

Customs

FBI

***Figure 10-4.*** *Organization of the NCMEC's Exploited Child Unit. Reprinted from the US General Accounting Office.*

Due to the experience with the CyberTipline and the handling of more than 100 000 child pornography reports, the ECU has become a leading resource on the identification of children victimized in the creation of child pornography. The mission of the CVIP is twofold:

1. Identify child victims featured in child pornography images.

2. Assist law enforcement agencies and prosecutors in enhancing the prosecutions of federal, state, and local cases involving child pornography and CSE.

The most beneficial resource contained within the CVIP is the broad knowledge base of child victims who have been identified by law enforcement in previous investigations. Despite the arduous nature of such a compilation, the NCMEC's strong relationship with domestic and international law enforcement agencies has developed into an ever-growing catalog of child pornography series containing known victims.

The ruling of the US Supreme Court in the case of *Ashcroft v Free Speech Coalition,* which stated that digitally created child pornography is legal, (2002) has led to new developments within the CVIP. This ruling created an explosion of requests from law enforcement and prosecution teams working vigorously to ensure convictions in child pornography cases. The expertise within the CVIP is solicited on a daily basis for assistance in securing convictions for those offenders charged with child pornography-related crimes.

In response to this court ruling, the NCMEC has taken on a new role by assisting law enforcement agencies and prosecutors with selecting child pornography images that contain children who have been identified as real children in past investigations. This information is provided to requesting law enforcement agencies on a case-by-case basis.

## Child Recognition & Identification System

The Child Recognition & Identification System (CRIS) is a computer application developed by the NCMEC to scan and select image files containing child victims who have been identified by law enforcement in past investigations. CRIS recognizes images based solely on the MD5 hash values (a mathematical algorithm) to verify that the content of a file exactly matches another.

In conjunction with the United States Postal Inspection Service (USPIS), CVIP analysts review seized child pornography images on a case-by-case basis. The questionable images are transferred via US mail to the postal inspector assigned to the NCMEC. The submitted images are controlled and secured by sworn law enforcement officials and provided to a CVIP analyst for review. All images are processed through CRIS for immediate selection of those files that contain child victims who have been identified by law enforcement agencies in previous investigations. In addition, images are visually reviewed by CVIP staff to ensure that all images of known children have been documented. Upon completion of the analysis, a Child Identification Report is generated for the submitting agency. This report provides law enforcement point-of-contact information for each child victim. The report specifies exact file names along with the contact information for the law enforcement agency that identified each child. This information allows the requestor to go directly to the police officer who interviewed the child and to obtain documentation for court purposes that the child is, indeed, a real child.

## Child Pornography Evidence Guide

The ECU has created a Child Pornography Evidence Guide to assist law enforcement in becoming familiar with many child pornography series containing identified children. This guide also assists investigators in selecting images that contain identified children. This guide is distributed to requesting law enforcement agencies only.

Pursuant to the NCMEC's concern in protecting against further victimization, the Evidence Guide does not contain any images of the child victims. The Child Pornography Evidence Guide contains the following information:

— Child pornography series name(s)

— Comprehensive series description (sexual activity, background, physical descriptions)

— Series identifiers (distinct items, clothing, tattoos)

— Partial file names

The Child Pornography Evidence Guide is continually being revised to reflect the newest child pornography series containing known victims. The NCMEC seeks continued cooperation with law enforcement to facilitate sharing information on investigations in which a child has been identified as being exploited in the production of child pornography. The information compiled from numerous law enforcement agencies is critical to continuing successful prosecutions all over the country.

## Methods of Identification

Identifying the children featured in child pornography images is a daunting challenge. The most critical impediment in the identification process is the lack of distinguishing features within the images themselves. The rapid proliferation of the images ensures that, within hours of a new image being posted on the Internet, hundreds or thousands of people will have downloaded the image and may already be trading it. Therefore, a basic assumption in online investigations is that the person who is trading the illegal images often was not involved in the creation of the image. This being the case, it is necessary that the child pornography images be analyzed for any items in the background that may assist in determining a jurisdiction where the child may be located. Some items that may assist in the identification process are electrical sockets, shopping bags, calendars, automobile license plates, telephone books, or television programs. As a leading resource on child pornography cases, the NCMEC has learned of multiple ways in which child victims have been identified by law enforcement.

It is quite common for a victim of child pornography to be "accidentally" rescued as a result of a police investigation into another crime. In one instance, an adult male traveled to a midwestern state to engage in sexual activity with what he thought was a teenage girl he had met online. Upon his arrival, the same undercover law enforcement agents who had been communicating with him arrested him. After his arrest, the perpetrator's home computer was seized and subjected to forensic analysis. Dozens of images showing him sexually molesting his daughter were found on his computer. Unfortunately, the images of this child are well known on the Internet and are practically a "staple" for most child pornography collectors. Realistically, had this perpetrator not been arrested for traveling to another state to have sex with a minor, his daughter may never have been identified and received the therapeutic help she so desperately needed.

Sometimes, victims of child pornography are rescued when a child discloses his or her abuse to a trusted adult. A young girl who had been molested over several years by her father summoned the courage to approach a school official and disclose the abuse. Law enforcement and social services were immediately notified, and the child was removed from her home that day. The child's biological father and stepmother were arrested and charged with child molestation and production of child pornography. What the authorities did not realize at the time of trial was that the images of this young girl had been posted to the Internet and could be found on countless Web sites, newsgroups, and message boards. Although the child was removed from the abusive situation, the long-term emotional scars for the child will include not only the sexual abuse but also the knowledge that pictures of her most traumatic experiences are actively traded and collected by pedophiles around the world.

Sometimes, clues found within an image will lead to the identification of a child victim. A certain child pornography series on the Internet contains one image that features an abuser wearing a long-sleeved shirt with a company logo on the front shirt pocket. Observant authorities noticed the logo and decided to pursue the lead. They took a photograph of the adult male's face to the company and requested assistance in his identification. Company officials revealed that this individual was an ex-employee. Law enforcement authorities immediately obtained a search warrant, and the search of the perpetrator's home revealed the child victim seen in the pornographic images. The child was rescued from the sexual abuse of her father and mother.

Several European nations have decided to take a proactive approach to identifying unknown child pornography victims. Law enforcement officials subject the images from child pornography series to intense analysis for information that may identify or locate the victim. This proactive approach has identified several child victims. In 2002, a new child pornography series attracted the attention of investigators in several countries. Authorities analyzed the images closely in an effort to determine the country of origin. Based upon electrical sockets and several items with brand names seen in the background, the investigators concluded that the images were produced in a specific European country. Authorities issued a wide- spread request to all law enforcement agencies in that country inquiring whether the child victim had been identified in any past criminal cases. When authorities were confident that the child victim had not yet been rescued from the abusive situation, they decided to solicit the help of the public. A headshot of the young child was featured on a nationwide television network along with a message that made no mention of the sensitive details of the case. Instead, authorities merely stated that pictures of the girl were found during a criminal investigation and that police wanted to know the identity of the child. More than 30 tips were phoned in from citizens offering information on the identity of the child. Within hours, the child's abuser went to a local police station and surrendered. He confessed to sexually molesting this child and was immediately arrested. Although this proactive approach involving media assistance is controversial in some countries due to legal constraints, several children have been rescued from sexually abusive situations because of this technique.

## EXPLOITED CHILD UNIT TECHNICAL ASSISTANCE SERVICES

In addition to providing many other services, the ECU serves as a technical and informational resource for more than 18 000 state and local law enforcement agencies in the United States and abroad. Investigating child exploitation cases may require specialized technical skills outside the scope of usual investigation methods. As a result of being the central clearinghouse on CSE and handling more than 120 000 CyberTipline reports and requests from law enforcement, ECU staff members have vast experience in CSE cases. Analysts are available to assist in any child exploitation case, not just those originating from the CyberTipline. The technical assistance services available from the ECU are listed in **Table 10-1**.

## LAW ENFORCEMENT PARTNERSHIPS

The NCMEC is not an investigative agency, so partnerships with law enforcement are critical to the success of the NCMEC and the ECU. The NCMEC is fortunate to have several federal agencies represented at its headquarters in Virginia. The FBI, the Bureau of Immigration and Customs Enforcement (formerly the United States Customs Service), the USPIS, the United States Secret Service, and the Bureau of Alcohol, Tobacco and Firearms each have personnel assigned to work at the NCMEC's headquarters. They serve as the liaisons to their respective agencies and assist NCMEC staff members with case analysis and investigative support. As a result of these partnerships, hundreds of arrests have resulted from reports received via the CyberTipline. The following 2 case studies are examples of this success.

**Case Study 10-1**

The CyberTipline received a report from an individual who had pretended online to be a 14-year-old boy. The suspect began communicating with the reporting person in private chat rooms and sent images of child pornography to the reporting party. The suspect claimed that he was the adult pictured in these child pornography images and stated that his 40-year-old friend was also molesting one of the boys depicted in the images. The ECU conducted various Internet and public record searches that confirmed the suspect's residential address in Akron, Ohio. The ECU contacted the Akron Police Department and the Ohio Attorney General's Office. Nine days later, the Akron Police Department arrested the suspect at work, and a search warrant was executed at his home. The suspect was charged with the rape of 2 boys, corruption of a minor (for a third boy), and pandering sexually oriented material on the Internet. The predator was sentenced to 2 life sentences.

**Case Study 10-2**

The Wisconsin Division of Criminal Investigation (DCI) received a tip from a woman in Iowa reporting a possible abduction in Madison, Wisconsin. The caller stated that she had information about a 53-year-old man from Indiana who had been communicating with a 14-year-old girl from Wisconsin via the Internet for 3 years. The caller stated that the suspect intended to have sexual relations with the child and that she wished to run away with him. Based on this CyberTipline report, law enforcement initiated an investigation and identified the 14-year-old child. The online identity of the child was assumed by law enforcement, and arrangements were made to meet the suspect in Madison. On June 16, 2000, the 53-year-old suspect was arrested when he traveled to Madison to meet the child. After his arrest, DCI agents conducted a search of his truck and found in his possession an unsheathed 12-inch axe, 4 pieces of rope, drug paraphernalia, and a bottle of Demerol painkillers. A criminal history records check revealed that in 1968, the suspect had been convicted of second-degree murder in Indiana. He was released on parole in October 1991. During a 1-week jury trial in Dane County Circuit Court, he was found guilty and sentenced to 14 years in prison, followed by 10 years probation.

**Table 10-1. Technical Assistance Services Available From the Exploited Child Unit Internet Searches**

ECU analysts have extensive training in data collection using the Internet. Analysts use Internet resources to gather information on Web sites, e-mail addresses, newsgroup postings, and suspect locations as well as other important pieces of information relevant to the case. Many times the ECU analyst is able to provide information to the requesting agency with a detailed list of the suspect's Internet activities.

PUBLIC RECORD DATABASE SEARCHES

The ECU has access to several public record databases that may yield critical information on suspects such as Social Security and/or drivers' license numbers, past criminal history, and recent addresses.

CYBERTIPLINE HISTORICAL SEARCHES

As of July 2003, there were more than 135 000 reports in the CyberTipline and technical assistance databases, and they continue to grow by more than 1000 reports a week. ECU analysts can search these databases for previous reports related to current investigations using various criteria such as suspect names, e-mail addresses, Web addresses, and even text phrases.

TECHNICAL EXPERTISE

The computer skills and knowledge of the ECU analysts are continually developing and expanding as the Internet continues to evolve. Analysts have a pool of expert knowledge on the various programs, software, and technology used on the Internet today in forums such as peer-to-peer networks, the World Wide Web, e-mail applications, Internet Relay Chat, and File Transfer Protocol.

LAW ENFORCEMENT CONTACTS

CyberTipline leads are received from all over the world; therefore, the ECU is continually establishing new contacts with domestic and international law enforcement agencies that specialize in child exploitation cases. These contacts may be beneficial for multijurisdictional and multinational cases.

INTERNET SERVICE PROVIDER (ISP) CONTACTS

Since 1999, ISPs have been required to report child pornography to the CyberTipline per 42 USC § 13032(B)(1). ISPs are able to provide law enforcement with evidence, subscriber information, and user history. The ECU has an extensive list of ISP contact names, telephone numbers, and e-mail addresses to assist law enforcement in accessing information.

PUBLICATIONS

The NCMEC has numerous publications available on Internet safety and preventing, understanding, and investigating child sexual exploitation. Copies of these publications are available online at www.missingkids.com or may be obtained by calling 1-800-843-5678.

TRAINING

The NCMEC, in conjunction with various partners, offers numerous courses several times a year all around the nation to train professionals on investigating and preventing child exploitation. The NCMEC Legal Resource Division offers training in specialized skills needed by prosecutors, judges, and law enforcement officers on how to adjudicate these cases successfully. In addition, it also provides technical assistance in the investigation and prosecution of violent crimes against children.

FEDERAL BUREAU OF INVESTIGATION
Crimes Against Children Program
In May 1997, FBI Director Louis Freeh ordered each of the 56 field offices to designate at least 2 agents as Crimes Against Children Coordinators (US GAO,

2002). These agents coordinate investigations for the FBI and serve as liaisons with local law enforcement agencies on crimes against children cases.

Innocent Images National Initiative

The FBI's Innocent Images National Initiative (IINI) identifies and investigates sexual predators who use the Internet to exploit children. The IINI program is run out of the CyberCrimes Division and focuses on 2 areas of CSE: individuals who indicate a willingness to travel interstate for the purpose of engaging in sexual activity with a minor and producers and/or distributors of child pornography (FBI, 2003).

BUREAU OF IMMIGRATION AND CUSTOMS ENFORCEMENT

The Bureau of Immigration and Customs Enforcement established the Cyber-Smuggling Investigations Center to focus resources more effectively on Internet crimes (US GAO, 2002). The center acts as a clearinghouse of investigations on cybercrimes. More specifically, it targets the illegal importation and trafficking of child pornography (US GAO, 2002).

UNITED STATES POSTAL INSPECTION SERVICE

The USPIS has been involved in the investigation of child pornography cases since the first federal law banning the sending of child pornography through the mail was passed in 1978. The USPIS has inspectors all over the country specially trained in handling CSE cases. Even though the use of the Internet has grown dramatically, the postal inspectors still find vast amounts of illegal material being sent through the US mail (US GAO, 2002). As a result of their many years working on child exploitation cases, USPIS inspectors can provide invaluable assistance to any requesting law enforcement agency.

INTERNET CRIMES AGAINST CHILDREN TASK FORCES

While federal programs for CSE have expanded over the past years, local law enforcement is a critical partner in combating CSE. In 1998, the US Department of Justice's Office of Juvenile Justice and Delinquency Prevention authorized the creation of the Internet Crimes Against Children Task Force Program to help state and local law enforcement agencies develop an effective response to Internet crimes against children (Medaris & Girouard, 2002). The funding has allowed law enforcement agencies to increase forensic and investigative resources and provide opportunities for training and technical assistance, victim services, and community education (Medaris & Girouard, 2002). Currently there are 36 regional task forces and 43 investigative satellites funded through this program.

MULTIJURISDICTIONAL CASES

Internet-related CSE cases can present unique jurisdictional challenges for local, state, federal, and international law enforcement agencies. The Internet knows no boundaries; therefore, in many instances, it is extremely difficult to determine one location for a particular incident. Consider this example: a commercial child pornography Web site has been established using a free Web-hosting company located in Country A. The individual who created the Web site resides in Country B. The billing company being used by this criminal is hosted in Country C. The customers who purchase access to the commercial site are located all over the world. Which law enforcement agency should lead this investigation? How many law enforcement agencies need to be involved? What are the laws in each country regarding the possession, manufacturing, and/or distribution of child pornography? Understandably, this type of scenario can create jurisdictional problems because numerous law enforcement agencies would need to be involved in such a case. Despite the seemingly overwhelming challenges, there have been several successful multijurisdictional investigations.

The USPIS conducted a joint operation (code-named "Operation Avalanche") with the Dallas Internet Crimes Against Children Task Force regarding a commercial child pornography Web site that was being run out of Texas but had customers from all over the world purchasing access. These 2 agencies used the network of Internet Crimes Against Children Task Forces to investigate targets within the United States. So far, 130 individuals have been arrested. Information regarding suspects in foreign countries was forwarded to the respective law enforcement agencies in each country, and numerous arrests have resulted. To date, this was the largest commercial child pornography enterprise ever encountered.

## CONCLUSION

In March 1998, the ECU's CyberTipline received a total of 450 reports. In contrast, during March 2003, more than 6700 CyberTipline reports were received. The astounding increase in the number of reports demonstrates the vast problem of child exploitation and the need for all law enforcement agencies to have a coordinated response. No longer can law enforcement agencies deny that these heinous events are occurring.

The sexual exploitation of children, online and offline, is an issue beyond any recognizable borders and requires a global response. Now more than ever, the coordination of efforts and agencies is necessary to apprehend those who commit these atrocious crimes. Virtually all computer-related child exploitation cases will require law enforcement officers to interact with agencies outside their jurisdiction. A strong network of capable investigators is critical for success. By continuing to address the ever-evolving needs of CSE investigators worldwide, the ECU will remain an international resource at the forefront of combating child sexual victimization.

## REFERENCES

*Ashcroft v Free Speech Coalition*, 535 US 234 (9th Cir 2002).

18 USC § 2256.

18 USC § 2423a.

18 USC § 2423b.

18 USC § 2425.

18 USC § 2431.

18 USCA § 1470.

Federal Bureau of Investigation (FBI). Online child pornography: Innocent Images National Initiative. FBI Web site. Available at: http://www.fbi.gov/hq/cid/cac/innocent.htm. Accessed February 2, 2003.

42 USCA § 13032.

Medaris M, Girouard C. *Protecting Children in Cyberspace: The ICAC Task Force Program: The Internet Crimes Against Children Program.* Washington, DC: Office of Juvenile Justice and Delinquency Programs; January 2002. NCJ 191213. Available at: http://www.ncjrs.org/pdffiles1/ojjdp/191213.pdf. Accessed September 28, 2004.

National Center for Missing & Exploited Children. The CyberTipline. 2003. Available at: http://www.cybertipline.com. Accessed September 19, 2003.

US General Accounting Office. *Combating Child Pornography: Federal Agencies Coordinate Law Enforcement Efforts, but an Opportunity Exists for Further Enhancement.* Washington, DC: US General Accounting Office; 2002. GAO-03-272.

# Chapter 11

# MEDICAL ANALYSIS OF CHILD PORNOGRAPHY

Sharon W. Cooper, MD, FAAP

The medical analysis of child pornography is an adjunct to the investigation process, although it is not an absolute requirement since most child sexual abuse images clearly depict children. At times, however, clarification becomes necessary, especially when teenagers are included in the evidence. The medical practitioner's input can be helpful when the question arises as to whether the images are consistent with a child of a certain age or with a child who is younger than a certain age. For example, some statutes call for different penalties if an image is consistent with a child younger than 18 years or 12 years.

## PROPER HANDLING OF EVIDENCE

During the investigation process, a medical analysis is most often sought when the ages of subjects in pornographic images are questionable (ie, do the images depict adults or children?). Practitioners may find the recommendations for handling child pornography beneficial (**Table 11-1**). When handling these images, practitioners should proceed with caution for the following reasons:

— To ensure there is no risk of courtroom confusion or possible exclusion of evidence as a result of confusion

— To ensure there is no risk of further exploitation of a child victim

### ELIMINATING THE RISK OF POSSIBLE COURTROOM CONFUSION OR EXCLUSION OF EVIDENCE

Practitioners must ensure there is no risk of courtroom confusion or possible exclusion of evidence as a result of confusion. For example, when documenting the pho-

---

**Table 11-1. Recommendations for the Proper Handling of Child Pornography Evidence**

— Properly label all images if there are not file names already assigned.

— Indicate the investigation case number and computer-based image file number for each image.

— Be able to verify that the images were secured while in the possession of the medical expert.

— Be able to verify that the evaluation of the images pertains specifically to the case in question and that there is no chance that images from another case were included during the expert evaluation.

— Be extremely sensitive and strive to ensure that the child victim is not further exploited by the court proceedings.

---

tographs of a child who has been physically abused and the bruises or injuries are pictured, if those images have not been properly labeled, then the evidence can be excluded since proof does not exist that the photographs were taken of that child. Similarly, if the investigation case number and computer-based image file number of an image are not indicated, it may be difficult to prove that the image pertains to a particular investigation. This attention to detail comes under the same consideration as chain of evidence.

The practitioner must also be able to verify that the images have been secured while in their possession to ensure that there has been no chance of mixing the images with those from other cases. Even if all images provided for analysis are copies of the original evidence, the onus rests on the medical expert to ensure that the review of these images is for a specific case and that images from another case have not been included.

### ELIMINATING THE RISK OF FURTHER EXPLOITATION OF THE CHILD VICTIM

The second important reason that images should be handled with care is to ensure that there is no risk of further exploitation of a child victim. The medical expert should be the most sensitive individual in respecting the child victim and protecting the child from further exploitation. When medical experts testify that they have made a significant effort to respect the privacy of the child victim, even if the identity of the child remains unknown to the examiner, a standard is created for the entire multidisciplinary team as well as the court with respect to the need to protect this victim. In a courtroom setting, the best scenario would be if the forensic medical analysis confirmed that pictured images were indeed consistent with children and that testimony could stand alone without the need for the jury to see the actual images. This scenario affords the least amount of further exploitation and allows a jury to understand that the dissemination of sexual abuse images is illegal.

## RECEIPT OF EVIDENCE

When contacted to review images, the practitioner should use the original source in order to avoid further reproduction of the images. This rule is especially pertinent if the images have been found on a computer or by another electronic means of storage (eg, CD-ROMs, floppy disks). If the images have been published in magazines or stored as photographs in an album or otherwise, an on-site review of the data is best to avoid the risk of further exploitation of the children in the images. When the images have been stored as videos, the review usually requires personal access because the time needed to conduct a review is significant since there are often multiple images and subjects to be analyzed.

### RECEIPT OF PHOTOGRAPHS AND VIDEOS

If the medical expert can not travel to review the images as a result of time or distance constraints, then the evidence must be delivered in a controlled manner. Within the law enforcement community, this delivery method is often described as "badge-to-badge" and involves coordination between law enforcement agencies. The Federal Bureau of Investigation (FBI), the US Customs and Border Protection, the Department of Homeland Security, and the US Postal Inspection Service frequently handle this form of contraband and are well versed in the appropriate manner of ensuring that the chain of custody is maintained within the United States. The International Criminal Police Organization (Interpol) and its affiliates throughout the world frequently facilitate these issues outside of the United States. The medical expert should be sure to document when and from whom the evidence is received (eg, certified mail, hand-delivered, commercial carrier), and this information should be included in the expert's case file.

As with most contraband received for evaluation, safekeeping is in order. Child pornography should be kept in a secure place during analysis so there is no risk of a legal challenge that the images were altered in any manner during evaluation. The return of evidence should also be tracked so clear documentation exists. The report of such cases should *not* be transmitted via electronic mail; rather, the report should be an original document with the signature of the person who evaluated the evidence and the tracking ability of the report provided. This procedure ensures that discovery can be provided in a timely fashion, as deemed by the court system.

## RECEIPT OF COMPUTER-BASED EVIDENCE

If copies of images have already been made available for review, the evidence should be provided on CD-ROM so that the medical analysis of individual images can be conducted and the examiner has the ability to enlarge the images if necessary. Evidence should be reviewed in a manner that avoids copying images to the reviewer's computer hard drive since storage of such contraband could constitute a violation of existing laws.

Sometimes copies of images are provided as printouts. At minimum, printouts should be made in color and should be larger than a typical ***thumbnail*** (ie, a file format used by imaging software, usually with a file extension of ".thn"). This enlargement is preferable so that analysis can be made with more ease. If this accommodation is not available, the reviewer may need access to magnification capabilities.

If possible, documentation of computer-based images should include the complete file name of each image. Information should be included regarding the investigation case number, the total number of images considered to have met the criteria of child pornography, and the total number of images provided for medical analysis. Frequently, the medical expert receives only a percentage of the total number of images since thousands or tens of thousands of images may have been discovered at the scene. In such instances, investigative agencies often select images that appear most like children.

*Ashcroft v Free Speech Coalition* (2002) placed the burden of proof on investigators to ensure that at least 1 image in a collection is of a known victim. Federal jurisdictions require that at least 1 image of child pornography be that of a known victim; state statutes vary, but there can not be less than 1 known image. Although this ruling made prosecution of child pornography cases more difficult, because most images presently seen on the Internet show unknown children, it did provide a greater motivation to identify children who have been sexually abused in this manner. Consequently, although a medical examiner of pornography may be providing information for the courts, there must have already been at least 1 identified child in order for the case to proceed.

In 2003, the federal statutes of the United States changed when President George W. Bush signed the **P**rosecutorial **R**emedies and **O**ther **T**ools to end the **E**xploitation of **C**hildren **T**oday (PROTECT) Act. This new bill was sponsored by Senator Orrin Hatch and cosponsored by Senator Patrick Leahy. This legislation includes in its definition of child pornography images that, to an ordinary observer, appear to be of an actual minor. The bill also allows the option for the accused to escape prosecution if they can prove that the images were not produced using a real child. The provisions of the bill have 4 components with respect to defining child pornography:

1. The ability to contest a virtual image is limited to digital, computer, or computer-generated images.

2. The images must strongly appear to depict real children (as compared to animated images).

3. The sexual content of the images must be explicit.

4. The accused may escape prosecution by convincingly contesting that the images are not of a real child.

At times, the medical expert may be asked whether digital modification of the images (a process often referred to as ***morphing***) exists. This determination requires advanced computer skills and the ability for an analysis to be made by forensic computer experts who have access to significant image magnification tools and the ability to analyze pixel definition, color variations, and other factors. Forensic medical analysis is specifically for determining the content of the image and not the image's quality. As a result, it is unwise for medical analysts to try to determine whether morphing was involved in production of the image unless they have received advanced training in the area of computer forensic analysis or have access to a prior report that addresses this issue at the time of medical analysis.

When morphing is obvious, it often includes the image of a well-known person's face being placed on the body image of someone else. Such images are obvious and can be commented on by the medical practitioner; however, such an inclusion is somewhat frivolous and not necessary for analysis. The medical analyst can use such an image in a trial as a demonstrative aid to ensure that the analysis is serious and does not include nonsensical images.

# PURPOSES OF MEDICAL ANALYSIS OF CHILD PORNOGRAPHY

Several purposes of a medical analysis of child pornography exist, including:

— Assessing the victim's age to determine whether the evidence meets the criteria of the law regarding child pornography

— Identifying the victim in the image in order to help locate that victim

— Gaining information about the collector to determine a specific fetish or behavioral pattern

— Assessing the images produced by the collector to find evidence that may be used in further investigation

— Determining if there is evidence of an elevated level of violence and possible physical danger to a child victim, which may necessitate a more aggressive means of identification

## ASSESSING THE VICTIM'S AGE

Medical analysis is most often used to assess the victim's age and determine whether the evidence meets the definition of the law, thereby constituting *child* pornography. According to US laws, the examiner assesses whether the images are consistent with a child younger than 12 years or between the ages of 13 and 18 years. Other countries may designate different age limits that determine whether images are illegal. It is important to note that a state's or country's age of consent may not necessarily be the same age as determined for pornographic production. For example, the age of consent in Canada is 14 years. However, if child sexual abuse images in Canada are consistent with youths less than 18 years of age, they are illegal and contraband.

In assessing the appearance of age consistency, the examination must be as objective as possible. The examiner must interpret the evidence only as it is presented. Speculation should be reserved only for victim identification and location so that all possibilities are considered. However, if the legal question is whether an image meets the definition of child pornography, one should not guess how a person came to appear as they did. One might speculate that a woman may have shaved her pubic hair, but unless the image is part of a video showing that action, an examiner must be objective and interpret only what is present in the image. If an image is presented with a significant variance in one aspect of sexual maturation (eg, breast development) in comparison to another part of the body (eg, absence of pubic hair), then the examiner must still interpret what is presented, rather than speculate about how the image came to look that way. The age consistency would then be cited as commensurate with the most mature aspect of the body rather than the least.

### IDENTIFYING THE VICTIM

The second goal of image analysis of child pornography is to identify the victim. In this circumstance, speculation could certainly be allowed, especially if there is an indication that manipulation of body hair could cause a child to appear older or younger than their actual age. Speculation regarding shaving would be permitted in this circumstance to allow the consideration of all possibilities that might help locate a child victim. If, however, the analysis is specifically to define whether the images are consistent with a child, such speculation should be avoided since there would be no objective evidence in the images to support such speculation. Identifying the victim becomes particularly important when there is evidence of possible physical danger to the victim.

### GAINING INFORMATION ABOUT THE COLLECTOR

A third goal of image analysis is to gain information regarding the collector. From a behavioral analysis perspective, it is helpful to note whether images have common features that might lead to the discovery that an offender has a specific fetish. This information is important since some collectors of child pornography use these images as a blueprint for action. For example, if most images of victims show a certain gender or ethnicity, that information can be used to conduct further investigations regarding possible contact offenses.

### ASSESSING IMAGES PRODUCED BY THE COLLECTOR FOR FURTHER INVESTIGATIVE EVIDENCE

A fourth reason for image analysis is to assess the images produced by the collector to find evidence that may be used in other investigations. For example, if the images indicate evidence of international travel to high-risk locations for child prostitution, and the offender has numerous images of children who appear to be from that part of the world, then a further investigation for child sex tourism might be needed since the images may have been personally produced by the suspect to memorialize a true sexual encounter.

## VIDEOTAPE EVIDENCE

When reviewing videotaped evidence, the examiner should use a videotape player with the ability to either freeze screens or display frames at a sufficiently slow enough rate to afford careful visualization of the images. Since child pornography may be inserted into videos of other subjects, the examiner must view the entire videotape.

The videotape identification number may be an investigation case file number. It is also important to identify the title of the videotape because it usually suggests the juvenile nature of the content. This information can lend support to the intent of the offender to collect contraband that is child pornography, as compared to a claim of ignorance about the videotape's subject matter.

### INSERTED PORNOGRAPHIC VIGNETTES

Viewing the entire videotape is extremely important since pornographic vignettes may be "sandwiched" within other benign materials. Crime scene investigations have revealed pornographic clips within children's cartoon videos as well as in the middle of an action movie. Such evidence will usually have been discovered before being given to the examiner, though the examiner may not be informed that a videotape includes more than one inserted vignette. Determining the amount of time that pornography is displayed via this form of media is helpful.

Since many tapes include several vignettes that last from 5 to 30 minutes or more, a brief description of the vignette by the examiner affords the triers of fact the opportunity to be familiar with the content without viewing the entire videotape. An examiner's description of the content is relevant because a judge may not allow the actual contraband to be viewed in the courtroom due to the video's potentially prejudicial nature. During a trial, such a report allows the jury or judge the opportunity to understand the explicit nature of the content and the degree of exploitation evident.

### UNUSUAL ANGLES SHOWN IN THE VIDEO

Videotaped images often show views of a child from unusual angles (eg, beneath the body). As a result, the examiner must discern whether any identifying aspects of those images exist that could indicate whether a child has been previously seen in the video. The examiner should ensure with a reasonable amount of certainty that these unusual views are also of the original child seen earlier in the videotape. Since these unusually angled views are often sexually explicit, they can help the examiner discern hair distribution on both the child's and perpetrator's bodies. The absence of axillary hair or the pubic hair distribution may also help determine the sexual maturity of the depicted child victim.

### PARTIAL IMAGE OF A PERPETRATOR

Videotaped evidence will frequently include partial images of a perpetrator. An example of this depiction may be seen when a child is forced to perform fellatio on a standing adult. In this typical profile view, only the adult's lower abdomen, genitalia, hips, upper thighs, lower arms, and hands are seen.

If there is an identified suspect in the case, then the analysis must be limited to those frames of the videotape that confirm the suspect's identity. On occasion, the suspect evaluation may include photos of the suspect's body, which may be used for comparison. If the hands are visible from the suspect detainment photographs, the examiner may be able to compare details (eg, fingernails, venous pattern on the dorsum of the hand, identifying body marks) to better determine whether that person's features are consistent with those of the person shown in the videotape. These photographs can be extremely helpful in identifying a suspect in a fellatio image in which the face may not be seen. Such identification would require that a suspect's detainment photographs document the hand's venous pattern in a similar state of downward arm extension. The examiner can superimpose an outline of the venous pattern noted on the dorsum of the hands of the suspect's photographs onto the pattern noted on the videotaped evidence. If the patterns match, it may provide supportive evidence of the suspect's role in the production of the child pornography.

### MULTIPLE SUBJECTS IN A VIDEO

Videotapes of child pornography may be commercially available and frequently include multiple child and teenaged subjects. Such evidence is especially time consuming for analysis purposes because there may be 40 or more subjects on one tape, which is often a compilation of several, short vignettes. These tapes frequently do not have an audio background, and they are commonly filmed in Europe, South America, or Central America.

In most of these videos, the teenaged subjects are initially clothed, but as the video continues, they often become naked and participate in sexual activity. The "actors" in these videotapes usually are believed to be homeless children and/or young people who have been coerced into juvenile prostitution.

When analyzing such a video, the examiner must be careful to describe each child or young person separately. One way to label the young subjects is according to the sequence of their appearance in the video. The examiner should provide a brief, body-identifying description (eg, race and hair color) that adequately indicates to another observer which young person is being analyzed. **Figure 11-1** provides a suggested model for a worksheet that may be used when identifying subjects according to their order of appearance in a video. First, each subject is assigned a letter according to their appearance in the video. A brief description of the subject (eg, blond male with red shirt) may be provided in an adjoining column. Sexual maturation ratings can be assigned, and other details (eg, presence of axillary hair, muscle development, head to body ratio) can be included. A final column exists for the examiner's determination of whether the subject is consistent with a youth younger than 18 years or a child younger than 12 years. This final column also allows space to designate whether the images meet the definition of child erotica in accordance with US laws.

*Figurre 11-1.* A worksheet like this can be helpful to organize the descriptions of multiple subjects in one video.

**Multiple Victim Child Pornography Analysis Sheet**

**VIDEO & TITLE:** _____

Vignette
#1 _____
_____
_____

| Subjects | PH | G | B | Other Findings | Meets Criteria |
|----------|----|----|----|----------------|----------------|
| A | | | | | |
| B | | | | | |
| C | | | | | |
| D | | | | | |
| E | | | | | |
| F | | | | | |
| G | | | | | |
| H | | | | | |
| I | | | | | |
| J | | | | | |

Vignette
#2 _____
_____
_____

| Subjects | PH | G | B | Other Findings | Meets Criteria |
|----------|----|----|----|----------------|----------------|
| A | | | | | |
| B | | | | | |
| C | | | | | |
| D | | | | | |
| E | | | | | |
| F | | | | | |
| G | | | | | |
| H | | | | | |
| I | | | | | |
| J | | | | | |

It is important to remember that in other international jurisdictions, images that are defined as erotica in the United States may not meet that country's legal criteria for child pornography.

### CONTENT OF VIDEO MAY PROVIDE INFORMATION ABOUT THE SEDUCTION OF CHILDREN

The content of commercially produced child pornography may provide important information about the seduction of young children for this form of sexual abuse. One example was noted in a large series of pornographic videos produced in Mexico. In these videos, young male children (approximately 12 or 13 years of age) were videotaped in a bedroom that appeared to be a hotel room. The children were seated on a bed, nude, and masturbating. The boys maintained fairly fixed gazes away from the camera. The filmmaker provided a brief, panoramic view of the room that revealed that adult pornography on the television was the source of sexual stimulation for the boys, reinforcing the idea that pornography is often used to stimulate participants in what may ultimately be a child sexual abuse or exploitation scenario.

Another *modus operandi* depicted in a child pornography videotape showed a comfortable, carpeted living room scene in which an adult onlooker encouraged 2 adolescent youths to wrestle. As the boys became sweaty, the adult encouraged them to remove their clothing to be more comfortable, assuaging their fears of indecency by stating that they were all male. Shortly thereafter, the subsequently nude wrestling boys began to tire and slow down. With strong encouragement from the adult, the boys began to caress and fondle each other. As their sexual stimulation increased, the boys became mutually sexually active. There have been reports made by teen males of these exact tactics while they were on camping trips with male counselors who eventually sexually abused them. This scenario suggests that at some times, pornography may provide a blueprint for action to a sex offender.

### INCEST SHOWN ON A VIDEOTAPE

At times, videotapes made available on the Internet have been made in a home and within a family (ie, **incest**). These tapes often include a sound track. On this sound track, a young child may interact with a family member, to whom the child may even refer as a parent. One frequently depicted scenario includes a 4- or 5-year-old white female who is encouraged to perform fellatio on a nude, supine, white adult male. Her verbal responses are appropriate for a young child, in that she laughs, questions the instructions, acquiesces, and makes intermittent comments regarding the performance of the act, which does not seem to be a first-time experience. Near the end of the video clip, the child asks about the anticipated physical ejaculation of the adult in childlike terms. These types of videotapes are important because they reiterate the fact that most sexual abuse of children occurs in a familiar setting and by a family member, friend, or acquaintance. Data from the Victim Identification Unit of the National Center for Missing & Exploited Children confirms that the majority of known victims are sexually abused and photographed by their own family members (M. Collins, oral communication, December 2004).

## PHOTOGRAPHS AND PUBLISHED MATERIALS AS EVIDENCE

When analysis is requested for photographs or published materials (eg, magazines, books), careful documentation of the evidence number is important to avoid confusion. If photographs for review have not been labeled by law enforcement officials or are given to the reviewer as a group or collection and labeled only by the date of the investigation, then the reviewer should assign a label to each image. Such labels should preferably describe the content in order to minimize problems when discussing specific photographs. Another way to define the images is to request that the investigators assign a specific name or number to each picture. An example of a situation in which the labeling of photographs would be beneficial would be if a case file includes a homemade photo album with combinations of child erotica and child pornography images inside. Initially, the reviewer would want to comment on the entire file and include the total number of pictures in the album. Further analysis would determine the number of images in the album that constitute child pornography, child erotica, or other details. The album would then be cited as part of the contraband in that specific case.

# WRITTEN CHILD PORNOGRAPHY

During the investigation of child pornography possessions, investigators sometimes discover collections of pornography written about adults and children on the suspect's hard drive or at the scene. This form of pornography is generally protected by the First Amendment of the US Constitution. The well-known, commercially available prototype of this form of pornography can be read in magazines such as *Penthouse Forum*, *Penthouse Letters*, or *Penthouse Variations*. In these venues, sexually explicit descriptions are frequently made using the scenario of perpetrator and victim role reversal. That is, there is usually a theme of a victim seducing a perpetrator, and that person succumbing to the irresistible temptation. The themes frequently include mutual sexual gratification between the participants. This written rationalization is an excellent example of the cognitive distortion that can exist in preferential sex offenders whose primary targets are children.

## EXAMPLE OF WRITTEN CHILD PORNOGRAPHY

The following example provides an abbreviated specimen of written child pornography. This sample story was found during a child pornography possession and dissemination investigation. Investigators found this written child pornography on the hard drive of a 34-year-old male who was actively engaged in an Internet chat with a 13-year-old teenager. During his chat, he transmitted child pornography to her to "teach her of the great feelings associated with sex":

One evening, I had the task of putting my lovely 7-year-old daughter to bed, while her mom was out at an evening class. I got her into her pajamas, though she struggled with me, trying to play with my [penis] as I told her to hurry. I really wanted to watch the Monday night football game. After I got her into bed, and settled down with a brew, the next thing that I saw was her, standing in the door of the living room. I said, "Get back to bed, sweetheart, Daddy's watching the game!" She responded in a low and husky voice, "I've got a game for you, Daddy, and it's right here!" She came over and climbed into my lap, rubbing herself back and forth, making me respond, even though I knew I shouldn't. She kept cooing and kissing my ear, and after a while, I couldn't even think of the game, because the real game was getting ready to start right in my living room!

## SIGNIFICANCE OF WRITTEN CHILD PORNOGRAPHY

Although written child pornography is not illegal in the United States, the presence of such stories in child sexual exploitation cases serves a number of purposes:

— Provides the sex offender with a rationalization for such behavior

— Allows the sex offender to fantasize about being seduced by a young child and trying to resist this seduction

— May memorialize an actual event in the form of "fiction" for some offenders

Sex offenders read and write child pornography in an effort to rationalize their reasons for committing a contact offense with a child. These stories allow offenders to play the role of being seduced by a young child, thereby expressing a fantasy about their efforts of resistance and their efforts to convince the child victim to turn away from prurient behaviors.

Another explanation is that these stories may represent a written version of a prior event and the offender wants to memorialize it in the form of "fiction." This is possible in incest-themed examples of child sexual abuse, which are often found accompanying personal collections of computer-based child pornography. Investigators will not know whether these incest-themed stories are autobiographical, self-written, or saved from other sources.

The presence of written child pornography has a similar significance to that of the presence of child erotica. Neither of them are illegal, but both imply a preferential interest in sex with children.

### OTHER INFORMATION COMMONLY FOUND WITH WRITTEN CHILD PORNOGRAPHY

When investigating the hard drive of an offender, investigators may find tables of international ages of sexual consent in addition to the written child pornography. The presence of such tables are especially noteworthy; even if the tables are inaccurate, they appear to provide "the collector" with another piece of the blueprint for child sex tourism or sexual fantasy. Investigators may also find information regarding various groups that advocate sex with children such as the North American Man/Boy Love Association (NAMBLA). Although not considered pornographic, these ancillary details may be included in a trial as evidence that the child pornography images that were found on the offender's computer were not coincidental findings.

## THE DEFINITION OF SEXUALLY EXPLICIT IMAGES IN THE UNITED STATES

Investigators and examiners must understand the legal definitions of sexually explicit images in the United States. Though the lay public may perceive images as being of a prurient nature, even if these images are only associated with nudity, the First Amendment to the US Constitution, which allows for free speech, permits a certain degree of expression within cyberspace.

The PROTECT Act defines sexually explicit conduct in the federal statute 18 USC § 2256 as:

(A) sexual intercourse, including genital-genital, oral-genital, anal-genital, or oral-anal, whether between persons of the same or opposite sex;

(B) bestiality;

(C) masturbation;

(D) sadistic or masochistic abuse; or

(E) lascivious exhibition of the genitals or pubic area of any person.

Another important term is "graphic," which, according to 18 USC § 2256(10), "means that a viewer can observe any part of the genitals or pubic area of any depicted person or animal during any part of the time that the sexually explicit conduct is being depicted."

Another means of defining child pornographic images has been described internationally by using a taxonomic system. This system allows individuals to communicate about the overall severity of a collection and, if necessary, transmit information to others in a more covert fashion. The use of such a system, however, should not encourage the practice of discounting the importance of less severe forms of pornography. One such system, the COPINE system (Taylor et al, 2001), is currently used in many European countries among law enforcement agencies.

## VICTIM IDENTIFICATION ANALYSIS

Since a significant amount of child pornography is made within the home and by family members, investigators must carefully question the children as well as their friends because delayed disclosure often occurs in child sexual abuse cases. A recent pilot project being conducted in Toronto, Canada, provides sex crime investigators who have found confirmed child pornography on a computer with the necessary manpower to carefully question all children in an offender's circle in an effort to establish a potential victim matrix. This project is a more proactive means of determining whether evidence of contact offenses exists. This effort is important in light of the high recidivism rate in child sexual offenders and the prevalence of delayed disclosure in child sexual abuse (Gillespie, 2003).

When reviewing images, the examiner must include all of the people shown in the images. This means that the examiner should also note and comment on the appearance of children who may appear in the background of the image. One example was noted in the analysis of a collection of child pornography with a sadism theme. In this case, a young, nude child of an undetermined gender was flexed at the waist in the forefront of the picture, and an adult male was penetrating the child's anus with his hand. Such an image was so aversive that the examiner could have failed to notice that in the background, a young boy was hanging on a wall, which appeared to be made of large stone blocks, by a 4-point chain with cuff wrist and ankle restraints. This child was prepubescent, nude, and wore a black hood over his head. Although neither child could be identified by facial features, the presence of the boy in the background and the clear sodomy of a child in the foreground could imply that the latter was also a male child. The stone wall led the examiner to suspect that the images were produced in a studio. Although the staging suggested role-playing of sadistic abuse in a medieval theme, the sexual abuse undoubtedly appeared quite real. For these children, and thousands of others, the primary focus of medical analysis should always be to ascertain possible identities of victims.

## GENDER

Historically, the most memorable child pornography magazines have featured predominately girls as their subjects. Although she was unknown to most of the world, one child pornography video star, 6-year-old Thea Pumbroek, died in Amsterdam in 1984 of a cocaine overdose (Taylor & Quayle, 2003). Years after Thea's death, female images continue to proliferate on the Internet. As the number of images dramatically increases, however, there has been a steady trend toward more male victims appearing in the images. The gender of a victim is an important factor, from both the victim and offender perspectives.

A common method of continued exploitation through prostitution is to begin with pornographic documentation of sexual abuse. Offenders show victims a combination of these child pornographic images and adult pornography with members of the same sex as the victim in order to normalize sexual contact between minors and adults. Victims who are shown pornography involving people of the same sex as the child may become desensitized to the nature of the act. From the perspective of the offender, the sex of victims in collections likely reflects a specific sexual preference and provides clues to a potential victim matrix in the circumstance of multiple victims.

The European Union-sponsored project Combating Paedophile Information Networks in Europe (COPINE) at the University of Cork College, Ireland, which specifically monitors Internet newsgroups for child pornography, has noted that from the year 2000 to the present, gender distribution of child pornography seems to be trending toward a more equal distribution between male and female child subjects. This change represents an increased number of male images as opposed to the historic preponderance of female images.

In the area of commercially produced video pornography, it is difficult to determine whether one gender predominates over another, although male child pornography seems to be in greater supply.

Generally, determining the gender of a child depicted in a sexual abuse image is not difficult. However, sometimes a child is photographed fully clothed, or possibly shown from the posterior so only the child's back and buttocks can be seen. In such cases, the examiner can state only what is visible in the image. If the child's body has evidence of waist definition, which is indicative of the deposition of fat typically found in adolescent females, or if the shoulder-to-hip ratio is 1.35 or more, which is indicative of maturation often seen in older adolescent males, then the examiner may make a tentative determination of gender. Deciding a child's gender according to hair length is obviously unreliable. Also, when an image is of a young child, clear designation of a gender is often difficult to discern unless the genitals are revealed; therefore, the examiner should only state the child's visible physical features to avoid speculation.

Another circumstance in which gender may be too difficult to determine is when pornographic images include only a child's head (usually in profile) performing fellatio on an adult male whose abdomen and genitalia may be the only body parts seen. In such circumstances, the examiner can not speculate about the child's gender; however, the relative size of the child's head next to an erect penis will usually be complete enough information to determine that the image is indeed that of a child.

Since videotape pornography often shows large groups of children, analysis of these tapes requires the ability to decrease the speed of the tape so that each subject can be completely evaluated. Even if a preponderance of one gender is seen, the examiner must view each child carefully since male and female cross-dressing is occasionally depicted in this medium.

## ETHNICITY

The ethnic origin of children (often referred to as *ancestry* in the field of forensic pathology) is especially relevant when attempting victim identification. Sexually abused and exploited children are commonly photographed in their country of origin. If children or teenagers have been transported to another country, the likelihood of human trafficking with subsequent prostitution becomes a greater consideration. In such situations, the possibility of a large-scale, commercial, organized crime operation may be a concern. The examiner's suspicion should increase if an ethnic business is the site of pornography production (eg, a Thai massage parlor, a Latino exotic dance club). Currently, meta-analysis of the background environment of Internet images plays a key role in victim identification for such children.

### CLINICAL INDICATIONS TO HELP DETERMINE A CHILD'S ETHNICITY

Several clinical indications are often present to give an astute clinician an indication of ancestry. The most reliable ancestry assignment is made with the adult skull, and the 3 most easily established groups with discernable skull differences are those of Asian, African, and European descent (**Figures 11-2-a, b,** and **c**). When a cadaver is discovered, determination of ancestry is extremely important to facilitate identification of the body. Forensic anthropologists establish ancestry either by osteological analysis of anthroposcopy or osteometry. ***Anthroposcopy*** entails the use of visually discernable differences noted in the skull's shape and the orientation of facial features. ***Osteometry*** uses metric measurements to compare a known victim to standard measurements within a culture.

Fortunately, visual review of the living human face requires far less knowledge than that of forensic pathology and anthropology. Racial differences are often more than just skin pigmentation. The shape of the eyes, the appearance of the hair, and often the nasal form qualities assist an examiner when establishing ancestry. Of course, examiners acknowledge that few pure ethnic groups exist. In fact, interracial/interethnic mixing over generations makes the establishment of ancestry based solely on visual facial perusal not completely accurate.

### General Characteristics of European Ancestry

Children of European ancestry have the most commonly recognizable facial features, such as:

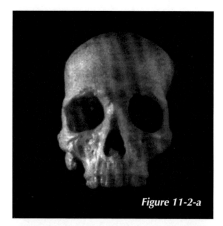

*Figures 11-2-a, b,* and *c. Racial differences shown in mid-face, frontal view of skulls of Asian (a), African (b), and European (c) descent. Burns, KR. Forensic Anthropology Training Manual, The. 1st Edition. © 1999. Reprinted with permission of Pearson Education, Inc., Upper Saddle River, NJ.*

*Figure 11-2-a*

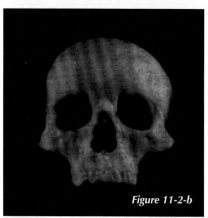

*Figure 11-2-b*

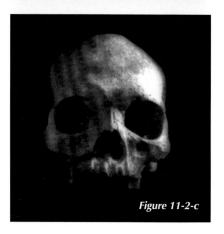

*Figure 11-2-c*

— Minimal projection

— Relatively small zygomatic arches, which give the face a relatively narrow appearance across the midface and a narrow nasal appearance

— A typically receding lower eye border

— Possible presence of hypertelorism or hypotelorism (increased or decreased distance between the eyes, respectively), though this is often genetic instead of an ancestry trait

### General Characteristics of Hispanic Ancestry

Children of Hispanic origin often have the following facial characteristics:

— Dark hair

— Almond-shaped eyes

— A somewhat darker complexion than those of European descent with a subjectively more olive tone; those of direct Spanish descent (ie, Spain) will still have the European characteristics

### General Characteristics of Asian Ancestry

Though children of Asian origin are usually easy to discern, their exact country of origin is more difficult to determine. Their common characteristics include:

— Characteristic body habitus (eg, typically shorter stature, small features in girls)

— Dark hair

— Almond-shaped, upward slanting eyes

— Upper and lower eyelids typically appear fuller than those of other races, an observation that led to actual high-resolution magnetic resonance imaging (MRI) evidence that the orbital fat projected further both anteriorly and superiorly to the inferior border of the tarsus (Carter et al, 1998)

— Skin pigment is less uniform than in other ethnic groups because based on country of origin, children may have darker pigment associated with more sun exposure, or may be even provided make-up to appear extremely fair, as is the custom in some Asian countries

— Children from certain parts of Eurasia (eg, India, Nepal, Bangladesh) may be as hyperpigmented as some children of African descent

### General Characteristics of African Ancestry

Common characteristics of children of African descent include:

— Skin tone and complexion with varying degrees of pigmentation

— Dark hair

— Round eyes

— Relatively broad nasal bridge

— Projection of the alveolar ridge

— Rarely crowded dentition, as is often seen in European children

The facial features of these children may vary tremendously based on the multiethnic background for many children of African descent. This is particularly true of African American children due to the prevalence of racial mixing in the United States. Children from certain African nations will have an appearance consistent with their specific country of origin (eg, Egyptian children compared to Ethiopian children). For unknown reasons, children of African descent are less often posed pornographically. These children are not often seen in multiple series of child pornography.

OTHER CLUES TO HELP DETERMINE A CHILD'S ETHNICITY
Other clues that may help an examiner determine a child's ethnicity include:

— Video titles and Internet Web site banners

— Stereotypical settings of the country of origin

— Background scenes

## Video Titles and Internet Web Site Banners

One clue to help examiners determine the likely ethnicity of the children shown in Internet images of child pornography or video pornography is the Internet Web site's announcing banner or the video's title. For example, the title "Juan and Carlos Boys" most likely indicates Hispanic children, and Internet banners such as "Thai Teens" and "Eastern Pedo-Sex" indicate children of Asian descent. As has been the case in other studies regarding the content and title of pornographic materials (Lebergue, 1991), Internet banners are often accurate regarding the subject matter of the associated images, with the possible exception of the cited age of the "models."

## Stereotypical Settings of the Country of Origin

Occasionally, stereotypical settings will be used in the image that can help an examiner determine a child's ethnicity. For example, Hispanic children may be pornographically photographed in exotic, tropical-appearing environments. In one large videotape series, Mexican children were depicted as if they were members of an Aztec or Inca tribe. These children were clothed in loincloths, and some wore headdresses. They were also shown standing on seaside cliffs and near beaches, which may imply that the images were taken in South America. Another example could include known European sites, such as a recognizable German river in the background of children on a boat. The tourist-like settings are occasionally preludes to eventual pornographic scenes.

## Background Scenes

Background scenes may provide clues as to the country in which the pornography production occurs. After the country of origin is determined for some pornographic pictures, some victims have been successfully located. Of the children identified so far, more than half were photographed in normal home settings or outside in parks or playgrounds near where they live. As a result, key features in the background can help lead investigators directly to the victims and the abusers. From a law enforcement perspective, background findings, particularly in a room, would constitute a crime scene.

# TODDLER PORNOGRAPHY

## DEVELOPMENT OF MATURATION OF TODDLERS

Many child pornography collections, whether on the Internet or videotape, show victims as young as infants or toddlers (approximately 12 to 36 months old) and preschool-aged children (approximately 36 to 60 months old). Different developmental stages may provide examiners with an indication of the degree of maturation present in younger children.

If there are videotapes or Internet video clips of sexual abuse images, an examiner can observe a child's gross motor skills to help identify the child's developmental level (**Table 11-2**). For example, toddlers who walk with their hands held above their head (often referred to as ***high-guard gait***) or at shoulder level (often referred to as ***mid-guard gait***) are just beginning to walk independently.

A high-guard and mid-guard hand stance is usually associated with a wide-based foot placement with each step, thereby providing a gait that attests to the child's lack of integration of motor skills. When such a pattern of walking is apparent, most toddlers are between 13 and 15 months old.

An early walker's integration of the hand stance from high-guard and mid-guard to the normal, reciprocating swing found in older children and adults can be affected by several factors. These factors include prematurity, motor strength, cognition, and general neurological tone (Bly, 1994).

Toddlers tend to develop the skill of walking backward when pulling an object between 12.5 and 21 months of age. This skill may be compared with a child who walks facing forward and uses one hand to pull an object behind their body, which is a motor skill that emerges at 15 months and is mastered by 18 months. The average age of a child who can carry a large object (eg, a ball) while walking is between 17 to 18.5 months old. A child's ability to squat while playing normally becomes apparent between 20 and 21 months of age.

A pose frequently seen in toddler pornography is that of a nude male child bending over and looking through his legs. This pose highlights the presence of the anus and testes since the penis is usually too small to be seen in much detail in this pose. The child's ability to stand in this way usually begins between 14.5 and 15.5 months old.

### Sadistic Toddler Abuse

Toddler pornography is increasingly associated with vaginal, anal, or oral penetration. Toddlers in such circumstance may wear additional "props" such as a spiked dog collar around the neck, a blindfold over the eyes, a gag in the mouth, or a rope tied around the ankles or wrists. In such images, these props are probably actual, sadistic paraphernalia, so the examiner should assume that the use of such props is likely a part of the commission of the sexual crime. In these images, the child's face is often shown, and grimaces of pain are apparent. This type of pornographic image is consistent with the most severe form of child pornography called ***sadistic abuse***. With sadistic abuse, the perpetrator is motivated by sexual gratification from the infliction of pain.

Some video clips of sadistic toddler abuse have been recovered with sound. These video clips help explain the reason a 3- or 4-year-old child may be able to suffer a penetrating, sexually abusive event yet appear to be able to smile. One such case, which involved child pornography produced by the grandfather of a young child,

---

**Table 11-2. Stages of Development of Gross Motor Skills in Toddlers**

— *Walking independently.* Toddler is probably between 11.5 and 13.5 months old and usually younger than 15 months old, which is the upper limit for normal development. (Note: African American children tend to walk 2 to 4 months earlier than other chidren.)

— *Walking backward when pulling an object (eg, a toy).* Toddler is probably between 12.5 and 21 months old.

— *Walking with high-guard or mid-guard stance with wide-based foot placement.* Toddler is probably between 13 and 15 months old.

— *Standing and looking through legs.* Toddler is probably older than 14.5 to 15.5 months.

— *Walking facing forward and pulling an object behind the body with one hand.* Toddler is probably between 15 and 18 months old.

— *Carrying a large object while walking.* Toddler is probably between 17 and 18.5 months old.

— *Squatting during play.* Toddler is probably older than 20 to 21 months.

revealed the grandfather's insistence that his granddaughter "smile for the camera" amidst her verbal protests about the pain she was experiencing. The victim was able to muster a brief, though weak, smile in the classic, conditioned response that children often demonstrate when given a firm and familiar command (T. Jones, oral communication, April 2003).

### IMPACT OF SADISTIC ABUSE ON INFANTS AND TODDLERS

For infants and toddlers, the impact of sadistic abuse, which is essentially sexual, physical, and emotional abuse, should be considered significant since penile-vaginal penetration at this age would typically be extremely painful and would probably result in direct tissue trauma. Depending on the size of the penetrating object, anal penetration could also cause physical injury and psychological trauma that is secondary to the pain. Although infants who have been penetrated may be preverbal, studies of pain management in infants reveal that an infant's perception of pain is as acute as that of adults. This means that blood pressure, heart rate, diaphoresis, and distress all increase.

Since sadistic images are often of children who appear to be younger than 5 years old, the victim's ability to verbalize the nature of the assault is greatly impaired. Recent trauma research supports evidence that sexual and physical abuse in young children influences the developing brain neuroarchitecture, which often results in cellular and structural changes in the limbic system that lead to a life-long impact (eg, post-traumatic stress disorder) (Teicher et al, 2002, 2003). This research helps contradict the commonly accepted belief that sexual and physical abuse in toddlers and young children will be forgotten and, therefore, not have a long-term impact.

Child sexual abuse is not necessarily an isolated event in a growing number of abusive experiences that adults relate. Children who are sexually abused commonly experience physical abuse and neglect as well. Many children who report that they have been sexually abused do not readily describe the chaotic neglect in which they live, though this may be apparent once a full investigation occurs. Children who are sexually abused and exploited (eg, in cases of human trading for illicit drugs), or who are provided commercially as pornographic subjects, have often suffered immensely frightening stresses such as coerced substance abuse or witnessing intimate partner violence.

Child sexual abuse in young toddlers may also lead to permanent behavioral, cognitive, and emotional changes. A detailed review of this subject matter by Glaser (2000) underscores the fact that the actual effects of child abuse may lead to numerous manifestations of the stress response, including dysregulation with sleep disturbance, mood lability, distractibility, increased motor activity, and angry outbursts. Such behaviors can be labeled "attention deficit hyperactivity disorder," "anxiety disorder," "episodic dyscontrol behavior," "oppositional defiant disorder," "aggression," or "dysthymia." These victims are also at risk of developing sexual offending behaviors, especially if they do not receive cognitive behavioral therapy during their preschool years, which is when sexual acting out may become more prevalent.

## PSYCHOSEXUAL MATURATION

Other aspects of developmental maturation include psychosexual maturation. Children in pornographic images are often shown participating in sexualized and explicit behaviors that are well outside their normal developmental schema. Dr. William Freidrich has contributed immensely to the field of knowledge regarding normative sexual behaviors in children. In 1991 Friedrich reported on the sexual behaviors of children living in the United States who were between the ages of 2 and 12 years and who did not have a history of sexual abuse. These behaviors revealed a wide variance within the sexual arena. The behaviors of highest frequency were typically self-stimulatory and somewhat suggestive of exhibitionism. In this study, the behaviors he found most unusual, though still within the normative data, were those which were more aggressive in nature or more imitative of adult sexual behavior (Friedrich et al, 1991).

Friedrich et al (1991) found that several factors increased sexualized behaviors in children: family violence, prolonged stays in daycare centers each week, stressful life circumstances, and family attitudes regarding sexual matters (eg, nudity, exposure to pornography in the home, co-bathing, co-sleeping). The types of behaviors that he found to have the highest frequency included self-stimulatory actions, exhibitionism, and behaviors related to the dissolution of personal boundaries. However, there was not an immense increase in the incidence of far more explicit behaviors. Such explicit behaviors are more consistently seen in those who have been abused and include:

— Placing of the child's mouth on someone else's sexual organ

— Inserting objects into the vagina or anus

— Imitating intercourse

— Mimicking sexual sounds verbally (eg, moans, groans, rhythmic grunts)

— Requesting permission to engage in sexual acts with another person

— Masturbating with an object

— French kissing (ie, seeking to kiss and insert the tongue into another person's mouth)

— Undressing another person

— Asking permission to watch sexually explicit shows on television

— Imitating sexual behaviors with dolls

The results of Friedrich's research led to the development of the Child Sexual Behavior Inventory (CSBI) (Friedrich 1993; Friedrich et al, 1992).

Subsequent research has revealed that sexually abused children are consistently reported to have more sexual behavioral problems than children who do not have a history of abuse (Friedrich et al, 2001; Mannarino & Cohen, 1996). Also, such behaviors were specific to children who had a history of sexual abuse in that these reported behaviors did not occur significantly in neglected or physically abused children or those children who had been diagnosed with psychiatric disturbances (Friedrich et al, 1997). Children who had a history of sexual abuse tended to engage in more sexualized behaviors associated specifically with genital sexual behavior (eg, mimicking intercourse, inserting foreign objects into the vagina or anus) (Friedrich et al, 2001).

## PORNOGRAPHY AND CHILD SEDUCTION

Exposure to pornography of any kind is inappropriate for a school-aged child. Graphic sexual experiences of this kind are outside the normal psychosexual developmental realm for this age group. In child sexual abuse prosecutions, the defense frequently tries to assert that the child's explicit sexual knowledge originated from living in a home in which pornography had been found. One phenomenon that negates this premise is the presence of ***sensory memory*** (ie, what the victims felt, saw, heard, tasted, or smelled), which the victims are frequently able to recount. When a child describes a painful, penetrating experience, the descriptions clearly indicate that they did not gain knowledge about this experience from watching pornography, because most video pornography portrays sexual encounters as pleasurable. A child's recollection of the tactile characteristic of body fluids is another sensory detail that strongly supports actual experience. In addition, a child may recount a common phrase that the perpetrator has spoken in the past to adult sexual partners, thereby

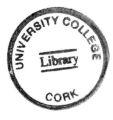

revealing that while in the act of sexual gratification with the child, the perpetrator slipped into repetitive behaviors that someone else could validate. Close attention to such details obtained during the medical evaluation and forensic interview is important to the presentation of this information should it be required before a judge or jury.

Early elementary-aged children who report that child and/or adult pornography was shown to them during their sexual victimization often describe at least 1 of the following 3 scenarios:

1. The pornography was used to instruct the child so they could mimic what they saw happening.

2. The pornography was used as a means of exciting the perpetrator.

3. The pornography was used to sexually stimulate and excite the child.

### PORNOGRAPHY USED TO INSTRUCT THE CHILD

In the first circumstance, children have reported being forced to watch pornography and then being told that it is normal behavior for children. Also, they are told that such behavior is fun and that they should not have reservations about doing the same things with the perpetrator. This is an excellent example of the use of pornography to desensitize a child or young person to sexual actions.

### PORNOGRAPHY USED TO EXCITE THE PERPETRATOR

When pornography has been used as a means of exciting the perpetrator, children have reported that the offender was either watching pornography online immediately before a sexual assault or that the offender was watching pornographic videos or looking at magazines before masturbating and then sexually assaulting the child. In this circumstance, some children have noted little verbal exchange with the perpetrator, and instead, endured forceful sexual contacts that were often followed by a threatening admonishment warning the child not to tell anyone about the event. This behavior is especially common among adolesent and young adult sex offenders. These young offenders may weave a competition scenario (eg, playing a computer video game in which the perpetrator has far superior skills to those of the victim) into the picture, which is almost always associated with the victim losing and the sexual encounter being the victim's penalty.

### PORNOGRAPHY USED TO EXCITE THE CHILD

At times, children and young people are shown pornography to sexually excite them and to encourage them in autoerotic stimulation. Pornography may be used when an offender is encouraging children and/or young people to enter into mutual sexual encounters. This is frequently the case in pornographic media when young children are demonstrating highly sexually explicit behaviors alone, with other children of the same age, or with an adult. The viewer can assume that such images are candid but probably not spontaneous. For example, if an image shows a 5- or 6-year-old child performing fellatio on an adult male, this would most likely be a coerced act but may represent a conditioned response to chronic sexual abuse. Another example would be a videotape of an 11- or 12-year-old male attempting to masturbate to ejaculation when he is being shown adult pornography as a stimulus.

### CHILDREN WHO APPEAR DRUGGED

Orchestrated child sexual abuse images in which the child appears to be drugged may be found on the Internet or at the scene of a crime in the form of videotapes or DVDs. A careful search should be performed to ensure that no potential date rape drugs are found in the home, particularly if young children are possible victims. The use of date rape drugs, sedatives, or alcohol can leave a child victim amnesic to the abusive events. These children are frequently shown in video clips as immobile participants in sexual assault encounters (eg, prepubescent boys or girls dressed in sexually provocative clothing while placing sex toys in or on their genitalia or anus).

Although these children may not remember such events, examiners who see the images immediately recognize that the normal course of psychosexual maturation is being short-circuited. The psychological impact of these acts, in addition to the child's knowledge of the memorialization of such acts through pictures, videos, or digital images, can not be seen as beneficial in any way.

# MUSCULOSKELETAL DEVELOPMENT

Musculoskeletal development is helpful in cases of child pornography for several reasons. It can be used for children in some images to help determine their approximate age, and for victims, once they are found, to verify that they are the children shown in the images. Some parameters may also prove useful for investigations involving children who are not able to communicate their true age and who have nothing documenting their true age.

## RADIOGRAPHIC STUDIES

When a sexually exploited child is identified and the actual age of that child is unknown, radiographic studies can be performed to determine bone age. This technique has been used in investigations involving foreign national children who have been trafficked into the United States for the purpose of prostitution and who have false documents regarding date of birth and other information. By using accepted standards that measure maturation of the carpal bones in the hands, clinicians can provide a more accurate, true age of children. This technique is also used when human remains of missing children are recovered and efforts must be made to establish the child's age.

## COMPARING HEAD HEIGHT AND TOTAL HEIGHT RATIO

Another means of determining whether an image is consistent with that of a child is to compare the ratio of the head height (ie, crown to chin) to the total height (ie, crown to sole of the feet). Typical results are as follows:

— Toddlers have a ratio of 1:5.

— School-aged children (ie, approximately 5 to 7 years old) have a ratio of 1:6.

— Young people of about 15 years old have an approximate ratio of 1:6.5.

— Adults have a ratio of 1:7.5 or 1:8.

These ratios help examiners determine whether an image of a child is consistent with a younger child, even though that child may be dressed up and made to appear older.

Although using these ratios is helpful to provide more supportive evidence that the image is of a child, this adjunct analysis information of head to total body height ratio must be used with caution, because an image may have been distorted with the use of programs that allow morphological changes. Also, a computer-based image does not always provide an examiner with an opportunity to fully assess a child's height because the child's body may not be fully exposed.

## OTHER SIGNS OF MUSCULOSKELETAL MATURATION

Other signs of maturation of the musculoskeletal system include actual muscular development, such as the muscular development seen with the pectoralis muscles as the androgens and estrogens become more available during maturation. The adolescent male's increase in gonadal steroids plays an important role in the pubertal growth spurt. In addition to muscular development, the body habitus changes in men as the shoulders broaden. Growth hormone, thyroid hormone, luteinizing hormone, gonadotropin-releasing hormone, estradiol, and testosterone all play a role in the pubertal process and its physical manifestation.

# DENTAL MATURATION

The eruption and shedding of teeth is a helpful parameter to use when analyzing images of young children. Tooth eruption occurs at a fairly predictable rate in infants and toddlers. When tooth eruptions are visible in a computer image, analysis may provide important victim identification information. For example, the maxillary deciduous incisors erupt after the mandibular incisors, that is, between 6 and 8 months old and between 5 and 7 months old, respectively. The presence of the maxillary cuspids, which are often referred to as the *canines*, is evident between 16 and 20 months old. Since toddler pornography may reveal a child's dentition, dental information is helpful when trying to determine the child's age.

When mandibular maturation begins, children begin to shed their teeth. The central incisors of the mandible are usually lost between 6 and 7 years of age, whereas the maxillary front teeth are usually shed between 7 and 8 years of age. The new eruption of permanent teeth occurs almost immediately after the deciduous shedding. As a result, if an image of a child reveals missing canines in conjunction with the presence of the larger, secondary central incisors, the examiner can reasonably assume that the child's age is consistent with that of a 9- to 11-year-old child. **Table 11-3** presents the chronology of human dentition for primary and secondary teeth.

Medical conditions or socioeconomic concerns may affect tooth shedding due to poor nutrition, poverty, and dental caries. These circumstances are associated with advanced tooth shedding; however, the presence of malnutrition would be apparent in more than a child's teeth, and in the absence of malnutrition, an examiner should feel comfortable that the standard ages of dental maturation apply.

## PHYSICAL SEXUAL MATURATION

Determining sexual maturation and a child's correlative age based solely on images involves a margin of error. The norms of sexual maturation are based on actual, physical examinations of children whose ages are known. In contrast, when an examiner is only able to review pictures of children, only certain aspects of information may be provided—the child's approximate height ratios, body habitus (as seen in the prepubescent child and pubescent adolescent), dentition, muscular development, dysmorphia (ie, any abnormality in facial or body appearance that may be consistent with a recognizable syndrome, such as Down's syndrome or a cleft lip and palate sequence), and physical sexual maturation.

### STAGES OF SEXUAL MATURATION

The Tanner stages of sexual maturation were described by James Tanner (1962) and continue to provide healthcare providers with a sequence for sexual maturation in males and females. Additional analyses have provided examiners with a means to use a sexual maturation rating (SMR) system when evaluating children and youths. In the original Tanner stages, a numeric rating system is assigned to pubic hair development (PH), breast development (B) in females, and the development of the gonads (testicles) and penis (G) in males. These levels of development are typically expressed from stage 1, which is consistent with a prepubertal child, to stage 5, which is consistent with a fully mature body (Marshall & Tanner, 1969, 1970) (**Figures 11-3, 11-4,** and **11-5; Tables 11-4** and **11-5**).

A compilation of data by Wu et al (2002) provides an equally important perspective of the sexual maturation of American girls found in the far more recent and thorough National Health and Nutrition Examination Survey III (NHANES III). The NHANES III study was done for 10 years per study group, looking at large and representative samples of American girls and boys of different ethnic groups. These latter components were not considered in the original Tanner study, which was completed nearly 4 decades before. The age ranges cited in the original Tanner research makes it unsuitable for child pornography analysis. In addition, the original Tanner stages were devised for the purpose of clinical medical investigation as compared to forensic analysis for victim assessment and possible identification (Marshall & Tanner, 1986). This point was emphasized in a letter to the editor of the journal

**Table 11-3. Chronology of Human Dentition for Primary (Deciduous) and Secondary (Permanent) Teeth**

| | CALCIFICATION | | AGE AT ERUPTION | | AGE AT SHEDDING | |
|---|---|---|---|---|---|---|
| PRIMARY TEETH | BEGINS AT | COMPLETES AT | MAXILLARY | MANDIBULAR | MAXILLARY | MANDIBULAR |
| Central incisors | 5th fetal month | 18-24 months | 6-8 months | 5-7 months | 7-8 years | 6-7 years |
| Lateral incisors | 5th fetal month | 18-24 months | 8-11 months | 7-10 months | 8-9 months | 7-8 months |
| Cuspids (canines) | 6th fetal month | 30-36 months | 16-20 months | 16-20 months | 11-12 years | 9-11 years |
| First molars | 5th fetal month | 24-30 months | 10-16 months | 10-16 months | 10-11 years | 10-12 years |
| Second molars | 6th fetal month | 36 months | 20-30 months | 20-30 months | 10-12 years | 11-13 years |
| SECONDARY TEETH | BEGINS AT | COMPLETES AT | MAXILLARY | MANDIBULAR | | |
| Central incisors | 3-4 months | 9-10 years | 7-8 years | 6-7 years | | |
| Lateral incisors | Maxillary, 10-12 months; Mandibular, 3-4 months | 10-11 years | 8-9 years | 7-8 years | | |
| Cuspids (canines) | 4-5 months | 12-15 years | 11-12 years | 9-11 years | | |
| First premolars (bicuspids) | 18-21 months | 12-13 years | 10-11 years | 10-12 years | | |
| Second molars (bicuspids) | 24-30 months | 12-14 years | 10-12 years | 11-13 years | | |
| First molars | Birth | 9-10 years | 6-7 years | 6-7 years | | |
| Second molars | 30-36 months | 14-16 years | 12-13 years | 12-13 years | | |
| Third molars | Maxillary, 7-9 years; Mandibular, 8-10 years | 18-25 years | 17-22 years | 17-22 years | | |

*Reprinted from Behrman RE, Kleigman RM, Jenson HB, eds.* Nelson's Textbook of Pediatrics. *16th ed. Philadelphia, Pa: WB Saunders Company, 2000, with permission from Elsevier.*

*Pediatrics* in December 1998, by Dr. Arlan Rosenbloom and Dr. James Tanner. Consequently, more recent sexual maturation ratings with the correlative ages provide an enhanced background for the analysis of sexual abuse images.

Stages 1 and 2
In a photograph or digital image, gonad and penis growth and pubic hair of a child at the SMR of stage 2 may be difficult to differentiate from that of a child at stage 1. Essentially, these children still appear to be prepubescent because of the scanty nature of hair distribution.

The associated breast development of girls in these stages will not be completely prepubescent since breast development and the growth of pubic hair are not always completely synchronous in rate of development.

In boys, the emergence of axillary hair and pigmentation of the scrotal sac is another important visual parameter of sexual maturation. This is important in child sexual abuse images since one can not visually measure the size of the testes, which

Table 11-4. Median Ages at Entry Into Each Maturity Stage and Fiducial Limits* in Years for Pubic Hair and Breast Development in Girls by Race

| STAGE | AGE AT ENTRY FOR GIRLS | | | | | |
|---|---|---|---|---|---|---|
| | Non-Hispanic White | | Non-Hispanic Black | | Mexican American | |
| | Median | FL | Median | FL | Median | FL |
| Pubic hair | | | | | | |
| PH2 | 10.57† | 10.29-10.85 | 9.43† | 9.05-9.74 | 10.39 | — |
| PH3 | 11.80† | 11.54-12.07 | 10.57† | 10.30-10.83 | 11.70† | 11.14-12.27 |
| PH4 | 13.00† | 12.71-13.30 | 11.90† | 11.38-12.42 | 13.19† | 12.88-13.52 |
| PH5 | 16.33† | 15.86-16.88 | 14.70† | 14.32-15.11 | 16.30† | 15.90-16.76 |
| Breast development | | | | | | |
| B2 | 10.38† | 10.11-10.65 | 9.48† | 9.14-9.76 | 9.80 | 0-11.78 |
| B3 | 11.75† | 11.49-12.02 | 10.79† | 10.50-11.08 | 11.43 | 8.64-14.50 |
| B4 | 13.29† | 12.97-13.61 | 12.24† | 11.87-12.61 | 13.07† | 12.79-13.36 |
| B5 | 15.47† | 15.04-15.94 | 13.92† | 13.57-14.29 | 14.70† | 14.37-15.04 |

*\* Calculated 98.3% FLs to adjust for multiple comparisons between races for an overall $\alpha$ of 0.05.*
*† Significant pair-wise racial difference, $P < 0.05$.*
*NOTE: FL indicates fiducial limit.*
*Reprinted from Sun SS et al, 2002. Reproduced with permission from Pediatrics, Vol. 110, Pages 911-919, Copyright © 2002 by the AAP.*

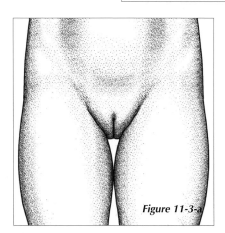

Figure 11-3-a

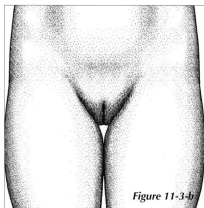

Figure 11-3-b

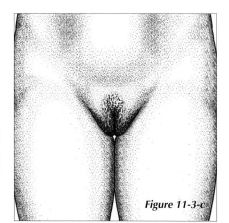

Figure 11-3-c

**Figures 11-3-a, b, c, d,** and **e.** *Tanner stages 1 through 5 of female pubic hair development.*

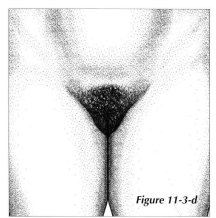

Figure 11-3-d

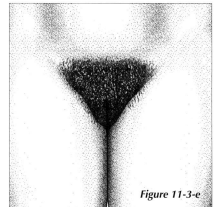

Figure 11-3-e

**Figures 11-4-a, b, c, d,** and **e.** Tanner stages 1 through 5 of female breast development

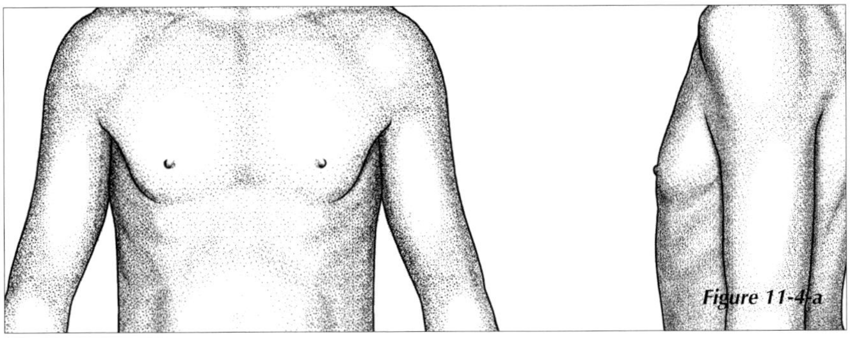

Figure 11-4-a

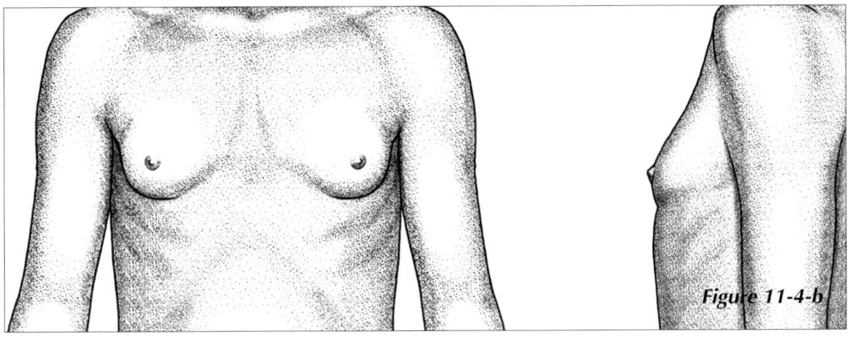

Figure 11-4-b

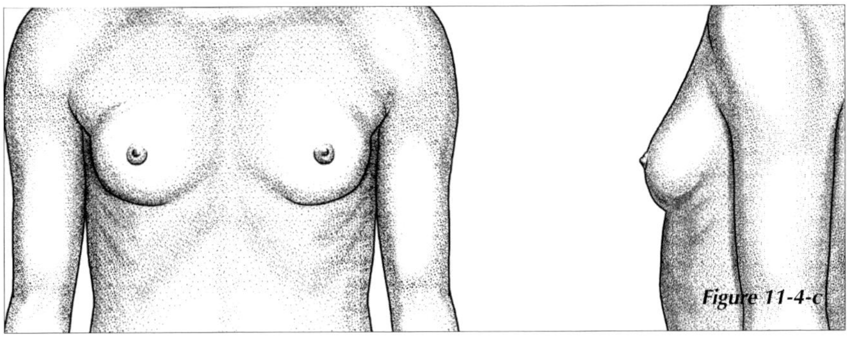

Figure 11-4-c

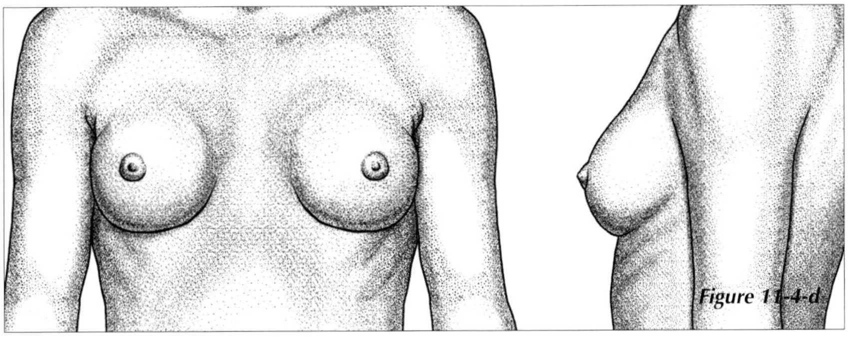

Figure 11-4-d

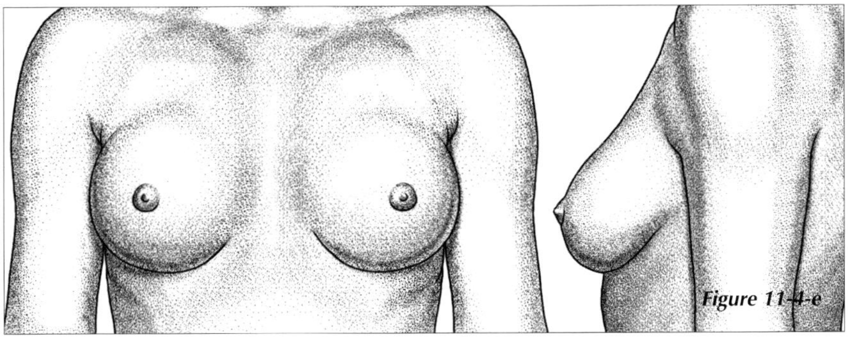

Figure 11-4-e

**Table 11-5. Median Ages at Entry into Each Stage and Fiducial Limits\* in Years for Pubic Hair and Genitalia Development in Boys by Race**

| STAGE | AGE AT ENTRY FOR BOYS | | | | | |
|---|---|---|---|---|---|---|
| | Non-Hispanic White | | Non-Hispanic Black | | Mexican American | |
| | Median | FL | Median | FL | Median | FL |
| Pubic hair | | | | | | |
| PH2 | $11.98^{†}$ | 11.69-12.29 | $11.16^{†}$ | 10.89-11.43 | $12.30^{†}$ | 12.06-12.56 |
| PH3 | 12.65 | 12.37-12.95 | $12.51^{†}$ | 12.26-12.77 | $13.06^{†}$ | 12.79-13.36 |
| PH4 | 13.56 | 13.27-13.86 | 13.73 | 13.49-13.99 | 14.08 | 13.83-14.32 |
| PH5 | 15.67 | 15.30-16.05 | 15.32 | 14.99-15.67 | 15.75 | 15.46-16.03 |
| Genitalia development | | | | | | |
| G2 | 10.03 | 9.61-10.40 | $9.20^{†}$ | 8.62-9.64 | $10.29^{†}$ | 9.94-10.60 |
| G3 | 12.32 | 12.00-12.67 | $11.78^{†}$ | 11.50-12.08 | $12.53^{†}$ | 12.29-12.79 |
| G4 | 13.52 | 13.22-13.83 | 13.40 | 13.15-13.66 | 13.77 | 13.51-14.03 |
| G5 | $16.01^{†}$ | 15.57-16.50 | $15.00^{†}$ | 14.70-15.32 | $15.76^{†}$ | 15.39-16.14 |

\* *Calculated 98.3% FLs to adjust for multiple comparisons between races for an overall $\alpha$ of 0.05.*
† *Significant pair-wise racial difference, $P < 0.05$.*
*NOTE: FL indicates fiducial limit.*
*Reprinted from Sun SS et al, 2002. Reproduced with permission from Pediatrics, Vol. 110, Pages 911-919, Copyright © 2002 by the AAP.*

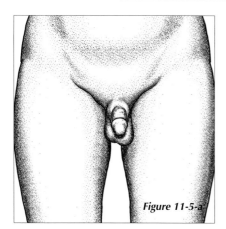

Figure 11-5-a

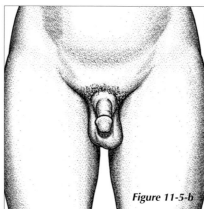

Figure 11-5-b

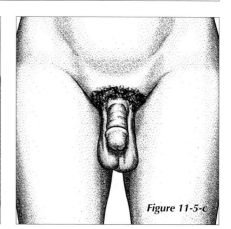

Figure 11-5-c

**Figures 11-5-a, b, c, d,** and **e.** Tanner stages 1 through 5 of male pubic hair and genitalia development.

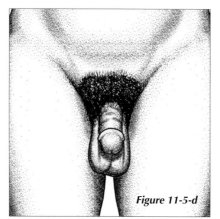

Figure 11-5-d

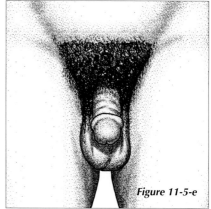

Figure 11-5-e

otherwise would require a juxtaposed orchidometer. However, pigmentation of the scrotal sac may be a reliable sign of emergence in puberty and is particularly obvious when the SMR approaches G4 or G5.

## Stage 3

An SMR of pubic hair at stage 3 is more important than one at stage 5 when seeking to confirm that images are consistent with child pornography. The reason is because stage 5 is consistent with an adult distribution and although a youth might be less than 18 years of age, one would not be able to make that determination visually. A child's development at SMR of pubic hair in stage 3 is much more apparent than that of children in stages 1 and 2, especially if a close-up or enhanced image has been provided.

For girls in the United States, the median age of entry into SMR stage 3 for pubic hair is 11.80 years for non-Hispanic, white girls; 10.57 years for non-Hispanic, black (ie, African American) girls; and 11.70 years for Mexican American girls. The median age of entry into SMR stage 3 for breast development is 11.75 years for non-Hispanic, white girls; 10.79 years for non-Hispanic, black (ie, African American) girls; and 11.43 years for Mexican American girls (Sun et al, 2002).

For boys in the United States, the median age of entry for a SMR of stage 3 for pubic hair is 12.65 years for non-Hispanic, white boys; 12.51 years for non-Hispanic, black (African American) boys; and 13.06 years for Mexican American boys. The median age of entry for stage 3 for gonad growth and enlargement of the penis is 12.32 years for non-Hispanic, white boys; 11.78 years for non-Hispanic, black (African American) boys; and 12.53 years for Mexican American boys (Sun SS et al, 2002).

## Stage 4

The average age for the onset of axillary hair growth is 14.36 years in boys and 12.90 years in girls (Marshall & Tanner, 1969, 1970). Based on the trends of puberty occurring slightly earlier since the 1960s, the ages of axillary hair growth are also clinically occurring earlier.

## Stage 5

In the 1960s, stage 5 occurred by the time a young person was 15 to 16 years old, and this did not vary until the 21st century. The most recent norms for children in the United States are in the NHANES III study, compiled over a 10-year period determining the prevalence of pubic hair, breast development, and menarche in 3 racial and ethnic groups of girls. The most revealing data is found in the work of Wu et al (2002). These norms reveal that the median age of entry into stage 5 for pubic hair distribution for non-Hispanic, white girls became 16.33 years; for non-Hispanic, white boys, the median age of entry became 15.67. This means that an SMR of stage 5 will not usually be reached for most non-Hispanic, white girls in the United States until 16 years old and for boys until 15 to 16 years old (Sun et al, 2002).

## USING THE SEXUAL MATURATION RATING TO DETERMINE A CHILD'S AGE

Unless the examiner has access to the birth certificate of a child who has been photographed, only an estimate of the child's age may be made. Such an estimate can be established by observing the child's developmental cues and comparing these observations with the most recent data available regarding the median age of each stage of development. For the purpose of medical analysis, the examiner should use the age of *entry* into a given stage of pubertal development in order to emphasize the greatest degree of potential immaturity that a child might possess.

Pubic hair distribution is the most obvious and reliable gauge of sexual maturation in child pornography. Breast development actually precedes the onset of pubic hair growth in female children, but usually only by a few months. When a significant discrepancy exists between a female child's breast development and the presence or absence of pubic hair, the examiner should err on the age of the more advanced SMR. For example, if an image demonstrated a pubic hair SMR stage of PH2 and a breast SMR of B4, then the examiner should evaluate the overall image as consistent with a child whose age is associated with B4. For an image of a girl from the United States, the examiner would assess the child's age to be consistent with a 13 year old for a non-Hispanic white girl, a 12 year old for a non-Hispanic black girl, and a 13 year old for a Mexican American girl since these represent the median ages of entry into this stage.

Practitioners should remember the accepted sequence of puberty changes in girls, which can be recalled by the acronym BPAM: **B**reast development, **P**ubic hair, **A**xillary hair, and **M**enses. Remembering this sequence may help the practitioner determine whether a child is developing according to appropriate hormonal stimuli. The examiner should also be aware that premature breast development (referred to as *thelarche*) and premature pubarche are clinical conditions that warrant further endocrinological evaluation, but these conditions rarely occur and should not be considered when analyzing child pornography.

Although child pornography images cause the practitioner to consider the onset and duration of various stages of sexual maturation, examiners must also remember that the cycle of puberty requires 5 to 6 years for completion (Grumbach & Styne, 1998). Consequently, if a photographed child has *not* obtained complete, adult sexual maturation, that child is almost certainly younger than 18 years old.

## Delayed or Early Sexual Maturation

Delayed or early sexual maturation may occur in persons with rare genetic conditions. For females, Turner's syndrome (1 in 2500 girls) would be the most likely diagnosis of delayed puberty. For males, the most likely genetic diagnoses for delayed puberty would be Noonan's syndrome (1 in 1000-2500 boys) or Klinefelter's syndrome (1 in 500-1000 boys). Noonan's syndrome and Turner's syndrome are associated with webbing of the tissues of the neck as well as other physical abnormalities. Boys with Klinefelter's syndrome have sterility, breast development, normal penis growth but small testes, incomplete puberty, and learning problems.

Other differential diagnoses for delayed puberty in children include chronic diseases, anorexia nervosa, and malnutrition. Children with these disorders are likely to have physical findings indicative of these problems. Also possible in delayed puberty is **hypopituitarism**, which is very rare and reflects an inadequate function of the pituitary gland in the brain.

Early sexual maturation, or precocious puberty, is another very rare occurrence in children. Defined as the onset of puberty before the age of 7 years in girls and 9 years in boys, the majority of cases are idiopathic. In the circumstance of child sexual abuse images, if a child exhibited precocious puberty, the child would be shorter and younger than the norms for maturation stages.

The differential diagnoses of early or late puberty should be considered when analyzing child sexual abuse images. However, in the absence of any physical findings supportive of the previously noted genetic disorders, it should not be assumed that the images portray children who are either genetically or hormonally abnormal.

## Sexual Maturation Rates and Children Who Are Not From the United States

Similar information regarding age correlations of SMR and the ages of children who are not from the United States have been documented in several countries. A compilation from various international studies regarding estimated age determinations is listed in **Table 11-6**.

**Table 11-6. International Estimates of the Timing of Sexual Maturation of Children Listed Chronologically by Study**

| Study | Females B2-B5/PH2-PH5 | Males G2-G5/PH2-PH5 |
|---|---|---|
| **England:** Marshall & Tanner, 1969,1970* | 11.1-15.3/11.7-14.4 | 11.6-14.9/13.4-15.2 |
| **France:** Roy,1972; Roy et al, 1972 | 11.4-14.0 /11.3-13.2 (PH4) | 12.2-14.3 (G4)/ 12.4-14.3 (PH4) |
| **Sweden:** Karlberg & Taranger, 1976 | 11.4-15.6/11.5-15.2 | 12.2-15.1/12.5-15.5 |
| **Switzerland:** Largo & Prader, 1983a,b | Not studied | 11.2-14.7/12.2-14.9 |
| **Mexico:** Villarreal, 1989 | 10.9-15.1/11.2-15.5 | 12.2-16.3/12.8-16.1 |
| **The Netherlands:** Roede, 1990 | Not studied | 11.3-15.3/11.7-14.9 |
| **Hungary:** Dober & Kiralyfalvi, 1993 | Not studied | 11.9-14.4/11.8-14.6 |
| **United States of America:** Roche et al, 1995 | 11.2-12.4 (B4)/11.0-13.1 | 11.2-14.3/11.2-14.3 |
| **Germany:** Willers et al, 1996 | Not studied | 10.8-15.9/11.4-15.6 |
| **China:** Huen et al, 1997 | 9.8 (B2)/12.4 (menses)† | Not studied |
| **United States of America:** Herman-Giddens et al, 1997 | 9.96-10.30 (B3, white)/ 10.51-11.53 (PH3, white) | 10.1-15.9 (white)‡/ 12.0-15.7 (white) |
| | 8.87-10.19 (B3, black)/ 8.78-10.35 (PH3, black) | 9.5-14.9 (black)‡/ 11.2-15.4 (black) |
| **United States of America:** Sun et al, 2002*; Wu et al, 2002* | 10.4-15.5/10.6-16.3 (white) | 10.0-16.0 (white)/ 12.0-15.7 (white) |
| | 9.5-13.9/9.4-14.7 (black) | 9.2-15.0 (black)/ 11.1-15.3 (black) |

*\* These studies have been used for normative data in the past.*

*† Menses occurs in 90% of females who have attained an SMR of B4/PH4.*

*‡ G2 may not have been staged accurately because of using visual assessment only.*

# Child Erotica Images

When examining images, the healthcare provider must also differentiate between child pornography and child erotica. **Child pornography** images depict child sexual abuse and constitute the scene of a crime. **Child erotica** images do not depict sexual abuse but may be highly suggestive and may ultimately serve the purpose of a fantasy source for a collector.

Child erotica images may often include images taken from store catalogues for children's clothing such as underwear or pajamas. These images may include photographs of children in nudist colonies or naturist communities, which are readily found on the Internet. **Internet child erotica** is any picture of a child that does not meet the standard for sexual abuse images, as based upon various country definitions, but which is included in a collection of images that often include child pornography. The juxtaposition of normal childhood scenes with pornography provides an investigator or a forensic psychiatrist an opportunity to discern the potential sexual preferences of an offender. Healthcare providers who analyze child pornography must understand the laws of the jurisdiction of the investigation so that they will include all valid images.

One example of child erotica in the United States is the distribution of images of a 14-year-old American girl who was photographed extensively for pornography production. Her presence was even included in a Russian video. Additionally, this child had numerous pictures on the Internet that were not pornographic in nature and could sometimes be obtained as a complement to the pornographic images, thereby making the child more "real" for potential collectors who might choose to fantasize over the erotic images instead (Taylor & Quayle, 2003).

Child erotica may be found on a computer and included for analysis. Even if a child is nude, prepubescent, dressed in adult or sexually explicit clothing, and posed to appear coy, demure, or coquettish, unless actual sexual abuse, including masturbation, is depicted, the image would likely constitute child erotica in the United States. However, the same image in other countries may meet the legal definition of child pornography.

## CONCLUSION

The role of the medical analysis of child sexual abuse images is important. Healthcare providers who examine children on a frequent basis are able to address questions of whether images are consistent with toddlers, children younger than 12 years old, children with disabilities, or children who appear to be under the influence of a drug that alters the central nervous system. Healthcare providers are also well-suited to determine whether images show young people who appear to have reached their complete sexual maturation levels or are consistent with a teenager who appears to be younger than 16 or 17 years old. Using developmental parameters, musculoskeletal criteria, dentition, fat distribution, and knowledge of sexual maturation, a healthcare provider is extraordinarily equipped to determine whether images are consistent with those of children. Additionally, knowing the long-term sequelae of child sexual abuse makes the practitioner an important team member and one who can facilitate the investigation and prosecution of those who take part in child sexual exploitation.

## REFERENCES

*Ashcroft v Free Speech Coalition*, 535 US 234 (9th Cir 2002).

Bly L. *Motor Skills Acquisition in the First Year: An Illustrated Guide to Normal Development*. San Antonio, Tex: The Psychological Corporation; 1994.

Carter SR, Seiff S, Grant PE, Vigneron DB. The Asian lower eyelid: a comparative anatomic study using high-resolution magnetic resonance imaging. *Ophthal Plast Reconstr Surg*. 1998;14(4):227-234.

Dober I, Kiralyfalvi L. Pubertal development in South Hungarian boys and girls. *Ann Hum Biol*. 1993;20:71-74.

18 USC § 2256.

Friedrich WN, Dittner CA, Action R, et al. Child sexual behavior inventory: normative, psychiatric and sexual abuse comparisons. *Child Maltreat*. 2001;6:37-49.

Friedrich WN, Jaworski TM, Huxsahl JE, Bengston BS. Dissociative and sexual behaviors in children and adolescents with sexual abuse and psychiatric histories. *J Interpers Violence*. 1997;12:155-171.

Friedrich WN, Brambsch P, Broughton D, Broughton K, Beilke RL. Normative sexual behavior in children. *Pediatrics*. 1991;88:456-464.

Friedrich WN, Grambsch P, Damon L, et al. The child sexual behavior inventory: normative and clinical findings. *Psychol Assess*. 1992;4:303-311.

Friedrich WN. Sexual victimization and sexual behavior in children: a review of recent literature. *Child Abuse Negl*. 1993;17:59-66.

Gillespie P. Toronto police sexual exploitation service pilot project. Presented at: 21st Meeting of the Interpol Specialist Group on Crimes Against Children; June 3-5, 2003; Lyon, France.

Glaser D. Child abuse and neglect and the brain: a review. *J Child Psychol Psychiatry*. 2000;41:97-116.

Grumbach MM, Styne DM. Puberty: ontogeny, neuroendocrinology, physiology, and disorders. In: Wilson JD, Foster DW, Kronenberg HM, Larsen PR, eds. *Williams Textbook of Endocrinology*. 9th ed. Philadelphia, Pa: WB Saunders; 1998:1509-1625.

Herman-Giddens ME, Slora EJ, Wasserman RC, et al. Secondary sexual characteristics and menses in young girls seen in office practice: a study from the Pediatric Research in Office Settings network. *Pediatrics*. 1997;99:505-512.

Huen KF, Leung SS, Lau JT, Cheung AY, Leung NK, Chiu MC. Secular trend in the sexual maturation of southern Chinese girls. *Acta Pediatr*. 1997;86:1121-1124.

Karlberg P, Taranger T. The somatic development of children in a Swedish urban community. *Acta Paediatr Scand Suppl*. 1976;258:1-148.

Largo RH, Prader A. Pubertal development in Swiss boys. *Helvitica Pediatr Acta*. 1983a;38:211-228.

Largo RH, Prader A. Pubertal development in Swiss girls. *Helvitica Pediatr Acta*. 1983b;38:229-243.

Lebergue B. Paraphilias in US pornography titles: "pornography made me do it" (Ted Bundy). *Bull Am Acad Psychiatry Law*. 1991;19(1):43-46.

Mannarino AP, Cohen J. A follow-up study of factors that mediate the development of psychological symptomatology in sexually abused girls. *Child Maltreat*. 1996;1:246-260.

Marshall W, Tanner JM. Puberty. In: Falkner F, Tanner JM, eds. *Postnatal Growth: Neurobiology*. 2nd ed. New York, NY: Plenum Press; 1986:171-209. *Human Growth. A Comprehensive Treatise*; vol 2.

Marshall W, Tanner JM. Variations in the pattern of pubertal changes in girls. *Arch Dis Child*. 1969;44:291-303.

Marshall W, Tanner JM. Variation in the pattern of pubertal changes in boys. *Arch Dis Child*. 1970;45:13-23.

Roche AF, Wellens R, Attie KM, Siervogel RM. The timing of sexual maturation in a group of US white youths. *J Pediatr Endocrinol Metab*. 1995;8:11-18.

Roede MJ. The secular trend in The Netherlands: the third nationwide growth study. *Arztl Jugendkd*. 1990;81:330-336.

Rosenbloom AL, Tanner JM. Misuse of Tanner puberty stages to estimate chronologic age. *Pediatrics*. 1998;102:1494.

Roy MP. Évolution clinique de la puberté du garçon (étude longitudinale somatique de 68 adolescents) [Clinical course of puberty in boys (somatic longitudinal study of 68 adolescents)]. *C.R. 11e Réunion des Equipes Chargées des Etudes sur la Croissance et le Développement de l'Enfant Normal*. London, England and Paris, France: C.I.E.; 1972:185-190.

Roy MP, Sempe M, Orssaud E, Pedron G. Evolution clinique de la puberté de la fille (étude longitudinale somatique de 80 adolescents) [Clinical course of puberty in girls (somatic longitudinal study of 80 adolescents)]. *Arch Fr Pediatr.* 1972;29:155-168.

Sun SS, Schubert CM, Chumlea WC, et al. National estimates of the timing of sexual maturation and racial differences among US children. *Pediatrics.* 2002;110(5): 911-919.

Tanner JM. *Growth at Adolescence.* 2nd ed. Springfield, Ill: CC Thomas; 1962.

Taylor M, Holland G, Quayle E. Typology of paedophile picture collections. *The Police Journal.* 2001;74(2):97-107.

Taylor M, Quayle E. *Child Pornography: An Internet Crime.* New York, NY: Brunner-Routledge; 2003.

Teicher MH, Andersen SL, Polcari A, Anderson CM, Navalta CP. Developmental neurobiology of childhood stress and trauma. *Psychiatr Clin North Am.* 2002;25(2): 397-426.

Teicher MH, Andersen SL, Polcari A, Anderson CM, Navalta CP, Kim DM. The neurobiological consequences of early stress and childhood maltreatment. *Neurosci Biobehav Rev.* 2003;27(1-2):33-44.

Villarreal SF, Martorell R, Mendoza F. Sexual maturation of Mexican American adolescents. *Am J Hum Biol.* 1989;1:87-95.

Willers B, Engelhardt L, Pelz L. Sexual maturation in East German boys. *Acta Pediatr.* 1996;85:785-788.

Wu T, Mendola P, Buck GM. Ethnic differences in the presence of secondary sex characteristics and menarche among US girls: the Third National Health and Nutrition Examination Survey, 1988-1994. *Pediatrics.* 2002;110:752-757.

# Chapter 12

# CHILD SEXUAL ABUSE AND THE PARAPHILIAS

Peter I. Collins, MCA, MD, FRCP(C)

Any discussion regarding child pornography (child sexual abuse images) and other sex crimes against children would be incomplete unless one considers the broader subject of paraphilias. **Paraphilia** is derived from the Greek word for love, *philia*, and the word for beyond the usual, *para*. It is defined as abnormal, unusual, or deviant sexual preferences. These preferences can be directed toward a particular target or to an abnormal activity (Freund et al, 1997). The purpose of this chapter is to explore the relationship between child pornography and the paraphilias.

The primary classification guide used by mental health professionals in North America is the *Diagnostic and Statistical Manual of Mental Disorders* (DSM-IV-TR), now in its fourth edition. The first 2 editions (in 1952 and 1965) classified sexual deviances as personality disorders. With the publication of the third edition (DSM-III), the concept of erotic preference was recognized and the sexual deviances were categorized as paraphilias.

The DSM-IV-TR states that (1) the diagnostic criteria for paraphilias require recurrent and intense sexually arousing fantasies, urges, or behavior directed toward body parts or nonhuman objects, suffering or humiliation of either partner in the sex act, or sexual activity with a nonconsenting person, and (2) that these fantasies, urges, and behavior cause clinically significant distress or impairment of functioning (American Psychiatric Association, 2000).

The DSM-IV-TR lists the most common types of paraphilias. These are summarized in **Table 12-1**. Some paraphilic activities are legal (such as transvestism); however, the type of paraphilia is not always an indicator of criminality. The fetishist might have to steal worn female underwear to be aroused, but consensual sexual partners who are willing to role-play may satisfy a sexual sadist, thereby satisfying their sexual urges through legal means. Pedophilia, the most common paraphilia assessed in treatment clinics, is illegal.

The true prevalence of paraphilic disorders is largely unknown because the majority of these individuals do not seek help. Therefore, accurate epidemiological studies are difficult to conduct. We do know that most paraphilics report becoming aware of their deviant sexual interests in and around puberty but may not act on their fantasies for years, if at all. If they end up in treatment, it is most often post-arrest and on a judicial order. On occasion, it is at the request of their sexual partner(s) who can not tolerate the unconventional sexual activities. The average time, from the onset of the paraphilia, to the receiving of treatment, is 12 years. Among criminal paraphilics, the average individual has committed 44 crimes a year before arrest (Abel et al, 1985).

Why some targets or activities are more likely to become paraphilic preferences is not fully understood (Seto & Barbaree, 2000). Certain "activity" paraphilias—voyeurism, exhibitionism, frotteurism, and rape preference—have been theorized to be disorders of courtship. Freund (1990) stated that there are 4 stages of courtship: searching for a

**Table 12-1. Common Paraphilias**

| PARAPHILIA | PREFERRED ACTIVITY OR TARGET |
|---|---|
| Exhibitionism | Exposing one's genitals to an unsuspecting woman or child |
| Fetishism | Erotic attraction to a nonliving object |
| Frotteurism | Rubbing up against a nonconsenting person |
| Pedophilia | Prepubescent children |
| Masochism | Being humiliated, bound, or made to suffer |
| Sadism | Psychological or physical suffering of the target |
| Transvestic fetishism | Cross-dressing |
| Voyeurism | Observing unsuspecting individuals who are disrobing, naked, or engaging in sexual activity |

partner; pre-tactile intervention; tactile intervention; and genital contact. Paraphilic behavior, by extension, is a distortion of one of these courtship stages. As an example, searching is replaced by voyeurism; pre-tactile involves exhibitionism; tactile is replaced by toucherism or frotteurism and genital contact is achieved through preferential rape.

There is substantial evidence for the co-occurrence of paraphilias. Most individuals who meet the criteria for a diagnosis of a paraphilia rarely "specialize" in one paraphilic interest but instead have multiple paraphilias. These are referred to as "crossover" sexual offenses because victims are from multiple age, gender, and relationship categories (Heil et al, 2003).

According to Abel et al (1988), in their examination of 561 men, only 10% had 1 diagnosis of a paraphilia. Upward of 37% were, at the same time or in the past, engaged in 5 to 10 distinct forms of paraphilic behaviors. In the paraphilic "career" of a sexual deviant, one paraphilia may take dominance, only to be replaced over time by another. Bradford et al (1992), in their sample of 443 men, found that of the 155 subjects who reported voyeuristic activity (the largest single paraphilic group in this study), 66% reported that they had engaged in frotteurism, 52% had engaged in exhibitionistic activity, and 47% had committed rape. Historically, this is supported by Yalom (1960), who described cases of co-occurrence of voyeurism, exhibitionism, and rape, while Gebhard et al (1965) noted that 1 in 10 incarcerated exhibitionists had committed rape.

Lesser occurring paraphilic activities are addressed in the DSM-IV-TR as paraphilias "not otherwise specified," but this list is not all-inclusive. Many examples of rare or more obscure forms of sexually deviant behaviors are known to exist. Many of these obscure paraphilias are described in literature (Money, 1984) and are found on the Internet. **Table 12-2** lists examples of more obscure paraphilias.

The Internet has allowed researchers and clinicians an opportunity to examine the wide array of paraphilic themes, fantasies, and fetish items that sexually deviant men are attracted to, some of the items being quite obscure. The Internet has allowed individuals, who were previously isolated regarding their interest in a rare paraphilic activity, to communicate and even meet like-minded individuals. As an example, pedophiles, prior to the Internet, remained relatively isolate but through the Internet formed larger social networks that have been referred to as "virtual communities" (O'Connell, 2001; Quayle & Taylor, 2002; Taylor & Quayle, 2003). Ironically, this sense of community is achieved, for the most part, by assuming anonymity.

The Internet provides paraphilics a high-tech way of pursuing their sexual activities and desires. Regardless of whether they use newsgroups, e-mail, thematic Web sites, chat rooms, Internet Relay Chat (IRC), or other Internet resources, the sexual preferences of paraphilic individuals are not different than before the Internet was available (Kim & Bailey, 1997).

### Table 12-2. Examples of Clinically Identified Paraphilias

| PARAPHILIA | STIMULUS |
| --- | --- |
| Acrotomophilia | Stump of an amputee and/or the desire to amputate someone's limb |
| Apotemnophilia | Self-amputation (or done in a hospital) |
| Asphyxiophilia | Self-induced asphyxiation almost to the point of unconsciousness; also known as auto-erotic asphyxiation |
| Autoassassinophilia | Managing the possibility of one's own masochistic death |
| Autonepiophilia | Impersonating a baby in diapers |
| Biastophilia | Rape-preference |
| Coprophilia | Handling, being smeared with, or ingesting feces |
| Klismaphilia | Receiving or giving enemas |
| Morphophilia | A particular body type or size |
| Mysophilia | Smelling, chewing, or otherwise using soiled (urine, fecal material, menstrual discharge) or sweaty clothing |
| Necrophilia | A corpse, or someone acting as though they were dead |
| Partialism | Particular body part (eg, feet, neck, abdomen) |
| Scotophilia | Watching others engage in masturbation or sexual intercourse |
| Stigmatophilia | A partner who has been tattooed, scarified, or pierced in the genital area |
| Triolism | Observing one's partner engaging in sex with another person |
| Urophilia | Being urinated on and/or drinking urine |
| Zoophilia | Engaging in sex with animals |

# PEDOPHILIA

It is beyond the scope of this chapter to present an in-depth examination of the etiology, assessment, and treatment of pedophiles. Despite the debate regarding the taxonomic adequacy of the DSM-IV-TR diagnosis of pedophilia (O'Donohue et al, 2000), the target choice, for the pedophile, is a prepubescent child.

To assign a chronological age to a prepubescent child is difficult because children can reach puberty over a wide age range. Boys and girls now experience puberty at younger ages than in previous generations. In general, girls enter puberty between ages 8 and 13 and reach menarche several years later, while boys enter puberty between ages 9 and 14 (Winter, 1982). The reasons for earlier menarche in girls are not well understood. Most of the changes are attributed to better health and nutrition, although the influence of estrogen triggers and even sexually charged media messages have been theorized as contributory (Herman-Giddens et al, 1997).

There are 2 age variants to pedophilia. Infantaphilia is the erotic attraction to children 5 years of age and younger. With the advent of the Internet, there have been a number of Web sites and chat rooms devoted to sex with toddlers and infants. Hebephiles, or ephebophiles, are men who are sexually attracted to children who have reached puberty and are in the early stages of adolescence.

The DSM-IV-TR describes ***exclusive pedophiles*** as men who can have sex only with children. ***Nonexclusive pedophiles*** comprise those men who are capable of having age-appropriate sexual relations but fantasize about sexual contact with children. The latter group explains why some pedophiles can hide in spousal relationships. Prior to the Internet, some pedophiles would target single mothers and would enter a relationship with the woman to abuse the children. This has continued on the Internet, with men intentionally meeting women in chat rooms and dating and singles sites to access children.

Although the majority of pedophiles are attracted to same sex or opposite sex children, a small percentage are equally attracted to boys and girls. Their target age group is usually younger children; it is as though the immature body parts sexually arouse them and gender is not an influence.

Pedophiles usually do have a specific fantasy choice regarding preferred age, body type, hair color, etc. However, if their preferred erotic choice is not available, they will target others who do not meet their fantasy. There have been some cases where pedophiles will target boys even though, through self-report and confirmed by phallometric testing, they are attracted to girls. Phallometric testing (penile plethysmography) is a procedure in which a subject's pattern of sexual responding to different categories of sexual stimuli is assessed. Responses are recorded in terms of changes of penile volume during the presentation of a stimulus. This form of testing is less susceptible to faking than self-report measures. See Chapter 14, Ethical Issues in Sexual Offender Assessments, for more information on this topic.

When considering multiple paraphilias among child molesters, Marshall et al (1991) found that 14% of extrafamilial molesters of girls, 12% of extrafamilial male child molesters, and 8% of incest offenders disclosed, on self-report, more than one paraphilia. In the author's clinical and investigative experience, most of the co-occurring paraphilias, of interest to the pedophile, are thematic of the attraction to pre-pubescent children. For example, a pedophile may also be a fetishist, but the object of erotic attraction is girls' underwear or boys' running shoes. If primarily voyeurs or exhibitionists, they will peep or expose with children as the victims. Bradford et al (1992), in their aforementioned study, found that among the pedophiles, 9% had sexually assaulted an adult, and 13% had attempted to sexually assault an adult. Hebephiles had a slightly higher crossover rate of 10% and 24%, respectively.

Heil et al (2003) conducted polygraph testing on 223 incarcerated and 266 paroled sexual offenders in treatment. The purpose of the polygraph was to elicit admissions of offending behavior. They found high rates of crossover sexual offences consistent, for the most part, with Abel et al (1988). They found, however, that 78% of inmates who were known to molest children admitted to sexually victimizing adults.

## PEDOPHILES AND CHILD PORNOGRAPHY

Pedophiles collect child pornography for various reasons (Durkin, 1997; Quayle & Taylor, 2002). First and foremost, the images are used to fuel their sexual fantasies or serve as a masturbatory aid or prelude to sexual activity. Even nonpornographic or nonsexualized images can be erotically arousing to the pedophile. Knowing that there are many thousands of individuals who access child sexual abuse images on the Internet validates that their shared sexual preference is common. Most images portray compliant and smiling children contributing to the supposed appropriateness and validation.

Whereas pedophiles are a heterogeneous group regarding age, sex, and type of sexual activity preferred, the majority of same sex and opposite sex pedophiles use the process of grooming to victimize the child. Grooming is analogous to courtship behavior. Pedophiles have a knack for targeting children who may be more receptive to their sexual advances. Some will employ threats or enough force to achieve the requested sexual activity. Inflicting pain and suffering actually arouses a minority of pedophiles.

Pornography can be shown to potential victims as part of the grooming process, to lower their inhibitions and as an example of what activity the offender wishes the child to do (Durkin, 1997). Lanning (2001) suggests that an image can be used as a trophy and, for some offenders, it can be used to blackmail children to ensure their silence and cooperation for future assaults.

The relationship between viewing child pornography and contact offenses is complex. Marshall (1988) found that 53% of a sample of child molesters deliberately used pornographic material as part of their planned preparation for offending. Carter et al (1987) found that child molesters were more likely to use pornography before offending but could be satiated by relieving the impulse to offend and would thus not offend. Some sex offenders have proposed this as a reason for legalizing the possession of child pornography. (*R. v Sharpe*, 2001). However, every pornographic image of a child is a permanent record of the child's exploitation and abuse. This, coupled with what may satiate an offender, on one occasion, may incite to offend on another occasion, obviously does not justify the legalization of possession of child pornography.

Since 1997, the United States Postal Inspection Service (USPIS) has kept figures regarding its child exploitation arrests. Data through May 2004 indicate that of the 1866 individuals arrested by the USPIS, 639 (34%) were identified as having contact offenses against children by history or as a result of the arrest. A small percentage of the individuals arrested were ***travelers***, traveling to meet a child for planned sexual activity, and these individuals were included in this group of contact offenders (R. Smith, oral and written communication, July 2004).

Hernandez (2000a, b), in his preliminary study, examined 54 former inmates who participated in a US federal penitentiary sex offender treatment program. All 54 had been convicted of crimes involving the production, receipt, and possession of child pornography. Before treatment, based on the pre-sentence investigation report, only 46% appeared to have had contact offenses. After treatment, 79.6% admitted to having previous contact sexual crimes after participation in the treatment program— an additional 1371 victims never detected by the criminal justice system.

In Marshall's (2000) review of the literature relating to pornography use by sex offenders, he concluded that the exposure to pornography may influence, but is not the sole cause of, offending in an individual who has developed an appetite for sexual deviance.

Internet sites allow the pedophile easier access to an array of child abuse images that were much harder to obtain before widespread use of the Internet. Durkin (1997) identified 4 possible ways pedophiles misuse the Internet: they send and receive child abuse images; locate children to molest; engage in inappropriate sexual communication with children; and, as noted above, communicate with other like-minded individuals. Kim & Bailey (1997) add that the Internet allows pedophiles to locate fetish objects.

The Internet allows pedophiles a safer way of joining groups that advocate sex with children. Individuals have also established Web sites, known as "blogs," devoted to promoting sex with children. The North American Man/Boy Love Association (NAMBLA) is an organization, originally modeled after a number of similar European groups, with its own Web site. NAMBLA was founded in 1978 in response to the arrests of 24 businessmen and professionals in Revere, Massachusetts. It is a political, "civil rights," and educational organization that promotes adult sexual behavior with boys. DeYoung (1989) examined the strategies used by NAMBLA to justify, rationalize, and normalize its members' beliefs and practices. These involve denial of injury (children are not injured or harmed by sexual activity), "condemning the condemners" (attacking the criminal justice, mental health and child welfare systems, and specific professionals), appealing to higher loyalties (children's rights), and denying any harm to the victims.

Regardless of whether they are promoted by individuals or organizations on the Internet, these sites assist in fueling the rationalizations and justifications these men possess regarding children as sexual objects. These cognitive distortions are offense-facilitating, deeply held beliefs that existed before the Internet and can include the following thoughts:

— Sex with children was practiced in ancient Greece, so it is just a hang-up of the modern age.

— Homosexuality, in Canada, was regarded against the law until late 1968; therefore, it is only a matter of time before it becomes legal for men to have sex with children.

— Children are sexually curious and are capable of giving consent to have sex.

— If children ask to see an adult's genitals, they really are interested in having sex.

A variant of cognitive distortions is the idealization of literary figures who are alleged to have been sexually interested in children—Charles Dodgson (Lewis Carroll), JM Barrie, and Walt Whitman, to name a few. It is no coincidence that the international child pornography ring, the Wonderland Club was named for Carroll's *Alice in Wonderland.*

# OTHER PARAPHILIAS

Some of the co-existing paraphilic themes and/or activities engaged in by child pornography collectors include zoophilia (bestiality), fetishism, urophilia, coprophilia, klismaphilia, sadism, hyperdominance, and necrophilia.

## ZOOPHILIA (BESTIALITY)

Zoophilia involves using animals as sexual objects, involving fellatio, cunnilingus, coitus, and masturbation. It is a behavior that can occur opportunistically (curiosity, novelty, or unavailability of an appropriate human partner) or as a preferred sexual practice. The preferential use of animals was termed by von Krafft-Ebing (1925) as "zooerasty." Like other forms of sexual deviances listed as "not otherwise specified" in the DSM-IV-TR, the actual incidence and prevalence is unknown but is felt to be under-reported. In the Cambridge study of sexual offenses, Radzinowicz (1957) reported that only 2% of the total 1985 sexual offenses examined involved bestiality. In their study of male sexual fantasies, Crepault & Couture (1980) reported that only 5.3% of their sample had fantasized about having sex with animals. Abel et al (1993), however, found that 72% of juvenile sex offenders, in their study group, had a paraphilic interest in bestiality.

Consistent with the concept of multiple paraphilias, Abel et al (1988) report that all the 14 zoophilic respondents in their study reported at least 1 other paraphilic attraction and that 50% had 5 or more with the co-occurring paraphilias. These were pedophilia, exhibitionism, voyeurism, frotteurism, telephone scatophilia, transvestic fetishism, fetishism, sexual sadism, sexual masochism, urophilia, and coprophilia. In the author's clinical practice, individuals who had zoophilia as part of their offending profile were sexual sadists, pedophiles, or both.

The cases that do come to the attention of psychiatrists usually involve individuals who are under the influence of alcohol or drugs, are psychopaths, or who are cognitively impaired. Few are psychotic (Bluglass, 1990). This does not explain the proliferation of Web sites thematic of bestiality available on the Internet. Many are available, with titles such as: "Zoo Partners," "Animal Passion," "Farm Girls," "Bestiality Live," and "Beasty Whores." There is even an anti-bestiality site, titled the "Animal Sexual Abuse Information and Resource Site," which is hosted by a self-identified "ex-zoophile."

There are no accurate statistics available regarding the number of child pornography collectors who have, on their arrest, animal sexual abuse images in their collection. Response to a question posed to members of a "restricted access" law enforcement listserve indicated that in 10% to 40% of the judicially ordered seizures, the offender had both child and animal abuse images.

Dewaraja & Money (1986) describe a rare variant of zoophilia referred to as formicophilia. The focus is on small creatures such as "snails, frogs, ants or other insects creeping, crawling, or nibbling on their body, especially the genitalia, perianal area, or nipples."

## FETISHISM

The term ***fetish***, from the Portuguese *fetisso*, originally described an object that had religious or magical significance for the holder. It has evolved to being a descriptor for an inanimate object or part of the body (partialism) that has great erotic meaning for the person (Binet, 1887).

In some cases, the use of a fetish item is so strong that it becomes requisite for any sexual activity. There is stability, over time, with some fetish items, such as clothing, but the erotic attraction to the type of clothing can change. Sometimes it is not the item, per se, but the texture of the material that can be arousing (vinyl, silk, leather). There has been a displacement of material more popular in the 19th century such as velvet or silk, with rubber, polyvinyl, and other late 20th century synthetic material (Mason, 1997).

Conceivably, anything can become a fetish item. The most common fetish items are female undergarments or lingerie. This holds true in the fetishism-associated pedophilia and child pornography collectors. Often, the worn undergarments that have been soiled with urine or feces are of great importance to the fetishist.

**Case Study 12-1**

A 24-year-old man who lived in a mid-sized city would write to families of girls who came to his attention through reading neighborhood newspapers that reported on middle school track meets. Representing himself as an executive for a well-known athletic shoe manufacturer, he would offer to send the child a new pair of shoes but they would have to, in exchange, send in their old shoes. The man was a pedophile with an erotic attraction to girls between the ages of 12 and 14 and who had a fetish for girls' athletic shoes.

There have been many cases in which panties or underwear have been labelled and kept in plastic bags by the offender or kept in open display, and readily available, to be used to masturbate with. There is a higher emotional significance if the underwear has been taken from a victim. This elevates the item to being a *souvenir*, an item taken from the victim as a reminder of a pleasurable encounter, and may be used for masturbatory fantasies.

With the widespread use of the Internet, many obscure or rarer forms of fetish items now have Web sites or chat rooms devoted to that particular fetish item whether it is balloons, feathers, or another object. Pictures of children or adults using the fetish items are available, and "fetters," as many of them will refer to themselves, can communicate with individuals with similar deviant interests.

The Diaper Pail Fraternity is one of a number of organizations with its own Web site that caters to individuals who are erotically aroused by wearing diapers and acting or being treated as babies. Preferring to call themselves "adult babies" or "diaperists," these individuals can order adult-size diapers, pacifiers, and other items. to act out their erotic fantasies. The behavior can consist of being disciplined, spanked, or restrained and often is associated with urophilia or coprophilia. A number of these men are pedophiles or specifically infantiphiles.

In 1995, New Scotland Yard, of the Metropolitan Police, made a link between a diaper club and a known pedophile organization. In November 2001, the Paedophile Intelligence Unit of Her Majesty's Customs and Excise Service in England intercepted 3 German nationals who were en route to a Diaper Pail conference in the United States. One of the travelers was a known pedophile, and the other 2 were suspected of having an erotic preference for children.

A variant of this fetish are individuals who have been known to break into residences, or steal the garbage from houses, where the individuals have first-hand knowledge or have determined by indicators outside the house (eg, baby carriages, car seats in vehicles) that a baby is in the residence. The soiled diapers are then used as masturbatory aids. These men do not report that they fantasize about being a baby or being treated like a baby.

Little has appeared in the psychiatric literature regarding infantilism. Tuchman & Lachman (1964) reported on an incest case involving the molestation of 4- and 6-year-old daughters. The molester would wear rubber pants over the diapers and would urinate and masturbate in them. Malitz (1966) reported a case of a 20-year-old college student who broke into a house due to a compulsion to wear diapers and defecate in them. Orgasm often accompanied defecation when he was wearing the diapers. Wearing rubber pants over the diapers erotically aroused him as well.

Recently, Pate & Gabbard (2003) reported on a case of a 35-year-old male with "adult baby syndrome." It is interesting to note that their case study concentrated on the psychodynamic aspects of the behavior with sexual deviance not being considered a major causal factor.

**Case Study 12-2**

Members of a Regional Police Service arrested a man who was planning to abduct a 7-year-old boy and "raise him like a baby." The man had disclosed this information to another pedophile who became concerned and contacted the authorities. A search of the residence revealed a crib that was built to accommodate the planned victim that would serve as a cage. The subject built an adult-sized crib that he slept in. Wearing diapers sexually aroused him.

## Urophilia, Coprophilia, and Klismaphilia

Urophilia, coprophilia, and klismaphilia are described in the DSM-IV-TR nomen-clature as lesser occurring paraphilias. As noted above, there is an association with urophilia, coprophilia, and to a lesser degree, klismaphilia, with pedophilic acting out. Erotic activities involving urine are known as undinism (after the water nymph, Undine). This term was coined in the 1930s by the sexologist Havelock Ellis, who was said to be a practitioner of this sexual deviance. Activities involve being urinated upon (golden showers), observing others urinating, drinking urine, drinking urine out of toilets where children have voided, or collecting the urine of victims. On oc-casion, it is associated with sadomasochistic behavior (Denson 1982) or as a way of demeaning the victim after a sexual attack. Newsgroups have existed since 1971, predating the World Wide Web by 22 years. Of the almost 85 000 newsgroups, a high percentage are devoted to these deviant sexual themes. Daily, one can find news-groups named alt.sex.toilettraining or alt.girlsex.goldenshowers.

**Case Study 12-3**

Over a 2-month period, 2 boys and 1 girl were sexually assaulted in a wooded area in separate incidents. The subject would forcibly pull them off the trail into a more isolated area, make the victims take off their clothes, and demand that they urinate into his hands. Despite the efforts of 3 police agencies, the cases remain unsolved.

Although some offenders may defecate on the victim in order to add insult to the sexual injury, individuals engaged in coprophilia have a sexual fascination with the use of feces in sexual activities. This typically involves the smelling, eating, or smearing of feces on the body. The author has been involved in cases in which the pedophiles have collected specimen bottles with labeled stool samples or have photo-graphed the bowel movements of their victims.

**Case Study 12-4**

RB, a 42-year-old man, broke into the apartment of a 28-year-old woman. Upon entering her apartment, he gained control of her with a knife he had brought to the scene. Forcing her to undress, he loosely blindfolded her with a T-shirt, and then digitally penetrated her vagina and rectum. The victim heard him smelling and licking his fingers after penetration. No penile penetration was attempted. Arrested a year later based on DNA evidence, the author interviewed the subject. His only previous charge was for mischief; a decade earlier, in another province, he was arrested after crawling out of an outhouse at a baseball field. He left the jurisdiction prior to trial. He admitted on interview, however, that he crawled down the outhouse to watch women and girls urinate and defecate. He regularly peeped into bathrooms of residences and often sat, undetected, in the women's restrooms of fast food restaurants to listen to women or girls use the facilities. He would hide in areas adjacent to where teenagers would have outdoor parties to hear the teenage girls urinate in bushes.

Practitioners of klismaphilia are erotically aroused by the giving or receiving of enemas. The focus of organizations such as the American Sphincter Society or Enema Buddies, is the use of enemas as a sexual object. This erotic focus sometimes includes the victimization of children.

## Sadism and Hyperdominance

Sadism takes its name from the writings of the Marquis de Sade (1740-1814). The sadist obtains his sexual pleasure through the infliction of pain and suffering on the victim. According to Marshall & Yates (2004), the important features of sexual sadism, not common in all sexual assaults, were cruelty and torture of the victim, the sexual mutilation of the victim, and sexual interests in sadistic acts as shown by self-reports or phallometric assessments.

Related to sadism is the hyperdominant sexual activity of bondage. Many child pornography images found on the Internet involve the bondage or "punishment" of children. Spanking sites have also emerged on the Internet. A child pornography pro-duction group based in Russia offered videotapes of boys being raped. Customers had a choice of ordering the tapes with the actual sounds of the victims being assaulted or with a music score playing in the background. The majority ordered the sounds of the children. Even nonpornographic pictures of children can be altered, through the drawing of ligatures on pictures of children, thereby creating an erotic image from a previously benign picture of a child.

Money (1990) states that

[i]n sexual sadism, there is an obsessive and compelling repetition of sexual thoughts, dreams, or fantasies that may be translated into acts in which the mental or physical suffering of a victim is intensely sexually arousing. Sexual sadism may involve retraining, blindfolding, or gagging as well as torturing by means of whipping, pinching, burning, electrical shocking, cutting, stabbing, mutilating, raping, strangulating, and killing.

Sadism and pedophilia is a frightening and often lethal combination of paraphilias. Storr (1990) correctly notes that sexually violent acts against children, "especially those which are incestuous, are sadistic in nature, and are prolonged because the child is threatened with even worse and more painful punishments if he does not comply." In the author's experience, although sadism can occur in cases involving incest, it is more prevalent in nonfamilial contacts.

Sexual homicides of children, despite all the media attention, are fortunately rare. Not all the killers are sadists; however, after being abducted by sadists, 44% of the victims are killed within an hour, 74% within 3 hours, and 91% within 24 hours of abduction (Hanfland, 1997).

The killing of a child is often the handiwork of a sadist but on occasion, nonsadistic pedophiles will knowingly kill a child, not because this is sexually arousing for them, but out of fear of being caught. If the body is subsequently dismembered by the nonsadistic pedophile, it is regarded as defensive dismemberment (Rajs et al, 1998).

*Picquerism* is the erotic arousal to the poking with a sharp object, or ritualistic stabbing of the victim, for sexual pleasure. Images of arrows, spears, or knives are sometimes drawn on pictures of children or videotapes of nude children having hypodermic needles inserted in their buttocks are made. In the world of pornography, a *snuff film* is a homemade movie or video allegedly depicting an actual murder for entertainment purposes. Adult snuff film Web sites (always involving the use of actors) often have links to other sadism, picquerism, and necrophilia sites.

### Case Study 12-5

A man was arrested for sexually assaulting his 9-year-old daughter. The sexual assault included the poking of the victim with a sharpened coat hanger, which was usually applied to her abdomen. He had a previous history of accosting women and teens on the street, demanding that they pull up their shirts so he could see their midriffs. Fantasy writings that he authored involved torturing a bound female with the application of a cattle prod to her abdomen.

### Case Study 12-6

In May 2000, Canada Customs intercepted a video mailed to a school vice principal residing in Montreal. The video showed a man brutally spanking 4 naked children. The videotape originated in the United States, which led the FBI and the USPIS to uncover a network of men who were erotically aroused by the brutal spanking of children. They had originally met through ads placed in publications such as the Domestic Discipline Digest and in Internet chat rooms. Ring members included an elementary school teacher, a nurse and former Boy Scout leader, a bank security guard, a Sunday school teacher, a railway worker, and a retired chauffeur. A number of children were rescued from abusive households where the spanking took place. One "club" member no longer had access to children. To obtain new material from other members, he photographed himself spanking a mannequin to fool others into thinking he was punishing a girl.

## NECROPHILIA

The term necrophilia is derived from the Greek word meaning "love of the dead" and was first introduced by the Belgian psychiatrist Joseph Guislain in the mid-19th century. Documented in literature and legends, von Krafft-Ebing (1925) associated the act with sadism. Essentially, there are 2 types of necrophilia. Rosman & Resnick

(1988) examined 122 accounts of **necrophilia**, the sexual attraction to corpses (n = 54), and **pseudo-necrophilia**, in which corpses act as a sexual substitute (n = 33). The subject suffered from a disorder of thought in only 11% of the cases.

The behavior of necrophiliacs varies. The sexual activity is not necessarily intercourse but can involve kissing, fondling, or performing cunnilingus on the body (Hucker, 1990). Others will steal pubic hair. Still others will mutilate the body and engage in **necrophagia**, the eating of corpses or body parts of corpses. Necrophilia is rare, but with no victim to complain, it is likely under-reported.

**Case Study 12-7**

A 22-year-old man was arrested, along with his father and 24-year-old brother, for purchasing access to child pornography Web sites. On a judicially approved search of their house, a framed photograph of a gravestone was found hanging in the subject's bedroom. Under the glass of the frame was a clipping of an obituary notice of the 12-year-old girl whose gravestone was in the photo. Taped to the glass were the previous 3 years worth of memorial announcements of her death. The deceased died in a motor vehicle accident and was previously unknown to the subject. He kept other obituary clippings in a coffin-shaped box on his desk. He was a frequent visitor to virtual memorial sites on the Web where the subject of the site was a deceased girl or teen. These are sites to permanently memorialize a departed member of the family with photographs and links to other sites that were of interest to them when alive—television shows, cartoon characters, sports teams, etc. On interview, the subject became visibly animated while discussing a summer job cutting lawns at the cemetery where the teenage victim of a well-known serial killer was buried.

## CONCLUSION

Investigators must always be cognizant that child pornography seizures may yield other deviances that should not be ignored. The concept of multiple paraphilias is recognized and should always be kept in mind when searching the premises and computers of child pornography collectors. As part of the collateral material found in the collection of sex offenders in general, and specifically pedophiles, it can augment hard evidence for investigators in presentation of their case for prosecution and by prosecutors in the use of expert testimony in educating the judges and juries (Hazelwood & Lanning, 2001).

## REFERENCES

Abel GG, Becker JV, Mittleman M. Sexual offenders: results of assessment and recommendations for treatment. In: Ben-Aron MH, Hucker SJ, Webster CD, eds. *Clinical Criminology: Current Concept*. Toronto, Canada: M & M Graphics; 1985:191-205.

Abel GG, Becker JV, Cunningham-Rather J, Mittleman M, Rouleau JL. Multiple paraphilic diagnoses among sex offenders. *Bull Am Acad Psychiatry Law*. 1988; 16:153-168.

Abel GG, Osborn C, Twigg D. Sexual assault through the lifespan: adult offenders with juvenile histories. In: Barbaree H, Marshall W, Hudson S, eds. *The Juvenile Sex Offender*. New York, NY: Guilford Press; 1993.

American Psychiatric Association. *Diagnostic and Statistical Manual of Mental Disorders*. 4th ed. Text Revision. Washington, DC: American Psychiatric Association; 2000.

Binet A. Du fétishisme dans l'amour. *Revue Philosphique*. 1887;24:142-167.

Bluglass R. Bestiality. In: Bluglass R, Bowden P, Walker N, eds. *Principles and Practice of Forensic Psychiatry*. London, England: Churchill Livingstone; 1990:671-676.

Bradford JMW, Boulet J, Pawlak A. The paraphilias: a multiplicity of deviant behaviors. *Can J Psychiatry*. 1992;37:104-108.

Carter D, Prentky R, Knight R, Vanderveer P, Boucher R. Use of pornography in criminal and developmental histories of sexual offenders. *J Interpers Violence*. 1987;2: 196-211.

Crepault C, Couture M. Men's erotic fantasies. *Arch Sex Behav*. 1980;9:565-581.

Denson R. Undinism: the fetishization of urine. *Can J Psychiatry*. 1982;27:336-338.

Dewaraja R, Money J. Transcultural sexology: formicophilia, a newly named paraphilia in a young Buddhist male. *J Sex Marital Ther*. 1986;12:139-145.

De Young, M. The world according to NAMBLA: accounting for deviance. *J Sociol Soc Welf*. 1989;16(1):111-126.

Durkin KF. Misuse of the Internet by pedophiles: implications for law enforcement and probation practice. *Fed Probat*. 1997;61:14-18.

Freund K, Seto M, Kuban M. Frotteurism and the theory of courtship disorder. In: Laws DR, O'Donohue W, eds. *Sexual Deviance: Theory, Assessment and Treatment*. New York, NY: Guilford Press; 1997:111-130.

Freund, K. Courtship disorder. In Marshall WL, Laws DR and Barbaree HE, eds. *Handbook of Sexual Assault: Issues, Theories, and Treatment of the Offender*. New York, NY: Plenum Press; 1990:195-207.

Gebhard PH, Gagnan JH, Pomeroy WB, Christenson CV. *Sex Offenders: An Analysis of Types*. New York, NY: Harper & Row; 1965.

Hanfland KA, Keppel RD, Weis JG. Case *Management for Missing Children Homicide Investigation*. Olympia: Attorney General of Washington; 1997.

Hazelwood RR, Lanning KV. Collateral materials in sex crimes. In: Hazelwood RR, Burgess AW, eds. *Practical Aspects of Rape Investigation: A Multidisciplinary Approach*. 3rd ed. Boca Raton, Fla: CRC Press; 2001:221-232.

Heil P, Ahlmeyer S, Simons D. Crossover sex offenses. *Sex Abuse*. 2003;15(4): 221-236.

Herman-Giddens ME, Slora EJ, Wasserman RC, et al. Secondary sexual characteristics and menses in young girls seen in office practice: a study from the Pediatric Research Office Settings network. *Pediatrics*. 1997;99:505-512.

Hernandez A. Self-reported contact offenses of federal inmates convicted of child pornography offenses. Poster session presented at: 19th Annual Research and Treatment Conference of the Association for the Treatment of Sexual Abusers; November 2000a; San Diego, Calif.

Hernandez A. Self-reported contact sexual offenses by participants in the Federal Bureau of Prisons' sex offender treatment program: implications for Internet sex offenders. Poster session presented at: the 19th Annual Research and Treatment Conference of the Association for the Treatment of Sexual Abusers; November 2000b; San Diego, Calif.

Hucker S. Necrophilia and other unusual philias. In: Bluglass R, Bowden P, Walker N, eds. *Principles and Practice of Forensic Psychiatry*. London, England: Churchill Livingstone; 1990:671-676.

von Krafft-Ebing R. *Psychopathia Sexualis*. Rebman FJ, trans. 12th German ed. London, England: Staples Press; 1925.

Kim PY, Bailey JM. Sidestreets on the information highway: paraphilias and sexual variations on the Internet. *J Sex Educ Ther*. 1997;22:35-43.

Lanning KV. *Child Molesters: A Behavioral Analysis*. Alexandria, Va: National Center for Missing & Exploited Children; 1986.

Lanning KV. *Child Molesters: A Behavioral Analysis*. 4th ed. Alexandria, Va: National Center for Missing & Exploited Children; 2001.

Malitz S. Another report on the wearing of diapers and rubber pants by an adult male. *Am J Psychiatry*. 1966;122:1435-1437.

Marshall WL, Barbaree HE, Eccles A. Early onset and deviant sexuality in child molesters. *J Interpers Violence*. 1991;6:323-335.

Marshall WL. The use of sexually explicit stimuli by rapists, child molesters, and nonoffenders. *J Sex Res*. 1988;25:267-288.

Marshall WL. Revisiting the use of pornography by sexual offenders: implications for theory and practice. *J Sex Aggress*. 2000;6:67-77.

Marshall WL, Yates P. Diagnostic issues in sexual sadism among sexual offenders. *J Sex Aggress*. 2004;10:21-27.

Mason F. Fetishism: psychopathology and theory. In: Laws DR, O'Donohue W, eds. *Sexual Deviance: Theory, Assessment and Treatment*. New York, NY: Guilford Press; 1997:75-93.

Money J. Paraphilias: phenomenology and classification. *Am J Psychother*. 1984;38:164-179.

Money J. Forensic sexology: paraphilic serial rape (biastophilia) and lust murder (erotophonophilia). *Am J Psychotherapy*. 1990;44:26-36.

O'Connell RT. Paedophiles networking on the Internet. In: Arnaldo CA, ed. *Child Abuse on the Internet: Ending the Silence*. New York, NY: Berghahn Books/UNESCO Publishing; 2001:65-79.

O'Donohue W, Regev LG, Hagstrom A. Problems with the DSM-IV diagnosis of pedophilia. *Sex Abuse*. 2000;12(No. 12):95-105.

Pate JE, Gabbard G. Adult baby syndrome. *Am J Psychiatry*. 2003;160:1932-1936.

Quayle E, Taylor M. Pedophiles, pornography and the Internet: assessment issues. *Br J Soc Work*. 2002;32:863-875.

Radzinowicz L. *English Studies in Criminal Science: Sexual Offences IX*. London, England: Macmillan; 1957.

Rajs J, Lundström M, Broberg M, Lidberg L, Lindquest O. Criminal mutilation of the human body in Sweden—a thirty-year medico-legal and forensic study. *J Forensic Sci*. 1998;43:563-580.

*R. v Sharpe*, 1 SCR 45 (2001).

Rosman J, Resnick P. Necrophilia: an analysis of 122 cases involving paraphilic acts and fantasies. *Bull Am Acad Psychiatry Law*. 1988;17:153-163.

Seto MC, Barbaree HE. Paraphilias. In: Van Hasselt VB, Hersen M, eds. *Aggression and Violence: An Introductory Text*. New York, NY: Allyn & Bacon; 2000:198-213.

Storr A. Sadomasochism. In: Bluglass R, Bowden P, Walker N, eds. *Principles and Practice of Forensic Psychiatry*. London, England: Churchill Livingstone; 1990:711-717.

Taylor M, Quayle E. *Child Pornography: An Internet Crime*. New York, NY: Brunner-Routledge; 2003.

Tuchmann WW, Lachman JH. An unusual perversion: the wearing of diapers and rubber pants in a 29-year-old male. *Am J Psychiatry*. 1964;120:1198-1199.

Winter JSD. Nutrition and the neuroendocrinology of puberty. In: Winick M, ed. *Adolescent Nutrition*. New York, NY: John Wiley & Sons; 1982:3-12.

Yalom ID. Aggression and forbiddenness in voyeurism. *Arch Gen Psychiatry*. 1960;3:305-319.

# ABUSIVE IMAGES OF CHILDREN AND THE INTERNET: RESEARCH FROM THE COPINE PROJECT

Max Taylor, PhD, C. Forensic Psychology
Ethel Quayle, BA, MSc, PsychD

Abusive images of children on the Internet constitute a major area of social concern. Surprisingly, however, understanding of this issue is limited. It is difficult to imagine that such an important area that commands enormous political and media attention is so lacking in basic policy development, supportive research, and conceptual inquiry. The COPINE Project has been at the forefront of developing understanding in this area through programs of action research and analysis and close relationships with law enforcement, probation, prisons, and child welfare communities. In the following chapter, we will describe the project's origins and nature and briefly summarize some of the results.

## THE ORIGINS OF COPINE

COPINE is an acronym that stands for **CO**mbating **P**aedophile **I**nformation **N**etworks in **E**urope. It was the name of the project that resulted in the first funding received from the European Commission for work to explore the nature of the problem of abuse images and images on the Internet and to hold what proved to be the first major international conference regarding abuse images in 1998 in Dublin. It has remained the overall title of the broad collection of activities now embraced under the label COPINE. In effect, the COPINE Project is not one project but a collection of projects. It would be intellectually satisfying, but rather dishonest, to describe the development of the COPINE Project in logical and systematic terms as a response to perceived policy and knowledge gaps. In reality, the project and its activities have been developed by individuals that have learned to appreciate the problem's complexity and scale.

The Internet increasingly impinged on public awareness in the late 1990s, and along with naïve optimism (perhaps illustrated by the dot-com boom), there was a growing recognition of a dark side to the Internet, exemplified by the sexual exploitation of children. While working with street children in developing countries, a collaboration with what was to become the COPINE Project and the Paedophile Unit of the London Metropolitan Police developed.* It was through this contact that the significance of abuse images as an element of child sexual exploitation became clear, as did the emerging role of the Internet as a medium for distribution.

The history of work in developing countries brought a clear action and child-centered focus to the COPINE Project. The origins of the project in applied psychology

---

\* The Paedophile Unit of the London Metropolitan Police played a critical role in the development of COPINE, through sharing knowledge and more general support, and we acknowledge in particular the contributions of Chief Inspectors Jim Reynolds and Bob McLachlan and DS Steve Quick.

provided a conceptual orientation (Veale & Taylor, 1997). In addition, the specific academic backgrounds of key project workers in clinical and forensic psychology gave the project a distinctive applied focus. From this context, the project has developed 4 distinct emphases:

— Images as evidential material

— The primacy of child victims

— The behavior of offenders in their engagement with abuse images

— The development of systematic assessment and intervention material

Work in each of these 4 areas remains ongoing. We will describe some results of the work so far. Much of this research activity derives from the ongoing program of offender interviews undertaken for this project, and as much as possible, we will place our work in the context of the wider academic literature. It should be noted, however, that to date there is little published material in this area.

Many people access images that may indicate sexual interest in children. However, it is important to note that not all images that attract adults with a sexual interest in children are necessarily illegal (Taylor et al, 2001). To understand this, think of the range of such images as lying along a continuum, which can be expressed in a degree or level of victimization (which may not necessarily relate to the capacity for an image to generate fantasies). Understanding the nature of victimization shown in abuse images is important, the significance of which has been reflected in the sentencing guidelines for offenses related to possession of abuse images in the UK (Court of Criminal Appeal Division, 2002). These guidelines for sentence length on conviction of charges related to possession of abuse images depend on the nature and qualities of the possessed images. A further reason for focusing on image qualities is because offenders' collections of images reflect their level of engagement with the material and provide visible evidence of sexual fantasy and, on occasion, sexual assault evidence.

Until recently, the term child pornography has been used to describe these images. Using the term pornography carries complex connotations, allowing comparison with the depictions of "consensual" sexual activity between adults. These depictions are widely available from newsagents and video retailers and are designed to titillate rather than harm. Such a view of pornography is contentious, and authors such as Itzin (2002) have presented a compelling argument that pornography per se is "instrumentally causal in the aetiology of sex offending." In the context of children, however, there can be no question of consent, and use of the word pornography may effectively allow us to distance ourselves from the material's true nature. A preferred term is *abuse images*, and this term is increasingly gaining acceptance among professionals working in this area. Using the term abuse images accurately describes the process and product of taking indecent and sexualized pictures of children, and its use is, on the whole, to be supported. However, it equally has to be recognized that in many countries, the term child pornography has a legal meaning (as is the case in Ireland), and at least within that context it will continue to be used.

## What Is Child Pornography?

Different jurisdictions have different legal definitions of child pornography. The COPINE categorization scale (Taylor et al, 2001) identifies 10 types (levels) of images attractive to adults with a sexual interest in children (see **Table 13-1** for a brief overview of the scale and **Table 13-2** for revised UK Sentencing Guidelines expressed as levels based on the scale). The scale describes an ascending series of categories that broadly reflect degrees of victimization. In most jurisdictions, levels 5 or 6 upward are illegal. However, amongst jurisdictions, critical judgments about what constitutes illegal material may differ depending on whether obscenity or sexual qualities are emphasized. Because of this, countries may take different positions on the illegality of some images, particularly those involving naked children (which might be categorized as level 5 or 6). In the UK, the Sentencing Advisory Panel (2004) established that a 5-level structure should be created for sentencing purposes, focusing on levels 5-10 of the COPINE scale. The UK Court of Appeals, with some compression of categories 4 and 5, adopted this, but levels COPINE 1-3 were dropped, suggesting that such categories of images could not be classed as illegal. These rulings draw our attention to an important distinction between psychological and legal perspectives on images that will be discussed later.

In the United States, a recent court ruling (*Ashcroft v Free Speech Coalition*, 2002) has required that evidence be produced demonstrating that the child in the image is real before an image can be judged child pornography (and, therefore, sexual abuse of a real child). The distinction drawn here is between a real child and one depicted by a computer-generated image (which is, of course, not evidence of a crime against a real child). One unintended consequence of this ruling may well be a potential increase in the computer-generated images created and circulated. It also raises serious conceptual

**Table 13-1. The COPINE Typology of Abusive Images of Children**

| LEVEL | DESCRIPTION |
| --- | --- |
| 1 | Indicative (nonerotic/nonsexualized images) |
| 2 | Nudist (naked or semi-naked children in legitimate settings) |
| 3 | Erotica (surreptitious images showing underwear/nakedness) |
| 4 | Posing (deliberate posing suggesting sexual content) |
| 5 | Erotic posing (deliberate sexual provocative posing) |
| 6 | Explicit erotic posing (emphasis on genital area) |
| 7 | Explicit sexual activity not involving adult |
| 8 | Assault (involving adult) |
| 9 | Gross assault (penetrative assault involving adult) |
| 10 | Sadistic/bestiality (sexual images involving pain or animals) |

*Adapted from Taylor M, Holland G, Quayle E. Typology of paedophile picture collections.* Police Journal. *2001;74(2):97-107.*

**Table 13-2. The UK Court of Appeals Sentencing Guidelines Scale Derived From the COPINE Typology**

| LEVEL | DESCRIPTION |
| --- | --- |
| 1 | COPINE levels 5 and 6 |
| 2 | COPINE level 7 |
| 3 | COPINE level 8 |
| 4 | COPINE level 9 |
| 5 | COPINE level 10 |

*Adapted from Taylor M, Holland G, Quayle E. Typology of paedophile picture collections.* Police Journal. *2001;74(2):97-107.*

issues about distinguishing an image of a real child from a pseudo-image or computer-generated image. For example, Akdeniz (2001) has noted that the typical pseudo-photograph is one or more photographs that are in some way altered, perhaps by a graphics manipulation package. But in objective terms, the definition of pseudo- or computer-generated images remains vague. Gillespie (2003) has given an interesting example of how problematic this might be:

Let us take an example of a sexually explicit photograph of a six-year-old girl. This image is scanned and stored in the computer. No difficulty arises with this: it is quite clearly an indecent photograph. Let us assume that the girl has a large birthmark on her face. Using a graphics program, this birthmark is airbrushed out. Is this now a photograph or a pseudo-photograph?

An examination of Irish law offers an opportunity to consider these general issues further. Under Irish law, the principal legal provision related to abuse images is the Child Trafficking and Pornography Act, 1998. A critical element of this act is the definition of child pornography:

Child pornography is … any visual representation … that shows … a person who is or is depicted as being a child and who is engaged in … explicit sexual activity, witnessing such activity, or an image whose dominant characteristic is the depiction for a sexual purpose of the genital or anal regions of a child.

In comparisons with legal provisions in other jurisdictions, Irish law is relatively precise. By emphasizing sexual qualities rather than drawing on concepts of obscenity or indecency, it avoids many of the problems of interpretation and social judgment that those terms present. However, difficulties may arise over what the term sexual might mean with respect to particular images (and, in particular, the relationship between sexual and nakedness) and what "depiction for a sexual purpose" might mean. The courts have yet to address this. This problem can be illustrated by reference to a particular Web site (which, when accessed, was part of the "zboys" group) that appears to offer access to images of clothed children. This site is advertised as legal, but is oriented to adults with a sexual interest in children. However, the individual images that might come from that site are probably of clothed children, which, when taken out of context, may well be judged to be nonsexual—yet they are clearly offered within in a sexual context and for a sexual purpose.

A distinction can be made between legal definitions of child pornography and images attractive to an adult with a sexual interest in children that may fall outside pornography statues. Many images can produce sexual arousal for a fantasizing individual, but those images need not be explicitly sexual and therefore illegal. The problem is that sexual arousal lies in the viewer's mind (and is closely related to and dependent on fantasy) rather than in the objective sexual (in legal terms) qualities of an image. This analysis is the foundation for the structure of the COPINE scale, and this problem will be exacerbated if sexual details rather than contextual features are considered.

It is presumably not appropriate to control or police individual legal or illegal fantasies that are not enacted. Therefore, images that might generate or enable sexual fantasy but do not require a child to be abused to produce them, or do not result in a child being abused, fall outside legal control. If the laws controlling child pornography are designed to protect children (rather than addressing some moral standard or as an assertion of inappropriateness), then, as in the *Ashcroft* judgment, nonabusive images, although they might be used to sustain illegal masturbatory fantasies, should not fall within legal constraints because children are involved in sexual fantasy rather than behavioral reality. Abusive images, on the other hand, regardless of their fantasy potential, have at some point required a child to be abused and, therefore, might fall into a different category.

These arguments change if a relationship can be demonstrated among images (of any kind), fantasy, and contact offending because, presumably, the fantasy activities may then move from to real life and contribute to contact offending. Research suggests that this seems to be the case, though, for any particular individual, the relationship may be complex and not even present. Considering each case on its own merits rather than relying on general rules is important.

Relatively little is known about the relationship between possession of abuse images of children and contact offending. However, what is becoming clear is that distinctions between individuals in terms of their probability of committing contact offenses (sometimes referred to as dangerousness) are necessary. Individuals who produce abuse images are involved in the commission of a contact offense, but individuals in possession of abuse images are less clearly dangerous in this sense. For some in this category, engagement with abuse images prompt contact offending; for others, this may not be the case. This emphasizes the need to treat each case on its own merits. This is clearly an area that requires more empirical research.

The complex relationship between sexual offending against children and possession of abuse images can validate the sense in which the process of trading and collecting abuse images constitutes one of the principal factors driving the production and distribution of new abuse images. In market terms, collecting abuse images generates the demand for more images met by photographing additional sexual abuse. This is perhaps one of the primary reasons why the trade in abusive images of children, and their possession, is rightly regarded as an aspect of the sexual abuse of children and should attract heavy penalties.

## How Do Images Circulate on the Internet?

The following seeks to describe what we have termed "the natural history of trading abusive images on the Internet" and exemplifies the complex behaviors associated with the circulation of images. Anyone on the Internet has to identify himself or herself in some way by specifying a user name. This may be a real name, but usually it is an assumed nickname, which may play a part in the individual's self-representation on the Internet. This nickname may indicate something about the individual (eg, kidlover) or may be a fictitious real name (eg, malcom3); the names used may change between different Internet activities or over time. People can be possessive about nicknames, and these names tend to be constant although individuals may possess multiple names. There is some evidence that the selection of nicknames is purposeful and reflects some sense of how the individual sees himself (Bechar-Israeli, 1995).

Mann & Stewart (2000) have suggested that the self-representation in real life and in (non-role-play) online communities are more similar than might be expected. What we see is the probability that self-representation online is an extension of the real individual into a different social environment. In Bechar-Israeli's (1995) study, 8% of online participants used their real names, 45% used "nicks" that related to themselves in some way, and only 6% chose nicks of a fanciful nature. In an unpublished replication of this study using text drawn from chat rooms dedicated to groups of people who share a sexual interest in children (taken from the COPINE archive), the categorization of nicknames was somewhat different. In this analysis, people were more likely to use names that represented aspects of their real or acquired identity as it related to sexual interest or perceived role within that community.

Trading images on the Internet takes place in various settings, employing different Internet protocols involving different degrees of interaction or communication with other people. Some protocols facilitate secret communication between people. **Table 13-3** and **Figure 13-1** illustrate a fictitious but perfectly plausible trading process where an image moves from the secret world of e-groups, via the more public protocol of Internet relay chat (IRC), to appear in the highly public newsgroups. The IRC is a more open form of a similar protocol, and newsgroups are forms of bulletin boards. The time scale over which this might occur varies but may occur within a few hours, days, or weeks, and the same image may appear many times in numerous arenas. The location of the people accessing the material at any point may be anywhere in the world.

One of the more potentially secret forms of communication on the Internet relates to e-groups. These are proprietary chat rooms that users can establish. The founder or owner of the e-group can specify the level of access to other people, forbidding access

---

### Table 13-3. A Fictional Trading Process Described (Illustrated in Figure 13-1)

**Trading stage 1.** In Stage 1, a user with the nickname "billboy" has an image of a child he has taken, which he trades with another member of a secret e-group whose membership is confined to people who produce abuse images. User "herbert" in turn trades that image with "lol" (both producers of images). The time taken for the image to pass among these 3 people may be a matter of minutes, days, or weeks.

**Trading stage 2.** Unlike billboy and herbert, user lol not only trades in the e-group but also is in contact with other people through Internet relay chat (IRC). This is a similar protocol to e-groups but is more generic and less secret. A number of chat rooms on different IRC networks enable trade in abusive images of children. In our example, lol communicates with "carl," who does not produce images but has a large collection. The image of billboy's child would be a highly attractive image to carl (given that it is new and not previously circulated on the Internet), and carl might allow lol open access to his large collection of images in return for trading the image. Note that at this point, the image moves out of the circle of people who have a direct stake in maintaining secrecy (because all are involved in the production of images, a highly illegal act) into a much more open environment.

**Trading stage 3.** Carl in turn trades with "furd" on the IRC (and in all probability many other people as well); thus, the image passes through more hands.

**Trading stage 4.** In addition to trading on the IRC, furd also places images on the newsgroups. This is an older Internet protocol, rather like bulletin boards. More than 70 000 newsgroups exist, with about 30 or so specializing in abusive images of children. Messages to newsgroups and image attachments can be posted anonymously, so identifying who has posted images is not always possible.

**Trading stage 5.** Anyone accessing the newsgroup that furd posted the image to can download that image. It is not possible to quantify how widely images are accessed in this way nor the spread of any given image throughout the network. User "majordom" accesses that image and downloads it onto his own computer. In this fictitious example, for the sake of completeness and a just ending, he then experiences a problem, sends his computer to be repaired, images are found during the repair and reported to the police, and majordom is arrested (a common route to detection).

Clearly, the trading process may be more complex than this, as it is highly likely traders have no single linear relationship; rather, they have a series of multiple exchanges. Because of this, images can move among large numbers of individuals rapidly, with the number of traders of any given individual image increasing exponentially. Tracing the image's origin to the original producer can be complex and frequently impossible, particularly with anonomyzing software. This example also illustrates the difficulty of eradicating abuse images from the trading network. The reality for the victimized child is that his or her image will continue to be used for sexual purposes by potentially many unknown adults.

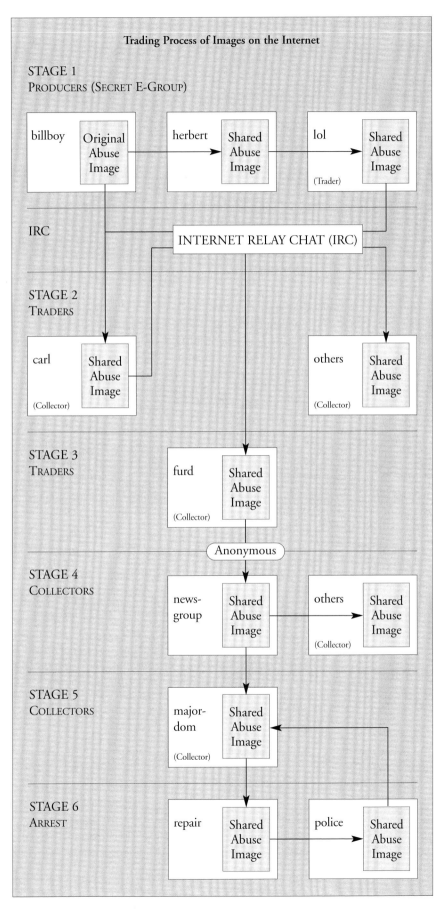

**Figure 13-1.** *The natural history of trading images on the Internet.*

unless permission is given. Many e-groups exist for trading abusive images of children, but are secret and often allow access only to individuals who can themselves prove that they are taking abusive images. (Evidence of this is seen in images of a child holding up a paper with a message, often in the form of a name and date.) The global nature of such e-groups can be seen in Operation Candyman. In 2001, the FBI initiated this investigation after an undercover agent identified 3 e-groups which were involved in the posting, exchanging, and transmitting of child pornography. This operation identified 7000 unique e-mail addresses, with 2400 from outside of the United States.

Three broad groups of individuals can be identified in the process of trading abusive images: the producer, the trader, and the collector. These catagories may overlap, and producers may be traders and collectors; the reverse, however, may not apply. Collectors may be active (they directly communicate with other people through, for example, the IRC) or passive (they access images through protocols that do not require direct access to other people, eg, through the newsgroups or through Web sites).

**Figure 13-2** (Taylor & Quayle, 2003) illustrates the probable relationship between producers, traders, and collectors of abuse images of children. Points to note are that collectors number more than producers, but many (if not all) producers are probably traders and collectors. However, it also seems likely that not all producers of abuse images necessarily trade their own images with other people and retain images for personal use. The various relationships are probably best seen as a reflection of a process, whereby individuals move among different roles as inclination and opportunity allow (Quayle & Taylor, 2003). It is important to stress that in general, no money changes hands in the trading activities described here. This trade is not driven by money; rather, it is often a form of barter. However, access to pay Web sites represents a different means of obtaining images, where money is central to the process, at least on the part of the Web site owner. For example, Landslide Productions Inc, was operated and owned by Thomas and Janice Reedy, who sold access to child pornography Web sites. Customers from around the world paid monthly subscription fees via a post office box address or the Internet for access to hundreds of Web sites, which contained extremely graphic abuse images of children (US Postal Inspection Service, 2004). Landslide Productions originally dealt with the sale of adult Web sites, but as the business grew, most of the profits came from child pornography Web sites, and in just one month the business grossed as much as $1.4 million.

## The Nature of Offending

The fictitious example shown in **Figure 13-1** and described in **Table 13-3** illustrates some of the offending behaviors associated with abuse images. In this context, there are 4 broad classes of offending: downloading, trading, production, and Internet seduction. These categories overlap, and they revolve around engagement with the Internet and the possession of abuse images. Downloading child abuse images is invariably a purposeful activity. While it is relatively easy to access adult pornography accidentally, this is rarely the case in relation to abuse images of children. For some people, we might conceptualize downloading as a largely passive way of collecting images, perhaps from Web sites or from newsgroups. Although downloading may involve searching for material (and, therefore, interaction with Internet processes), such passive collecting is unlikely to include substantial direct social engagement with other people engaged in similar activities. However, it may heighten the justification of such activities for the individual involved because of the evidence that large numbers of people are similarly engaged.

Not all collectors of abuse images move from passive collection to contact or communication with others. But social contact

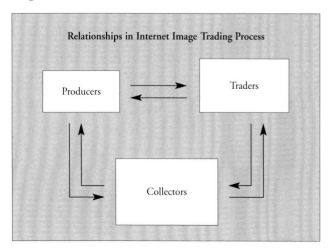

***Figure 13-2.*** *A possible relationship between trading, collecting, and producing abuse images of children.*

can be important in legitimizing and normalizing sexual interests. Taylor & Quayle (2003) have suggested that

for those … who traded or distributed images, the notion of images as currency appeared to be important. They are currency in terms of trading for new material, but they are also currency in maintaining existing online relationships and giving credibility. An important aspect of this is the notion of a community of collectors serving to normalize the process of collecting but also legitimizing the downloading and saving of images that in other contexts may have been aversive to the respondent.

The drive for new material to trade may provide the stimulus for the production of new material. Most highly abusive Internet images are largely produced in a domestic context. Research from the COPINE Project suggests that where child victims have been identified, they are almost invariably part of the offender's real or acquired family or are on the receiving end of a caregiving relationship. When offending takes place in these circumstances, such offenses may relate to the need to sustain and increase credibility among others and may serve as a way of gaining access to other desired images of child abuse, as well as an expression of sexual behavior. It is significant that newness of images is central in ensuring status within a trading community, and providing access to such images is a source of power to the producer. He can decide what material to release, when, and to whom. Images may be created according to the personal fantasies of the producer or his perception of the market. Indeed, in some circumstances, images can be "commissioned" by others, who may express preference for certain types of sexual activities. (See Quayle and Taylor, 2003, for case study examples.)

As we have already suggested, pornography per se heightens sexual arousal and disinhibition and, with the Internet, may aid Internet seduction of children through fantasy manipulation and masturbation. This is largely accomplished through chat rooms. A study by Finkelhor et al (2000) suggested that 1 in 5 children between the ages of 10-17 received sexual solicitations over the Internet and, of those, 1 in 33 received an aggressive solicitation. This involved being asked by an adult to meet, being contacted on the telephone, or being sent regular mail, money, or gifts. Durkin (1997) suggested 4 ways in which people with a sexual interest in children may misuse the Internet in this context: to traffic child pornography, to locate children to molest, to engage in inappropriate sexual communication with children, and to communicate with other pedophiles. Chat rooms may provide a perfect vehicle for all of these. For those with a sexual interest in children, the Internet facilitates the abuse of children online and offline, either in the production and exchange of abuse images or in attempted sexual engagement. Quayle & Taylor (2001) have presented a case history of the development of Internet seduction, which emphasizes Talamo & Ligorio's (2001) suggestion that "activities in cyberspace produce outputs for real life and vice versa."

Cyberspace is an interactive arena, and tools such as chat rooms offer new interactive resources. People are able to self-represent in different ways (DiMarco, 2003), and where the purpose of self-representation is specifically sexual, as in the online seduction of children, then the absence of nonverbal cues greatly increases the possibility of deception (see Quayle & Taylor, 2001). When children are already vulnerable, they provide easy targets for such deception and serve as perfect victims, online and offline, for those who wish to exploit them (Wolak et al, 2003).

## ABUSE IMAGES AND THE OFFENDING PROCESS

We have no clear understanding of how many people access abuse images. We rely on data derived from convictions, and many people who operate within private Internet networks are by definition inaccessible to monitoring. However, from the limited evidence we have, it would appear that people with a sexual interest in children and who access Internet abuse images are a heterogeneous group. They include people of all ages and from all social backgrounds who display various degrees of technical sophistication. They may include people who have a known history of sexual offending and others who have no previously acknowledged sexual interest in children. To date, other than media reports, there have been no published accounts of female offending on the Internet (although there are anecdotal accounts), and this is apparently a largely male activity. However, our knowledge of this may change over time. Although research in this area is limited, the available evidence suggests that in a general sense, the problems associated with Internet child pornography are the following:

— Its production (as distinct from viewing) involves the sexual abuse of a child

— A photograph preserves abuse.

— Sexual fantasy may become reality.

— Images can act as instruments in the grooming process.

— It may sexualize other aspects of child and family life.

This last point is perhaps the most pervasive and worrisome although quantifying the threat is diffuse and difficult (for a discussion of some of the broader issues relevant to this, see Kincaid, 1998). However, it must be emphasized that the function of abuse images and their relationship to the commission of contact offenses remain unclear. Research in this area is often conflicting and mostly predates the advent of the Internet. Goldstein (1999) had suggested that child pornography could be understood as a by-product of contact offenses. On the other hand, authors such as Itzin (1997) have described such images as central to child abuse:

Pornography, in the form of adult and/or child pornography used to season/groom/initiate/coerce children into agreeing to be abused, or the production of child pornography (the records of children being sexually abused), is implicated in every form of child abuse, however it is organised.

In many ways, this is difficult to substantiate as children who are victimized through the production of images remain largely silent (Svedin & Back, 1996). Furthermore, many offenders appear never to have been questioned (at least in times past) about their use of pornography in the commission of a contact offense. However, from our research in the COPINE Project, it seems many aspects of the sexual victimization of children, whether through the production or viewing of images or through Internet child seduction, have the use of abuse images as a central component.

Earlier research by Goldstein (1999) had differentiated between pornography and erotica. Any material that stimulates sexual arousal may be described as erotic, regardless of its content, and in the context of the Internet may include images that are legal. Lanning (1992) and Goldstein (1999) have emphasized that abuse images function as an aid to fantasy and masturbation and serve the following purposes:

— Symbolically keep the child close

— Remind the offender of what the child looked like at a particular age

— Make the child feel important or special

— Lower the child's inhibitions about being photographed

— Act as a memento that might give the offender status with other people

— Demonstrate propriety by convincing children that what the offender wants them to do is acceptable because he has engaged in similar acts with other children

— Provide a vehicle for blackmail

— Act as an aid to seduce children by misrepresenting moral standards and by depicting activities that the offender wishes the child to engage in

A problem with this analysis is that these functions seem to relate to the planned commission of a contact offense, and collections of images and memorabilia primarily obtained for that purpose may be qualitatively different from those secured from the Internet. Given this, a significant point to consider is that Internet abuse images are, in their entirety, less likely to relate to a child known to the offender. In developing our understanding, therefore, thinking of how the availability of Internet pornography and erotica create additional factors is better for us to consider rather than seeking to absorb the Internet within our existing models of offending. That pornography and its use leads to the objectification of the people within the pictures has been argued. This is seen most clearly in the context of abuse images where offenders make objects of the children photographed. Evidence of this is seen in chat about the images, where they are referred to as being part of a collection with little or no reference to content. Offenders talk about the images as if they were other collectibles and, in some instances, they edit the images themselves to remove features (for example, the child's face) that are of no interest to them.

Internet abuse images lead to the fragmentation of the viewer's own sexuality. The Internet allows for the expression of sexual behavior with others that otherwise is unlikely to find expression in the offline world. It is important to note that this extends beyond the use of abuse images to other forms of sexual activities and pornographies. Most people have sexual fantasies, some of which are shared with a consenting adult partner and are acted upon. The ability to enact sexual fantasies, either through solitary masturbatory behavior or ***cybersex*** (ie, sexual stimulation and gratification by use of the Internet), becomes possible through a stimulus or audience accessible only in the online world. All sexual preferences are catered for in the anarchy that is the Internet. Sexual behavior in general is less inhibited online (Cooper et al, 1999), and though this may be seen in a positive light in the newfound ability of adults to explore their sexual feelings and behaviors, this becomes problematic when the objective of the sexual exploration involves the abuse of children.

Such a disinhibiting effect might lead to the emergence of otherwise dormant antisocial inclinations. We can not answer why so many adults are expressing a sexual interest in children through the use of Internet abuse images. One disturbing prospect may be that we have grossly underestimated the numbers of potential sex offenders or, at least, adults with a sexual interest in children, within our societies. In relation to the new technologies, many people are involved in accessing and distributing child pornography who have no apparent history of pursuing sexual contact or relationships with real children (Quayle et al, 2000). This raises the frightening possibility that the Internet is facilitating an interest in children that may not have found expression.

As we have considered, the Internet can have a marked disinhibiting effect on behavior. Demetriou & Silke (2003) established a Web site to examine whether people, who visited for the purposes of gaining access to legal material, would also attempt to access illegal and/or pornographic material. Over an 88-day period, 803 visitors entered the site, and the majority of visitors accessed those sections purporting to offer illegal and/or deviant material. The combination of opportunity, ease, perceived anonymity, and the immediacy of personal rewards created a situation where such behavior is "not simply common, it actually becomes the norm." This is similar to the findings of Cooper et al (2000), which discussed the triple A engine (access, affordability, anonymity) in the context of problematic online sexual behavior.

An analysis of offenders that use abuse images identifies 6 principal discourses (Quayle & Taylor, 2002) that distinguish their engagement with the Internet:

— An aid to sexual arousal

— Collectibles

— A way of facilitating social relationships

— A way of avoiding real life

— A form of therapy

— Abuse images and the Internet

Within the COPINE sample of interviewed offenders, all of the discourses are common among offenders, with the exception of abuse images facilitating social relationships. This discourse is largely confined to offenders who chat online with others through protocols such as the IRC. Abuse images function for the offender in many ways depending on the involvement with the Internet. This involvement seems to be best characterized as a process within which offenders may move between different aspects depending upon circumstances and opportunity.

The primary function of abuse images is as an aid to sexual arousal, where many of the images accessed (but not all) are used for masturbatory purposes. Offenders may be selective in the images used, and the selection process may relate to specific age groups, physical types, gender, or to a particular sexual activity. Images may be selected to concur with earlier contact offenses or to new offending fantasies.

Abuse images function as collectibles and as a medium for exchange and trading. Offenders often call themselves collectors and use this term to differentiate themselves from pedophiles. In this sense, collecting abuse images can be no different than collecting any other artifacts, except that their content is illegal and functions as an aid to sexual arousal. Offenders can build up large collections of images quickly, and rapid acquisition is often accompanied by the ability to trade or exchange images while maintaining relative anonymity. For some offenders, this undoubtedly facilitates the building of community networks. On the Internet, abuse images of children are often presented within a framework, as a part of a numbered or named series. Inevitably, as with other collections, status is gained from having a complete collection, and the acquisition of new material is a prioritized goal among collectors. To supply collectors' demands for new material, more photographs have to be taken that depict the ongoing abuse of children. In some cases, this may directly lead to the production of new material through the abuse of children in the offender's immediate social network.

For many people with a sexual interest in children, abuse images can be used to facilitate social relationships with like-minded individuals. Child abuse images and social relationships are almost exclusively seen in offenders who trade images and who use synchronous or asynchronous communication forms to link with others. The exchange of images and the discourse surrounding this practice (which may or may not be sexually related) enable social cohesion and rapid acquisition of images through trading networks. Such networks appear to have their own social hierarchies, associated with the number of images, the ability to complete picture series, and access to new or unusual material.

For some people, the Internet and access to of abuse images is used to avoid real-life relationship and social problems. For many offenders, establishing online relationships provides important social support that often replaces unsatisfactory relationships in the offline world. This is similar to the findings of Morahan-Martin & Schumacher (2000) who described the Internet as providing an attractive alternative to a mundane or unhappy life. Prolonged engagement with the Internet may result in a change of mood (Kennedy-Souza, 1998). This may be construed as a form of displacement activity:

Therefore for whatever reason the Internet is initially accessed, there is every inducement to end up doing something else that promises to be more interesting or pleasurable. ... Individuals engage in these alternative activities because they are readily available, attractively presented and appear to be more immediately interesting and gratifying than completing the work originally in hand (Hills & Argyle, 2002).

It is likely that many who use the Internet would identify with this and would readily acknowledge that we use the Internet on occasions to reduce mild negative emotional states, such as boredom. What is more problematic, in the context of excessive or compulsive Internet use for sexual purposes, is the likelihood not only that the individual is using the Internet to change or avoid negative mood states but also that the material accessed is highly reinforcing, particularly as access often culminates in masturbation (Quayle & Taylor, 2002).

While the primary focus for concern is the images, research also suggests that the Internet can influence individuals with problematic sexual behavior, emphasizing again the significance of a notion of process in understanding engagement with abusive images and the Internet. For such people, the Internet is not just a passive means of communication. In summary the Internet may change beliefs and behavior in any of the following ways:

— Alter mood

— Lessen social risk and remove inhibitions

— Enable multiple self-representations

— Show evidence of group dynamics

— Validate, justify, and offer an exchange medium

— Challenge old concepts of regulation

— Disrupt and challenge conventional hierarchies

— Empower traditionally marginalized people and groups

In understanding the function of abuse images for the offender and how this relates to the Internet, we can build on a conceptual model that allows us to examine offending activities related to abuse images as such a process. (For a discussion of a process model within a CBT framework, see Quayle & Taylor, 2003.) This is important because, as we noted at the beginning of this chapter, adult sexual interest in children on the Internet embraces both legal and illegal activities. Many offenders move through various offending behaviors, and we need to be open to some moving away from illegal activities to those that we may consider undesirable but are still legal. This may, for example, relate to adult pornography and involve the collection of sadomasochistic images or the access of sites showing murder victims. While most readers would think of these as being inappropriate sexual stimuli, they do not, in the current climate, involve any illegal activity.

Regardless of what sense we make of the images' function, the problems related to child abuse images on the Internet are growing. In the 6-week period from August to mid-September 2002, the COPINE Project downloaded a total of 140 917 child image files from the Usenet newsgroups monitored by the project. More than 35 000 of these images were images not contained within the COPINE archive of more than 500 000 images. Almost 30 000 of the new images were from identifiable Web sites (containing reference to a Web site in the image). In the remaining images, 20 new children (9 girls, 11 boys) were categorized at level 7 or above (COPINE categorizing scale). This represents a considerable increase from previous years in amount of abusive images and the number of children involved in highly abusive images. This level of activity was largely sustained in 2003.

In 1999, when the COPINE research project prepared data on the nature of abusive images on the Internet for the US/EU Conference,* the majority of available material consisted of scanned hard copy images of old magazines and poor quality video captures from cine or video film. In 2003, images were primarily high quality, tended to

---

* *Taylor M. Congress introductory paper: the nature and dimensions of child pornograhpy on the Internet. Paper presented at: US/EU International Conference: Combatting Child Pornography on the Internet; September 1999; Vienna, Austria.*

show new children, and contained a relatively high incidence of images of toddlers and babies. The images produced in domestic settings tended to be more abusive, some-times showing bondage or other sadistic qualities. An enormous growth in images has come from Eastern Europe, many from Web sites with probable links to organized crime. However, it is important to stress that the images accessed through the COPINE Project represent the tip of the iceberg of circulated material. An enormous (but unquantifiable) amount of material is circulated privately, only some of which emerges in due course into the public locations monitored by COPINE.

This leads to an important conclusion. There has been no effective control or reduction of abusive images of children on the Internet. Perhaps acknowledgement of this problem might prompt the development of more focused and effective policy in this area.

Victims

The focus of research within the COPINE Project is child protection and the primacy of child victims. But the sad reality is that there is very little published research that relates to victimization through the production of abuse images. Indeed, the few studies that have been conducted in this area predate the Internet. In the absence of anything more substantial, we have to draw on the findings of such studies and extrapolate their significance for children who are victims of abuse images. In the COPINE Project, we have been attempting to explore the response of law enforcement and child protection agencies to the discovery of children abused through image production. We have also been examining the accounts of offenders who have produced abuse images to provide some conceptual framework for understanding the victimization process.

One of the fundamental problems in understanding victimization consequences through the production of abuse images relates to our ability to distinguish these effects from the consequences of other sexually exploitative practices. This is problematic because of the close connections between abuse images, intrafamilial and extrafamilial abuse, and studies of ritualized abuse. Also, the little data we have comes from various sources and is analyzed through different methodologies. What we can conclude is no single response pattern to sexual abuse occurs and that this is likely the case for the consequences of image victimization.

Earlier work by Finkelhor & Berliner (1995) provided a conceptual framework for an understanding of the impact of child sexual abuse. They described 4 trauma-causing factors: traumatic sexualization, betrayal, powerlessness, and stigmatization. These authors suggested that although these factors could be present in other traumatic experiences, the way they intersected within a given set of circumstances made the sexual abuse trauma unique. Kelly et al (1995) used this framework and expanded it to include notions of shame and enforced silence that had been derived from previous research.

In the context of abuse images, 4 substantial studies (all of which predate the Internet) have sought to examine the impact of child pornography:

— Burgess et al (1984) examined children's involvement in pornography and sex rings.

— Silbert (1989) examined child pornography production in the context of child prostitution.

— Svedin and Back's (1996) sample was drawn from a group of children exposed to both the production of pornography and intrafamilial and extrafamilial abuse.

— Scott's (2001) study was in the context of ritual abuse.

The populations in each of these studies vary.

All 4 of these studies are similar in the accounts they give of the children's symptoms produced during the abuse. Again, it is difficult to disentangle the consequences of the abuse (physical symptoms, such as urinary infections and genital soreness, as well as behavioral symptoms, such as sexualized behaviors) from the consequences of being photographed. However, Svedin & Back (1996) give examples of behaviors among their sample of restlessness, depression, hunger, exhaustion, concentration difficulties, and aggressive behaviors—problems not immediately associated with sexual exploitation. Silbert's (1989) study also suggested children who were exposed to longer periods of exploitation suffered more intense emotional reactions, such as feelings of isolation, fear, anxiety, and emotional withdrawal.

A pattern of enforced silence becomes apparent. The children in Svedin & Back's (1996) study were reluctant to disclose the abuse, and these authors suggested that the recording of the abuse exacerbated, and in some cases prevented, disclosure. Even when confronted with the visual evidence of their abuse, children continued to limit disclosure, telling people only what they thought the adults knew. Silbert (1989) had earlier coined the phrase "silent conspiracy" to describe this silence.

It is unclear whether the sense of shame and humiliation, often reported in these studies, relates to the photography itself or disclosing it to others. Children may fear being thought complicit in the abuse or photography through the evidence of, for example, their smiling faces. Scott (2001) reinforced this idea in the description of how abusers had shown children films they had made of them as a way of demonstrating their level of engagement and enjoyment.

Silbert (1989) indicated that the long-term effects of being photographed were more debilitating than those short-term or medium-term effects and that these effects are compounded when children are involved in more than one form of sexual exploitation. This may be exacerbated by the knowledge that others may see or distribute the films. One account given to the COPINE Project by a victim of abuse images talked of feeling fearful every time the mail arrived, overwhelmed with anxiety that the photographs would be in the post and that her mother would see them. Silbert (1989) described such feelings as psychological paralysis. This is accompanied by the knowledge that such photographs may be used to exploit other children (Svedin & Back, 1996).

This research has implications for children involved in Internet abuse image production. They are confronted by the knowledge that the images can never be destroyed and that they may continue to be viewed and used by thousands of people. The age of the child at the time of the production of the abuse images may be relevant. In an interview through the COPINE Project with a now adult victim, the images, which covered up to when she reached pubescence, had now been scanned and distributed through the Internet. As an adult woman, she was probably still identifiable from these images. When images are taken of young children, the radical physical changes that take place as a result of growth and physical development may offer at least some protection from future identification when such children reach adulthood.

With our analysis of offender accounts from the COPINE Project, we examined in detail what actually happened to children who were photographed. As yet, no published accounts relate to the Internet, and we felt this was a valuable source of information. We were aware that it would be inappropriate to privilege such information over the accounts of children and have attempted to protect these victims, who have largely remained silent. Through this analysis, different levels of Internet victimization through photography emerged related to the degree of child involvement in the process. Expressing this seemed important because it focused on issues in addition to, or perhaps compounding, the actual sexual abuse. We can think of such engagement as occurring on 4 levels:

— *Level 1*. A child is photographed without their knowledge (for example, on a beach, at a swimming pool, or at a children's playground). The child is not aware of being photographed, and no direct engagement is in the process. In a sense, the child and caretakers have no knowledge of victimization unless they become aware of the presence of these images on the Internet. Photographs of this kind are extensively distributed through the Internet and used for sexual purposes. In this sense, they are clearly abusive, even if the particular child has no knowledge of the event and can not be identified.

— *Level 2.* A child is sexually abused and the act is surreptitiously photographed. These images may be distributed through the Internet, but these are hidden photographs, and the child has no knowledge that they have been taken. Sexual victimization of which the child was aware may have taken place, but the child may have no awareness of the added photographic element involving distribution to other adults.

— *Level 3.* A child is sexually abused and openly photographed during that abuse. He or she is shown images of the abuse, as a means of further engagement or perhaps as a form of blackmail. However, the child is not involved in the distribution of these images and may not be aware that the images are shown to other adults.

— *Level 4.* A child is sexually abused and photographed during the abuse. The child is aware of being photographed and is shown the images; the child is involved in creating more images, Internet distribution, and selecting which images to send and whose commissions to respond to. In this case, there is a sense in which the child is placed in a position of an active rather than passive participant in the photographic activities. This may also implicitly be the case in Level 3 situations, but in Level 4 the child is aware and explicitly engaged in the abuse, distribution of images, and perhaps contact with other adults.

We found all of these forms of victimization in our offender interviews, but as yet we have no empirical knowledge of the implications of such involvement for these children. In Level 1, there may be no victim because the child is not aware of having been photographed. Yet, such images are used in exactly the same ways as the other images. They are used for masturbatory purposes and may form part of collections of abuse images. In the future these children may become aware that their photographs have been distributed and used in this way. The specific psychological sequelae of the other victimization levels, if they exist, are not understood. However, intuitively, these levels may represent an increasing degree of victimization with long-term negative outcomes.

The evidence we have suggests that any psychological sequelae may relate to the child's age during the abuse and when disclosure occurs. We know that the emergence of such sequelae to victimization may be distant in time from the actual event; involvement in photography may be an exacerbating factor in this.

These proposed levels may focus attention on systematically evaluating the effects of photography in sexual abuse. they might serve as a parallel scale to the COPINE image typology and give an objective framework to establish the extent and nature of victimization for sentencing purposes.

Unfortunately, the COPINE research suggests that the resources available to such victims (at least for the UK and Ireland) are often inconsistent and poor. Studies such as those of Svedin & Back (1996) emphasized the need for long-term support and the destruction of materials. Destruction is impossible because of the Internet, and this alone may be a major obstacle to closure. Child protection workers need more training in this area, and more resources should be made available to explore and to generate appropriate therapeutic strategies and contexts in which they can be used.

Victims who are reticent or in denial present challenges to law enforcement. In Svedin & Back's (1996) study, some children acknowledged the abuse only when they were confronted by the photographs that depicted sexual acts between themselves, other children, and the abusers. These children were not given a choice about this disclosure nor to whom the information was to be disclosed. Although such practices may be justified for acquiring evidence and other information for prosecution purposes, this highlights how legal and law enforcement priorities can exclude or override children's needs. In addition, the child's knowledge that others have witnessed the abuse may increase feelings of humiliation and shame. Other related ethical issues arise when an adult abused as a child is confronted with pictures discovered in a seizure of Internet abuse images.

## CONCLUSION

Understanding the nature and role of abuse images of sexually exploited children is complex. At one level, this is not an area that lends itself to simple-minded solutions in terms of understanding processes or in terms of management of offenders. On the other hand, whatever the complexities, it is quite clear that the production of abusive images of children feeds, sustains, and generates sexual exploitation of children. It results in countless children being drawn into a form of the sex trade and fuels at a societal level a corrosive and dangerous blurring of boundaries regarding what constitutes appropriate behavior involving children. While making distinctions between offenders is reasonable in terms of the degree of victimization a child is exposed to in the production of images, the actual victimization of a child, or the sense of dangerousness of the individual offender, these distinctions should not diminish the gravity of the offense in an absolute sense. There are no good and bad offenders with respect to the trade of abuse images of children.

## REFERENCES

Akdeniz Y. Governing pornography and child pornography on the Internet: the UK approach. *Univ West Law Rev*. 2001:247-275.

*Ashcroft v Free Speech Coalition*, 535 US 234 (9th Cir 2002). Available at: http://a257.g.akamaitech.net/7/257/2422/16apr20021045/www.supremecourtus.gov/opinions/01pdf/00-795.pdf. Accessed February 17, 2004.

Bechar-Israeli H. From <Bonehead> to <cLoNehEAd>: nicknames, play, and identity on Internet Relay Chat. *Play Perform Comput-Mediated Commun*. 1995;1(2). Available at: http://www.ascusc.org/jcmc/vol1/issue2/bechar.html. Accessed February 17, 2004.

Burgess AW, Hartman CR, McCausland MP, Powers P. Impact of child pornography and sex rings on child victims and their families. In: Burgess AW, ed. *Child Pornography and Sex Rings*. Lexington, Mass: Lexington Books; 1984.

Child Trafficking and Pornography Act, Ireland (1998)

Cooper A, McLoughlin IP, Campbell KM. Sexuality in cyberspace: update for the 21st century. *Cyberpsychol Behav*. 2000;3(4):521-536.

Cooper A, Scherer CR, Boies SC, Gordon BL. Sexuality on the Internet: from sexual exploration to pathological expression. *Prof Psychol Res Pr*. 1999;30(2):154-164.

Court of Criminal Appeal Division. *Regina v Mark David Oliver, Michael Patrick Hartney, Leslie Baldwin*, Neutral Citation Number (2002), EWCA Crim 2766; 2002.

Demetriou C, Silke A. A criminological Internet "sting." *Br J Criminol*. 2003;43: 213-222.

DiMarco H. The electronic cloak: secret sexual deviance in cybersociety. In: Jewkes Y, ed. *Dot.cons: Crime, Deviance and Identity on the Internet*. Portland, Ore: Willan Publishing; 2003.

Durkin KF. Misuse of the Internet by pedophiles: implications for law enforcement and probation practice. *Fed Probat.* 1997;61(3):14-18.

Finkelhor D, Berliner L. Research on the treatment of sexually abused children: a review and recommendations. *J Am Acad Child Adolesc Psychiatry.* 1995;34:1408-1423.

Finkelhor D, Mitchell KJ, Wolak J. *Online Victimization: A Report on the Nation's Youth.* Alexandria, Va: National Center for Missing & Exploited Children; 2000.

Gillespie AA. Sentences for offences involving child pornography. *Crim Law Rev.* 2003;81-93.

Goldstein SL. *The Sexual Exploitation of Children: A Practical Guide to Assessment, Investigation, and Intervention.* 2nd ed. Boca Raton, Fla: CRC Press; 1999.

Hills P, Argyle M. Uses of the Internet and their relationship with individual differences in personality. *Comput Hum Behav.* 2002;19(1):59-70.

Itzin C. Pornography and the construction of misogyny. *J Sex Aggress.* 2002;8(3):4-42.

Itzin C. Pornography and the organization of intra-familial and extrafamilial child sexual abuse: developing a conceptual model. *Child Abuse Rev.* 1997;6:94-106.

Kelly L, Wingfield R, Burton S, Regan L. *Splintered Lives: Sexual Exploitation of Children in the Context of Children's Rights and Child Protection.* London, England: Barnardos; 1995.

Kennedy-Souza BL. Internet addiction disorder. *Interpers Comput Technol.* 1998; 6:1-2.

Kincaid JR. *Erotic Innocence: The Culture of Child Molesting.* Durhan, NC and London, England: Duke University Press; 1998.

Lanning KV. *Child Molesters: A Behavioural Analysis.* 3rd ed. Washington, DC: National Center for Missing & Exploited Children; 1992.

Mann CC, Stewart FF. *Internet Communication and Qualitative Research: A Handbook for Researching Online.* London, England: Sage Publications; 2000.

Morahan-Martin J, Schumacher P. Incidence and correlates of pathological Internet use among college students. *Comput Hum Behav.* 2000;16:13-29.

Quayle E, Taylor M. Child pornography and the Internet: perpetuating a cycle of abuse. *Deviant Behav.* 2002;23(4):331-362.

Quayle E, Taylor M. Child seduction and self-representation on the Internet. *Cyberpsychol Behav.* 2001;4(5):597-608.

Quayle E, Taylor M. Model of problematic Internet use in people with a sexual interest in children. *Cyberpsychol Behav.* 2003;6(1):93-106.

Quayle E, Holland G, Linehan C, Taylor M. The Internet and offending behaviour: a case study. J *Sex Aggress.* 2000;6(1/2):78-96.

Sentencing Advisory Panel. The panel's advice to the court of appeal on sentences involving child pornography. London, England: Sentencing Advisory Panel; 2002.

Scott S. *The Politics and Experience of Ritual Abuse: Beyond Disbelief.* Buckingham, England: Open University Press; 2001.

Silbert MH. On effects on juveniles of being used for pornography and prostitution. In: Zillman D, Bryant C, eds. *Pornography: Research Advances and Policy Considerations.* Hillside, NJ: Lawrence Erlbaum; 1989.

Svedin CG, Back K. *Children Who Don't Speak Out.* Stockholm, Sweden: Swedish Save the Children; 1996.

Talamo A, Ligorio B. Strategic identities in cyberspace. *Cyberpsychol Behav.* 2001; 4(1):109-120.

Taylor M, Quayle E. *Child Pornography: An Internet Crime.* Hove, England: Brunner-Routledge; 2003.

Taylor M, Holland G, Quayle E. Typology of paedophile picture collections. *Police J.* 2001;74(2):97-107.

US Postal Inspection Service. The US Postal Inspection Service teams with Internet Crimes Against Children Taskforce in Operation Avalanche. 2003. Available at: http://www.usps.com/postalinspectors/avalanch.htm. Accessed February 17, 2004.

Veale A, Taylor M. Street kids as abandoning or abandoned? In: Panter-Brick CA, ed. *Anthropological and Historical Perspectives on Child Abandonment.* Cambridge, England: Cambridge University Press; 1997.

Wolak J, Mitchell KJ, Finkelhor D. Escaping or connecting? Characteristics of youth who form close online relationships. *J Adolesc.* 2003;26:105-119.

Chapter 14

# ETHICAL ISSUES IN SEXUAL
# OFFENDER ASSESSMENTS*

Elizabeth J. Letourneau, PhD
David S. Prescott, LICSW

In the wake of recent sexual abuse legislation, sex offender assessments have gained new importance in the prosecution and treatment of male offenders. Clearly, the consequences of such assessments have always been serious, particularly given the frequency with which sex offender assessment results are introduced during the guilt (or sentencing) phase of judicial hearings. Balancing the rights and well-being of the community, victim, and offender remains a challenge to all who practice in legal settings. However, with the introduction of consequences based specifically upon the potential future risk of an individual, such as community notification and civil commitment, the stakes are higher than ever before.

Given the scope of these issues, it is no surprise that researchers, practitioners, policy-makers, and other interested parties have all attempted to better understand and identify those at high risk for re-offense. With the emerging evidence-based tools now available come new concerns about their ethical use. Understanding their construction, proper use, and application to diverse legal frameworks continues to challenge those attempting to reduce the harm of sexual abuse.

Fortunately, the majority of professionals conducting such assessments appear to do so in a thoughtful and ethical manner, usually after taking part in the substantial training necessary to work with this select clinical population. For example, a review of ethics complaints filed with the Association for the Treatment of Sexual Abusers (ATSA), an organization of approximately 2000 professionals who work with sex offenders, revealed that only 12 complaints were made between 2001 and 2003. Of these, only 3 ended with recommendations of sanctions for behavior.

Certainly, the actual rate of ethics violations is higher than this figure represents. Many violations are never reported, and only complaints from current organization members are accepted. Nevertheless, these numbers suggest that, by and large, members of this organization go about their business, which includes conducting sex offender assessments, with an appropriate degree of professionalism. However, there is no aspect of a sex offender assessment that is exempt from potential abuse, misuse, or simple misunderstanding.

This chapter will review the development of assessment standards and guidelines resulting, in large part, from concerns regarding the appropriate execution and interpretation of sex offender evaluations. We will review assessment measures that have generated the most controversy due to ethical concerns, and assessment conditions under which misinterpretation of results appears most likely.

---

*The information in this chapter pertains to adult male sex offenders and not to juvenile offenders or female offenders. Data indicate that juvenile sex offenders bear little resemblance to their adult counterparts (Miranda & Corcoran, 2000). There is little empirical information on the assessment of female sexual offenders, who consistently comprise 5% or fewer of sex offenders in any given study sample (Finkelhor & Russell, 1984).

# STANDARDS AND GUIDELINES FOR SEX OFFENDER ASSESSMENTS

The goals of psychosexual assessments depend on the intended use of the assessment results. For example, assessments are commonly performed just before the start of sex offender-specific treatment with the goal of assisting therapists in developing individual treatment plans. Assessment results can serve as a blueprint for treatment crafted to meet the offender's individual needs. Assessments are frequently requested during the initial prosecution, or guilt phase hearings, of an individual charged with a crime. Under these conditions, the often unstated goal of the assessment is to help determine guilt or innocence. Potential ethical problems with pretrial assessments, particularly assessments conducted in the absence of a guilty plea, are addressed later in this chapter.

Additionally, sex offender assessments are often requested following decisions of guilt, but before sentencing or before sentence completion. The goal of presentencing assessments can be to help determine the most appropriate level of supervision and treatment needs. The goal of prerelease assessments is also frequently to address supervision needs. Paradoxically, the options for post-incarceration supervision of convicted sex offenders have increased and decreased in recent years. So-called "truth in sentencing" laws require certain offenders to complete the entirety or majority of their sentences, with no chance for parole. One effect of such legislation is that without parole, there can be no additional supervision of sex offenders once they complete their sentences and transition back into the community. On the other hand, recent legislation has been enacted at both the federal and state levels to increase the supervision of sex offenders (SEARCH, 1998). Registration, community notification, and civil commitment are all means by which the supervision of known sex offenders has increased. Whether the lack of parole and supervision of some offenders reduces community safety or whether registration, community notification, and/or civil commitment increase community safety are empirical questions that remain unanswered. Nevertheless, many sex offender assessments are now conducted as part of civil commitment proceedings and to determine whether certain offenders warrant placement on sex offender registries and/or subjection to community notification procedures.

Although sex offender assessment remains a relatively small specialty within the mental health field, the number of professionals working with sex offenders has increased markedly since the 1980s (McGrath et al, 2003). Growing national awareness of the extent of sexual abuse and a demand for the prosecution and treatment of sex offenders have contributed to this growth. In retrospect, awareness of the harm of sexual abuse has been particularly hard-won. By all accounts, sex offenders have been around since time immemorial. Indeed, the Bible refers to the "seduction" of Lot by both of his daughters (see Genesis 19:31-38). This passage is interesting because it appears to provide an early example of child sexual abuse, and a common cognitive distortion employed by child molesters (ie, seduction by the child victim).

Cultural differences notwithstanding, modern victim advocacy groups have only recently gained sufficient political power (based in part on empirical evidence of the effects and extent of sexual assault) to change long-held notions about the rarity of sexual assault against women and children. In 1995, distinguished sociologist David Finkelhor discussed the "extraordinary successful social movement" that produced changes in the way institutions, professionals, and laypersons view assaultive and neglectful behavior against children (Finkelhor, 1995). The success of this still-ongoing movement hinged largely on the success of the women's movement (Brownmiller, 1975), and it was first realized in the 1980s. It was during this time that sex offender treatment organizations first began to coalesce as more professionals became involved in the assessment and treatment of this population.

Another major influence in the growth of professionals working with alleged and convicted sex offenders was the development of reliable, easy-to-use sexual arousal measures. These will be discussed later. Thus, interest in the assessment of sex offenders and growth in this specialized area within the field of mental health occurred not in a vacuum but in the context of improved assessment devices, growing understanding and acknowledgment of the problem of sexual abuse, and the increased prosecution of offenders that resulted from such awareness. However, as this small specialty field grew, so did concerns about occasions of misuse and misinterpretation of assessment measures and their results.

# THE ASSOCIATION FOR THE TREATMENT OF SEXUAL ABUSERS

Organizations for practitioners and researchers developed out of the perceived need for standardization of assessment and treatment practices as used with alleged and convicted sex offenders. By a considerable margin, the largest and most geographically diverse of these is the Association for the Treatment of Sexual Abusers (ATSA). ATSA was established by a small group of practitioners in Oregon who were concerned about the proper use of penile plethysmography (PPG) (see section titled Measures Used in Sexual Offender Assessments), and were motivated to exchange information regarding assessment and treatment of sex offenders (Prescott, 2002). Headed by Robert Freeman-Longo, then director of a unit at the Oregon State Hospital in Salem, this group held informal brown-bag luncheon meetings in the early 1980s to share information and address concerns specific to the misuse of the plethysmograph. Concerns included use of plethysmography for determining guilt or innocence, evaluators' lack of experience and training, and apparently abusive assessment practices (eg, evaluations lasting 8 hours) (Prescott, 2002). After one such meeting, the idea of developing an organization that could unite professionals and develop standards of ethical practice was promoted, and the ATSA (originally the Association for the Behavioral Treatment of Sexual Aggressives) was born.

Meanwhile, Drs. Gene Abel and Judith Becker had worked with a grant from the National Institute of Mental Health (NIMH) since the mid-1970s to research sexually abusive behavior, including the use of plethysmography to assess sexual arousal. The NIMH grant also provided funding for 5 national conferences, the first of their kind in the United States. Although small, these conferences were significant because they allowed researchers and practitioners to meet one another. The last of the NIMH-funded conferences occurred in Tampa, Florida, in February 1986, as a part of a grant awarded to Dr. Richard Laws. After that meeting, the ATSA assumed sponsorship of the conferences, and annual professional conferences have been held each year since that date, with increasing attendance. Informal luncheons grew into comprehensive professional conferences. The most recent have drawn upwards of 1200 attendees, with hundreds of individual speakers presenting the latest in sex offender research and clinical applications. (See www.ATSA.com for organization details, including conference information.)

Many of the concerns that sparked the development of the ATSA continue to exist today. For example, though few question the need for standards of care to guide ethical practice, disagreement exists among individual practitioners about how these standards should best be developed and executed. While other organizations have attempted to develop standards for assessment and treatment, none have been as widely distributed as those of the ATSA.

## ATSA STANDARDS

In 2001, ATSA published the most comprehensive set of standards and guidelines for conducting sex offender assessment and treatment (ATSA, 2001). The *Practice Standards and Guidelines for Members of the Association for the Treatment of Sexual Abusers* (ATSA standards) is a "living" document that undergoes revision as needed.

(Indeed, the latest revision was released by ATSA in March 2005.) However, the ATSA standards might be considered the "gold standard" for psychosexual evaluations given the size of ATSA's membership (all members are subject to these standards) and that these standards have been formally adopted by numerous state and local agencies. According to the 2001 ATSA standards, sex offender assessments should include information in 15 distinct areas of behavior and functioning (**Table 14-1**). A thorough assessment addresses each of these subject areas, regardless of the specific assessment goal. Likewise, the standards require that data be gathered from several sources and that no assessment rely upon a single source for information. Sources for assessment information include client interviews and self-report measures (or psychometric tests), interviews with collateral informants, psychophysiological testing, and review of official documents (eg, victim statements). The degree to which examiners attempt to access all 5 sources of data suggested by the standards varies depending upon the goals of the assessment. However, when information on the same psychological construct (eg, deviant sexual interest) is gathered from multiple sources that result in similar conclusions, the examiner and those using the assessment results have much more confidence in the results (Campbell & Fiske, 1959).

---

**Table 14-1. Information to Be Included in All Sex Offender Assessments**

CONSTRUCT OR BEHAVIOR

— Internet access

— Antisocial behavior

— Developmental history & family background

— Deviant sexual interests & behaviors

— Educational & employment histories

— Cognitive functioning

— Medical & mental health histories

— Sexual & nonsexual crimes

— Peer & romantic relationship histories

— Psychopathy

— Relevant personality traits

— Sexual fantasies, urges, & behaviors

— Sexually abusive behavior

— Substance use

— Use of sexually arousing materials

*Adapted from Association for the Treatment of Sexual Abusers (ATSA).* Practice Standards and Guidelines for Members of the Association for the Treatment of Sexual Abusers. *Portland, Ore: ATSA; 2001:8.*

---

## MEASURES USED IN SEXUAL OFFENDER ASSESSMENTS

Of the 15 constructs and behaviors listed in **Table 14-1**, a few have received considerable attention pertaining to risk of misuse in sex offender assessments. These include physiological measures of sexual arousal and interest (ie, penile plethysmography and viewing time devices), measurement of dissimulation (ie, polygraphy), and measurement of psychopathy (ie, the Hare Psychopathy Checklist). Thus, each of these constructs and related measurement tools is addressed below.

### PHYSIOLOGICAL MEASURES OF SEXUAL AROUSAL AND INTEREST: PENILE PLETHYSMOGRAPHY

Working for the Czechoslovakian government in the 1950s, Dr. Kurt Freund developed a device designed to determine sexual orientation. The "volumetric penile plethysmograph" (**Figure 14-1**) developed by Freund (and subsequently applied to the more general measurement of sexual arousal) involved measuring air or water displaced from a glass tube during penile tumescence (Freund, 1981). Specifically, a glass cylinder was placed over the examinee's penis and sealed at the base with an inflatable rubber ring. Penile tumescence forced air or water through a tube affixed to the top of the cylinder, and the displaced air or water was then measured. The Czechoslovakian government used Freund's initial research to detect those attempting to feign homosexuality to avoid military service. Freund was also one of the first scientific researchers to argue that homosexuality could not be "cured." His later work, conducted after he immigrated to Canada, included investigation into understanding some harmful sexual behaviors in the context of "courtship disorder" (Freund & Seto, 1998).

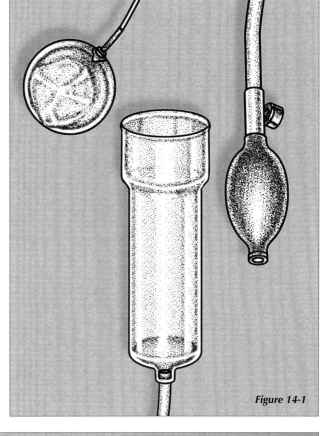

*Figure 14-1*

By the 1980s, Freund and a handful of others had researched the volumetric device for several decades. However, these devices were clumsy, fragile, and expensive (Freund, 1981) and required the direct involvement of a technician—the subject could not place the tube himself. Thus, as might be imagined, the volumetric plethysmograph never gained wide appeal with practitioners. However, in the late 1970s, researchers adapted the volumetric device by replacing the tube with a "strain gauge"—either a metal or rubber band that fit around the penis (Bancroft et al, 1966; Barlow et al, 1970) (**Figure 14-2**). Small electrodes placed in the metal strain gauge, or a small electrical current passing through a filler substance such as mercury or indium gallium in the rubber strain gauge, measure changes in minute electrical currents that occur due to changes in penile circumference.

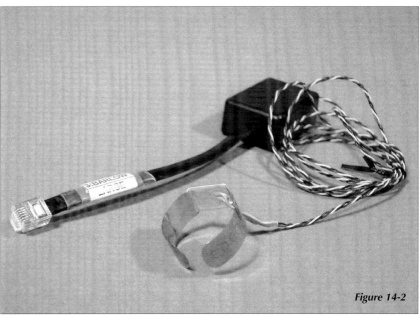

*Figure 14-2*

These "circumferential strain gauges" were less expensive and less fragile than the volumetric device and, perhaps most important, did not require a "hands-on" approach to placement. Subjects were easily instructed in the placement of the ring and could then do so in the privacy of the testing laboratory. Further, data from several laboratories suggested that the newer circumferential devices produced results that were in general accordance with results from the volumetric device (Kuban et al, 1999).

*Figure 14-1. Volumetric plethysmograph.*

*Figure 14-2. Circumferential Strain Gauge. Contributed by Peter Byrne, PhD, President, Behavioral Technology, Inc, Salt Lake City, Utah.*

As the more user-friendly circumferential strain gauges and related software programs became commercially available, more practitioners began to employ this assessment method. At present, between 25% and 34% of adult community and residential treatment programs utilize PPG (McGrath et al, 2003).

As previously noted, PPG techniques have been in use for decades to provide information on patterns of male sexual arousal (Bancroft et al, 1966; Barlow et al, 1970; Freund, 1965; McConaghy, 1989). Adequate internal consistency and test-retest reliability for plethysmography have been demonstrated in several studies (Abel et al 1998; Day et al, 1989). Classification accuracy of PPG with child molesters has been demonstrated (Miner et al, 1995). However, several reviews have noted significant and ongoing problems with plethysmography, including lack of normative data (ie, plethysmography data from nonoffenders), lack of method standardization, and few comparison studies that include other measures of sexual arousal (Laws, 2003; Marshall & Fernandez, 2003; O'Donohue & Letourneau, 1992).

Despite these concerns, many consider plethysmography the most effective method for assessing deviant sexual arousal. It is the single best predictor of recidivism risk in child molesters (Hanson & Bussiere, 1998).

### Ethical Issues in the Use of Penile Plethysmography

Despite the promise demonstrated by PPG, several ethical issues are associated with its use. The principal ethical concerns stem from the previously common use of nude stimuli, the inappropriate application of plethysmography to certain populations, and the inappropriate interpretations of the data. The development of alternatives to plethysmography occurred, in part, during the aftermath of legal inquiries regarding the use of nude stimuli during plethysmography testing (Abel et al, 1998).

#### *Inappropriate Use of Nude Stimuli*

Several ethical problems are inherent in using images of nude children. First, nude photos were often obtained from seizures of pornography—thus, the children were abused during the making of the stimulus materials. Second, it is difficult to determine how "consent" could be obtained for use of even nonabusive pictures (eg, the harmless family photo of children bathing). Parents may give examiners consent to use such pictures, but children and preteens are generally considered too young even to provide assent (permission). In the event that parental consent and child assent were obtained, the question remains whether children should be asked for their permission annually until they are adults and can provide consent. The time, effort, and cost to obtain updated assent and, eventually, consent from child models would be unmanageable for all but the largest of companies. Because of these and other concerns, the use of nude stimuli has become uncommon in the United States.

Other stimulus modalities commonly used with PPG include pictures or video clips of clothed minors, audiotapes, and combinations of these stimulus modalities. Thus, the elimination of nude stimuli in no way impedes the use of PPG. Indeed, for some uses, audiotapes may be better suited. In particular, when portraying an action (eg, rape) or an emotion (eg, fear, disgust) rather than a static feature of a target (eg, age or gender), audiotapes may be better suited than pictures, nude or otherwise. Furthermore, there are no readily identifiable ethical concerns with the use of audiotaped descriptions of sexual interactions, except insofar as PPG is used with minors, when exposure to deviant sexual stimuli of any modality is ethically suspect.

#### *Inappropriate Application to Certain Populations*

A second significant concern with plethysmography is its use with populations where data on reliability and/or validity are limited or lacking altogether. For example, approximately 10% of juvenile sex offender community and residential treatment programs employ plethysmography (McGrath et al, 2003). However, research indicates that juvenile sex offenders demonstrate highly variable patterns of sexual arousal, as measured by PPG (Hunter et al, 1994) that do not correlate with other important clinical characteristics (Becker, 1998). Of particular concern is that no published studies examine the arousal patterns of non-offending adolescents. Thus, no scientifically validated "norms" exist for the arousal patterns of boys. Given this lack of normative information, one may ask how it is possible to examine an arousal pattern and determine whether it is deviant. What constitutes "deviant" if what constitutes "normal" is completely unknown? Concerns also exist regarding the use of plethysmography with mentally retarded or developmentally delayed (MR/DD) adult men. Though research is limited, it has been reported that MR/DD subjects are more likely to produce deviant arousal patterns, perhaps due to a lessened ability to fake arousal or poorer understanding of when such faking might be advantageous (ATSA, 2001). In general, larger, normative studies that include normative samples and representative samples of important subgroups (eg, non-offending adolescents, MR/DD adult men) are needed. Until such studies are completed, plethysmography with subjects or clients with understudied characteristics should be avoided, or results from such examinations should be treated with great caution.

### Inappropriate Use of Results

A third area of concern is the inappropriate use of plethysmography results. Practitioners and researchers have long voiced serious concerns about the misuse of plethysmography results (Adams, 1989; Annon, 1992; Marshall & Eccles, 1991; Marshall & Fernandez, 2003). As noted by Marshall & Fernandez (2003), professionals and technicians employing plethysmography often receive little formal training. This may account for the misinterpretation of plethysmography results. Plethysmography is sometimes viewed as a sexual "lie detector" with powers to determine whether someone is sexually attracted to children. In a recent show broadcasted nationally, a live demonstration of plethysmography was presented. The segment begins with the announcer stating, "[f]or the first time ever on TV, a lie detector test for sex" (Introduction, 2003). The clear message from this show was that negative results from the plethysmograph exonerated the alleged offender of sexually molesting children.

This simplistic view of plethysmography ignores important limitations to its use. First and foremost, no test or combination of tests can determine guilt or innocence. Men can commit sexual assaults in the absence of clear patterns of arousal to those targets (eg, children) or situations (eg, rape). Men can also avoid the commission of crimes even when highly aroused by inappropriate targets or situations. Indeed, several studies reported that arousal patterns of incest offenders were more similar to those of nonoffenders than to arousal patterns of extrafamilial offenders (Marshall et al, 1986; Quinsey et al, 1979). Thus, the expectation that a sex offender assessment can indicate guilt or innocence is completely inappropriate and to offer assessment results as evidence is unethical.

### Lack of Standardized Procedures

A final concern regarding plethysmography is the lack of standardized procedures for plethysmographic assessment. Though not necessarily an ethical concern, the lack of standardization likely contributes to a host of problems, including the apparently infrequent use of inappropriate stimuli, the inappropriate application of plethysmography to poorly studied populations, and the inappropriate interpretation of plethysmography results. By comparison, readers of this text may be familiar with intelligence testing and that only a few highly standardized and very well-validated measures of intellectual ability, such as the Stanford-Binet, are in wide use. These measures are highly standardized because of the need for consistency in evaluation of results and because of the grave implications that low and high intelligence quotients can have for an individual. Despite a few attempts to standardize plethysmography testing (Laws et al, 1995), many examiners employ idiosyncratic methods, and thus, their procedures vary along many factors, including stimuli, stimulus modality, data reduction methods, and level of data considered appropriate for interpretation. Lack of standardization of any test causes results to differ across examiners and across examinations, reducing confidence in any single set of test results.

## PHYSIOLOGICAL MEASURES: VIEWING TIME

Current viewing time (VT) measures have been developed to avoid some of the specific concerns that plague plethysmography testing. It has long been hypothesized that VT may serve as an indicator of sexual interest (Rosenzweig, 1942), and several studies have reported that sexual interest is significantly correlated with amount of time spent viewing congruent slides (Abel et al, 1994; Harris et al, 1996; Ware et al, 1972). Consequently, a new measure of sexual interest has been developed based on the length of time in which subjects view slides of models who differ in age and gender (Abel et al, 1998). Of the commercially available VT devices, the best studied is that created by Gene Abel. Several studies have indicated good reliability of the Abel VT as well as significant correlations between offense-specific characteristics (eg, young male child victim) and response time to slides of models representing those characteristics (Abel et al, 1994, 1998; Letourneau, 2002; however, cf Fischer & Smith, 1999). In several studies, VT has performed as well, or in some cases as poorly, as plethysmography in identifying specific subgroups of sex offenders (Abel et al, 1998; Letourneau, 2002).

These measures tend to be highly standardized and include only non-nude stimuli. Abel's VT measure is the most widely used in North America and will be the focus of this section. Raw VT data from all user sites are sent to a central location for scoring. This procedure has 2 obvious benefits: first, considerably less variability should be in scoring procedures if all scoring is conducted at a single site; second, copies of the raw and scored data for all assessments are retained at the centralized location, permitting research on large samples. Consequently, Abel currently possesses data on more than 8000 adult male child molesters and more than 3000 juvenile sex offenders with younger victims (Abel, 2003). He and his colleagues have used these data to examine and refine the validity of this VT measure (Abel, 2003; Abel et al, 1998, 2001).

Concerns with the central warehousing of data collection and scoring include the continued cost of such scoring and the limited access to raw data by researchers. Neither concern is purely ethical in nature, but each deserves mention. The first concern is primarily economic: Some practitioners may be unable to use the Abel VT due to the continued cost of scoring. Expense is always a concern, regardless of the measure being considered for use, and is certainly not unique to the Abel VT. Limited access to raw data by researchers comes closer to ethical concerns in that it limits the external verification of the reliability and validity of this measure. To our knowledge, only a single study has been published in which raw (ie, unadulterated) data were provided to the author (Letourneau, 2002). Independent evaluation of instruments is an important step in the validation process (Hanson, 2002).

### Ethical Issues in the Use of Viewing Time Measures

The principal ethical concerns with VT stem from misinterpretation of VT results and use of this measure with subjects from understudied populations. Misinterpretation of VT data seems principally related to a lack of normative data (ie, VT data on nonsexual offenders) and the lack of data linking VT results with recidivism (ie, longitudinal studies).

Included with the scored results of VT examinations are "probability scores." These scores indicate the degree to which the pattern of results from the subject matches the average pattern of results from incest offenders or child molesters (Abel et al, 2001). However, there appears to be no published research on the pattern of results from non-offending men. Instead, the research establishing response patterns for child molesters and incest offenders has compared these groups with men who have committed other sexual crimes (eg, rape of adult women). Thus, the ability of the VT to distinguish offenders from non-offenders, and not simply from offenders against adults, remains to be determined.

Indeed, in a recently published study, researchers did not find differences in viewing time between a group of juvenile sex offenders and a group of delinquent youth who had no official record of sexual offending (Smith & Fisher, 1999). Abel has disputed the results of this study (Abel, 2000) but has not yet published data on non-offending (or nonsexual offending) juveniles with which to counter Smith and Fisher's assertions.

### Misinterpretation of Results

As noted above, practitioners receive "probability scores" with scored VT reports. The use of the term "probability" implies action or the probability that someone did something (ie, is guilty or not guilty of a specific crime) or will do something in the future (ie, the recidivism risk of an individual). Neither interpretation has been subjected to empirical testing. Thus, probability scores *in no way* indicate the probability that the examinee committed the crime for which he was evaluated or the probability that the examinee will commit a new sexual offense in the future. At the October 2003 ATSA conference, Abel presented data on juvenile sex offenders who had completed the VT. During his presentation, only 2 questions were asked, one of which was whether a probability score of 75% meant that the examinee had a 75% chance of having committed the sexual offense for which he was being assessed. Clearly, the professional posing the question misunderstood the meaning of the VT probability scores, and we believe such misconceptions are common among users of this technology.

Another common misinterpretation of the VT probability scores is the idea that these scores indicate the probability that the subject will commit a sexual offense in the future. While plethysmography results have been linked with recidivism, no longitudinal studies have examined the recidivism rates of men with deviant (versus nondeviant) VT scores. Thus, despite apparent similarities between the constructs assessed by plethysmography (sexual arousal) and VT (sexual interest), it can not be assumed that VT results are indicative of recidivism risk. Longitudinal studies must be conducted to examine whether sexual interest in children is related to a greater risk of re-offending against children in the future.

The use of probability scores to determine whether a person's responses are similar to those of known offenders may be ethical. Abel has amassed information on a huge and constantly growing sample of child molesters that provides a rich source of data on the characteristics of these men and, more recently, their adolescent counterparts. However, the limitations of VT seem to be misunderstood by many practitioners. Though the development of VT measures is obviously beneficial to the field, the use of language in communicating the meaning of results, and the limitations to those results, seems all the more important in situations where personal liberty, as well as proper assessment and treatment, may hang in the balance.

### Use With Understudied Populations

The second principal concern noted with the VT is its use with understudied populations. In particular, evidence for the accuracy of VT with juvenile offenders is limited and contested (Abel, 2000; Smith & Fischer, 1999) and little evidence exists that VT accurately identifies men sexually interested in rape or other criminal activities (eg, voyeurism or exhibitionism). Yet the VT is marketed for use with juveniles, and the adult version includes scoring for interest in sadism, which appears to be used by many practitioners to assess men interested in rape. Slides that assess interest in voyeurism and exhibitionism are included, though these are identified as "experimental." As noted in the section on PPG, it may be difficult for an individual slide to represent an action, such as the sadistic abuse of a woman, or to identify the emotions (eg, fear) that women might experience upon discovering someone peering through their windows. The VT includes slides that attempt to discern such actions and emotions. Buyers simply must beware that just because a measure exists does not mean that it is reliable or valid. The best strategy is to wait until independent evidence from multiple studies indicates an adequate level of reliability and validity for any measure. Furthermore, marketing practices should make clear any limitations or experimental aspects of a measure. Given the wide use of the Abel VT with under-studied populations, it appears such practices would benefit from additional empirical support.

## MEASUREMENT OF DISSIMULATION: POLYGRAPHY

An obvious problem in the assessment of sex offenders is dissimulation. Increasingly, probation officers and mental health professionals have turned to the polygraph for help in managing sex offenders. For example, between 1992 and 2002, the percentage of community-based sex offender treatment programs that regularly employed polygraphy increased from 29% to 70% (McGrath et al, 2003). An overview of polygraphy techniques is beyond the scope of this chapter. (See the thorough review of polygraphy by the National Research Council [2002] and the Handbook of Polygraph Testing [Kleiner, 2002]).

### Ethical Issues in the Use of the Polygraph

Of all the measures reviewed in this chapter, the polygraph is the most controversial, perhaps because of its wider applicability. Within the subgroup of professionals working with sex offenders, the polygraph has generated sufficient interest that specific recommendations for its use with sex offenders have been developed by individuals (Wilcox, 2000) and by organizations such as ATSA (2001) and the American Polygraph Association (Consigli, 2002). Indeed, in some parts of the US, polygraph use is required in the community management of sex offenders (Ahlmeyer et al, 2000). However, several researchers have voiced serious concerns regarding the reliability and validity of the polygraph, particularly when used outside of specific, preconviction criminal investigations (Cross & Saxe, 2001; Fiedler et al, 2002; National Research Council, 2002; Saxe & Ben-Shakhar, 1999). Principal concerns include the limited theory upon which polygraph testing is based, the difficulty in testing the validity of the polygraph due to the inherent difficulty in ascertaining the actual "truth" regarding any given question, and the application of the polygraph to situations for which there is limited evidence of validity.

### Limited Theoretical Basis

Regarding the first concern, lie detection via polygraphy is loosely based on the "arousal theory," which holds that persons will experience greater physiological arousal when lying about issues of greater perceived relevance than when lying about issues of less perceived relevance (National Research Council, 2002; Saxe & Ben-Shakhar, 1999). Saxe and his colleagues have been particularly vocal about concerns regarding the lack of theoretical basis to support the notion that humans present a consistent physiological pattern when lying and the lack of data indicating that physiological responses are unique to lying (Cross & Saxe, 2001; Saxe & Ben-Shakhar, 1999). Rather, the physiological indices measured during polygraphy (breathing rate, skin conductivity, and heart rate) manifest changes to a host of other stimuli besides lying (eg, changes in these indices occur when subjects are anxious, stressed, or excited) (Cross & Saxe, 2001; Fielder et al, 2002). Researchers note that even if humans did produce relatively stable patterns of arousal across multiple physiological indicators when lying, little evidence supports the related hypothesis that the degree of arousal parallels the perceived relevance of the lie (Fielder et al, 2002; Kleiner, 2002). Further, these authors note that the entire process hinges upon the examiner's ability to create "white lie" questions, known as control questions, against which to compare physiological data from more relevant questions. Interestingly, there is apparently agreement between polygraph proponents and critics that no specific "lie response" exists (Kleiner, 2002).

## Lack of Validity

Regarding the second concern, supporters and critics of polygraph testing admit the difficulty in constructing validity studies for this measure. Mock situations in which subjects know they are participating in a research study bear little resemblance to real-life scenarios, in which subjects know that the results of a polygraph examination can carry grave consequences (Fielder et al, 2002; National Research Council, 2002). Further, there is the problem of determining, in advance of testing, the correct or "truthful" response to questions. Proponents of polygraph testing have pointed to the spontaneous admissions of offenders during or following testing as evidence that polygraph testing is valid. There are 2 problems with this method. First, use of spontaneous admissions to validate polygraph testing necessarily limits the validity pool to those people who provide such admissions. Subjects who "pass" a polygraph and who do not make spontaneous admissions are "true misses" or "false misses," and it is almost impossible to tell which is correct. This means that the actual "hit rate" of polygraph testing is impossible to determine. The second problem with spontaneous admissions is that researchers have no way to determine whether the person is being truthful. The consequences of "failing" polygraph testing are often severe, and it may well be the case that some examinees fabricate admissions of guilt to pass the test. Further, it seems likely that the most vulnerable populations, such as juveniles and MR/DD adults, are at greatest risk for fabricating deviant behaviors or fantasies to pass examinations.

Apart from issues of validity are concerns about the reliability of polygraph testing. There is little information about the reliability of polygraph testing as used with sex offenders or other subject populations. However, one study of sex offenders reported substantial decreases in the number of disclosures from the first to the second polygraph test, suggesting poor test-retest reliability (Ahlmeyer et al, 2000).

## Application to Inappropriate Situations

The third concern involves the application of polygraph testing to situations for which there is little empirical evidence of validity. The most common type of polygraph assessment involves the comparison of physiological data between a subject's responses to "relevant" questions and that subject's responses to "control questions," known as the control question technique or CQT (Kleiner, 2002). When CQT testing involves highly specific relevant questions (eg, "Did you touch Julia's vagina on May 13, 2000?"), there is some evidence supporting the validity of polygraphy (National Research Council, 2002). Highly specific questions are most likely to occur during preconviction investigations (Wilcox, 2000). However, professionals working with sex offenders are more likely to be involved in postconviction polygraph testing. As noted by Wilcox, postconviction, clinical, or monitoring polygraph examinations are more likely to involve nonspecific questions regarding "What have you been doing?" rather than the preconviction "Did you do it?" types of questions (Wilcox, 2000). Few, if any, validity or reliability studies specifically examine the results of polygraph testing when used with less specific questions. Rather, most research of the psychometric properties of polygraph testing involved specific questions. However, a recent review of polygraph testing was conducted that specifically examined the evidence for use of the polygraph in screening questions procedures for federal jobs. Screening examinations are less likely to include specific questions and more likely to include hypothetical or nonspecific questions (eg, "Would you ever do it?"), which seem more similar to the nonspecific questions employed in postconviction/monitoring examinations of sex offenders. The NRC review concluded that data do not support the use of polygraph testing in screening assessments.

*Use of Deception*
Finally, concerns have been expressed in many quarters that the polygraph is intrusive and deceptive. In other words, the examinee must believe that the polygraph will detect lies and thus, the examinee will experience considerable anxiety as a result. While these concerns are related more to the underlying values of those working with sex offenders than with the polygraph itself, the authors recommend that practitioners explore their own values around the use of this measure.

It must be acknowledged that several studies report increases in abuse disclosures by sex offenders in response to polygraph testing. Specifically, several studies have tracked offenders' disclosures from self-report measures to clinical interview to polygraph testing. Results generally indicate that, at each step, the number of disclosures increased (Abrams et al, 1991; Ahlmeyer et al, 2000; Emerick & Dutton, 1993). Polygraphy results in more admissions of deviant sexual behavior, cognitions, and fantasies and, therefore, polygraph testing may have utility when used to enhance information on the sexual history of clients for the purposes of clinical treatment (Wilcox, 2000). However, as noted, clinicians still can not be certain that additional information offered during polygraph testing is accurate. It is our conclusion that the use of polygraphy be limited to those situations for which there is empirical support (ie, specific question testing) or for which the risk of harm from "failing" the test is low, relative to the potential "benefit" to be gained from the test. The only situation that meets the latter criterion is when polygraph testing is used to enhance the clinical picture of the subject and when results will not be used to justify negative consequences, such as expulsion from treatment or reports to probation.

## MEASUREMENT OF PSYCHOPATHY: THE HARE PSYCHOPATHY CHECKLIST
*"Antisocial personality disorder (ASPD) is defined as a personality disorder characterized by 'a pervasive pattern of disregard for, and violation of, the rights of others that begins in childhood or early adolescence and continues into adulthood'" (American Psychiatric Association, 2000).*

Numerous studies have established differential rates of ASPD between criminal and noncriminal comparison groups (Cloninger et al, 1997). However, the criteria for ASPD cover such broad ground that most incarcerated male subject samples (50% to 80%) meet diagnostic criteria for ASPD (see Hart & Hare [1997] for a brief review of this literature). Further, the assessment of ASPD has serious limitations. For example, some measures of ASPD appear to greatly overestimate the presence of this disorder in noncriminal, nonforensic samples (Lilienfeld et al, 1997). It appears that conceptual and methodological limitations reduce the usefulness of this particular diagnosis (Lilienfeld et al, 1997). By comparison, the construct of psychopathy, as assessed by the Hare Psychopathy Checklist-Revised (PCL-R) (Hare, 1991) and its screening version (Hart & Hare, 1997) is more discriminating, conceptually and methodologically, and has greater predictive validity. Psychopathy is defined as a personality disorder and describes individuals who are callous, lack empathy, and engage in destructive behaviors with no apparent concern for the rights of others.

The psychometric properties of the Hare scales (ie, indicators of reliability and validity) perform well among raters who have attained minimum test criteria, that is, raters who have completed specific training and whose scoring of several test scales is judged to be accurate. Substantial training and familiarity with the literature is necessary before examiners may score assessment results (Hart & Hare, 1997), but the resulting skills are worth the time and expense. PCL-R scores, particularly in the presence of established sexual deviance, are strong predictors for sexual and nonsexual recidivism (Quinsey et al, 1995). Thus, men with high scores are more likely to commit additional sexual and nonsexual offenses. Indeed, although not intended as a measure of recidivism risk, the PCL-R and its screening version perform as well or better than actuarial measures designed specifically for this purpose (Hanson, 2000; Salekin et al, 1996; Serin, 1996).

Ethical Issues in the Use of the Psychopathy Checklist

The principal ethical issues regarding the use of the PCL-R concern the appropriate training of examiners and the application of personality diagnoses to minors. Hare and his colleagues spent the past 2 decades refining and validating the PCL-R to identify key features that distinguish psychopathy from other disorders. Importantly, normative data from non-offenders and from forensic patients (ie, patients who are prisoners or detainees) are provided in the assessment manual (Hare, 1991). However, because the PCL-R relies upon a combination of official records with a semi-structured interview, adequate training of examiners is essential and should be revisited periodically by professionals who utilize this measure. Hare and his colleagues have been vigilant regarding the qualifications of professionals requesting training in the use of the PCL-R. Typically, trainees must be willing to provide evidence they are qualified to provide mental health diagnoses within their jurisdictions. Hare and his colleagues further offer credentialing for professionals who seek additional training. This consists of taking a written test that reviews the literature, and scoring the PCL-R revised and screening versions on 8 cases for whom background information and videotaped interviews are provided. Extensive individual feedback is provided by Hare and his colleagues, who recommend keeping abreast of new research and completing such exercises as joint scoring of 5 cases with experienced colleagues in order to improve inter-rater agreement.

The measurement of psychopathy in juveniles is especially troubling. There has been great anticipation in the juvenile sex offender field of the release of the Hare Psychopathy Checklist: Youth Version (PCL-YV), a modification of the PCL-R for use with juvenile populations (Forth et al, 1997). However, in their critique of the application of the psychopathy construct to juvenile offenders, Seagrave & Grisso (2002) contend that many of the elements descriptive of the psychopath are elements of normal adolescent development. Hart et al (2002) echo these concerns, noting that personality is a developing process not yet crystallized in adolescence (Kernberg et al, 2000). Second, if psychopathy does exist in juveniles, it is unlikely to present across different stages of development (childhood, early adolescence, and late adolescence) in the same manner, suggesting that a single measure of psychopathy would inadequately capture this construct for differently aged minors.

Adolescence is a time for considerable change. For example, in a longitudinal study, Müller et al (2001) found that conditional reasoning—the ability to discern cause-effect relationships—shows considerable improvement from 11 to 16 years of age. Additionally, the ability to understand how others feel and think (ie, empathy) develops throughout childhood and adolescence (Piaget, 1972). Adolescence is a time of dramatic changes in identity and social relationships, during which youth may "try on" different personalities (Erikson, 1968; Harter, 1990). This experimentation with various behaviors, personas, and social approaches is frequently shaped by important interpersonal relations, including those with parents, friends, and significant adult figures (Harter et al, 1996). Other authors (eg, Kernberg et al, 2000) have described a process of "heterotypic continuity," in which the expression of personality pathology can change across childhood and adolescence. For some portion of youth, offending, including sexual offending, may be an unfortunate part of the process of development rather than an indication of a stable personality trait. Furthermore, risk factors for juvenile sex offending parallel those for juvenile delinquency and include many factors beyond individual characteristics, such as parental monitoring, parental conflict, association with delinquent peers, and poor school adjustment (Blaske et al, 1989). Thus, individual characteristics play only a part of the role in determining delinquency, and labeling minors as having stable personality traits related to future offending may unnecessarily limit treatment and other options for these youths.

# CONDITIONS CONTRIBUTING TO THE LIKELIHOOD OF MISINTERPRETATION

There are some situations under which the risk for misinterpretation of sex offender assessment results appears to increase. These include assessments conducted before findings of guilt, in the absence of guilty pleas, and assessments conducted with vulnerable subjects (eg, minors and MR/DD clients). Many examiners have conducted psychosexual assessments for clients charged with sexual crimes who are not yet adjudicated. The potential for benefit and harm can occur from such assessments.

Numerous potential benefits come from conducting a thorough psychosexual assessment. Such assessments may (a) help clients better understand their own sexual arousal patterns, (b) help lawyers better understand the extent to which their clients pose a risk to the community, including children in a client's home, (c) address issues of appropriate supervision level and treatment readiness, and (d) provide direction for treatment, such as indicating areas of deviant sexual arousal that should be targeted.

Risks are associated with conducting psychosexual assessments if the results will be introduced into court during the guilt phase of criminal trials, for example, the case of a client who has been charged with a crime but who is not guilty and pleads not guilty. If the client completes a PPG examination as part of an assessment, there is a chance that he will demonstrate deviant sexual arousal, even though he has never engaged in deviant sexual behaviors. For example, Barbaree & Marshall (1989) reported that 15% of their non-offender comparison group demonstrated greater or equal arousal to child stimuli as compared with adult consenting stimuli. Thus, an adult man who agrees to PPG testing at pre-trial has a substantial risk of "looking like" a child molester even in the absence of such behavior—potentially biasing a jury to convict an innocent person.

In the case of someone who is guilty and who pleads not guilty, test results may be used to sway a jury toward a "not guilty" finding. For example, if the client completes PPG as part of an assessment, there is a chance that he will not demonstrate deviant arousal, even though he has engaged in deviant sexual behaviors. In the same study, Barbaree & Marshall (1989) reported that 52% of nonfamilial child molesters and 72% of incest offenders did not show deviant profiles. Thus, someone who is guilty may "look like" he is not guilty, based on assessment information.

Though presumably least likely to occur, there are documented instances of persons who are not guilty but who pled guilty. Further, it seems likely that the more vulnerable members of society—minors and the mentally disabled—are most likely to land in this category. Imagine the case of a 14-year-old boy who is charged with molesting 2 younger boys. If results from the psychophysiological testing (eg, VT or PPG testing) indicate interest in and/or arousal to young boys, the boy's lawyer may recommend that he plead guilty for a reduced sentence or to avoid adult court.

The primary benefits derived from psychosexual evaluations (eg, statements regarding risk for future recidivism, identifying individual treatment goals) can be accomplished from assessments conducted post-adjudication. Given the risks inherent in conducting assessments whose results may be used during the guilt phase of a trial, the question becomes, "Why conduct psychosexual assessments before adjudication?"

Occasionally, there are pragmatic reasons. For example, the cost of the exam might be covered by the judicial system if the client agrees to participate prior to adjudication. Clients pleading guilty and who know or are reasonably sure they will be ordered by the court to receive treatment may, in these circumstances, save a substantial sum of money. Certainly clients may have other reasons for requesting an examination after being charged with a sexual crime and, if they do not intend to use the assessment results in their defense, there is no apparent reason for denying such services.

Occasionally, a defense lawyer may want to have a more complete picture of his or her client. For example, a lawyer may use assessment results in deciding whether to argue for less restrictive supervision of a specific client awaiting trial. Again, if the results will not be entered as evidence during the guilt phase of the trial, the client has few risks outside the cost of the exam.

Many pre-adjudication assessments are requested by lawyers or clients who intend to use the results in defense or prosecution of the client. This is where problems may arise and where the potential risks to the client or to society may outweigh the potential benefits. The most recent version of the ATSA standards was amended to address the issue of pre-adjudication psychosexual evaluations. These specific standards fall under section 9: "Members *shall* be balanced, fair, and honest in their professional communications" (ATSA, 2001). In particular, Standard 9.02 reads "Members *shall not* knowingly provide court testimony during the guilt phase of a criminal trial from which a reasonable person would draw inferences about whether the client did or did not commit a specific [sexual] crime" (ATSA, 2001).

This standard leaves wide discretion regarding how a "reasonable person" might interpret psychosexual testing results. Recently, the ATSA's Ethics Committee, with assistance from the advisory board and executive board of directors, determined that members presenting testing results during the guilt phase of a criminal trial should, at minimum, clearly state that such testing results do not indicate the client's guilt or innocence.

It is difficult to imagine a reasonable person (eg, a member of a jury or a judge) listening to results from a psychosexual evaluation and then completely discounting those results when making a determination of guilt or innocence. Thus, some argue that future standards should be modified to prohibit ATSA members from presenting assessment results as part of the guilt phase of a trial. This prohibition may be established easily but would not answer questions about how evaluators might best be helpful in the guilt phase of legal proceedings. For example, it is easy to imagine professionals not bound by ATSA standards conducting assessments containing erroneous information. Examples could include statements such as "the client's Minnesota Multiphasic Personality Inventory (MMPI) profile was inconsistent with those of known child molesters and suggests the client is not guilty of molesting his daughter," or "in my clinical opinion, based on 25 years of experience, this is a truly dangerous man." However, it is also easy to envision how these evaluations might be helpful, such as in providing education around the uncertain role of sexual arousal in adolescence (Hunter & Becker, 1994), the absence of empirically validated risk assessment measures for youth (Prescott, In press), or "counterfeit deviance" in the developmentally delayed (Blasingame, 2001). The ATSA is reviewing the current standards to determine whether revision is warranted and, if so, how best to modify these standards. The issue, to be clear, is not whether to conduct such assessments but how results of psychosexual assessments may be used in the best interests of our clients and society.

## CONCLUSION

In the past half century, and particularly the past few years, enormous growth has occurred in the recognition, assessment, and treatment of harmful sexual behavior. This growth has occurred across diverse professions (eg, legal, medical, clinical) in the public and private sectors. Sexual aggression is better understood across the lifespan and as arising from many potential domains (such as sexual deviance, antisociality, personality). Social (eg, women's movement), legal (eg, Megan's Law), and technological factors (eg, plethysmography, polygraphy, viewing time) have all contributed to this growth. As many have observed, with this growth comes awesome responsibilities in protecting the rights of all, including perpetrators, whose lives are impacted by sexual abuse.

Many concerns have rightfully accompanied the technological advances in sex offender assessment. For many, these measures have an initial allure that quickly diminishes to confusion and disappointment when the measures are used improperly. The above ethical considerations are, of course, only a small part of what evaluators will wish to bear in mind upon entering the field. However, it is our hope that by outlining portions of our field's history, current status, and work yet to be done, others may better contribute to its future and more effectively reduce the harm of sexual abuse.

# REFERENCES

Abel GG. The importance of meeting research standards: a reply to Fischer and Smith's articles on the Abel Assessment for Sexual Interest®. *Sex Abuse.* 2000; 12:155-161.

Abel GG. Usefulness of visual reaction time with adolescents. Paper presented at: Association for the Treatment of Sexual Abusers' 22nd Annual Research and Treatment Conference; October 2003; St. Louis, Mo.

Abel GG, Huffman J, Warberg B, Holland CL. Visual reaction time and plethysmography as measures of sexual interest in child molesters. *Sex Abuse.* 1998;10: 81-96.

Abel GG, Jordan A, Hand CG, Holland LA, Phipps A. Classification models of child molesters utilizing the Abel Assessment for child sexual abuse interest. *Child Abuse Negl.* 2001;25:703-718.

Abel GG, Lawry SS, Karlstrom EM, Osborn CA, Gillespie CF. Screening tests for pedophilia. *Crim Justice Behav.* 1994;21:115-131.

Abrams S, Hoyt D, Jewell C. The effectiveness of the disclosure test with sex abusers of children. *Polygraph.* 1991;20:197-203.

Adams HE. Is the penile plethysmograph an adequate clinical assessment procedure or a harmless toy for clinical researchers? Paper presented at: Association for the Advancement of Behavior Therapy Annual Convention; November 1989; Washington, DC.

Ahlmeyer S, Heil P, McKee B, English K. The impact of polygraphy on admissions of victims and offenses in adult sexual offenders. *Sex Abuse.* 2000;12:123-138.

American Psychiatric Association. *Diagnostic and Statistical Manual of Mental Disorders.* 4th ed. Text Revision. Washington, DC: American Psychiatric Association; 2000:701-702.

Annon JS. Misuse of psychophysiological arousal measurement data. Memorandum sent to: members of the Court of the First Circuit (Hawaii), Hawaii probation staff, and Hawaii sex offender treatment team staff. October 1992.

Association for the Treatment of Sexual Abusers (ATSA). *Practice Standards and Guidelines for the Evaluation, Treatment, and Management of Adult Male Sexual Abusers.* Portland, Ore: ATSA; 2005.

Association for the Treatment of Sexual Abusers (ATSA). *Practice Standards and Guidelines for Members of the Association for the Treatment of Sexual Abusers.* Portland, Ore: ATSA; 2001:8.

Bancroft J, Jones HG, Pullan BR. A simple transducer for measuring penile erections with comments on its use in the treatment of sexual disorders. *Behav Res Ther.* 1966; 4:239-241.

Barbaree HE, Marshall WL. Erectile responses amongst heterosexual child molesters, father-daughter incest offenders, and matched nonoffenders: five distinct age preference profiles. *Can J Behav Sci.* 1989;21:70-82.

Barlow DH, Becker R, Leitenberg H, Agras WS. A mechanical strain gauge for recording penile circumference change. *J Appl Behav Anal.* 1970;3:73-76.

Becker JV. What we know about the characteristics and treatment of adolescents who have committed sexual offenses. *Child Maltreat.* 1998;3:317-329.

Blasingame GD. *Developmentally Delayed Persons with Sexual Behavior Problems: Treatment, Management, Supervision.* Oklahoma City, Okla: Wood'N'Barnes; 2001.

Blaske DM, Borduin CM, Henggeler SW, Mann BJ. Individual, family, and peer characteristics of adolescent sex offenders and assaultive offenders. *Dev Psychol.* 1989; 25:846-855.

Brownmiller S. *Against Our Will: Men, Women and Rape.* New York, NY: Simon and Schuster; 1975.

Campbell DT, Fiske DW. Convergent and discriminant validation by the multitrait-multimethod matrix. *Psychol Bull.* 1959;56:81-105.

Cloninger CR, Bayon C, Przybeck TR. Epidemiology and Axis I comorbidity of anti-social personality. In: DM Stroff, J Breiling, JD Maser, eds. *Handbook of Antisocial Behavior* (12-21). New York, NY: John Wiley & Sons; 1997.

Consigli JE. Post-conviction sex offender testing and the American Polygraph Association. In: Kleiner M, ed. *Handbook of Polygraph Testing.* San Diego, Calif: Academic Press; 2002: 237-250.

Cross TP, Saxe L. Polygraph testing and sexual abuse: the lure of the magic lasso. *Child Maltreat.* 2001;6:195-206.

Day D, Miner M, Sturgeon V, Murphy J. Assessment of sexual arousal by means of physiological and self-report measures. In: Laws DR, ed. *Relapse Prevention With Sex Offenders.* New York, NY: Guilford; 1989:115-123.

Emerick RL, Dutton WA. The effect of polygraphy on the self report of adolescent sex offenders: implications for risk assessment. *Ann of Sex Res.* 1993;6:83-103.

Erikson EE. *Identity, Youth and Crisis.* New York, NY: Norton; 1968.

Fiedler K, Schmid J, Stahl T. What is the current truth about polygraph lie detection? *Basic Appl Soc Psych.* 2002;24:313-324.

Finkelhor D. The backlash in sociological perspective. *APSAC Advisor.* 1995;8(3): 1-2,18-22.

Finkelhor D, Russell D. Women as perpetrators: review of the evidence. In: Finkelhor D, ed. *Child Sexual Abuse: New Theory and Research.* New York, NY: The Free Press; 1984:171-187.

Fischer L, Smith G. Statistical adequacy of the Abel Assessment for Interest in Paraphilias. *Sex Abuse.* 1999;11:195-205.

Forth AE, Kosson DS, Hare RD. *The Hare Psychopathy Checklist: Youth Version (PCL-YV)—Rating Guide.* Toronto, Canada: Multi-Health Systems; 1997.

Freund K. Diagnosing heterosexual pedophilia by means of a test for sexual interest. *Behav Res Ther.* 1965;3:229-234.

Freund K. Assessment of pedophilia. In: Cook M, Howells K, eds. *Adult Sexual Interest in Children.* London, England: Academic Press; 1981:139-173.

Freund K, Seto MC. Preferential rape in the theory of courtship disorder. *Arch Sex Behav.* 1998;27:433-443.

Hanson RK. Introduction. *Sex Abuse.* 2002;14:205.

Hanson RK. *Risk Assessment.* Prepared for: the Association for the Treatment of Sexual Abusers. Beaverton, Ore: ATSA; 2000.

Hanson RK, Bussier MT. Predicting relapse: a meta-analysis of sexual offender recidivism studies. *J Consult Clin.* 1998;66:348-362.

Hare RD. *The Hare Psychopathy Checklist-Revised.* Toronto, Canada: Multi-Health Systems; 1991.

Harris GT, Rice ME, Quinsey VT, Chaplin TC. Viewing time as a measure of sexual interest among child molesters and normal heterosexual men. *Behav Res Ther.* 1996;34:389-394.

Hart SD, Hare RD. Psychopathy: assessment and association with criminal conduct. In: Stoff DM, Maser JB, Maser JD, eds. *Handbook of Antisocial Behavior.* New York, NY: John Wiley & Sons; 1997:22-35.

Hart SD, Watt KA, Vincent GM. Commentary on Seagrave and Grisso: impressions of the state of the art. *Law Hum Behav.* 2002;26:241-245.

Harter S. Processes underlying adolescent self-concept formation. In: Montemayor R, Adams G, Gullata T, eds. *From Childhood to Adolescence: A Transitional Period? Advances in Adolescent Development.* Vol 2. Thousand Oaks, Calif: Sage Publications; 1990:205-239.

Harter S, Marold DB, Whitesell NR, Cobbs G. A model of the effects of perceived parent and peer support on adolescent false self behavior. *Child Dev.* 1996;67:360-374.

Hunter JA, Becker JV. The role of deviant sexual arousal in juvenile sexual offending: etiology, evaluation, and treatment. *Crim Justice Behav.* 1994;21:32-149.

Hunter JA, Goodwin DW, Becker JV. The relationship between phallometrically measured deviant sexual arousal and clinical characteristics in juvenile sexual offenders. *Behav Res Ther.* 1994;32:533-538.

Introduction [transcript]. Primetime Live. *ABC News.* October 16, 2003.

Kernberg PF, Weiner AS, Bardenstein KK. *Personality Disorders in Children and Adolescents.* New York, NY: Basic Books; 2000.

Kleiner M, ed. *Handbook of Polygraph Testing.* San Diego, Calif: Academic Press; 2002:106.

Kuban M, Barbaree HE, Blanchard R. A comparison of volume and circumference phallometry: response magnitude and method agreement. *Arch Sex Behav.* 1999; 28:345-359.

Laws DR. Penile plethysmography: will we ever get it right? In: Ward T, Laws DR, Hudson SM, eds. *Sexual Deviance: Issues and Controversies.* Thousand Oaks, Calif: Sage Publications; 2003:82-102.

Laws DR, Gulayets MJ, Frenzel RR. Assessment of sex offenders using standardized slide stimuli and procedures: a multisite study. *Sex Abuse.* 1995;7:45-66.

Letourneau EJ. A comparison of objective measures of sexual arousal and interest: visual reaction time and penile plethysmography. *Sex Abuse.* 2002;14:207-224.

Lilienfeld SO, Purcell C, Jones-Alexander J. Assessment of antisocial behavior in adults. In: Stoff DM, Maser JB, Maser JD, eds. *Handbook of Antisocial Behavior.* New York, NY: John Wiley & Sons; 1997:60-74.

Marshall WL, Barbaree HE, Christophe D. Sexual offenders against female children: sexual preferences for age of victims and type of behaviour. *Can J Behav Sci.* 1986; 18:424-439.

Marshall WL, Eccles A. Issues in clinical practice with sex offenders. *J Interpers Viol.* 1991;6:68-93.

Marshall WL, Fernandez YM. *Phallometric Testing with Sexual Offenders: Theory, Research, and Practice.* Brandon, Vt: Safer Society Press; 2003.

McConaghy N. Validity and ethics of penile circumference measures of sexual arousal: a critical review. *Arch Sex Behav.* 1989;18:357-369.

McGrath RJ, Cumming GF, Burchard BL. *Current Practices and Trends in Sexual Abuser Management: the Safer Society 2002 Nationwide Survey.* Brandon, Vt: The Safer Society Foundation; 2003.

Miner MH, West MA, Day DM. Sexual preference for child and aggressive stimuli: comparison of rapists and child molesters using auditory and visual stimuli. *Behav Res Ther.* 1995;33:545-551.

Miranda AO, Corcoran CL. Comparison of perpetration characteristics between male juvenile and adult sexual offenders: preliminary results. *Sex Abuse.* 2000;12: 179-188.

Müeller U, Overton WF, Reene K. Development of conditional reasoning: a longitudinal study. *J Cogn Devel.* 2001;2:27-49.

National Research Council. *The Polygraph and Lie Detection.* Committee to Review the Scientific Evidence on the Polygraph. Division of Behavioral and Social Sciences and Education. Washington, DC: The National Academies Press; 2002.

O'Donohue WT, Letourneau EJ. A review of the psychometric properties of the penile tumescence assessment of child molesters. *J Psych Behav Assess.* 1992;14(2): 123-175.

Piaget J. Intellectual evolution from adolescence to adulthood. *Hum Dev.* 1972;15: 1-12.

Prescott DS. The History of ATSA. *Forum* (newsletter). Association for the Treatment of Sexual Abusers. Winter 2002.

Prescott DS. Emerging strategies for risk assessment of sexually abusive youth: theory, controversy, and practice. In press.

Quinsey VL, Chaplin TC, Carrigan WF. Sexual preferences among incestuous and non incestuous child molesters. *Behav Ther.* 1979;10:562-565.

Quinsey VL, Rice ME, Harris GT. Actuarial prediction of sexual recidivism. *J Interpers Viol.* 1995;10:85-105.

Rosenzweig S. The photoscope as an objective device for evaluating sexual interest. *Psychosom Med.* 1942;4:150-157.

Salekin R, Rogers R, Sewell K. A review and meta-analysis of the Psychopathy Checklist and Psychopathy Checklist-Revised: predictive validity of dangerousness. *Clin Psychol Sci Pract.* 1996;3:203-215.

Saxe L, Ben-Shakhar G. Admissibility of polygraph tests: the application of scientific standards post-Daubert. *Psychol Public Policy Law.* 1999;5:203-223.

Seagrave D, Grisso T. Adolescent development and the measurement of juvenile psychopathy. *Law Hum Behav.* 2002;26:219-239.

SEARCH. *National Conference on Sex Offender Registries: Proceedings of a BJS/ SEARCH Conference.* Washington, DC: US Dept of Justice, Office of Justice Programs, Bureau of Justice Statistics; April 1998.

Serin RC. Violent recidivism in criminal psychopaths. *Law Hum Behav.* 1996; 20:207-217.

Smith G, Fischer, L. Assessment of juvenile sexual offenders: reliability and validity of the Abel Assessment for Interest in Paraphilias. *Sex Abuse.* 1999;11:207-216.

Ware E, Brown M, Amoroso D, Pilkey D, Breusse M. The semantic meaning of pornographic stimuli for college males. *Can J Behav Sci.* 1972;4:204-209.

Wilcox DT. Application of the clinical polygraph examination to the assessment, treatment, and monitoring of sex offenders. *Sex Aggress.* 2000;5:134-152, 138.

# THE COMMERCIAL SEXUAL EXPLOITATION OF CHILDREN IN NORTH AMERICA*

Richard J. Estes, DSW, ACSW
Elena Azaola, PhD
Nicole Ives, MSW, PhD (Candidate)

Recent estimates from the US government indicate that approximately 600 000 to 800 000 people worldwide are trafficked across international borders annually, and between 14 000 and 18 000 of these victims are trafficked to the United States (USDOS, 2004). According to US law, ***trafficking*** is "the transport, harboring, or sale of persons within national or across international borders through coercion, force, kidnapping, deception or fraud, for purposes of placing persons in situations of forced labor or services, such as forced prostitution, domestic servitude, debt bondage, or other slavery-like practices" (18 USC § 1589 et seq.). Most of the victims of trafficking are women and children. Most come from less economically advanced countries or countries characterized by social chaos, such as certain countries in Asia, areas with recurrent civil and intra-regional wars, such as certain areas in Africa, or countries experiencing profound political and economic transformations, such as those in Central America, South America, and the successor states to the former Soviet Union (Bales, 1999; Barr, 1996; Basu, 2003; Budapest Group, 1999; Caldwell et al, 1997; Cockburn, 2003; Hughes, 2000; Hughes & Roche, 1999; Lederer, 2001; Shelly, 2000; United Nations, 1995, 1999; USDOS, 2003d; Williams, 1999; Yoon, 1997). However, some trafficking victims, such as Native American girls and Canadian women, are citizens or permanent residents of more economically advanced countries. Like those from less economically advanced countries, the individuals become victims of the brutality associated with forced prostitution, domestic servitude, debt bondage, and even slavery.

International trafficking in human beings is just one aspect of the commercial sexual exploitation of children (CSEC) and youth throughout the world. The commercial sexual exploitation of children includes the ***domestic trafficking*** of children (ie, the trafficking of citizens or permanent residents of a nation within their own country), child pornography, the prostitution of juveniles, and ***child sex tourism*** (ie, travel, usually across international borders, with the intention of engaging in a commercial sex act with a child) (Barnitz, 1998; Calcetas-Santos, 1999; De Albuquerque, 1999; Estes & Weiner, 2001; Klain, 1999; Pettman, 1997; Simmons, 1996; Spangenberg, 2001; UNICEF, 1996; United Nations, 1994; USDOL, 1996; WHO, 1996). These additional dimensions of CSEC are especially widespread, and child victims have extraordinary risks including physical and emotional violence.

* Partial funding in support of the research reported for the US portion of this chapter was received from the National Institute of Justice of the US Department of Justice (Grant #1999-IJ-CX-0030), the William T. Grant Foundation, the Fund for Nonviolence, the Research Foundation of the University of Pennsylvania, and the Dean's Discretionary Fund of the University of Pennsylvania School of Social Work. Additional information on the topics in this chapter can be accessed at http://caster.ssw.upenn.edu/~restes/CSEC.htm.

In an effort to understand more fully CSEC exploitation phenomenon in the 3 countries of the North American region—Canada, Mexico, and the United States (which are collectively referred to as *the region* in this chapter)—the following regionwide research and planning initiatives were undertaken between 1999 and 2003:

— The launching in 1999 of a cooperative research project in the region that focused on identifying the nature, extent, and severity of CSEC in each country and within the region as a whole

— The identification of social, political, and economic factors within the region that contribute to CSEC

— An assessment of the role of international crime and criminal units in promoting CSEC in the region

— An assessment of the national and regional capacity for responding to the needs of child victims of commercial sexual exploitation

— The development of a general framework for a regional strategy to combat CSEC in North America

— The framing of recommendations for strengthening the national and regional capacity for preventing CSEC

The following show the considerable progress that has been made since 1999 in attaining each of these goals:

— Studies were completed detailing the nature, extent, and seriousness of CSEC in Mexico (Azaola, 2001, 2003a,b) and the United States (Estes & Weiner, 2001, 2003).

— Considerable understanding exists concerning the seriousness of CSEC in Canada (CISC, 2003; Senate of Canada, 1999; Tremblay, 2003).

— All 3 countries in the region have stronger and more comprehensive laws that make the earlier apprehension and prosecution of adults involved in CSEC possible, including those who benefit sexually or economically from child pornography, juvenile prostitution, and trafficking of children.

— All 3 countries have a richer array of primary, secondary, and tertiary preventive services for child victims of commercial sexual exploitation, albeit these services require additional elaboration, more secure funding, and better integration.

— All 3 countries are at least signatory members of major international agreements, declarations, and covenants relating to combating CSEC.

— All 3 countries participated in the First World Congress Against Commercial Sexual Exploitation of Children held in Stockholm in August 1996 (see http://www.csecworldcongress.org/en/stockholm/).

— All 3 countries participated actively in the First Tri-National Regional Consultation on CSEC in North America held in Philadelphia in December 2001 (Ives, 2001).

— As a follow-up to the Tri-National Regional Consultation on CSEC in North America, all 3 countries prepared national reports on CSEC and contributed to the regional report on CSEC in North America for presentation at the Second World Congress Against Commercial Sexual Exploitation of Children held in Yokohama, Japan, in December 2001 (see http://www.csecworldcongress.org/en/yokohama/).

— A series of recommendations have emerged concerning strategies for strengthening national and regional efforts to combat CSEC.

This chapter is divided into 3 parts: (1) a brief analysis of the social, political, and economic situation of the region related to CSEC; (2) the nature, extent, and seriousness of CSEC in each country in the region and a summary of the major strategies currently being used by each country to combat the epidemic; and (3) the key principles for use in framing effective national and regional strategies for combating CSEC using the Tri-National Regional Consultation on CSEC in North America as the frame of reference.

# NORTH AMERICA: THE PARADOX OF AFFLUENCE AND POVERTY

North America consists of 3 sovereign states—Canada, Mexico, and the United States. Though the structure of the economies of these countries varies, the sociopolitical structures of all 3 are remarkably similar (**Table 15-1**). For example, all 3 countries are open market democratic societies with bicameral legislatures and multiple political parties. They are all former colonies of European powers and as a result, the judicial systems reflect a mixture of Old World and New World legal principles and practices. Administratively, each country is divided into a series of states, provinces, counties, and territories, all of which develop and enforce their own laws and legal procedures. The governance structure of the United States consists of 52 separate legislative bodies (50 state legislatures, the Council of the District of Columbia, and the federal government), whereas Canada's government consists of the federal government and the legislatures of 10 provinces and 3 territories. Mexico's governance structure is organized around a strong central government, 31 states, and a federal district—Mexico City—in and around which approximately 30% of the nation's total population resides.

**Table 15-1. Selected Political and Economic Characteristics of Canada, Mexico, and the United States***

| SELECTED INDICATORS | CANADA | MEXICO | UNITED STATES |
|---|---|---|---|
| POLITICAL CHARACTERISTICS | | | |
| **Official country name** | Canada | United Mexican States | United States of America |
| **Independence date** | July 1, 1867 (from the United Kingdom) | September 15, 1810 (from Spain) | July 4, 1776 (from Great Britain) |
| **Constitution date** | April 17, 1982 (Constitution Act) | February 5, 1917 | September 17, 1787, effective March 4, 1789 |
| **Government type** | Confederation with parliamentary democracy | Federal democratic republic | Constitution-based federal republic; strong democratic tradition |
| **Administrative divisions** | 10 provinces and 3 territories | 31 states and 1 federal district | 50 states and 1 district |
| **Branches of the central government** | Bicameral legislative Parliament, judicial, and executive | Bicameral National Congress, judicial, and executive | Bicameral legislative Congress, judicial, and executive |

*(continued)*

**Table 15-1. Selected Political and Economic Characteristics of Canada, Mexico, and the United States\*** *(continued)*

| SELECTED INDICATORS | CANADA | MEXICO | UNITED STATES |
|---|---|---|---|
| **POLITICAL CHARACTERISTICS** | | | |
| **Legal system** | Based on English common law, except in Quebec, where civil law system is based on French law | Mixture of US constitutional theory and civil law system; judicial review of legislative acts | Based on English common law; judicial review of legislative acts |
| **Politically dependent territories and areas** | None | None | Multiple, mostly located in the South Pacific |
| **Political party system** | Multiple | Multiple | Multiple |
| **Suffrage** | 18 years; universal | 18 years; universal and compulsory (but not enforced) | 18 years; universal |
| **ECONOMIC CHARACTERISTICS** | | | |
| **Dominant type of economy** | Market oriented | Market oriented | Market oriented |
| Currency | Canadian dollar ($, CAD) | Mexican peso ($, MXN) | US dollar ($, USD) |
| Currency exchange rate to USD (December 2004) | 1.23 | 11.23 | 1.00 |
| **Gross domestic product (GDP) in purchasing power parity (PPP) (in USD billions, 2002 estimates); regional total = 12 308.5** | 934.1 | 924.4 | 10 450.0 |
| Inflation rate (%); regional average = 3.4 | 2.2 | 6.4 | 1.6 |
| GDP real growth rate (%); regional average = 2.1 | 3.3 | 0.7 | 2.4 |
| Per capita PPP in (USD); regional per average = 24 833 | 29 300 | 8900 | 36 300 |
| **Structure of economy by sector (%, 2002 estimates)** | | | |
| Agriculture; regional average = 3 | 2 | 5 | 2 |
| Industry; regional average = 23.7 | 27 | 26 | 18 |
| Services; regional average = 73.3 | 71 | 69 | 80 |
| **Patents granted to residents (per 100 000 population, 1999); regional average = 114.3** | 44 | 1 | 298 |

*(continued)*

**Table 15-1.** *(continued)*

| SELECTED INDICATORS | CANADA | MEXICO | UNITED STATES |
|---|---|---|---|
| ECONOMIC CHARACTERISTICS | | | |
| **Central government budget expenditures (in USD billions, 2002 estimates); regional total = 2353** | 161 | 140 | 2052 |
| Health (%); regional average = 5 | 6.6 | 2.5 | 5.8 |
| Education (%); regional average = 4.9 | 5.5 | 4.4 | 4.8 |
| Defense and military (%); regional average = 1.6 | 1.2 | 0.5 | 3.1 |
| Total debt service (%) | NA | 7.9 | NA |
| **Population below poverty line (%, 2001 estimates); regional average = 17.6** | NA | 40 | 12.7 |
| **Labor force (in millions, 2001 estimates); regional total = 198** | 16.4 | 39.8 | 141.8 |
| Unemployment rate (%, 2002 estimates); regional average = 5.5 | 7.6 | 3 | 5.8 |
| Youth unemployment rate (2002 estimates); regional average = 9.2 | 12.8 | 4.1 | 10.6 |

*\* Estimates are for the year 2003 unless otherwise indicated.*

*Data from USDOS, 2003b,c,d; United Nations Development Programme, 2003; World Bank, 2003.*

The region's population exceeds 430 million, half of which is 33 years of age or younger; the median age of Mexico's population is even younger—24 years. Children younger than 14 years currently comprise approximately 24% of the region's total population—approximately 103 million boys and girls. Unfortunately, a disproportionate number of the region's children live in poverty. Official child poverty rates for the United States and Canada are 16.7% (Proctor & Dalaker, 2003) and 16.5% (Campaign, 2000; Sarlo, 2001), respectively. Child poverty rates for Mexico are higher, with 36% of children in urban areas and 70% of children in rural communities living in poverty (E. Azaola, written communication, April 2004). According to the United Nations Development Programme (UNDP), at least 24% of Mexico's total population subsists on less than 2 American dollars (2 USD) per day (UNDP, 2003). Mexican national estimates are higher, with 57% to 65% of the population living in poverty (E. Azaola, written communication, April 2004). In all 3 countries, child poverty rates are especially high for children living in single-parent and female-headed households. Aboriginal, Native American, and other children who are ethnic or racial minorities are at high risk of poverty and are especially vulnerable to economically driven sexual exploitation.

The region's racial and ethnic mix is one of the world's most heterogeneous. Certainly, North America is more diverse than other economically advanced regions (Estes, 2004, In press[a]). The region's cultural mix is a product of the first peoples who inhabited the land long before European settlers arrived in the New World, reproduction between settlers and the first peoples, and since at least 1880, large waves of migration into North America from Asia, Africa, South America, and Europe (Fairchild, 2004; Higham, 1971). The majority of new arrivals in Mexico are from

Central America and South America. (See **Table 15-2** for an overview of the population, health, and social characteristics of the countries in the region.)

In addition to differences in culture, language, and religion, each new group to arrive in North America brought with it extraordinarily innovative ways of dealing with the physical, social, and economic challenges confronting its new world. As a result, the level of technological innovation that characterizes North America, which is measured by the number of patents granted to residents, is unparalleled compared with other world regions. The region's wealth, moderate rates of inflation, and by European standards, comparatively low levels of unemployment are also remarkable. However, youth unemployment and underemployment remain significant problems for out-of-school youth who lack the skills needed to compete in the region's technologically and service-based economies.

**Table 15-2. Selected Population, Health, and Social Characteristics of Canada, Mexico, and the United States***

| SELECTED INDICATORS | CANADA | MEXICO | UNITED STATES |
|---|---|---|---|
| POPULATION CHARACTERISTICS | | | |
| **Population (in millions); regional total = 427.4** | 32.2 | 104.9 | 290.3 |
| Population growth rate (%); regional average = 1.1 | 0.94 | 1.4 | 0.92 |
| Birth rate (%); regional average = 15.7 | 11.0 | 21.9 | 14.1 |
| Total fertility rate (children born per woman); regional average = 2.1 | 1.6 | 2.5 | 2.1 |
| Net migration rate per 1000 population; regional average = 2.3 | 6.01 | -2.7 | 3.52 |
| Median age (years); regional average = 32.5 | 37.8 | 23.8 | 35.8 |
| **Age structure (%)** | | | |
| 0-14 yr; regional average = 23.9 | 18.5 | 32.3 | 20.9 |
| 15-64 yr; regional average = 66.1 | 68.6 | 63.1 | 66.7 |
| ≥65 yr; regional average = 10 | 12.9 | 4.6 | 12.4 |
| **Racial and ethnic mix**[†] **(%)** | | | |
| White | NA | 9 | 77 |
| *British Isle origin* | 28 | NA | NA |
| *French origin* | 23 | NA | NA |
| *Other European* | 15 | NA | NA |
| Black | NA | NA | 12 |
| Mestizo (Amerindian-Spanish) | NA | 60 | NA |
| Amerindian and Alaska Native | 2 | 30 | 2 |
| Asian | NA | NA | 4 |
| Other (primarily Asian, African, and Arab) | 6 | NA | NA |
| Native Hawaiian and Pacific Islander | NA | NA | <1 |
| Other | 26 | 1 | 4 |

*(continued)*

**Table 15-2.** *(continued)*

| SELECTED INDICATORS | CANADA | MEXICO | UNITED STATES |
|---|---|---|---|
| HEALTH AND SOCIAL CHARACTERISTICS | | | |
| **Infant mortality rate per 1000 live births; regional average = 12.1** | 4.9 | 23.7 | 7.8 |
| **Life expectancy at birth (Years)** | | | |
| Females; regional average = 79.6 | 83.4 | 75.5 | 80 |
| Males; regional average = 73.4 | 76.4 | 69.3 | 74.4 |
| **Number of physicians per 100 000 population (2002 estimates); regional average = 195.3** | 186 | 130 | 276 |
| **Per capita health expenditures (in USD) (PPP, $, 2000 estimates); regional average = 2503.3** | 2534 | 477 | 4499 |
| **HIV/AIDS (2001 estimates)** | | | |
| HIV/AIDS adult prevalence rate (%); regional average = 0.4 | 0.3 | 0.3 | 0.6 |
| Number of people living with HIV/AIDS; regional total = 1 105 000 | 55 000 | 150 000 | 900 000 |
| Number of HIV/AIDS deaths; regional total = 19 700 | <500 | 4200 | 15 000 |
| **Literacy rate (%); regional average = 95.3** | 97 | 92 | 97 |
| **Crime victimization rate (% of total population)** | | | |
| All crimes (%); regional average = 22.5 | 23.8 | NA | 21.1 |
| Sexual assaults (%); regional average = 0.6 | 0.8 | NA | 0.4 |
| **Gender equality measure (GEM); regional average = 0.87** | 0.93 | 0.79 | 0.94 |

*\* 2003 estimates unless otherwise indicated.*

*† A separate listing for Hispanics is not included for the United States, because the US Census Bureau considers a **Hispanic** person to be a person of Latin American descent—of Cuban, Mexican, or Puerto Rican origin—living in the United States who may belong to any race or ethnic group, such as white, black, or Asian.*

*Data Sources: USDOS, 2003b,c,d; United Nations Development Programme, 2003; World Bank 2003.*

With the exception of certain sectors of development in Mexico, social development in the region is comparable to that found in Europe, Australia and New Zealand, Japan, and other economically advanced countries and regions (Estes, 2004, In press[a]). For the majority of the region's residents, access to primary healthcare and at least primary education explains the region's highly favorable patterns of life expectancy, comparatively low rates of infant and child mortality, and high levels of youth and adult literacy. However, poverty, income inequality, and gender inequality remain 3 issues on the region's social agenda (Estes, 2002; UNDP, 2003). Certainly, the concentration of such a disproportionate share of the region's annually generated wealth in the hands of a relative minority of its population—24% of household income earners in Canada, 41% in Mexico, and 31% in the United States—remains an anomaly among economically advanced regions.

The paradoxes associated with the region's pattern of extreme wealth and extreme poverty is known to play a role in CSEC, especially in Mexico, where the majority of children who engage in pornography, prostitution, and trafficking use survival sex and other sex-for-money exchanges because of familial poverty (Azaola, 2001; 2003a,b; Azaola & Estes, 2003). Poverty is a major factor that contributes to CSEC in Canada and the United States though a history of sexual abuse, family breakdown, recurrent school failure, chronic drug use, running away from home, and other factors combined with poverty can increase the risk for sexual victimization for many children (Azaola & Estes, 2003). The role of nonfinancial factors is especially important for understanding the sexual exploitation of children from middle-income and upper-income households in the United States and Canada.

# COMMERCIAL SEXUAL EXPLOITATION OF CHILDREN IN THE REGION

Knowledge concerning the extent of CSEC in the region is derived from various sources, including the following:

— Reviews of the relevant studies pertaining to CSEC in North America (Estes, 2001; Estes & Weiner, 2001)

— Reports of original research conducted by the chapter's authors in each of the region's countries (Azaola, 2001; 2003a,b; Azaola & Estes, 2003; Estes, 2002; Estes & Weiner, 2001, 2003; Tremblay, 2003)

— Background papers and other formal analyses prepared by representatives of governmental and nongovernmental organizations (NGOs) in preparation for the Stockholm (1996) and Yokohama (2001) world summits on CSEC (F/P/T Working Group on Prostitution, 1998; Hecht, 2001; Davidson, 1996, 2001, 2004; Senate of Canada, 1999)

— Background reports prepared by representatives of governmental and nongovernmental organizations in preparation for the 2001 Tri-National Regional Consultation on CSEC in Philadelphia

— An executive summary of the Tri-National Regional Consultation (Ives, 2001)

— Anecdotal reports concerning CSEC in North America provided by youth who are child victims of CSEC, human service workers, law enforcement officials, field investigators, and others working directly with commercially sexually exploited youth and their families

## COMMERCIAL SEXUAL EXPLOITATION OF CHILDREN IN CANADA

Precise estimates of the number of child victims of CSEC are unavailable for Canada. However, child pornography, the prostitution of juveniles, and domestic and international trafficking of children for sexual purposes are known to represent serious problems for the country (F/P/T Working Group on Prostitution, 1998; Senate of Canada, 1999). As a result, important initiatives have been launched by the Canadian authorities with the dual goals of identifying child victims of sexual exploitation and apprehending the adults that prey on these children (CISC, 2003). Indeed, Canada's recent CSEC-related legislative reforms and service innovations have influenced similar developments in the United States and Mexico.

### Profiles of the Children

As with other sexually exploited children, a prior history of sexual abuse, family dysfunction, poverty, drug use, and poor school performance are recurring themes in the lives of sexually exploited children in Canada (F/P/T Working Group on Prostitution, 1998; Kingsley, 2000; Senate of Canada, 1999). Homeless youth in Canada, referred to as "street children," are particularly vulnerable to sexual exploitation, especially youth who live on the streets in the country's larger cities, such as Montreal, Toronto, Vancouver, and to a lesser extent, Windsor (F/P/T Working Group on Prostitution, 1998; Senate of Canada, 1999). Recent stories in the media have focused on the problem of juvenile prostitution in these cities (Guilty 'john,' 2002; Lopinto, 2002; Quebec City sex trial, 2003). As in the United States, survival sex is common among Canadian homeless children. Regardless of the socioeconomic status of their family of origin, once children are living on the streets, they have no predictable means of financial support and, therefore, are considered poor. In Montreal, data confirm the existence of networks of gay men who recruit and refer sexually exploited children to other members of the network and organized sex crime rings (Tremblay, 2003). Nationally and internationally organized crime groups appear to play a significant role in the commercial sexual exploitation of Canadian children (CISC, 2003; F/P/T Working Group on Prostitution, 1998).

National estimates of the numbers of commercially sexually exploited children and youth in Canada do not exist, and no specific data are available regarding the various subgroups of children at the national level who are believed to be especially vulnerable to sexual exploitation, such as runaway and abandoned children, other homeless children, and children who are members of racial, ethnic, or sexual minority groups (eg, gay boys, transgender boys and girls, boys and girls with confused sexual identities). However, the national incidence rates are available for 8 separate categories of child sexual abuse in Canada (Publications—incidence studies, 2004). The number of Canadian children apprehended for prostitution is difficult to estimate because prostitution-related activities can be categorized as other types of crimes to protect children from the stigma associated with prostitution (F/P/T Working Group on Prostitution, 1998). However, some studies suggest that certain Canadian children become involved in commercial sexual exploitation at as young as 6 to 8 years old though the vast majority become involved in prostitution after puberty. The average age of entry of Canadian youth into prostitution is between 13 and 15 years (Ouimet, 1997). Other reports confirm that at least 10% to 15% of all street persons engaging in prostitution in Canada are youth younger than the age of 18 (Senate of Canada, 1999).

## Profiles of the Exploiters

Sexual exploiters of children in Canada encompass the full spectrum of people as identified by Davidson (1996, 2001, 2004), including pedophiles, preferential child sex abusers, **_situational child sex abusers_** (ie, persons who take advantage of selected situations to sexually exploit children, usually while in transit during which a high level of anonymity may be possible), transients (eg, military personnel, seamen, truckers, migrant laborers, traveling businesspeople, sex tourists), expatriates, local clients, aid workers, and employers of domestic workers. Exploiters are not just men. Women and other children, including runaway and homeless children, are exploiters of Canadian children (Kingsley, 2000). Sexual exploiters of children in Canada include members of virtually all social classes, educational and income levels, and occupational groups; some are even married men that have children who are the same ages as their child victims (Ives, 2001; Senate of Canada, 1999).

The Canadian federal government is in the process of upgrading the databases used by the Canadian Police Information Centre (CISC, 2003). Once completed, these upgrades should make possible the construction of more complete pictures of the many types of adult sex offenders known to police authorities. At a minimum, the databases will provide detailed information concerning the sociodemographic profiles of adult sex offenders, their records of convictions, and their recidivism rates after being released. The databases should identify the subset of adult sexual offenders that targets children and youth for sex crimes including CSEC.

## Trafficking

The sexual trafficking of children in Canada is a problem. Trafficking involves nationals of Canada as well as the citizens of other countries who are trafficked into Canada (Kingsley, 2000). The majority of people trafficked into Canada for sexual purposes come from China, Thailand, Cambodia, the Philippines, Russia, Korea, and Eastern Europe (USDOS, 2003a). Sexual trafficking of children appears to be an especially serious problem in Canada's larger cities. Reports in the media indicate that small numbers of children from the United States are abducted and taken into

Canada, albeit the dominant trafficking pattern involves the use of Canada as a transit country into the United States for the nationals of other countries (USDOS, 2003a).

In June 2002, Canada implemented a new Immigration and Refugee Protection Act (IRPA) that significantly enhances the ability of the central government to apprehend and prosecute traffickers. The IRPA imposes tougher sentences for those convicted of participating in trafficking activities. The law references the "best interests of the child," expands the definition of dependent child, and clarifies certain provisions related to international adoptions in which children could be at risk for sexual and other forms of exploitation. The trafficking provisions of the IRPA provide for penalties ranging up to $1 million and imprisonment for life (CHHD, 2004).

## National Legislation

Child welfare legislation in Canada is province based, and criminal law has national applications; therefore, offenses pertaining to CSEC are criminal offenses throughout Canada (CISC, 2003). All cases involving child sexual exploitation carry steep legal sanctions, and repeat offenders face large fines and long jail sentences. These penalties apply to crimes of a sexual nature that involve children under the age of 18 years. Furthermore, penalty severity is directly related to the age disparity between the child victims and their adult exploiters; for example, a more substantial penalty is imposed on a 30-year-old exploiting a juvenile than on an exploiter who is younger than 25 years. Similar offense and age disparity penalties are reflected in the statutes of most Canadian provinces. Some jurisdictions, such as Ontario as of April 2001, mandate registration of sexual offenders with local police.

Canadian federal law prohibits profiting from the commercial sexual exploitation of individuals 18 years of age and younger. Recent laws have expanded and prohibit aiding, abetting, counseling, compelling, or luring those younger than 18 years into prostitution. The penalties are especially severe for those who use coercion, force, or threats to compel children to engage in prostitution, pornography, and sexual trafficking.

Canadian law prohibits Canadian citizens and permanent residents from participating in international sex tourism. Recently adopted laws related to CSEC, including Bill C-15A, contain extraterritorial and extradition provisions that make it possible for Canadian federal authorities to cooperate with police authorities of other nations to apprehend Canadian nationals who travel abroad and engage in sex with persons younger than the legal age of sexual consent of the host country (IBCR, 2000).

The Canadian criminal code offers legal protection to children 14 years of age or older who engage in nonexploitative sexual behavior (eg, people below the age of legal sexual consent engaged in noncommercial sexual relationships with one another). The code delineates the circumstances under which a child may legally consent to sexual activity and identifies the types of defenses that may be applicable to such offenses.

Almost all of Canada's sweeping legislative and programmatic reforms regarding CSEC are consistent with the nation's commitment to implement as fully as possible the 1996 Stockholm Declaration and Agenda for Action to Combat the Commercial Sexual Exploitation of Children and its own recently developed National Strategy to Combat CSEC (CHHD, 2004; Senate of Canada, 1999).

## Law Enforcement

Reliable estimates of the numbers of child victims of sexual exploitation are difficult to obtain because different ages are associated with each type of sexual offense. For example, according to the Young Offenders Act, a ***young person*** is defined as younger than 18 years, a guideline consistent with Parliament's view that prostitution of children younger than age 18 constitutes sexual exploitation. However, the comparatively few children who are charged formally with prostitution-related offenses, even when arrested for engaging in commercial sexual activities, likely reflects preferences on the part of arresting officials to assign a reduced stigma-evoking arrest code to children younger than 18 years of age. Such practices are consistent with the Canadian view that youth engaging in commercial sex work are victims, not criminals; therefore, children engaging in prostitution should not be arrested unless it is the only way to keep them safe. The net result of these policies is an underestimation of the number of children involved in prostitution and other types of sex-for-money exchanges.

To coordinate efforts at the national and provincial levels, the Criminal Intelligence Service of Canada (CISC) initiated a nationally coordinated law enforcement strategy relating to CSEC. Made up of about 380 law enforcement member agencies, the CISC strategy assigns priority to child pornography, prostitution of children, and sex tourism. Implementation of the strategy is carried out through partnerships with the Royal Canadian Mounted Police (RCMP), the Canada Customs and Revenue Agency (CCRA), other federal departments, provincial and municipal police forces, and American and international agencies, including the International Criminal Police Organization (Interpol). To date, these coordinated efforts have proven effective in identifying and apprehending adult offenders in all areas associated with CSEC.

### Prevention, Prosecution, and Protection Programs

Educational programs explain that using youth for sexual purposes is child sexual abuse. These programs have had a positive impact on changing public attitudes toward exploited youth in Alberta, British Columbia, Nova Scotia, Ontario, and Saskatchewan. Specialized Police Prostitution Units have been established in British Columbia and Ontario and have contributed to the development of training modules for use with police and judges in other provinces. These modules seem to be changing the attitudes of judicial authorities toward sexually exploited children; many authorities have classified children as victims of CSEC rather than as criminals. In Victoria, British Columbia, an effective NGO—the Prostitute Empowerment, Education, and Resource Society (PEERS)—provides peer-based outreach, support, advocacy, and educational services to children and youth who want to leave sex work. Child-focused programs in Nova Scotia have developed witness protection program models for youth who want to leave prostitution and are willing to provide evidence against their pimps and traffickers.

In addition to educating Canadian youth and the general public about the dangers of CSEC, numerous human service organizations in Canada address child sexual exploitation issues. Many of these programs have developed outreach services for street youth and offer emergency housing, healthcare, and other types of temporary assistance to youth at high risk for exploitation. Increasingly, human service organizations with more secure funding can offer sexually exploited children a more comprehensive spectrum of long-term services to help them reestablish themselves in society, including chemical addiction and psychiatric rehabilitation services, long-term housing, education, job training, and when appropriate and possible, family reunification services. A listing of organizations that serve sexually exploited children in Canada is continuously updated by Child Find Manitoba and can be accessed at http://www.cybertip.ca/childfind/cybertip/1230.html.

### Child Pornography and Online Sexual Victimization

Child pornography is defined in Canada's criminal code as (1) a photographic, a film, a video, or another visual representation that advocates or counsels on sexual activity with a person younger than 18 years, regardless of whether the image was made by electronic or mechanical means, or (2) any written material or visual representation that advocates or counsels sexual activity with a person younger than 18 years. Individuals can be prosecuted for producing, distributing, selling, or being in the possession of child pornography, as well as for sending these materials to others through the postal mail or the Internet.

In March 2001, Bill C-15A, an Act to amend the Criminal Code and other Acts, was introduced into the House of Commons and became effective in July 2002. The bill strengthens Canada's national capacity to carry out the following tasks:

— Combat cyber crime

— Create a new offense that targets the luring and exploitation of children for sexual purposes via the Internet

— Make it a crime to transmit, make available, export, or access child pornography on the Internet

— Allow judges to order the deletion of child pornography on the Internet

— Authorize the seizure of materials or equipment used in the creation of electronic child pornography

— Enable judges to keep known sex offenders away from children through prohibition orders and 1-year peace bonds for offenses relating to electronic child pornography

— Amend the sex tourism law to make it easier to prosecute Canadians who sexually assault children abroad

Anticipation of the bill's adoption led to a sharp increase in the number of requests to Canadian federal authorities for assistance in investigating electronic and other forms of child pornography—from 245 in 2000 to 419 in 2001 to more than 900 in 2002. The majority of these requests for investigative assistance originated from national and international law enforcement agencies and hotlines that have been established in Canada for reporting suspected sex crimes against children (CISC, 2003). Suspected cases of child pornography or child sexual exploitation may be reported for investigation to the CyberTip at http://www.cybertip.ca. The bill amends the law regarding written child pornography for personal use and strengthens the range of sentencing options available to judges in cases involving child pornography.

### The Private Sector

Canada's private sector plays an important role in combating CSEC. CSEC-related activities of Canada's private sector include public education (eg, Beyond Borders, Manitoba; N'Dah Yah Win, Winnipeg; Project Intervention Prostitution Quebec, Quebec); advocacy and lobbying (eg, Beyond Borders, Manitoba; Horizons for Youth, Toronto); research (eg, Beyond Borders, Manitoba; Children and Youth Protection Strategy, Vancouver; Save the Children Canada, Toronto); training (eg, Children and Youth Protection Strategy, Vancouver), and most importantly for child victims of sexual exploitation, the provision of psychosocial and other supportive services (eg, Covenant House, Vancouver; PEERS, Victoria; Maison Marie Frederic, Quebec; Phoenix House, Halifax). The Beyond Borders Web site home page (http://www.beyondborders.org), which is the Canadian affiliate of End Child Prostitution, Child Pornography and Trafficking of Children for Sexual Purposes (ECPAT) International, includes links to many types of Canadian organizations involved in protecting children from sexual exploitation.

The majority of Canada's CSEC services are provided by private organizations and, in turn, are through private, often sectarian, resources. However, given the complex and generally long-term care needs of sexually exploited children, many private organizations have found it necessary and beneficial to partner with Canada's large public child welfare and health sectors to provide for these children. Thus, many of Canada's private programs for child victims of sexual exploitation receive a substantial share of their total funding from public sources, as do programs in the United States and Mexico.

COMMERCIAL SEXUAL EXPLOITATION OF CHILDREN IN MEXICO
Recent studies of CSEC in Mexico found that a minimum of 16 000 children per year are commercially sexually exploited (Azaola, 2001, 2003a,b). This number of identifiable cases of CSEC has been traced to familial poverty, a history of exploitation by family members or family friends, juvenile participation in survival sex, recruitment of children into sex-related work by organized criminal networks, and trafficking of children for sexual purposes into Mexico from less developed regions and countries, including Central and South America. The combination of the following other factors in cities such as Ciudad Juarez and Tijuana create an environment that encourages the local sex trade:

— The flow into urban centers of people who have no or few job skills but need an income

— The demand for sexual services from children by locals and people who are in transit and not with their families

— Tourists who cross international borders into Mexico with the specific intention of engaging in sex with children

The human service and law enforcement infrastructures of these cities are insufficient to meet the needs of the sexually exploited children who often are abandoned and left to live on the streets (Azaola, 2001, 2003a).

Sexually exploited children are at considerable risk for contracting sexually transmitted diseases (STDs). STDs are common among street youth in Mexico and typically are the result of repeated unprotected sexual experiences in settings other than legally registered adult brothels. The unregulated nature of juvenile prostitution in Mexico compounds the ability of local health officials to track and treat infected youth, the majority of whom receive little or no medical attention for STDs or other acute or chronic illnesses.

Profiles of the Children
Boys and girls involved in commercial sexual exploitation have been found as young as 8 years old though the majority range in age from 12 to 17 (Azaola 2001, 2003a,b; IIN, 2000). The background and status of children who are being exploited have several factors in common in the categories of abuse history, familial circumstances, at-risk status, and socioeconomic status (Calcetas-Santos, 1998; CDHDF, 1996). For example, the Observation Centre for Young Offenders in Guadalajara found the most important predictor of child sexual exploitation to be having at least one alcoholic parent, often a stepfather, in combination with recurrent violent behavior within the home. In many cases, the prostitution of children is actively promoted by family members (Azaola, 2001, 2003a).

The pervasiveness of drug use among street youth has become a central component of the exploitation of children in Mexico. Children who have become addicted to drugs before being exploited often become prostitutes to make enough money to support their addictions (Azaola, 2003a,b; Negrete, 2001). Poverty plays an important role in exploitation, especially in rural and urban poor families, who must struggle daily with deteriorating living conditions (Leñero, 1998). Regardless, many prostituted children are from middle-class backgrounds (Azaola, 2001, 2003a). For example, in cities throughout Mexico, groups of adolescent girls from higher socioeconomic backgrounds are routinely exploited by organizations and tour group operators who arrange private parties that include sex between the children and the visitors.

Profiles of the Exploiters
Child sexual exploiters in Mexico include temporary farm workers, illegal immigrants, ***polleros*** (traffickers of illegal immigrants over the border), truck drivers, traveling businessmen, military personnel and seamen, and men who have no fam-

ilies or are not with their families. Indeed, some of these men and many child victims have been brought to Mexico as illegal migrants or victims of trafficking via various transit zones on Mexico's southern border (Azaola, 2001, 2003b). Thus, the absence of social roots, a manifestation of social anomie, contributes to the contemporary child exploitation situation in Mexico (Azaola, 2001). The majority of men belonging in these groups are situational abusers and include tourists and conventioneers (Ruiz Torres, 2003).

Pedophiles and *preferential child sex abusers*, those who specifically target children as their preferred sexual "partners," frequently come to Mexico as tourists so that they can have sex with children (Azaola, 2003b). Though they are not authorized to provide sexual services, massage parlors, escort services, and modeling agencies promote sex with children and do so openly in the media (CDHDF, 1996). In Puerto Vallarta and Guadalajara, researchers found evidence of organized sex tourism involving boys (Azaola, 2001). Sex tourists, the majority of whom are male, often are more affluent than the children they exploit and take advantage of the destitute, abandoned, and neglected children.

Third-party exploiters benefit from the sexual exploitation of children. For example, taxi drivers play an important role in child exploitation, serving as a link between tourists and the various sex workers in their local areas. For example, they know which girls engage in sex work in the local community and are paid to transport the girls and their customers to hotels, brothels, and other locations. Some taxi drivers correctly classify themselves as pimps, whereas others claim they are protectors of children because they are helping the children economically.

## Trafficking

Mexico is an origin and a destination for victims of human trafficking. The majority of trafficking victims are Mexican nationals or the nationals of other countries in Central America. Mexico is used as a transit country on the way to the United States or Canada. Belize, El Salvador, Guatemala, and Honduras are among the primary countries of origin of those trafficked to North American cities from Central America. In addition, Mexico is a frequent point of entry for victims trafficked into the United States and Canada from Asia and Eastern Europe (Estes, In press[b]; USDOS, 2004).

Trafficking for sexual purposes is especially serious in Mexico City and the major cities and Mexican states that border the United States, such as Ciudad Juarez, Laredo, Nuevo Laredo, Tijuana, and Baja, California. People trafficked to Mexico from Central America or South America typically enter Mexico through Tapachula, Chiapas, and other southern border communities. In 2001, authorities along Mexico's southern borders turned back more than 15 000 undocumented aliens and hundreds of migrant smugglers (USDOJ, 2003). In 2002, federal police arrested the head of an international alien smuggling network (USDOS, 2003a).

Laws prohibiting international trafficking in people are in place in Mexico but are poorly enforced. Numerous binational trafficking agreements exist between Mexico and the United States and between Mexico and Canada. In some cases, they have been considerably effective; however, the majority of such cases involve the deportation back to Mexico of people who illegally enter the United States or Canada.

Services for the victims of sexual trafficking in Mexico are limited and are used by only a few of the thousands of Mexican children who become entrapped in trafficking each year. Widespread poverty, unstable public sector resources, a comparatively weak human service infrastructure, and alleged links of some local police with organized crime groups interfere with the development of a more comprehensive range of protective services for trafficking victims in Mexico.

## National Legislation

Mexico has various articles of legislation pertaining to CSEC. The federal penal code declares that procuring, facilitating, or forcing a child younger than 18 years to perform acts relating to pornography, prostitution, or consumption of narcotics or to commit criminal acts are criminal offenses punishable by at least 5 years in prison. Furthermore, the trafficking of children was recently characterized as a crime though it is not included in the legislation of all 31 Mexican states. In fact, children older than 16 years are not protected by most of Mexico's laws. A law to combat sex tourism was recently incorporated into the federal penal code. For example, an article of Mexico's criminal code makes it a criminal offense for any person to promote, advertise, invite, facilitate, or negotiate in any way the movement of a person inside or outside Mexico's national territory for the purpose of engaging in sexual relations with children younger than 18 years.

## Law Enforcement

During 1998, the Attorney's Office for Justice in Guadalajara carried out 186 preliminary investigations of the corruption of children. In 1999, 133 cases were investigated for a wide range of motives though not all investigated cases were linked to child sexual exploitation. Of a total of 319 investigations undertaken over 2 years, only 1 person was remanded for the corruption of children and 2 for luring children to prostitution (E. Azaola, written communication, April 2004). The Mexican legal system prosecutes few child sexual exploiters and brings to trial even fewer. In cases in which children press charges, the children often drop the cases because the exploiters threaten them or their families; in some instances, the exploiters pretend they are the children's benefactors. The prosecution's difficulties are compounded by the complicity of some local law enforcement officials in the sexual exploitation (Azaola, 2001, 2003a). In addition, considerable inequalities exist in the application of Mexican federal and state laws. Local law enforcement authorities, for example, can be more willing to involve themselves in halting the sex trade in poor areas than in the country's more lucrative tourist hotel zones, especially those in Acapulco, Cancun, Cozumel, and Mexico City.

## Prevention, Prosecution, and Protection Programs

The major Mexican cities where CSEC has been found to be thriving lack programmatic and institutional resources for sexually exploited children. Comparatively few public institutions exist in most Mexican communities to address the needs of homeless, street, or sexually exploited children. A few programs are helping exploited children, including the Attorney's Office for the Defense of the Child and the Woman and the Family and the Attention Centre for Border Children in Ciudad Juarez, which provides legal and psychological services for child victims who have experienced a wide range of abuse. The office and the center have collaborated to prosecute cases and together have participated in various follow-up activities with authorities in the central government to bring closure to cases involving the sexual exploitation of children. For example, El Caracol is a program in Mexico City that offers street children and youth an educational alternative by providing workshops where young people attempting to leave prostitution can acquire the knowledge, values, and skills needed to obtain mainstream employment. Casa Alianza in Mexico City offers a program designed to meet the particular needs of street children by providing outreach services, crisis centers, transition homes, and as a last resource, group homes. Comparatively few programs in Mexico offer the full range of support and treatment services needed by sexually exploited children.

## Child Pornography and Online Sexual Victimization

The use of children in pornographic material is widespread throughout Mexico (Ruíz Torres, 2003). The major players in Mexico's child pornography industry are expatriates, particularly American* and Canadian nationals, who systematically visit tourist spots for the purpose of sexually exploiting children through pornography. These expatriates collaborate with local exploiters in organized networks in which they buy children from the poorest areas of the country and then move them from one place to another, keeping the children under the influence of illegal substances to inhibit their ability to run away.

The Private Sector

The private travel and tourism industry plays a key role in Mexico's challenges with CSEC. A great deal of CSEC occurs in tourist areas, and Mexico's tourism industry is a logical source of activity. Following the international trend, 93% of CSEC activities in Mexico take place in hotels. Research on Mexican tourist areas revealed that hotel managers and other employees ignored the prostitution of children taking place in and near their own hotels. In some areas, exploited children work and live in the same hotel, as do some in Cancun's tourist zone (Azaola, 2001).

Though some advertisers in print media overtly market sex with children, some media organizations have attempted to halt such practices. Evidence shows that tolerance for child sexual exploitation is decreasing in Cancun, a major center for child sex tourists and pedophiles. Around the city, billboards and taxis display signs reading "No sex with children."

In an effort to galvanize support from the legal sector to combat CSEC, Bruce Harris, the former Latin American regional director for Casa Alianza, spoke at the November 2001 conference of the International Bar Association, which was held in Cancun. Approximately 2500 lawyers representing 158 countries, including 500 delegates from the United States, heard Harris's presentation on the international trafficking of children in Central America. He called for lawyers at the conference to make an effort to eliminate the trafficking of infants and children. Though the message was effective, considerable progress must be made to halt the flow of sexually exploited children into Mexico from Central America and from Mexico into Canada and the United States.

## COMMERCIAL SEXUAL EXPLOITATION OF CHILDREN IN THE UNITED STATES

Estes (2002) refers to the number of American children involved in commercial sexual exploitation as a "silent emergency," a largely unseen but significant problem that affects all aspects of social life in the United States. Estimates of the number of commercially sexually exploited children in the United States range from as few as 2000 to more than 300 000. The lower estimates are the result of combined national survey data obtained from Federal Bureau of Investigation (FBI) juvenile arrest records (Snyder, 2003) and preliminary results from the *Second National Incidence Studies of Missing, Abducted, Runaway, and Thrownaway Children* (NISMART-2). The NISMART-2 comprised 4 separate studies: (1) the National Household Survey of Adult Caretakers, (2) the National Household Survey of Youth, (3) the Juvenile Facilities Study, and (4) the Law Enforcement Study (Hammer et al, 2002; OJJDP, 2002; Sedlak et al, 2002). The higher estimates were generated by Estes & Weiner's (2001, 2003) national survey of American children and youth who were at high risk for being commercially sexually exploited, such as those who were runaways, thrownaways, otherwise homeless, or victims of domestic and international trafficking. Consistent with other local and national studies of child homelessness and CSEC (Goldman & Wheeler, 1986; Greene et al, 1999; Hofstede, 1999; Jaffe & Rosen, 1996; Lucas & Hackett, 1995; NCH, 1999, 2001; NCMEC, 2002; US Conference of Mayors, 2003), Estes and Weiner found that a very high proportion of children

---

* The term American *is used to refer to citizens or permanent residents of the United States.*

living in vulnerable and unstable situations used survival sex and other types of sex-for-money exchanges to obtain money for material needs, including food, shelter, clothing, transportation, and drugs.

## Profiles of the Children

In chapter 5 of this volume, The Commercial Sexual Exploitation of Children in the United States, Estes and Weiner identified 14 groups of American children at special risk of commercial sexual exploitation (**Table 15-3**). Though poverty is a significant factor in the commercial sexual exploitation of particular groups of American children—especially children from impoverished homes and children who run away from middle-income and high-income households and become poor when they begin living in the streets—other factors can be associated with the sexual exploitation of other groups of children. For example, the following factors are closely associated with the commercial sexual victimization of sexually abused children who continue to live in their own homes; children self identified as "gay" who engage in sex-for-money exchanges; American children who cross international borders in pursuit of alcohol, drugs, and sex; and foreign children who were brought into the United States legally but whose visas expired, subsequently causing them to join the ranks of the street children:

— Family dysfunction, including parents who are unstable, have a serious mental illness, or abuse drugs or alcohol

— A history of being physically or sexually abused or sexually assaulted as a child, which may encompass family child sexual abuse, serious depression, substance abuse, and recurrent mental illnesses

— The promotion of the prostitution of children by individuals such as parents, older siblings, and boyfriends or girlfriends

— Immaturity and poor sexual decision making by vulnerable children and youth, many of whom abuse drugs or alcohol

— Participation in criminal and other deviant behaviors that place children at higher risk of sexual exploitation

— The use of survival sex and prostitution to obtain money for their subsistence needs

— Preexisting adult prostitution markets in communities with numerous street youth

— Males without regular sexual partners living in the community or transiting between communities (eg, members of the military, truckers, conventioneers, tourists)

— For some girls, relationships with boyfriends who later reveal that they are pimps or traffickers

— Organized criminal networks that engage in numerous illegal activities—primarily drug involvement, thefts, and money laundering—as well as prostitution and the trafficking of children and women for sexual purposes

— The organized trafficking of domestic children and women for sexual purposes within countries (when trafficked, men appear to be used more for the conveyance of drugs or as laborers in sweat shops and other unregulated businesses)

— The trafficking of children and women for sexual purposes across international borders

— For some girls, membership in gangs

**Table 15-3. Children from Mexico and the United States\* Assessed to be at Special Risk for Commercial Sexual Exploitation (2000-2001)**

| AT-RISK GROUPS | STATISTICAL ESTIMATES OF CHILDREN AT RISK OF CSEC | |
|---|---|---|
| | MEXICO[†] | UNITED STATES[‡] |
| **GROUP A:** **SEXUALLY EXPLOITED CHILDREN NOT LIVING IN THEIR OWN HOMES** | | |
| A-1   Runaway children (from home) | A survey of 100 cities,[§] found approximately 114 000 children working in the streets in Mexico, of which 9000 were living in the streets. | 121 911 |
| A-2   Runaway children (from group foster homes or juvenile and other institutions) | | 6793 |
| A-3   Thrownaway children | | 51 602 |
| A-4   Homeless children (not elsewhere counted) | | 27 972 |
| **GROUP B:** **SEXUALLY EXPLOITED CHILDREN LIVING IN THEIR OWN HOMES** | | |
| B-1   Children ages 10-17 living in the general population | In 2000, 1044 cases of sexual abuse were reported to and substantiated by Mexican authorities, of which 110 were confirmed to be CSEC.[‖] | 72 621 |
| B-2   Children ages 10-17 living in public housing | | 4447 |
| **GROUP C:** **OTHER GROUPS OF SEXUALLY EXPLOITED CHILDREN** | | |
| C-1   Female gang members | Not available | 5400 |
| C-2   Transgender street youth | Not available | 3000 |
| **GROUP D:** **INTERNATIONAL DIMENSIONS OF SEXUALLY EXPLOITED AMERICAN CHILDREN IN THE UNITED STATES AND TRAVELING ABROAD** | | |
| D-1   Foreign children ages 10-17 brought into the United States *legally* who become victims of sexual exploitation | Not applicable | 3000 |
| D-2   Foreign children ages 10-17 brought into the United States *illegally* who become victims of sexual exploitation | Not applicable | 8500 |
| D-3   Unaccompanied minors entering the United States on their own who become victims of sexual exploitation | Not applicable | 2500 |

*(continued)*

**Table 15-3.** *(continued)*

| At-Risk Groups | Statistical Estimates of Children At Risk of CSEC | |
| --- | --- | --- |
| | Mexico | United States |

**GROUP D:**
**INTERNATIONAL DIMENSIONS OF SEXUALLY EXPLOITED AMERICAN CHILDREN IN THE UNITED STATES AND TRAVELING ABROAD**

| | | | |
| --- | --- | --- | --- |
| D-4 | Nonimmigrant children ages 10-17 crossing into a neighboring country for sexual purposes | Approximately 2500 | 2500 |
| D-5 | American youth ages 13-17 living within driving distance of a Mexican or Canadian city | Not applicable | 14 329 |
| D-6 | Nonimmigrant American youth ages 13-17 trafficked from the United States to other countries for sexual purposes | Not applicable | 1000 |
| | TOTAL ALL CASES | 16 000 | 244 181 |

*\* A national incidence study of CSEC in Canada has yet to be undertaken; however, see Tremblay (2003) for a detailed report of current patterns of child recruitment and sexual exploitation among adult pedophiles residing in Quebec province. In addition, numerous official studies of CSEC have been conducted by selected Canadian federal work groups (Senate of Canada, 1999). Data concerning juvenile prostitution are available for selected Canadian cities (CISC, 2003; F/P/T Working Group on Prostitution, 1998). Also, as noted by Kingsley (2000), disproportionate numbers of Canadian aboriginal children become victims of commercial sexual exploitation (Senate of Canada, 1999).*

*† Numerical data reported are based on field research in 7 Mexican cities: Acapulco, Cancun, Ciudad Juarez, Guadalajara, Mexico City, Tapachula, and Tijuana. However, the national incidence of CSEC in Mexico is known to be higher than that reported for these cities (Azaola, 2001, 2003a,b; Azaola & Estes, 2003).*

*‡ The estimates are based on a combination of in-depth surveys of 17 US metropolitan areas—Chicago, Dallas-Ft. Worth, Detroit, El Paso, Honolulu, Las Vegas, Los Angeles, Miami, New Orleans, New York, Oakland, Philadelphia, San Antonio, San Diego, San Francisco, San Jose, and Seattle—and statistical generalizations using national data sets of runaway, thrownaway, and otherwise homeless children and youth (Estes & Weiner, 2001, 2003; NRS Statistics, 2000; RHYMIS, 2004; Sedlak et al, 2002; US Conference of Mayors, 2003).*

*§ Comisión Nacional de Accion en Favor de la Infancia, 2001.*

*|| According to Azaola (written communication, April 2004), these "official numbers" must be regarded as preliminary inasmuch as "very few cases [of child sexual abuse, including the CSEC] come to the knowledge of authorities and because the registers [of suspected cases of child sexual abuse] are poor ... and not trustful."*

## Profiles of the Exploiters

From interviews with child victims, law enforcement officials, and human service professionals, Estes & Weiner (2001) identified groups of people who are more frequently associated with the sexual exploitation of children. It is useful to distinguish between (1) sexual exploiters of children living in their own homes (ie, exploitation associated primarily with child sexual abuse\* and child sexual assaults†) and (2) sexual exploiters of children not living in their own homes (ie, commercial sexual exploitation associated with runaway, thrownaway, and other homeless children who engage in survival sex and other types of commercial sexual exchanges).

---

*\* **Child sexual abuse** refers to illegal sexual activity involving persons younger than 18 years of age. The abusers are often adults, and the abuse includes activities such as rape and molestation, pornography, and the intentional exposure of children to the sexual acts of others (Goldstein, 1999; USDHHS, 2003a,b).*

*† **Child sexual assault** refers to any sexual act with a person younger than 18 years of age. The act is (1) forcible, against the person's will, or both or (2) not forcible or against the person's will but that occurs when the victim is incapable of giving consent because of a temporary or permanent mental or physical incapacity. Child sexual assault includes forcible rape, forcible sodomy, sexual assault with an object, and forcible fondling (National Incident-Based Reporting System [NIBRS] as cited in Snyder 2000; USDOJ, 2003).*

*Sexual Exploiters of Children Living in Their Own Homes*
— Though the numbers are beginning to decrease (Jones & Finkelhor, 2001), approximately 87 000 confirmed cases of child sexual abuse occur in the United States each year (USDHHS, 2003b).

— Almost all substantiated child sexual abuse occurs in the child's own home (84%).

— The majority of substantiated child sexual abuse is perpetrated against children 12 years of age or younger.

— In the majority of substantiated cases of child sexual abuse (96%), the child or the child's family knows the abuser, and the abuser may be a member of the child's own family (USDHHS, 2003a).

— Forty-nine percent of all cases of child sexual abuse involve exploitation by a neighbor, a friend of the family, a sports team coach, a religious leader, or other people known by the child or the child's family.

— Forty-seven percent of all cases of child sexual abuse involve exploitation by members of the child's own family, such as fathers, stepfathers, uncles, grand-fathers, or older siblings.

— Contrary to widely held beliefs, only 4% of substantiated child sexual abuse cases involve people who are strangers to the child.

— People older than age 18 are responsible for more substantiated cases of child sexual abuse and child sexual assaults than those younger than age 18 (USDOJ, 2003); however, perpetrators who are 18 years or older and sexually abuse young children living in their own homes are more likely to be members of the child's family.

— Perpetrators of child sexual abuse and child sexual assaults include men, women, and other juveniles (USDHHS, 2003a; USDOJ, 2003).

— Males initiated 62% of all confirmed cases of sexual abuse against children.

— Males and females acting together were responsible for 29% of all confirmed cases of child sexual abuse.

— Women were responsible for 9% of all confirmed cases of child sexual abuse.

— Comparatively few cases of child sexual abuse or child sexual assault have a commercial nexus and rarely involve commercial sexual exchanges (USDHHS, 2003a,b).

*Sexual Exploiters of Children Not Living in Their Own Homes*
Though their precise numbers are unknown, in Canada, Mexico, and the United States, the primary perpetrators of sexual victimization of children not living in their own homes include the following (Loeber & Farrington, 1998; Righthand & Welch, 2001; Snyder, 2000):

— Pedophiles

— Transient males, including members of the military, truck drivers, seasonal workers, conventioneers, and sex tourists

— Opportunistic exploiters

— Pimps

— Traffickers

— Other juveniles, including other runaway, thrownaway, and homeless youth

The sexual victimization of children not living in their own homes almost always involves strangers to the children and is usually commercial in nature; for example, the child exchanges sex with customers for money or something else commercially valuable to the child, the child's pimp, the child's traffickers, or organizations that benefit economically from CSEC, such as hotels, nightclubs, escort services, and taxi drivers.

In all 3 situations involving the sexual exploitation of children in the United States—child sexual abuse, child sexual assaults, and CSEC—the underlying dynamics of the exploitation are fundamentally the same: The exploitation is initiated by a more powerful offender, typically an adult, who exerts his or her will over a child to secure some sexual, economic, or other benefit. In situations involving CSEC, the relationship between the child victim and the exploiter is essentially economic. However, the impact on children of all 3 types of sexual exploitation is devastating. Their dignity, rights, and physical and emotional well-being are severely compromised.

Thus, child sexual abuse, child sexual assault, and CSEC form a continuum of abuse, one that is reflected in the personal histories of child victims of commercial sexual exploitation (Cauce et al, 2000; Molnar et al, 2001; Tyler & Cauce, 2002) and the children and youth who become adult prostitutes (Farley, 1998; Farley & Kelly, 2000; Ferrara, 2001; Nadon et al, 1998).

## Trafficking

The US Department of State estimates that between 14 000 and 18 000 persons, including children, are trafficked into the country each year from countries in developing Asia, Africa, Latin America, and the successor states to the former Soviet Union in Central Europe, Eastern Europe, and Central Asia (USDOS, 2004). International trafficking into the United States has become so troublesome that the State Department, as required by the Trafficking Victims Protection Act (TVPA) of 2000, has classified countries of origin—primarily Asian, African, Latin American, and Eastern European countries—*and* destination countries—primarily North American and Western European countries. They are classified into a 3-tier system that reflects each country's degree of compliance with basic laws of the United States regarding trafficking and the treatment of trafficking victims. Currently, 140 countries with a minimum of 100 confirmed internal cases of trafficking with a US nexus are included in the 3-tier classification system (USDOS, 2004):

— *Tier 1.* Countries that fully comply with the TVPA's minimum standards for the elimination of trafficking

— *Tier 2.* Countries that do not fully comply with the TVPA's minimum standards but are making efforts to bring themselves into compliance

— *Tier 2 Watch List.* Countries on Tier 2 requiring special scrutiny because of a high or increasing number of victims; failure to provide evidence of increasing efforts to combat trafficking in persons; or an assessment as Tier 2 based on commitments to take action over the next year

— *Tier 3.* Countries that neither satisfy the minimum standards nor demonstrate a significant effort to come into compliance; countries are subject to potential non-humanitarian and nontrade sanctions

Though still in its initial stages of development, the system has proven highly effective as a diplomatic tool for the State Department as it works with other governments to reduce trafficking worldwide (Bishop, 2003). Significant sanctions can be imposed by the State Department on tier 3 countries of origin and transit countries that consistently fail to take measures to halt international trafficking from their territories into the United States. Sanctions include withholding non-humanitarian, non–trade-related assistance from the United States and international financial institutions including the World Bank and International Monetary Fund.

The United States spends more than $70 million annually to halt the influx of trafficking victims from other countries (USDOS, 2004). The majority of this money is awarded to private organizations that serve trafficking victims directly, albeit increasingly higher levels of funding are being allocated to investigations and prosecutions.

The United States is in the early stages of eliminating the trafficking of women and children into the country. Indeed, during 2003 the majority of people officially certified as victims of severe forms of trafficking were men—54%, or 81 of 151 certifications granted; only 4% of such certifications were granted to minors (International Rescue Committee, 2004). Those certified as victims by the US Department of Health and Human Services are entitled to the same services and financial benefits available to refugees other than the Reception and Placement Program. Certification is required for receiving a *T-visa*, which permits trafficking victims to remain in the United States. Current enforcement efforts appear to be hampered by a serious lack of information about trafficking overall and information concerning the various ways in which trafficked women and children are moved across the United States once they enter the country. A better understanding is needed concerning the role of foreign organized crime units in national and international trafficking (Hughes, 2000; Interpol, 2003; Richard, 1999; Shelly, 2000). A continuing series of national and international conferences, news media stories, high-profile arrests, and formal public education efforts have helped bring the issues of child sexual exploitation and child sexual trafficking to the nation's attention (Cockburn, 2003; Critchell, 2003; Landesman, 2004; Smalley, 2003). However, only a comparatively small percentage of the American population appears to have an appreciation for the nature or extent of trafficking in the United States or of the profound levels of physical violence to which trafficking victims are exposed (Bump & Duncan, 2003; FSU, 2003).

In an effort to strengthen the nation's capacity to combat international trafficking of people, the federal government recently established the following program offices:

— The Office to Monitor and Combat Trafficking in Persons of the US Department of State was established in October 2001. The office leads American antitrafficking efforts and provides assistance to the President's Interagency Task Force to Monitor and Combat Trafficking in Persons.

— The President's Interagency Task Force to Monitor and Combat Trafficking in Persons was established in February 2002 through the TVPA of 2000. Charged with the responsibility for monitoring and combating trafficking, the task force's chairperson is the Secretary of State and the group comprises the Attorney General, the Secretary of Labor, the Secretary of Health and Human Services, the Secretary of Homeland Security, the Director of Central Intelligence, and others.

— The Trafficking in Persons Report Section of the State Department collects information and corresponds with governments throughout the year to assess their progress in combating trafficking. The section issues the annual Trafficking in Persons (TIP) Report, which monitors countries worldwide to assess their compliance with the requirements of the TVPA.

— The International Programs Section of the US Department of State promotes and coordinates US antitrafficking efforts in more than 75 countries.

— The Public Diplomacy and Outreach Section of the US Department of State works to develop public-private partnerships with American and international NGOs working to eliminate international trafficking of people.

Specialized antitrafficking units are a part of the US Department of Justice, the recently established US Department of Homeland Security, the US Department of Health and Human Services, the US Agency for International Development, and the US Department of Labor. See the Web site of the President's Interagency Task Force to Monitor and Combat Trafficking in Persons (http://www.state.gov/g/tip) for descriptions of the antitrafficking activities of these departments.

## National Legislation

The United States has a large and comprehensive body of criminal law pertaining to child sexual exploitation. These laws address the minimum age of sexual consent, child pornography, the prostitution of juveniles, trafficking of children, and in recent years, sex tourism. The majority of the nation's child sexual exploitation laws involve stringent penalties, including mandatory sentencing, and in almost all states, mandatory registration for convicted sexual offenders, or **Megan's Law**. However, the number of cases successfully prosecuted under the nation's federal juvenile prostitution, child trafficking, and child sex tourism laws remains relatively low though numerous cases involving electronic child pornography have been prosecuted.

## Law Enforcement

A sharp contrast exists between the numbers of juveniles engaged in commercial sexual exploitation and the numbers of juveniles arrested for having engaged in commercial sexual activities. For example, the US Department of Justice reported that in 2001, only 1400 youths were apprehended for crimes involving prostitution (Snyder, 2003). An additional 4600 youths were arrested in the same year on charges of forcible rape, and 18 000 more were arrested for "other types" of sexual offenses not including forcible rape and prostitution.

These arrest patterns differ sharply from what local law enforcement and other juvenile authorities acknowledge to be the high incidence of survival sex that occurs among street youth and other groups of homeless youth. Unclear definitions of CSEC, inadequate service arrangements for its victims, high costs of delivering comprehensive services to child victims of sexual exploitation, and significant public deficits in many local communities—combined with problems of inadequate staffing and unclear policies and procedures for dealing with the complex legal and human service needs associated with CSEC—result in a significant underestimation of the national incidence of CSEC (Estes & Weiner, 2001).

## Prevention, Prosecution, and Protection Programs

Prevention, prosecution, and protection are the central goals of the US campaign against CSEC. This tripartite commitment is reflected in the country's attempts to (1) increase public awareness about the existence of CSEC; (2) increase societal intolerance for all forms of CSEC; (3) initiate cooperative law enforcement activities among Canada, Mexico, and the United States for dealing with cross-border and regional aspects of CSEC; and (4) create a steadily more comprehensive system of local, state, and federal protection for child victims of commercial sexual exploitation and their families. These commitments are reflected in the country's extensive antitrafficking activities, which in recent years have resulted in substantial financial support from the federal government, state governments, and private organizations that are working to rescue women and children from trafficking, slavery, and debt bondage.

American efforts to combat CSEC have been especially apparent in the area of electronic child pornography. For example, Crimes Against Children units have been established across the country, and the CyberTipline Unit of the National Center for Missing & Exploited Children (NCMEC) functions as the national resource to which all suspected cases of electronic child pornography are referred. The US Customs Service, the US Postal Service, the FBI, and other units of the federal government have well-developed programs for apprehending producers and distributors of electronic child pornography.

In contrast, children involved in prostitution, survival sex, and other types of sex-for-money exchanges have received comparatively modest attention from the central government. The reasons for this are at least threefold: (1) prostitution at any age in the United States is defined primarily as a local rather than federal issue and, therefore, is handled by local law enforcement officials; (2) the prostitution of juveniles is not perceived to be as widespread or potentially harmful as child pornography; and (3) the law enforcement and human service resources required to solve the local, state, and national dimensions of the prostitution of juveniles are complex, expensive, and currently allocated to other policing functions. Even so, recognition of the prostitution of juveniles as a serious issue in the United States did result in the passage of new laws and the strengthening of existing laws that increased the age of sexual consent for juveniles, imposed stringent age disparity penalties on adults convicted of engaging in sexual relations with juveniles, and classified sex tourism a crime.

National conferences have been convened under the auspices of the White House, the US Department of Justice, and the US Department of Health and Human Services. Various private child advocacy and service agencies, including the Child Welfare League of America (CWLA), the NCMEC, the Bilateral Safety Corridor Coalition in San Diego, and the US Campaign Against CSEC are cooperating with state and federal governmental departments to educate their staff members about the realities of CSEC, including juvenile prostitution, and to create more comprehensive protective, legal, and treatment services for child victims of sexual exploitation and their families.

The recently adopted Prosecutorial Remedies and Other Tools to end the Exploitation of Children Today (PROTECT) Act of 2003 is one outgrowth of increasing public recognition of the seriousness of child pornography and child prostitution in the United States and in countries visited by American sex tourists. In addition to expanding the AMBER Alert system into a national program—a system designed to hasten the recovery of missing and abducted children—the PROTECT Act makes it a crime for citizens or legal residents of the United States to engage in sexual acts with a child younger than age 18 years in a foreign country. The PROTECT Act removed previous legal requirements relating to proof of intention to engage in such acts before travel, strengthened sentencing guideline provisions for offenders, and added a "two strikes and you're out" provision for repeat offenders of sex crimes against children (in such situations, convicted repeat offenders are subjected to mandatory minimum sentencing requirements). The PROTECT Act provides law enforcement authorities with new tools for dealing with prostitution of children, trafficking of children for sexual purposes, and child pornography, including the introduction of constitutionally contested prohibitions on "virtual" child pornography that depicts electronically created images of children engaged in obscene acts.

## Child Pornography and Online Sexual Victimization

Child pornography is a multimillion-dollar industry in the United States. Though the possession of child pornography is illegal, the advent of the Internet and the exponential growth of pornography accessibility have made law enforcement authorities even more rigorous in their attempts to identify and apprehend child pornography producers and consumers (Finkelhor et al, 2000). Regardless of the increased efforts, recent sting operations organized by federal agencies in cooperation with local communities expose increasing numbers of electronic child pornography sites in the United States and other countries. In August 2001, the FBI, the US Customs Service, the US Postal Inspection Service, and the Dallas Police Department worked cooperatively to shut down a child pornography Internet site based in Ft. Worth, Texas. Approximately 250 000 subscribers to the site worldwide were identified, and 100 people were arrested. US postal authorities estimated that the monthly fees generated by this individual site exceeded $1 million.

According to the CyberTypline Unit of the NCMEC, the Internet puts children at serious risk for sexual victimization, and the frequency with which children are being exposed to such risks is increasing exponentially (NCMEC, 2004; PR Newswire, 2004). Child sexual exploitation via the Internet is associated with children's use of interactive electronic chat rooms, in which children can have conversations with anyone, including unknown sexual predators. The potential exists for the exchange of pornographic photographs and occasionally the arrangement of children and adult predators meeting in person (Taylor & Quayle, 2003). Children with unsupervised access to the Internet are at higher risk of sexual exploitation than children whose access to the Internet is supervised or limited; for example, parents can place computers that have Internet access in more open areas of the house rather than a child's bedroom.

The Private Sector

Many private agencies and organizations are involved in combating CSEC in the United States. Some of these organizations are national groups, such as the NCMEC and the Office of Migration and Refugee Services of the US Catholic Conference of Bishops, and others are local offices of national efforts, such as Girls Town and Boys Town, the Paul & Lisa Program, and the Salvation Army. Other organizations originated and continue to operate in metropolitan areas, such as Breaking Free in Minneapolis, Girls Educational and Mentoring Services (GEMS) in New York, Helping Individual Prostitutes Survive (HIPS) in Baltimore, Standing Against Global Exploitation (SAGE) in San Francisco, Sisters Offering Support (SOS) in Honolulu, and Youth Care in Seattle. All share a commitment to working with sexually exploited children and their families to eliminate all aspects of child sexual exploitation. Almost all the groups work cooperatively with agencies in the public sector that address the same issues, such as child protective services (CPS) units, various Departments of Human Service (DHS), Crimes Against Children units of local police departments, and federal agencies engaged in halting international trafficking of persons (US Department of State), child pornography (US Department of Justice), and the prostitution of juveniles (Department of Health and Human Service and Department of Justice).

The vast majority of private agencies serving sexually exploited children and youth are small and underfunded. Most lack adequate numbers of staff members to achieve the high levels of program integration and service coordination required to serve the needs of sexually exploited youth adequately. Many private agencies have had to abandon their street outreach efforts because of decreasing budgets and escalating demands for services from children who are referred to them by other agencies. Serious service shortages are especially acute in the housing, education, vocational training, health, and mental health sectors (Estes & Weiner, 2001).

A growing number of private organizations in the United States are engaged in public education and advocacy activities on behalf of sexually exploited children: Captive Daughters, ECPAT-USA, Project HOPE International, the Protection Project, the US Campaign Against CSEC, and Youth Advocate Program International. Though the campaigns of these organizations are quite expansive, they are experiencing severe resource shortages that compromise their effectiveness in advancing the legislative reforms, service integration, and program enhancements needed to serve sexually exploited children and youth more adequately (Estes & Weiner, 2001).

# ELIMINATING THE COMMERCIAL SEXUAL EXPLOITATION OF CHILDREN IN NORTH AMERICA

Child sexual exploitation is a serious problem worldwide, especially in Canada, Mexico, and the United States. The crisis in North America is more extensive than previously thought and includes (1) child pornography; (2) the prostitution of juveniles, including survival sex and other types of sex-for-money commercial exchanges; (3) sex tourism; and (4) domestic and international trafficking of children for sexual purposes, often in combination with debt bondage, servitude, and in the most extreme cases, slavery. Every day, hundreds of thousands of children and youth in North America confront the horrors associated with sexual exploitation. No longer do the region's leaders assert that child sexual exploitation is only a problem in areas with impoverished economies, corrupt policies, or failed social systems—in other words, that child exploitation is only a problem in developing and Third-World nations. World leaders recognize that child sexual exploitation exists in all countries—rich and poor, developed and developing, north and south of the equator—including North America.

The North American countries are only beginning to come to terms with the magnitude of the child sexual exploitation problem in their areas. They are gradually implementing the broad-based social, political, and legal changes needed to solve the problem of CSEC (**Tables 15-4** and **15-5**), but the resources currently allocated for establishing a protective network of preventive and treatment services are inadequate for current needs. Regardless, at least several steps have been taken toward eliminating child sexual exploitation:

— The existence of child sexual exploitation in North America is recognized as a serious problem for all 3 of the region's countries.

— The region's governments, private sectors, and individual citizens have demonstrated a genuine willingness to cooperate with one another to prevent and protect children from sexual exploitation.

— Appreciable levels of public and private resources have been allocated to protect children from commercial sexual exploitation though these resources do not meet current needs.

— The region's governments have strengthened their child sexual exploitation and CSEC laws by imposing higher monetary and sentencing penalties on adults who sexually exploit children.

— All of the region's countries have established discrete performance objectives to combat child sexual exploitation though most of these performance objectives need to be more specific and require additional resources.

— All of the region's governments have established mechanisms for monitoring national progress and failure in protecting children from sexual exploitation.

The nations of North America have arrived at a new crossroads. Much progress has been made, but much more needs to be done to protect its children.

**Table 15-4. Ratification of International Agreements Relating to the Commercial Exploitation of Children and Women (2003)**

| SELECTED INTERNATIONAL AGREEMENTS* | CANADA | MEXICO | UNITED STATES |
|---|---|---|---|
| *Convention on the Elimination of Forced and Compulsory Labour* of the International Labour Organization: Optional Protocol #29 (Forced Labor Convention, 1930) | No | Yes | No |
| *Convention on the Elimination of Forced and Compulsory Labour* of the International Labour Organization: Optional Protocol #105 (Abolition of Forced Labor Convention, 1957) | Yes | Yes | Yes |
| *Convention on the Abolition of Child Labor* of the International Labour Organization: Optional Protocol #138 (Minimum Age Convention, 1973) | No | No | No |
| United Nations *Convention on the Elimination of All Forms of Discrimination Against Women* (1979) | Yes | Yes | No |
| United Nations *Convention on the Rights of the Child* (1989) | Yes | Yes | No |

*(continued)*

**Table 15-4.** *(continued)*

| SELECTED INTERNATIONAL AGREEMENTS | CANADA | MEXICO | UNITED STATES |
|---|---|---|---|
| *Convention on the Abolition of Child Labour* of the International Labour Organization: Optional Protocol #182 (Worst Forms of Child Labour Convention, 1999) | Yes | Yes | Yes |
| United Nations *Convention Against Transnational Organized Crime* (2000) | Yes | Yes | Yes |
| To the United Nations *Convention Against Transnational Organized Crime*: Optional Protocol to prevent, suppress, and punish trafficking in persons, especially women and children | Yes | Yes | No |
| To the United Nations *Convention on the Rights of the Child*: Optional Protocol relating to the sale of children, child prostitution, and child pornography | Ratification pending | Yes | Yes |

* See Appendix G in the electronic version of Estes & Weiner (2001) for a more detailed description of the content and requirements of these international agreements.

Data from ECPAT International, 2001; UNICEF, 2003; United Nations Development Programme, 2003; United Nations Office the High Commissioner for Human Rights, 2003.

---

**Table 15-5. National and Regional Efforts to Prevent the Commercial Sexual Exploitation of North American Children (2001-2003)\***

PRIMARY PREVENTION: INCIDENCE-FOCUSED EFFORTS TO PREVENT CSEC

**Prevention Goal**

— Strengthening of societal values and norms to protect children from sexual abuse and exploitation

— Introduction of new values, thinking, processes, and relationship skills that are incompatible with CSEC

— Promotion of healthy, nonviolent, and sexually nonexploitive relationships between children and adults

**Prevention Focus**

— Identification of the continuum of abuse formed by child sexual abuse, sexual assault, sexual exploitation, and CSEC

— Education of the general public about CSEC

— Education of parents, teachers, and others with direct responsibilities for children of CSEC

— Education of children at risk of CSEC about its existence and dangers

— Passage of comprehensive and more protective CSEC legislation, such as age of sexual consent, mandatory reporting, minimum sentencing standards, and sex offender registration

— Establishment of stronger sanctions and punishments for those who have committed sexual crimes against children

— Enforcement of existing and new laws regarding perpetrators of CSEC

— Research of the epidemiology and dynamics of CSEC

— Advocacy efforts directed at the passage of anti-CSEC legislation at the national, state, and local levels

*(continued)*

**Table 15-5. National and Regional Efforts to Prevent the Commercial Sexual Exploitation of North American Children (2001-2003)\*** *(continued)*

PRIMARY PREVENTION: INCIDENCE-FOCUSED EFFORTS TO PREVENT CSEC

**Examples in the North American Region**

Canada[†‡]

*For the General Population*
— National and local media campaigns portraying CSEC as child sexual abuse and as a crime

— Stolen Innocence: A National Education Campaign Against CSEC

— Out from the Shadows and Into the Light, a program designed to raise awareness and change public attitudes toward child victims of sexual exploitation

— Alliance Against Child Commercial Sexual Exploitation (Vancouver)

*For Caregivers*
— National Child Exploitation Coordination Centre to focus on public awareness and prevention of CSEC

— Illegal and Offensive Content on the Internet (booklet)

*For Children at Risk*
— Family Violence Prevention Project, a federal initiative focused on First Nations (ie, Native American) families

Mexico[§]

*For the General Population*
— National media campaigns portraying procurement of youth for sexual purposes as child sexual abuse

— National media awareness campaigns educating public that CSEC is a crime

— More stringent CSEC laws

*For Children at Risk*
— Adoption of the National Plan of Action to Combat the CSEC, coordinated by the nation's lead child protection and service agency, Sistema Nacional para el Desarrollo Integral de la Familia (DIF)

— Regular evaluations of activities in support of DIF's National Plan of Action

United States[||]

*For the General Population*
— Media stories and exposés concerning the nature, extent, and seriousness of CSEC (eg, Cockburn [2003], Critchell [2003], Landesman [2004], Smalley [2003])

— "Sexual Touching" and "Just Say 'No'" campaigns of national advocacy groups

— ECPAT-USA for research and advocacy

— US Campaign Against CSEC for advocacy and coordination

— Youth Advocates Program International for research and advocacy

— National and international conferences on CSEC, including programs sponsored by the US Departments of Justice and Health & Human Services

*For Caregivers*
— CSEC-focused international conferences and summits

— CSEC-focused national, state, and local conferences on CSEC, such as the annual Crimes Against Children conference held in Dallas

— Specialized CSEC content for inclusion in the basic curricula of core childcare professions

*(continued)*

**Table 15-5.** *(continued)*

PRIMARY PREVENTION: INCIDENCE-FOCUSED EFFORTS TO PREVENT CSEC

**Examples in the North American Region**

United States

*For Children at Risk*
— CSEC-focused school assemblies, community meetings, and similar types of programming in schools and community centers

Examples of Region-Wide Innovations Related to CSEC

— Regional summits and meetings focused on the nature, extent, and severity of CSEC in the North American Region (Ives, 2001)

— International and regional declarations, covenants, and agreements relating to regional aspects of CSEC

— Cooperative border and cross-border surveillance activities

— Cooperative training of police, human service workers, and others who come into direct contact with child victims of commercial sexual exploitation

SECONDARY PREVENTION: PREVALENCE-FOCUSED EFFORTS THAT TARGET INDIVIDUALS AT SIGNIFICANT RISK OF CSEC OR THOSE WHO ARE IN THE EARLY STAGES BECOMING VICTIMS OF CSEC

**Prevention Goal**

— Early case finding and detection

— Early diagnosis

— Early and successful intervention

**Prevention Focus**

— Education and other forms of prevention directed at children concerning types of maltreatment known to be associated with CSEC

— Outreach to groups of children at an early stage of experimenting with CSEC, such as those beginning to view adult and child pornography or those engaging in prostitution

— Outreach to groups of children engaged in survival sex strategies associated with CSEC

— Outreach to groups of children frequently associated with commercial sex, such as runaways, thrownaways, and other homeless and street children

**Examples in the North American Region**

Canada[†‡]

— Establishment of a National Committee Against CSEC

— Framing of a National Strategy to Combat CSEC in cooperation with the Criminal Intelligence Service Canada

— Through a partnership with Industry Canada, an online reporting site for suspicious Internet activities

— Creation of a Royal Canadian Mounted Police unit focused on disrupting and eradicating the global slave trade

— Within the National Child Exploitation Coordination Centre, a unit that focuses on the development of training tools for front-line law enforcement officers handling CSEC

— Establishment of the Canadian Border Security Agency to address illegal immigration and trafficking into Canada

— Implementation of the National Aboriginal Consultation Project

*(continued)*

## Table 15-5. National and Regional Efforts to Prevent the Commercial Sexual Exploitation of North American Children (2001-2003)* *(continued)*

SECONDARY PREVENTION: PREVALENCE-FOCUSED EFFORTS THAT TARGET INDIVIDUALS AT SIGNIFICANT RISK OF CSEC OR THOSE WHO ARE IN THE EARLY STAGES BECOMING VICTIMS OF CSEC

### Examples in the North American Region

Mexico[§]

— Municipality-based child protective services via DIF-administered programs

— Establishment of federal and local offices of sex and other crimes; includes national hotline numbers and official registries

— Establishment of a free hotline to report cases of missing, runaway, and potentially exploited children

United States[||]

— New federal, state, and local offices of child protective services

— Establishment of federal, state, and local offices of Crimes Against Children units and Interagency Crimes Against Children Task Forces

— In the National Center for Child Abuse and Neglect, a special focus on CSEC

— Establishment within the National Center for Missing & Exploited Children of the Exploited Child Unit (ECU) with a special focus on electronic child pornography

— Ongoing crisis intervention services of the National Runaway Switchboard (NRS)

— Nationwide implementation of the AMBER Alert for rapid reports of missing and potentially abducted children

Examples of Region-Wide Innovations Related to CSEC

— Memoranda of Understanding between North American Free Trade Agreement (NAFTA) member states relating to apprehension and extradition of suspected perpetrators of CSEC, sharing of evidence, and participation in judicial inquiries

— Joint training of NAFTA investigative and prosecutorial staff members

— Regionwide cooperation in collaborative CSEC-related research efforts

— Interpol and its several levels of national and international alerts

TERTIARY PREVENTION: INTERVENTION-FOCUSED EFFORTS TO MINIMIZE OR LIMIT THE IMPACT OF CSEC AFTER IT HAS OCCURRED

### Prevention Goal

*For Child Victims*
— Protection

— Comprehensive care and treatment

— Restoration to highest possible level of functioning

*For Exploiters*
— Detection

— Prosecution

— Punishment

— Judicial and legal supervision

*(continued)*

**Table 15-5.** *(continued)*

TERTIARY PREVENTION: INTERVENTION-FOCUSED EFFORTS TO MINIMIZE OR LIMIT THE IMPACT OF CSEC AFTER IT HAS OCCURRED

**Prevention Focus**

— The development of specialized treatment protocols focused on limiting the damage done by CSEC and helping to restore children to their highest possible level of functioning

— Strengthening of the existing network of services provided to child victims of sexual exploitation

— Establishment of comprehensive services to highly vulnerable groups of exploited children

— More rapid identification and control of perpetrators of CSEC

— Long-term supervision of adjudicated perpetrators of CSEC

**Examples in the North American Region**

Canada[†‡]

*Child-Focused Interventions*
— Prostitute Empowerment, Education, and Resource Society (PEERS; Victoria, British Columbia)

— Youth Witness Protection Program (Nova Scotia)

— Covenant House (Vancouver)

— Exit Routes, a program providing assistance to youth attempting to leave commercial sex work

*Perpetrator-Focused Interventions*
— Establishment within the Royal Canadian Mounted Police of a national youth strategy focused on apprehending repeat sexual exploiters

— The Immigration and Refugee Act of 2002, which strengthens federal efforts in apprehending international traffickers

Mexico[§]

In general, a severe shortage currently exists in Mexico for specialized CSEC services.

*Child-Focused Interventions*
— Specialized services of the DIF

— Municipality-based, DIF-sponsored programs and services

— Casa Alianza (Mexico City)

— Federacion Mexicana de Asociaciones Privadas (FEMAP Foundation), Ciudad Juarez

— Reto a La Juventud (Ciudad Juarez)

— Toll free telephone number for reporting missing and runaway children

*Perpetrator-Focused Interventions*
— Rapid response of the Prosecutors General Association of Mexico

United States[‖]

*Child-Focused Interventions*
— Covenant House at multiple locations

— GEMS in New York City

— Paul & Lisa Program

*(continued)*

**Table 15-5. National and Regional Efforts to Prevent the Commercial Sexual Exploitation of North American Children (2001-2003)\*** *(continued)*

TERTIARY PREVENTION: INTERVENTION-FOCUSED EFFORTS TO MINIMIZE OR LIMIT THE IMPACT OF CSEC AFTER IT HAS OCCURRED

**Examples in the North American Region**

United States

*Child-Focused Interventions*
— SAGE in San Francisco

— SOS in Honolulu

— Trafficking in Persons Program of the State Department, including the T-visa program

*Perpetrator-Focused Interventions*
— Mandatory participation in "john" schools in San Francisco, Las Vegas, and elsewhere for adult offenders arrested for purchasing sex services from prostituted women

Examples of Region-Wide Innovations Related to CSEC

*Child-Focused Interventions*
— San Diego "safety corridor" between Mexico and the Western US targeting runaway, thrownaway, and trafficked children

*Perpetrator-Focused Interventions*
— Memoranda of Understanding concerning regional cooperation in the identification, apprehension, arrest and prosecution of adults engaging in CSEC of children from neighboring countries¶

— Memoranda of Understanding related to trafficking of children and for sexual purposes (USDOS, 2004)

— Memoranda of Understanding concerning sex tourism in the region and elsewhere by nationals of the region's countries

*\* See Wolfe & Jaffe (1999) for a more detailed discussion of prevention in public health and in preventing violence toward children and youth.*

*† A comprehensive list of Canadian anti-CSEC efforts is available at http://sen.parl.gc.ca/lpearson/htmfiles/hill/17_htm_files/Committee-e/2001-ECPAT-EN1.pdf.*

*‡ The authors acknowledge with appreciation the assistance provided in preparing the Canadian portion of this table received from the office of Senator Landon Pearson of the Senate of Canada, Andrea Greig of the Strategic Policy and Research Team of Health Canada's Population and Public Health Branch, and Robin Perry of the Institute for Health and Human Services Research of the Florida State University.*

*§ Activities directed at combating CSEC in Mexico are not centralized, therefore, related information is not easily obtained. The various programs and other initiatives identified in this table are illustrative of types of CSEC-related initiatives in Mexico (E. Azaola, written communication, April 2004).*

*‖ For additional information see the electronic version of Estes & Weiner (2001): Appendix G for a compendium of US federal laws relating to CSEC, Appendix H for a partial listing of the most important international agreements relating to CSEC, and Appendixes I and K for examples of organizations in the United States serving child victims of sexual exploitation.*

*¶ See http://www.guadalajarareporter.com for an example of this type of international cooperation. In Guadalajara, Mexico, 13 adults engaged in pornography and sexual exploitation involving children were arrested, 10 of whom were American citizens. The Americans were extradited by Mexican authorities to the United Stated for prosecution.*

# REFERENCES

Azaola E. La explotación sexual comercial de niños en México: situación general de la infancia. In: Azaola E, Estes RJ, eds. *La Infancia Como Mercancía Sexual. México, Canadá, Estados Unidos.* Mexico City, Mexico: Siglo Veintiuno Editores; 2003a:140-155.

Azaola E. La explotación sexual de niños en las fronteras. In: Azaola E, Estes RJ, eds. *La Infancia Como Mercancía Sexual. México, Canadá, Estados Unidos.* Mexico City, Mexico: Siglo Veintiuno Editores; 2003b:240-322.

Azaola E. *Stolen Childhood: Girl and Boy Victims of Sexual Exploitation in Mexico.* Mexico City, Mexico: United Nations Children's Fund (UNICEF); 2001.

Azaola E, Estes RJ, eds. *La Infancia Como Mercancía Sexual. México: Canadá, Estados Unidos.* Mexico City, Mexico: Siglo Veintiuno Editores; 2003.

Bales K. *Disposable People: New Slavery in the Global Economy.* Berkeley, Calif: University of California Press; 1999.

Barnitz LS. *Commercial Sexual Exploitation of Children: Youth Involved in Prostitution, Pornography, and Sex Trafficking.* Washington, DC: Youth Advocate Program International; 1998.

Barr CW. *Child Sex Trade: Battling a Scourge.* Boston, Mass: Christian Science Publishing; 1996.

Basu K. The economics of child labor. *Sci Am.* October 2003;289:84-91.

Bishop C. The Trafficking Victims Protection Act of 2000: three years later. *Int Migration.* 2003;41(6):219-231.

Budapest Group. *The Relationship Between Organized Crime and Trafficking in Aliens.* Austria: International Centre for Migration Policy Development; 1999.

Bump MN, Duncan J. Conference on identifying and serving child victims of trafficking. *Int Migr.* 2003;41(5):201-218.

Calcetas-Santos O. *Report of the Special Rapporteur on the Sale of Children, Child Prostitution, and Child Pornography on the Issue of Commercial Sexual Exploitation of Children to Mexico.* Sales No #E/CN.4/1998/101/Add.2. New York, NY: United Nations; 1998.

Calcetas-Santos O. *Report of the Special Rapporteur on the Sale of Children, Child Prostitution, and Child Pornography.* Sales No E/CN.4/1999/71. New York, NY: United Nations; 1999.

Caldwell G, Galster S, Steinsor N. *Crime & Servitude: An Expose of the Traffic in Women for Prostitution From the Newly Independent States.* Moscow, Russia: Global Survival Network; 1997.

Campaign 2000. Poverty Amidst Prosperity: Building a Canada for All Children, 2002 Report Card on Child Poverty. Campaign 2000 Web site. Available at: http://www.campaign2000.ca/rc/rc02/NOV02reportcard.pdf. Accessed November 3, 2004.

Cauce AM, Paradise M, Ginzler JA, et al. The characteristics and mental health of homeless adolescents: age and gender differences. *J Emotional Behav Disord.* 2000;8:230-239.

Centre for Health and Human Development (CHHD). *Progress Report to the Organization of American States on Implementation of the 1996 Stockholm Declaration and Agenda for Action to Combat the Commercial Sexual Exploitation of Children.* Ottawa: Division of Childhood and Adolescence, Centre for Healthy Human Development, Population and Public Health Branch, Health Canada; 2004.

Cockburn A. 21st-century slaves. *Natl Geogr Mag.* September 2003;204:2-20.

Comisión de Derechos Humanos del Distrito Federal (CDHDF). *Al Otro Lado de la Calle: Prostitución de Menroes en La Merced.* Mexico City, Mexico: CDHDF-UNICEF; 1996.

Comisión Nacional de Accion en Favor de la Infancia. *Mexico: Programa Nacional de Accion en Favor de la Infancia. Evaluacion, 1990-2000.* Mexico City, Mexico: UNICEF; 2001.

Criminal Intelligence Service of Canada (CISC). Annual report on organized crime in Canada, *2002*. Ottowa, Canada: CISC; 2003. Available at: http://www.cisc.gc.ca/ AnnualReport2002/Cisc2002/frontpage2002.html. Accessed December 20, 2004.

Critchell D. Inside the teen-hooker factory. *Rolling Stone*. October 16, 2003;78-80.

Davidson JO. *The Identification and Management of Child Sexual Abusers as a Means of Protecting Children From Sexual Exploitation and Abuse: Moving Toward a Public Health Model?* Copenhagen, Denmark: Red Barnet; 2004.

Davidson JO. *The sexual exploiter*. Paper presented at: World Congress Against Commercial Sexual Exploitation of Children; August 28, 1996; Stockholm, Sweden.

Davidson JO. *The sexual exploiter*. Paper presented at: World Congress Against Commercial Sexual Exploitation of Children; December 17-20, 2001; Yokohama, Japan.

De Albuquerque K. Sex, beach boys, and female tourists in the Caribbean. In: Dank B, Refinetti R, eds. *Sex Work and Sex Workers: Sexuality & Culture*. Vol 1. New Brunswick, NJ: Transaction Publishers; 1999.

18 USC § 1589 et seq.

End Child Prostitution, Child Pornography, and Trafficking of Children for Sexual Purposes (ECPAT) International. Europe and North America regional profiles. Regional report prepared for: World Congress Against the Commercial Sexual Exploitation of Children; August 1996; Stockholm, Sweden.

End Child Prostitution, Child Pornography, and Trafficking of Children for Sexual Purposes (ECPAT) International. *Five Years After Stockholm: 2000-2001*. Bangkok, Thailand: ECPAT International; 2001.

Estes RJ. *At the Crossroads: Development Challenges of the New Century*. Dordrecht, Netherlands: Kluwer Academic Publishers; In press(a).

Estes RJ. Development challenges of the 'New' Europe. *Soc Indic Res*. 2004;69(2): 123-166.

Estes RJ. *The Sexual Exploitation of Children: A Working Guide to the Empirical Literature*. Philadelphia: University of Pennsylvania School of Social Work; 2001. Available at: http://caster.ssw.upenn.edu/~restes/CSEC_Files/CSEC_Bib_August_ 2001.pdf. Accessed December 20, 2004.

Estes RJ. The silent emergency: the commercial sexual exploitation of children in the US, Canada, and Mexico. In: Walker NE, ed. *Prostituted Teens: More Than A Runaway Problem*. Briefing Report No. 2002-2. Lansing: Michigan State University, Institute for Children, Youth and Families; 2002:15-22.

Estes RJ. *Social Development in Hong Kong: The Unfinished Agenda*. London & New York: Oxford University Press; In press(b).

Estes RJ, Weiner NA. The commercial sexual exploitation of children in the US, Canada, and Mexico. September 2001. Available at: http://caster.ssw.upenn.edu/~ restes/CSEC.htm. Accessed December 20, 2004.

Estes RJ, Weiner NA. La explotación sexual comercial de niños en Estados Uunidos. In: Azaola E, Estes RJ, eds. *La Infancia Como Mercancía Sexual. México, Canadá, Estados Unidos*. Mexico City, Mexico: Siglo Vientiuno Editores; 2003:44-90.

Fairchild AL. Policies of inclusion: immigrants, disease, dependency, and American immigration policy at the dawn and dusk of the 20th century. *Am J Public Health*. 2004;94(4):528-539.

Farley M. Prostitution in five countries: violence and post-traumatic stress disorder. *Fem Psychol*. 1998;8(4):405-426.

Farley M, Kelly V. Prostitution: a critical review of the medical and social science literature. *Women Crim Justice*. 2000;11(4):29-64.

Federal/Provincial/Territorial (F/P/T) Working Group on Prostitution. *Report and Recommendations in Respect of Legislation, Policy and Practices Concerning Prostitution-Related Activities*. Ottawa, Canada: F/T/P Working Group; 1998.

Ferrara FF. *Childhood Sexual Abuse: Development Effects Across the Life Span*. Pacific Grove, Calif: Brooks/Cole; 2001.

Finkelhor D, Mitchell KJ, Wolak J. *Online Victimization: A Report on the Nation's Youth*. Alexandria, Va: National Center for Missing & Exploited Children; 2000.

Florida State University. *Florida Responds to Human Trafficking*. Tallahassee: Center for the Advancement of Human Rights, Florida State University; 2003.

Goldman R, Wheeler V. *Silent Shame: The Sexual Abuse of Children and Youth*. Danville, Ill: The Interstate; 1986.

Goldstein SL. *The Sexual Exploitation of Children: A Practical Guide to Assessment, Investigation, and Intervention*. 2nd ed. Boca Raton, Fla: CRC Press; 1999.

Greene JM, Ennett ST, Ringwalt CL. Prevalence and correlates of survival sex among runaway and homeless youth. *Am J Public Health*. 1999;89(9):1406-1409.

Guilty 'john' alerts police to teen sex ring. *Ottawa Citizen*. April 6, 2002:A9.

Hammer H, Finkelhor D, Sedlak AJ. *Runaway/Thrownaway Children: National Estimates and Characteristics*. Washington DC: US Dept of Justice, Office of Justice Programs, Office of Juvenile Justice and Delinquency Prevention; October 2002. NCJ 196469.

Hecht ME. The role and involvement of the private sector. Paper presented at: World Congress Against Commercial Sexual Exploitation; December 17-20, 2001; Yokohama, Japan.

Higham J. *Strangers in the Land*. New York: Atheneum; 1971.

Hofstede A. *The Hofstede Committee Report: Juvenile Prostitution in Minnesota*. Minneapolis: Office of the Minnesota Attorney General; 1999.

Hughes DM. The "Natasha" trade: the transnational shadow market of trafficking in women. *J Int Aff*. 2000;53(2):625-652.

Hughes D, Roche C, eds. *Making the Harm Visible: Global Sexual Exploitation of Women and Girls*. Kingston, RI: Coalition Against Trafficking in Women; 1999.

Instituto Interamericano del Niño (IIN). *Violencia y Explotación Sexual contra Niños y Niñas en América Latina y el Caribe*. Montevideo, Uruguay: IIN; 2000.

International Criminal Police Organization (Interpol). *International Crime Statistics, 2003*. St. Cloud, France: Interpol; 2003.

International Rescue Committee. ORR trafficking persons program. *Trafficking Watch*. 2004;3:3.

International Tribunal for Children's Rights (ITCR). *International Dimensions of the Sexual Exploitation of Children*. Montreal, Canada: IBCR; 2000.

Ives N. *Final Report From the North American Regional Consultation on the Commercial Sexual Exploitation of Children*. Philadelphia: University of Pennsylvania School of Social Work; 2001.

Jaffe M, Rosen S, eds. *Forced Labor: The Prostitution of Children*. Upland, Pa: Diane Publishing Co; 1996.

Jones L, Finkelhor D. The decline in child sexual abuse cases. *OJJDP Bulletin*. Washington, DC: US Dept of Justice, Office of Justice Programs, Office of Juvenile Justice and Delinquency Prevention; January 2001:1-12.

Kingsley C, Mark M. *Sacred Lives: Canadian Aboriginal Children and Youth Speak Out About Sexual Exploitation*. Vancouver, Canada: Save the Children Canada; 2000.

Klain EJ. *Prostitution of Children and Child-Sex Tourism: An Analysis of Domestic and International Responses*. Alexandria, Va: National Center for Missing & Exploited Children; 1999.

Landesman, P. Sex slaves on main street: the girls next door. *New York Times Magazine*. January 25, 2004;30-39,66-67,72,75.

Lederer L. *Human Rights Report on Trafficking of Women and Children*. Baltimore, Md: Johns Hopkins University, The Paul H. Nitze School of Advanced International Studies; 2001.

Leñero L. *Los Niños de y en la Calle*. Mexico City, Mexico: Academia Mexicana de Derechos Humanos; 1998.

Loeber R, Farrington D, eds. Serious and violent juvenile offenders. *Juvenile Justice Bull*. May 1998;1-8.

Lopinto N. Working girls squeezed. *Montreal Mirror*. November 28, 2002. Available at: http://www.montrealmirror.com/ARCHIVES/2002/112802/news4.html. Accessed December 20, 2004.

Lucas BM, Hackett L. *Street Youth: On Their Own in Indianapolis*. Indianapolis, Ind: Health Foundation of Greater Indianapolis; 1995.

Molnar BE, Buka SL, Kessler RC. Child sexual abuse and subsequent psychopathology: results from the National Comorbidity Survey. *Am J Public Health*. 2001; 91(5):753-760.

Nadon SM, Koverola C, Schludermann EH. Antecedents to prostitution: childhood victimization. *J Interpers Violence*. 1998;13:206-221.

National Center for Missing & Exploited Children (NCMEC). *Female Juvenile Prostitution: Problem and Response*. Alexandria, Va: NCMEC; 2002.

National Center for Missing & Exploited Children (NCMEC). *Child Safety on the Information Highway*. Alexandria, Va: NCMEC; 2004.

National Coalition for the Homeless (NCH). *Homeless Families With Children, NCH Fact Sheet #7*. Washington, DC: NCH; 2001.

National Coalition for the Homeless (NCH). *Homeless Youth, NCH Fact Sheet #11*. Washington, DC: NCH; 1999.

National Runaway Switchboard (NRS) Statistics, 2000. NRS Web site. Available at: http://www.nrscrisisline.org/2000stat.asp. Accessed December 20, 2004.

Negrete N. *Explotación Sexual Comercial de la Niñez en el sur de México y Centroamérica*. San José, Costa Rica: ECPAT-Casa Alianza; 2001.

Office of Juvenile Justice and Delinquency Prevention (OJJDP). Highlights from the NISMART Bulletins. *NISMART Fact Sheet*. US Department of Justice, Office of Justice Programs, Office of Juvenile Justice and Delinquency Prevention; October 2002.

Ouimet M. *Sexual Offences and Offenders*. Montreal, Canada: School of Criminology, University of Montreal; 1997.

Pettman JJ. Body politics: international sex tourism. *Third World Q*. 1997;18(1):93-108.

PR Newswire. National Center For Missing and Exploited Children announces dramatic increase in reports of child sexual exploitation; up 750% in five-year period. *PR Newswire*. February 9, 2004.

Proctor BD, Dalaker J. *Current Population Reports: P60-222: Poverty in the US, 2002*. Report #P60-222. Washington, DC: US Government Printing Office; 2003.

Publications—incidence studies. Centre of Excellence for Child Welfare Web site. September 28, 2004. Available at: http://www.cecwcepb.ca/Pubs/PubsIncidence. shtml. Accessed November 3, 2004.

Quebec City sex trial moving to Montreal. Online News CBC Montreal Web site. November 7, 2003. Available at: http://montreal.cbc.ca/regional/servlet/View? filename=qc_trial20030711. Accessed December 20, 2004.

Richard AO. *International Trafficking in Women to the US: A Contemporary Manifestation of Slavery and Organized Crime*. Washington, DC: US State Dept Bureau of Intelligence and Research; 1999.

Righthand S, Welch C. *Juveniles Who Have Sexually Offended: A Review of the Professional Literature*. Washington, DC: US Dept of Justice, Office of Juvenile Justice and Delinquency Prevention; 2001.

Ruíz Torres MA. La explotación sexual de niños en dos ciudades turísticas: Cancún y Acapulco. In: Azaola E, Estes RJ, eds. *La Infancia Como Mercancía Sexual. México, Canadá, Estados Unidos*. Mexico City, Mexico: Siglo Vientiuno Editores; 2003: 156-239.

Runaway and Homeless Youth Management Information System (RHYMIS). US Department of Health and Human Services Web page. Available at: http://www.acf. dhhs.gov/programs/fysb/rhypage/homepage.htm. Accessed December 20, 2004.

Sarlo C. *Measuring Poverty in Canada*. Vancouver, Canada: The Fraser Institute; 2001.

Sedlak AJ, Finkelhor D, Hammer H, Schultz DJ. National estimates of missing children: an overview. *OJJDP NISMART Bulletin Series*. Washington, DC: US Dept of Justice, Office of Justice Programs, Office of Juvenile Justice and Delinquency Prevention; October 2002. NCJ 196465.

Senate of Canada. *Report on the 1997-99 Activities: Canadian Strategies Against Commercial Sexual Exploitation of Children and Youth. Follow-up to the 1996 First World Congress*. 1999; Stockholm, Sweden.

Shelley L. *Trafficking in Women and Children: Trafficking and Organized Crime*. Paper presented to: staff of the Protection Project; October 4, 2000; Washington, DC.

Simmons MJ. *Hookers, Hustlers, and Round-Trip Vacationers: The Gender Dynamics of Sex and Romance Tourism*. Knoxville, Tenn: Society for the Study of Social Problems; 1996.

Smalley S. This could be your kid. *Newsweek*. August 18, 2003:44-45,47.

Snyder HN. *Juvenile Arrests, 2001*. Washington, DC: US Department of Justice, Office of Juvenile Justice and Delinquency Prevention; 2003. NCJ 21370.

Snyder HN. *Sexual Assault of Young Children as Reported to Law Enforcement: Victim, Incident, and Offender Characteristics—A Statistical Report Using Data From the National Incident-Based Reporting System*. Washington, DC: US Dept of Justice, Office of Justice Programs; 2000.

Spangenberg M. *Prostituted Youth in New York City: An Overview*. New York, NY: ECPAT USA; 2001.

Taylor M, Quayle E. *Child Pornography: An Internet Crime*. New York, NY: Brunner-Routledge; 2003.

Tremblay P. Interacciones sociales entre pedofilos Canadienses. In: Azaola E, Estes RJ, eds. *La Infancia Como Mercancía Sexual: México, Canadá, Estados Unidos*. Mexico City, Mexico: Siglo Veintiuno Editores; 2003:91-139.

Tyler KA, Cauce AM. Perpetrators of early physical and sexual abuse among homeless and runaway adolescents. *Child Abuse Negl*. 2002;26:1261-1274.

United Nations. *Sale of Children, Child Prostitution and Child Pornography*. Doc. New York: United Nations General Assembly; January 14, 1994. E/CN.4/1994/84.

United Nations. *World Situation With Regard to International Traffic in Minors*. Costa Rica: UN Latin American Institute for the Prevention of Crime and the Treatment of Offenders; 1995.

United Nations. *Global Programme Against Trafficking in Human Beings: An Outline for Action*. Vienna, Austria: United Nations; 1999.

United Nations Children's Fund (UNICEF). *The State of the World's Children, 2003*. New York, NY: Oxford University Press; 2003.

United Nations Children's Fund (UNICEF). *The Stockholm Declaration and Agenda for Action*. Paris, France and New York, NY: United Nations; 1996.

United Nations Development Programme (UNDP). *Human Development Report, 2003: Millennium Development Goals—A Compact Among Nations to End Poverty*. New York, NY: Oxford University Press; 2003.

United Nations Office of the High Commissioner for Human Rights. Status of ratifications of the Optional Protocol to the Convention on the Rights of the Child on the sale of children, child prostitution and child pornography. 2003. Available at: http://www.unhchr.ch/html/menu2/6/crc/treaties/status-opsc.htm. Accessed December 20, 2004.

US Conference of Mayors. *Hunger and Homelessness Report, 2003: A 25-City Survey*. Washington, DC: US Conference of Mayors; 2003.

US Department of Health and Human Services (USDHHS). Perpetrators of child maltreatment, 1997-2001. Washington, DC: USDHHS, Administration for Children & Families; 2003a. Available at: http://www.acf.hhs.gov/programs/cb/publications/cm01/chapterfour.htm. Accessed December 20, 2004.

US Department of Health and Human Services (USDHHS). *Victims of Child Maltreatment, 1997-2001*. Washington, DC: United States Dept of Health and Human Services, Administration for Children and Families; 2003b. Available at: http://www.acf.hhs.gov/programs/cb/publications/cm01/chapterthree.htm. Accessed December 20, 2004.

US Department of Justice (USDOJ). *Juvenile Offenders and Victims: 2002 National Report*. Washington, DC: USDOJ, Office of Juvenile Justice and Delinquency Prevention; 2003.

US Department of Labor (USDOL). *Forced Labor: The Prostitution of Children*. Washington, DC: Government Printing Office; 1996.

US Department of State (USDOS). *Trafficking in Persons Report, 2003*. Washington, DC: USDOS, Office of the Under Secretary for Global Affairs; 2003a.

US Department of State (USDOS). *Trafficking in Persons Report, 2004*. Washington, DC: USDOS, Office of the Under Secretary for Global Affairs; 2004.

US Department of State (USDOS). *The World Factbook: Canada*. Washington, DC: USDOS, Central Intelligence Agency; 2003b.

US Department of State (USDOS). *The World Factbook: Mexico*. Washington, DC: USDOS, Central Intelligence Agency; 2003c.

US Department of State (USDOS). *The World Factbook: United States*. Washington, DC: USDOS, Central Intelligence Agency; 2003d.

Williams P, ed. *Illegal Immigration and Commercial Sex: The New Slave Trade*. London, England: Frank Cass Publishers; 1999.

Wolfe DA, Jaffe PG. Emerging strategies in the prevention of domestic violence. *Future Children*. 1999;9(3):133-144.

World Bank. *World Development Report, 2003: Sustainable Development in a Dynamic World*. New York, NY: Oxford University Press; 2003.

World Health Organization (WHO). *Commercial Sexual Exploitation of Children: The Health and Psychological Dimensions*. Geneva, Switzerland: WHO; 1996.

Yoon Y. *International Sexual Slavery*. Washington, DC: CG Issue Overviews; 1997.

# PSYCHOSOCIAL CONTEXT LEADING JUVENILES TO PROSTITUTION AND SEXUAL EXPLOITATION

James A. H. Farrow, MD, FSAM

This chapter reviews the psychosocial and health risks that place youth in jeopardy for sexual exploitation. Unless stated otherwise, "youth" refers to adolescents and young adults aged 12 to 21 years. The discussion will be primarily limited to youth whose first language is English and will reflect the experiences of young people in North America. There has been a limited amount of research in the United States on adolescent sexual exploitation and the prostitution of juveniles compared to studies of the phenomenon in other parts of the world. Studies reviewed in this chapter have provided a better understanding of the problem. The discussion of the antecedents and contexts for the prostitution of juveniles and sexual exploitation in other forms is based on a central theme of youth alienation and marginalization experienced by significant numbers of young persons in this society.

## YOUTH ALIENATION AND VICTIMIZATION

*Alienation* may be defined as a withdrawal or separation of a person from the values of one's society or family. Of the approximately 30 million youth aged 12 to 20 years in the United States, substantial numbers have become withdrawn or separated from the values of their families or society. *Marginalization*, as it is sometimes called, means being relegated to the outer limits of social standing. It is a result of the process of alienation; it is precipitated by a variety of psychological and social factors, including childhood abuse and victimization within the family, homelessness, and early onset of serious mental illness (Ringwalt et al, 1998a,b; Sleegers et al, 1998; Widom & Kuhns, 1996). All of these circumstances lead to greater risk for sexual exploitation of young people.

Youth who are marginalized in American society include the homeless, runaways, street youths, school dropouts, counterculture youth, and delinquent and institutional youth who are in and out of juvenile justice centers, foster care, or psychiatric facilities. They are more likely to affiliate with deviant peer groups such as gangs and engage in delinquent behavior (Waters, 1999). While immigrant youth in North America make up a sector of the marginalized youth population, most are members of the main-stream culture. Few of these youth are employed or receive regular educational or health services (Gerber, 1997; Klein et al, 2000). Young people who find themselves living in circumstances without adult supervision are at additional risk to be drawn into prostitution and other activities where they are sexually exploited as a method of survival (Deisher & Farrow, 1986; Greene et al, 1999).

Not all youth at risk come from deprived or abusive families. It is an overgeneralization to say that all of these young people come from homes where they have been neglected, abused, or have had poor relationships with parents. While research supports that this is true in many cases, there are substantial numbers of children who have had no such experiences but who become alienated through deviant peer associations (Whitbeck et al, 1997). Their socialization needs may be met through gang affiliation or association with young adults with alternative lifestyles. These youth appear to be running to a more intriguing and comfortable lifestyle rather than running from an intolerable home situation. Nonetheless, this socialization trajectory appears to be a common pathway to victimization and exploitation for many. This pathway may be especially applicable to sexual minority youth (ie, gay, lesbian, and transgendered youth) who seek out affiliations where personal and social expression is outside of society's mainstream but more acceptable to them (Gonsiorek & Rudolf, 1991; Hetrick & Martin, 1987; Noell & Ochs, 2001).

Regardless of the reasons young people find themselves in a marginalized position in our society, given their young age, lack of life experience, and absence of responsible adult supervision, the risks of victimization and sexual exploitation are high.

## A HISTORICAL PERSPECTIVE

As discussed in chapter 1, A Brief History of Child Sexual Exploitation, prostitution and involvement of juveniles in the sex trade are ancient phenomena (de Mause 1974; Weisberg 1987). Even in a predominantly Judeo-Christian society that condemns or ignores this type of involvement, the visibility of this pervasive social problem has increased significantly (Deisher et al, 1982) due to a number of social movements or forces over the last 40 years. Throughout the 1990s, for example, the visibility of child exploitation in the form of child pornography increased substantially because of child and adolescent sexual depictions on the Internet (O'Connell, 1999). Other forces contributing to the emergence of a youth culture susceptible to juvenile prostitution and child sexual exploitation include such social movements as the counterculture movement of the 1960s (flower children, free sex, and the hippie movement) and the subsequent problem of runaway youth, and street youth in particular, in the late 1960s and early 1970s (Melville, 1972; Suddick, 1973). These developments took place against a backdrop of efforts in the 1970s and 1980s to protect the rights of minors and to ensure their rights of free expression (Weisberg, 1987).

In the United States, the visibility and the increased recognition of child abuse and sexual abuse, particularly in the 1970s and 1980s, led to protective state and federal legislation. Advocacy efforts increased for homeless and abused children by governmental social and health agencies such as the Children's Bureau (Weisberg, 1984) and later the Agency for Children, Youth, and Families.

The children's rights movement in the United States translated into legislation and court decisions expanding the rights of juvenile offenders. There was a broad move in the early 1980s for states to use the same standards of proof for juveniles as for adults and to abandon status offenses (those offenses committed by minors, for which there are no comparable adult charges, such as truancy, incorrigibility, or runaway behavior) (Wooden, 1976). In the 1990s, however, many states and municipalities, under pressure from school districts and parents' rights groups, reinstated status offenses and curfews in the name of protecting juveniles who were out of school and "out of parental control."

The cross-cutting features of all of these historical social changes involve an increasing number of youth moving to the margins of society, adopting alternative lifestyles, being at odds with the law, and experiencing social alienation, homelessness, and exploitation. Urban homelessness and attempts to survive on the streets have put youth at special risk for entrance into prostitution, survival sex, and sexual exploitation (Deisher & Farrow, 1986; Hutchinson & Langlykke, 1997).

# Typology of Homeless Youth Involved in Survival Sex

The largest number of youth in the United States and Canada involved in prostitution and Internet exploitation come from the ranks of runaway and homeless youth (Greene et al, 1999; MacDonald et al, 1994; Whitbeck & Simons, 1993).

Several factors contribute to the origins of youth homelessness. Unlike their counterparts in developing countries, children and youth on the streets in the United States and Canada are not generally homeless because of poverty, parental loss due to disease, or war. The types of runaway and homeless youth at risk for sexual exploitation fall into 4 categories, as summarized in **Table 16-1**.

## Situational Runaways

The largest group of runaway youth, ***situational runaways***, leave home for short periods of time generally because of a disagreement with parents. They usually return home within a few days. The runaway behavior is often repeated. Most of the time, these young people temporarily reside with friends and extended family. A small number spend brief periods on the street, become attached to a more alienated group, and join the chronic runaway population. Because most are younger adolescents with a variety of family supports for survival, sexual exploitation in the community is relatively low. In addition, the chronic and more severe family dysfunction which typifies the experiences of repeat runaways is not usually part of the picture. These youth are not generally running from an abusive family situation or repeatedly running away to cope with family stresses (Whitbeck et al, 1997).

## Runaways

***Runaways*** are youth who leave home because of neglect, abuse, or serious conflicts with adult caregivers. Many of these young people become chronic runaways and denizens of the streets in urban centers. They may live in transitory housing and may repeatedly be in juvenile detention centers for short periods of time for minor status

**Table 16-1. Typology of Homeless Youth Involved in Survival Sex**

| Type | Description | Risk for Sexual Exploitation |
|---|---|---|
| **Situational runaways** | — Short periods away from home<br>— Minor disputes with parents<br>— Runaway behavior often repeated | Low-Moderate |
| **Runaways** | — Longer periods away from home<br>— Major disputes with parents<br>— Histories of abuse and neglect<br>— Delinquency history | Moderate-High |
| **Thrownaways** | — Younger age<br>— Parental neglect and rejection high<br>— In and out of youth shelters | Very high |
| **Systems youth** | — Histories of childhood group foster care and institutionalization<br>— History of mental illness and conduct disorders<br>— Vulnerable to dysfunctional living situations on the streets | Very high |

or misdemeanor offenses. Once on the street, they may reside in groups without shelter, in cheap hotels, or in abandoned buildings or "squats." These youth are at significant risk for physical violence and sexual victimization if they are without any resources necessary for survival (Kipke et al, 1997a). Sexual minority youth are over-represented among these runaways. It is difficult to know the actual number of gay adolescents on the streets, particularly because many heterosexual males will engage in same-sex relations for money. In a 1988 study, 20% of New York male runaways identified themselves as gay (Stricof et al, 1991). Another study in 1988 found a gay or bisexual identification in 16.5% of males in the Hollywood area of southern California (Yates et al, 1991). Other providers of services to gay, lesbian, and transgender street youth place the numbers in some urban areas as high as 40% (Kruks, 1991).

## Thrownaways

**Thrownaways** are youths who have been abandoned by their adult caretakers or who have been subjected to extreme levels of abuse or neglect. Many of these young people have spent time with relatives or in foster care and are known to child protective services. They are generally homeless at a very young age, usually by the time of early adolescence (Ryan et al, 2000). As with runaways in general, they are at exceptional risk for sexual exploitation and victimization once away from protective adult supervision (Brannigan & Van Brunschot, 1997). For these youth especially, sexual, physical, and emotional abuse are significant cofactors that make them vulnerable to exploitation.

## Systems Youth

**Systems youth** have a long history of institutionalization or group foster placement. They have a history of repeated runaway behavior from institutional care, and at some point in their adolescence, they became a part of the runaway and street subculture. Many suffer from clinically diagnosed mental disorders, are developmentally disabled, and often commit minor criminal offenses, prompting further institutionalization (McCaskill et al, 1998; Whitbeck et al, 2000). Pre-adolescent children are usually returned to their foster care living situations, but by the time they are early adolescents (11 to 14 years of age), most are unwilling to return and will remain on the streets in highly vulnerable and dysfunctional living situations (Durant et al, 1995; Ennett et al, 1999; Robertson, 1992).

For runaways and other young people living on the streets there are few legitimate or acceptable means of survival. Most try various kinds of illegal or illicit activities, such as selling drugs, panhandling, or stealing. One of the most common means of obtaining funds, however, is through "survival sex." **Survival sex** constitutes a less formal exchange of sex for money, shelter, drugs, or protection from someone who is older and more streetwise (Greenblatt & Roberston, 1993). Studies now show that substantial numbers of young women and young men who are on the streets for any period of time become involved in survival sex although young males appear to have more options available to them for survival. In studies conducted in Los Angeles, about one third of young women and men living on the streets reported involvement in sex work (Kipke et al, 1997b). Similar findings were reported in a study of street youth in Seattle (Wagner et al, 2001). Research has repeatedly shown that a history of incest or sexual abuse is an important determinant of engagement in prostitution or survival sex (James & Meyerding, 1977; Widom & Kuhns, 1996).

Prostitution or hustling for young men is not a homogenous phenomenon. Unlike young women involved in prostitution, young men are generally not organized by pimps or other adult leaders. Boys engage in other common forms of prostitution, such as becoming call boys or securing customers through advertisements in gay newspapers or Web sites or by hanging out in predominantly gay neighborhoods or near gay bars and clubs. Some become hardcore street hustlers, and a few work out of gay bath houses (Deisher et al, 1982; Rosenthal et al, 1994; Ryan & Futterman 1998; Weisberg, 1987). These young, mostly gay men are at risk for recruitment into video and Internet pornography, especially as they reach their 18th birthday.

## GENDER COMPARISONS

Additional ethnographical and sociological research has shown some interesting differences and similarities between male and female youth involved in prostitution. In general, the mean age for boys and girls involved is around 17 years of age; these youth come from all socioeconomic backgrounds (Clements et al, 1997; Ringwalt et al, 1998a), unlike their counterparts in developing countries, where sexual exploitation occurs for boys and girls at younger ages against a significant backdrop of poverty (Lalor, 1999; UNICEF, 1995). Studies of adolescent female prostitutes in North America reflect a large middle-class composition with a surprising number of youth from more affluent families (Deisher et al, 1982; Farrow et al, 1992; Hutchinson & Langlykke, 1997; Weisberg, 1987). In the United States and Canada, some young women who engage in prostitution have parents who are college-educated and lead professional lives. Most juvenile prostitutes in North America are Caucasian, with African American youth comprising the second largest racial group for male and female youth engaged in the sex trade. As stated earlier, many young women have a significant childhood history of sexual abuse and most young men have a significant childhood history of physical abuse (Brannigan & Van Brunschot, 1997; Widom & Kuhns, 1996). Estimates of the incidence of early intrafamilial sexual abuse among female prostitutes are high, ranging from 31% to 67% (Hutchinson & Langlykke, 1997). Juvenile male prostitutes also report having been sexually abused by family members. For young males, estimates of sexual abuse by family members range from 10% to 30% (Weisberg, 1987).

Entrance into prostitution is not always coerced. Peer influences on the entrance into prostitution are powerful for males and females. James (1980) reports that 13% of her female respondents first learned of prostitution from a girlfriend, and other studies note similar patterns for both boys and girls (Greene et al, 1999). For example, when a boy complains that he needs money and an older friend suggests that the youth can make quick money by prostitution, the older friend describes where and how sex for money is accomplished and usually accompanies the younger boy for at least the first encounter as protection (Bittle, 2002).

The formation of a sexual identity is a challenging developmental task for adolescents. Any coercive sex can negatively impact the healthy exploration of sexuality and sexual identity in particular. Once outside the home, these adolescents experience additional coercive sexual practices. Coercive same-sex relationships are more common among young men than women. Where young women might first engage in prostitution with an older man, so might a young man, serving to exacerbate sexual identity confusion.

Unlike their adult counterparts, juvenile sex industry workers who have the ability to earn large sums of money rarely retain much of their earnings. Few accumulate any savings or other material assets, and few have bank accounts. Most of their earnings are spent quickly on clothes, drugs, and entertainment (Bittle, 2002). When one ethnographical researcher asked a group of young prostituted males to count the money in their pockets at the time of the interview, more than half of the group had less than $1, and only 7 boys possessed more than $5 (Luna, 1997). Most of these youth depend on others, such as friends or "customers," to provide them with places to sleep and free meals. The significant difference between male and female adolescents with respect to finances is that females turn over much of their earnings to their pimps. Even though the adolescent male prostitute is more often self-employed, he still may not be able to retain any substantial portion of his earnings because of his chaotic lifestyle, which is often aggravated by drug abuse (Greene et al, 1999).

An additional difference between males and females entering prostitution is the element of homosexuality. As mentioned earlier, a homeless or prostituting boy's early, coerced, or negative sexual experiences are more likely than girls' to be homosexual in nature. James & Meyerding (1977) suggest that such early victimization may aggravate the youth's negative self-image and sexual identity confusion. This has been shown in other studies of young male victimization (Luna, 1997). Homosexual identity is also important at a subsequent stage in the process of exploitation. For gay youth, whether homeless or not, the decision to turn to prostitution may constitute an attempt to interact socially with other gay men. When a questioning male youth frequents venues where hustling is prominent, he may be attempting to explore whether or not he is homosexual or seeking some social acceptance within the gay community (Gonsiorek & Rudolph, 1991; Kruks, 1991). Nonetheless, because of the circumstances and the usual age differences, most of his sexual experiences are going to be exploitative, further aggravating his negative self-image. Many of these young men who "dabble" in prostitution within the gay community have a great deal of difficulty in their 20s becoming employable and self-sufficient, and many remain at considerable risk for human immunodeficiency virus/acquired immunodeficiency syndrome (HIV/AIDS) and substance abuse (Clatts et al, 1998; Gleghorn et al, 1998; Luna, 1997).

## HEALTH CONSEQUENCES OF SEXUAL EXPLOITATION

In terms of the health consequences associated with sexual exploitation and involvement in prostitution, several studies have noted significant increases in the medical and psychosocial consequences for youth involved in these activities compared to youth who are not involved in prostitution or the Internet sex trade. For example, a 1991 study by Yates et al of 620 self-identified homeless youth compared medical and psychosocial consequences for youth who were and who were not involved in prostitution (**Table 16-2**). For those youth involved in prostitution, twice as many reported having had a sexually transmitted disease, and all were at significant risk for HIV infection. There are no reliable HIV seroprevalence studies carried out in North America that focus exclusively on juvenile prostitutes; however, the HIV seroprevalence rates among homeless and street youth may be an indicator. Several studies have shown infection rates to be between 2% and 15% (Allen et al, 1994; Pfeifer & Oliver, 1997; Sweeney et al, 1995). Fewer youth who were involved in prostitution used family planning services. Three times as many had drug abuse problems, 3 times as many reported coercive sexual situations such as rape, and nearly 100% of those involved in prostitution reported significant risk behaviors for acquisition of HIV (**Table 16-2**) (Yates et al, 1991).

The demographic and psychosocial data reported in this research showed that youths engaged in prostitution dropped out of school at an earlier age and had fewer constructive hobbies and less sports participation. For youth involved in prostitution or survival sex, sexual exploitation and exposure to violence often produces depression, posttraumatic stress disorder, drug abuse, and other symptoms of psychological distress (Rohde et al, 2001; Smart & Walsh, 1993). A study of Los Angeles youth found significantly higher rates of self-reported depression and suicidal tendencies among those youth with histories of prostitution. Likewise, those youth who had engaged in prostitution had significantly higher rates of substance abuse, most notably injectable drug use (**Table 16-3**) (Yates et al, 1991).

Lastly, young women engaged in prostitution report a high incidence of pregnancy (Deisher et al, 1989; Greene & Ringwalt 1998). Deisher et al (1989) studied the pregnant adolescent prostitute. The study reported on pregnancy outcomes among 61 adolescent women with histories of homelessness, street involvement, and prostitution. The study found that pregnant adolescent prostitutes rarely requested pregnancy termination. The majority continued their pregnancy to term. Adoption or

**Table 16-2. Medical Diagnoses of Homeless Youths Involved (n = 153) and Not Involved (n = 467) in Prostitution**

| DIAGNOSES* | INVOLVED (%) | NOT INVOLVED (%) |
|---|---|---|
| Sexually transmitted disease | 19.0 | 9.9 |
| Pelvic inflammatory disease | 5.8 | 0.4 |
| Pregnancy | 18.3 | 6.5 |
| Uncontrolled asthma | 2.6 | 1.5 |
| Infectious disease | 13.1 | 9.4 |
| Dermatology problems | 5.9 | 7.1 |
| Family planning services | 23.1 | 30.9 |
| Drug abuse | 74.5 | 36.0 |
| Trauma | 3.3 | 4.5 |
| Rape | 2.6 | 0.9 |
| HIV risk | 100.0 | 7.7 |

* Patients were given as many as 6 diagnoses; approximately 300 different diagnostic categories were available to clinicians. This table represents only a portion of all diagnoses given; percentages will not equal 100%.

Reprinted with permission from Elsevier Science. Yates GL, Mackenzie RG, Pennbridge J, Swofford A. A risk profile comparison of homeless youth involved in prostitution and homeless youth not involved. J Adolesc Health. *1991;12(7):545-548.*

**Table 16-3. Psychosocial Interview Information on Homeless Youths Involved (n = 153) and Not Involved (n = 467) in Prostitution**

| PSYCHOSOCIAL INFORMATION | INVOLVED (%) | NOT INVOLVED (%) |
|---|---|---|
| **Home** | | |
| Relatives | 0.0 | 3.0 |
| Friends | 11.1 | 6.6 |
| Shelter | 61.4 | 77.9 |
| Streets | 24.8 | 11.1 |
| Other/unknown | 2.6 | 1.3 |
| **Education** | | |
| College | 2.0 | 2.4 |
| Trade/vocational college | 3.4 | 2.4 |
| High school | 34.2 | 48.5 |
| Junior high | 4.7 | 11.4 |
| Drop-out | 53.0 | 34.1 |
| Other/unknown | 2.7 | 1.3 |

*(continued)*

**Table 16-3. Psychosocial Interview Information on Homeless Youths Involved (n = 153) and Not Involved (n = 467) in Prostitution** *(continued)*

| PSYCHOSOCIAL INFORMATION | INVOLVED (%) | NOT INVOLVED (%) |
|---|---|---|
| **Activity** | | |
| Sports | 13.7 | 26.9 |
| Job | 12.4 | 9.5 |
| Hang out | 52.3 | 50.3 |
| Hobbies | 29.4 | 29.0 |
| Other/unknown | 22.1 | 19.8 |
| **Drugs** | | |
| Intravenous use | 21.7 | 3.7 |
| Hallucinogens | 39.2 | 15.0 |
| Stimulants | 57.9 | 27.6 |
| Inhalants | 17.1 | 8.5 |
| Narcotics | 25.0 | 7.6 |
| Marijuana | 70.4 | 47.8 |
| Alcohol | 78.3 | 59.6 |
| Cigarettes | 70.4 | 58.0 |
| Drug problem | 12.5 | 7.0 |
| No drug use | 3.3 | 22.4 |
| **Suicidality and depression** | | |
| Depressed | 54.6 | 50.1 |
| Suicide attempt | 47.4 | 26.7 |
| Suicidal | 7.2 | 4.5 |
| Mental health | 5.9 | 2.8 |
| **Sexual behavior** | | |
| Sexual orientation | | |
| — Heterosexual | 68.6 | 92.2 |
| — Homosexual | 15.7 | 2.9 |
| — Bisexual | 12.4 | 2.5 |
| — Undecided | 0.0 | 2.5 |
| Age at first sex | | |
| — Never | 0.0 | 12.7 |
| — 0-9 | 24.8 | 7.8 |
| — 10-14 | 49.0 | 54.1 |
| — 15-18 | 22.2 | 24.9 |
| — 19+ | 0.006 | 0.5 |
| — Unknown | 3.3 | 5.9 |
| **Sexual behavior** | | |
| Problems with sex | | |
| — Patient states yes | 3.3 | 1.5 |
| — Survival sex | 100.0 | 0.0 |
| **Physical abuse** | 24.2 | 12.9 |
| **Satanic abuse** | 11.1 | 3.2 |

*Reprinted with permission from Elsevier Science. Yates GL, Mackenzie RG, Pennbridge J, Swofford A. A risk profile comparison of homeless youth involved in prostitution and homeless youth not involved.* J Adolesc Health. *1991;12(7):545-548.*

relinquishment was almost totally rejected by the study group; many were glad to be pregnant and felt that childbearing would improve their lives. Some saw their pregnancy as a means to exit prostitution. None of the young women in the study had childcare skills or any realistic notion of where they would live or how they would support their children. As a result, they received late prenatal care or none at all, lived in unhealthy environments, and were unreliable contraceptive users. Also noted in this study was the challenge these young women presented to social service and healthcare professionals. These girls were suspicious of these adults' motives because of manipulation and exploitation by adult men and past experiences with the juvenile justice system. Also, their transient and often violent lifestyles, dependence on drugs, and need to drop out of sight for periods of time further isolated them. For many of these young women, access to helpful professionals was often barred by a controlling adult figure, most often a pimp, an abusive boyfriend, or an adult relative (Deisher et al, 1989).

## RECOMMENDATIONS

An understanding of the psychosocial context for youth involvement in prostitution and their subsequent sexual exploitation provides professionals with strategies for assisting children and youth to repair the damage to their lives and to reenter society from the margins.

Health and social services for youth involved in the sex trade or who have been sexually exploited outside the home expanded throughout the 1980s and 1990s. Provision of preventive healthcare and social services for this population remains difficult. Treatment compliance for psychiatric and substance abuse conditions is poor unless youth are provided with safe and secure shelter and other needed social services (Smart & Ogborne, 1994). Likewise, compliance with health maintenance visits and HIV/AIDS treatment depend on similar assurances of safe and reliable shelter and trusted adult support (Allen et al, 1994).

Community-based case-management approaches have been expanded. Streetside medical services appear to be effective in reaching vulnerable youth. Health and social services are offered in a manner that builds trust and eliminates access barriers. Health screening and patient education are best provided through an outreach effort that engages these young women and young men in the community, in institutions, and on the street. As mentioned, many of these young people require emotional support and safe shelter (Farrow et al, 1992). Criminal justice and legislative strategies alone are insufficient to reduce the problem to the degree they focus solely on the juvenile victim and not the adult exploiter (Bittle, 2002).

## REFERENCES

Allen DM, Lehman JS, Green TA, Lindegren ML, Onorato IM, Forrester W. HIV infection among homeless adults and runaway youth, United States, 1989-1992. Field Services Branch. *AIDS*. 1994;8(11):1593-1598.

Bittle S. *Youth Involvement in Prostitution: A Literature Review*. Ottawa, Canada: Research and Statistics Division of the Dept of Justice Canada. April 2002. rr2001-13e.

Brannigan A, Van Brunschot EG. Youthful prostitution and child sexual trauma. *Int J Law Psychiatry*. 1997;20(30):337-354.

Clatts MC, Davis WR, Sotheran JL, Atillasoy A. Correlates and distribution of HIV risk behaviors among homeless youths in New York City: implications for prevention and policy. *Child Welfare*. 1998;77(2):195-207.

Clements K, Gleghorn A, Garcia D, Katz M, Marx R. A risk profile of street youth in northern California: implications for gender-specific human immunodeficiency virus prevention. *J Adolesc Health*. 1997;20(5):343-353.

Deisher RW, Farrow JA. Recognizing and dealing with alienated youth in clinical practice. *Pediatr Ann.* 1986;15(11):759-764.

Deisher RW, Farrow JA, Hope K, Litchfield C. The pregnant adolescent prostitute. *Am J Dis Child.* 1989;143:1162-1165.

Deisher RW, Robinson G, Boyer D. The adolescent female and male prostitute. *Pediatr Ann.* 1982;11:812-825.

Durant RH, Getts A, Cadenhead C, Emans SJ, Woods ER. Exposure to violence and victimization and depression, hopelessness, and purpose in life among adolescents living in and around public housing. *J Dev Behav Pediatr.* 1995;16(4):233-237.

Ennett ST, Bailey SL, Federman ED. Social network characteristics associated with risky behaviors among runaway and homeless youth. *J Health Soc Behav.* 1999;40(1): 63-78.

Farrow JA, Deisher RW, Brown R, Kulig JW, Kipke MD. Health and health needs of homeless and runaway youth. *J Adolesc Health.* 1992;13:717-726.

Gerber GM. Barriers to health care for street youth. *J Adolesc Health.* 1997;21(5); 287-290.

Gleghorn AA, Marx R, Vittinghoff E, Katz MH. Association between drug use patterns and HIV risks among homeless, runaway, and street youths in Northern California. *Drug Alcohol Depend.* 1998;51(3):219-227.

Gonsiorek JC, Rudolph JR. Homosexual identity: coming out and other developmental events. In: Gonsiorek J, Weinrich J, eds. *Homosexuality: Research Implications for Public Policy.* Newbury Park, Calif: Sage Publications; 1991:161-176.

Greenblatt M, Robertson MJ. Lifestyles, adaptive strategies, and sexual behaviors of homeless adolescents. *Hosp Community Psychiatry.* 1993;44(12):1177-1180.

Greene JM, Ennett ST, Ringwalt CL. Prevalence and correlates of survival sex among runaway and homeless youth. *Am J Public Health.* 1999;89(9):1406-1409.

Greene JM, Ringwalt CL. Pregnancy among three national samples of runaway and homeless youth. *J Adolesc Health.* 1998;23(6):370-377.

Hetrick ES, Martin AD. Developmental issues and their resolution for gay and lesbian adolescents. *J Homosex.* 1987;14(1-2):25-33.

Hutchinson J, Langlykke K. *Adolescent Maltreatment: Youth as Victims of Abuse and Neglect.* Washington, DC: Health Resources & Services Administration, Maternal and Child Health Bureau, Tech Info Bulletin; 1997.

James J. *Entrance Into Juvenile Prostitution.* Washington, DC: National Institute of Mental Health; 1980.

James J, Meyerding J. Early sexual experiences as a factor in prostitution. *Arch Sex Behav.* 1977;1:31-42.

Kipke MD, Simon TR, Montgomery SB, Unger JB, Iversen EF. Homeless youth and their exposure to and involvement in violence while living on the streets. *J Adolesc Health.* 1997a;20(5):360-367.

Kipke MD, Unger JB, O'Connor S, Palmer RF, La France SR. Street youth, their peer group affiliation and differences according to the residential status, subsistence patterns, and use of services. *Adolescence.* 1997b;32:655-669.

Klein JD, Woods AH, Wilson KM, Prospero M, Greene J, Ringwalt C. Homeless and runaway youths' access to health care. *J Adolesc Health.* 2000;27(5):331-339.

Kruks G. Gay and lesbian homeless/street youth: special issues and concerns. *J Adolesc Health.* 1991;12(7):515-518.

Lalor KJ. Street children: a comparative perspective. *Child Abuse Negl.* 1999;23(8): 759-770.

Luna GC. *Youths Living with HIV: Self-Evident Truths.* New York, NY: Harrington Park Press; 1997.

MacDonald NE, Fisher WA, Wells GA, Doherty JA, Bowie WR. Canadian street youth: correlates of sexual risk-taking activity. *Pediatr Infect Dis J.* 1994;13(3):690-697.

de Mause L. The evolution of childhood. In: de Mause L, ed. *The History of Childhood.* New York, NY: Harper and Row; 1974;1-74.

McCaskill PA, Toro PA, Wolfe SM. Homeless and matched housed adolescents: a comparative study of psychopathology. *J Clin Child Psychol.* 1998;27(3):306-319.

Melville K. *Communes in the Counter Culture: Origins, Theories, Styles of Life.* New York, NY: Morrow; 1972.

Noell JW, Ochs LM. Relationship of sexual orientation to substance use, suicidal ideation, suicide attempts, and other factors in a population of homeless adolescents. *J Adolesc Health.* 2001;29(1):31-36.

O'Connell R. An analysis of paedophile activity on the Internet from a structural and social organizational perspective and the implications for investigative strategies. Paper presented at: 14th BILETA Conference: "CYBERSPACE 1999: Crime, Criminal Justice and the Internet"; March 29, 1999; York, England.

Pfeifer RW, Oliver J. A study of HIV seroprevalence in a group of homeless youth in Hollywood, California. *J Adolesc Health.* 1997;20(5):339-342.

Ringwalt CL, Greene JM, Robertson MJ. Familial backgrounds and risk behaviors of youth with thrownaway experiences. *J Adolesc.* 1998a;21(3):241-252.

Ringwalt CL, Greene JM, Robertson MJ, McPheeters M. The prevalence of homelessness among adolescents in the United States. *Am J Public Health.* 1998b;88(9): 1325-1329.

Robertson MJ. The prevalence of mental disorders among homeless persons. In: Jahiel RI, ed. *Homelessness: A Prevention-Oriented Approach.* Baltimore, Md: Johns Hopkins Press; 1992:57-86.

Rohde P, Noell J, Ochs L, Seeley JR. Depression, suicidal ideation and STD-related risk in homeless older adolescents. *J Adolesc.* 2001;24(4):447-460.

Rosenthal D, Moore S, Buzwell S. Homeless youths: sexual and drug-related behaviour, sexual beliefs and HIV/AIDS risk. *AIDS Care.* 1994;6(1):83-94.

Ryan C, Futterman D. *Lesbian and Gay Youth.* New York, NY: Columbia University Press; 1998.

Ryan KD, Kilmer RP, Cauce AM, Watanabe H, Hoyt DR. Psychological consequences of child maltreatment in homeless adolescents: untangling the unique effects of maltreatment and family environment. *Child Abuse Negl.* 2000;24(3):333-352.

Sleegers J, Spijker J, van Limbeek J, van Engeland H. Mental health problems among homeless adolescents. *Acta Psychiatr Scand.* 1998;97(4):253-259.

Smart RG, Ogborne AC. Street youth in substance abuse treatment: characteristics and treatment compliance. *Adolescence.* 1994;29(115):733-745.

Smart RG, Walsh GW. Predictors of depression in street youth. *Adolescence.* 1993; 28(109):41-53.

Stricof RL, Kennedy JT, Nattell TC, Weisfuse IB, Novick LF. HIV seroprevalence in a facility for runaway and homeless adolescents. *Am J Public Health.* 1991;81(suppl): 50-53.

Suddick DE. Runaways: a review of the literature. *Juvenile Justice.* 1973;24:47-54.

Sweeney P, Lindegren ML, Buehler JW, Onorato IM, Janssen RS. Teenagers at risk of human immunodeficiency virus type 1 infection. Results from seroprevalence surveys in the United States. *Arch Pediatr Adolesc Med.* 1995;149(5):521-528.

UNICEF. The Convention on the Rights of the Child. London, England: UK Committee for UNICEF; 1995.

Wagner LS, Carlin PL, Cauce AM, Tenner A. A snapshot of homeless youth in Seattle: their characteristics, behaviors and beliefs about HIV protection strategies. *J Community Health.* 2001;26(3):219-232.

Waters T. *Crime and Immigrant Youth.* Thousand Oaks, Calif: Sage Publications; 1999.

Weisberg DK. The "discovery" of sexual abuse: experts' role in legal policy formulation. *UC Davis Law Rev.* 1984;18:1-54.

Weisberg DK. *Children of the Night: A Study of Adolescent Prostitution.* Lexington, Mass: DC Heath and Co Press; 1987.

Whitbeck LB, Hoyt DR, Ackley KA. Families of homeless and runaway adolescents: a comparison of parent/caretaker and adolescent perspectives on parenting, family violence, and adolescent conduct. *Child Abuse Negl.* 1997;21(6):517-528.

Whitbeck LB, Hoyt DR, Bao WN. Depressive symptoms and co-occurring depressive symptoms, substance abuse, and conduct problems among runaway and homeless adolescents. *Child Dev.* 2000;71(3):721-732.

Whitbeck LB, Simons RL. A comparison of adaptive strategies and patterns of victimization among homeless adolescents and adults. *Violence Vict.* 1993;8(2):135-152.

Widom CS, Kuhns JB. Childhood victimization and subsequent risk for promiscuity, prostitution, and teenage pregnancy: a prospective study. *Am J Public Health.* 1996; 86(11):1607-1612.

Wooden K. *Weeping in the Playtime of Others: America's Incarcerated Children.* New York, NY: McGraw-Hill; 1976.

Yates GL, MacKenzie RG, Pennbridge J, Swofford A. A risk profile comparison of homeless youth involved in prostitution and homeless youth not involved. *J Adolesc Health.* 1991;12(7):545-548.

# Chapter 17

# Medical Care of the Children of the Night

Nancy D. Kellogg, MD

*Children of the night* is a term that refers to children and adolescents involved in a variety of adverse circumstances: being a runaway, homelessness, survival sex, sex for drugs, sexually transmitted diseases (STDs), substance abuse, crime, and violence. Medical care for such children typically begins with a medical emergency or with a compulsory examination after incarceration. When runaway behavior and prostitution are linked, the risk of medical problems escalates significantly. In one comparison study of runaway/homeless prostitutes and runaway/homeless nonprostitutes, prostitutes were about twice as likely to abuse drugs (74.5%) or have an STD (19%) and uncontrolled asthma (2.6%); about 3 times more likely to be pregnant (18%) or a victim of rape (2.6%); and about 12 times more likely to have pelvic inflammatory disease (PID) (5.8%) (Yates et al, 1991). In addition, prostitutes' risk of human immunodeficiency virus (HIV) approaches 100%, whereas in nonprostitutes it is less than 8% (Yates et al, 1991).

Despite these compelling medical problems and risks, most adolescent prostitutes consider their health "excellent" or "good," and more than half reported no change in their health since they became homeless or a runaway (Unger et al, 1998). This lack of concern may reflect denial, ignorance, or inability to understand the consequences of their lifestyle. Adolescents generally think in concrete rather than abstract terms such that a comprehensive understanding of intermediate- and long-term risks of their behavior is usually lacking. As discussed in Chapter 19, Community and Mental Health Support of Juvenile Prostitute Victims, these children and adolescents are reluctant to seek help and unwilling to give information that may result in their arrest, placement in a shelter, or return to their families. The medical care provider confronts the challenge of gathering information that is critical, accurate, and as complete as possible from mistrustful, sometimes hostile children who generally underreport and underestimate their health problems.

All suspected victims of child or adolescent sexual abuse should be evaluated by a pediatrician or mental health provider so that treatment and safety needs, particularly the degree of parental support, are comprehensively assessed (American Academy of Pediatrics [AAP] Committee on Child Abuse and Neglect, 1999b). When a child presents to a medical setting as a victim of prostitution or pornography, there are a number of clinical management options to consider. Depending on the resources available within the community, the need for forensic evidence collection, and the clinician's comfort level, the clinician may either refer the child to a specialized child abuse evaluation center or elect to conduct part or all of the medical evaluation. For example, if a patient states that sexual assault occurred 2 weeks ago, an interview and assessment may be conducted within an office setting; a victim presenting within a few hours of a sexual assault may best be cared for in a center equipped to evaluate more extensive trauma and to gather forensic evidence. Many communities have established multidisciplinary teams for evaluating all child and adolescent victims of sexual abuse and exploitation; referrals to such teams may provide the best care for all victims of acute and chronic sexual abuse. Specialized child abuse clinics are generally found within hospital settings or at child advocacy centers. If such resources are unknown, a child advocacy center can be contacted to provide referrals and assistance.

## CLINICAL APPROACH

When sexual abuse, physical injuries, and other health risks are suspected, the clinician should approach the child with concern and empathy while remaining nonjudgmental and maintaining confidentiality to the extent that the law allows. Although many victims do not fully disclose their victimization or risky health behavior in a clinical setting, the clinician may still acquire useful information in the short term and begin a relationship of trust in the longer term.

Many states have established definitions for "statutory rape" based on the ages of the individuals engaged in sexual contact, regardless of whether such activity is consensual or not. For example, in Texas any sexual contact with a child younger than 17 years old is statutory rape; however, an affirmative defense may apply to sexual contact among adolescents who are between 14 and 17 years old if one individual is not more than 3 years older than the other individual and the contact is consensual (Texas Penal Code § 22.011(e) (2002)). While confidentiality is generally a critical concern to the adolescent who reluctantly seeks healthcare for the consequences of his or her risky health behaviors, the clinician is nonetheless required by law to report "consensual" but illegal sexual contact to law enforcement or child protective services (CPS) agencies. The risks of reporting such illegal sexual contact include patient noncompliance and loss of patient trust; the benefits of reporting include a possibility that system intervention may address and reduce health risky behavior, including sexual contact with older individuals. When an adolescent is a victim of a rape by a stranger or an acquaintance who is unlikely to assault the same adolescent again, a report may prevent such perpetrators from assaulting another victim. The clinician should explain this rationale for reporting when victims are angry or distressed that such a report is required.

## "TEAMSTAT" APPROACH

The "TEAMSTAT" approach is one that may be followed when assessing children who have been abused. It is summarized in **Table 17-1**.

### TELL THEM YOUR AGENDA

The clinician should begin the interview by discussing with the child or adolescent the types of questions that will be asked and why. For example, the clinician may say, "I am going to ask you some questions about how your body is doing, how your feelings are doing, how your life is going, and about any hurtful or uncomfortable things that may have happened to you. The reason I am asking these questions is so I can figure out what I need to check you for, what tests I might need to do, and how I can best help you with your health."

The clinician should discuss the limits of confidentiality at the beginning of the interview. If child abuse is suspected, the clinician is obligated by law to report this. If the child states that he or she intends to hurt himself or herself or others, the clinician is obligated to notify other individuals.

### EXPRESS CONCERN

The clinician should state his or her concern for various medical conditions in a clear, direct, and empathetic way: "I am concerned about the painful sores you describe; have you ever been checked for sexual infections?" When an adolescent presents with abdominal pain and symptoms of gastritis, the clinician may state, "I am concerned about your stomach pain and would like to ask you a few questions about alcohol and drugs that may help me determine why you have this pain." It is best to link concern with the presenting medical complaint initially. This non-

**Table 17-1. The "TEAMSTAT" Approach**

**T**ell them your agenda

**E**xpress concern

**A**ssure normalcy of feelings

**M**edical issues

— Sexual/physical victimization

— Drug and alcohol use

— Psychiatric symptoms and diagnoses

**S**afety issues

— Family history, support

— Runaway tendencies

**T**est and treat presumptively

— Sexually transmitted diseases (STDs)

— Pregnancy prophylaxis, birth control

**A**ccess appropriate psychological and legal assistance

— Psychiatric assessment

— Reporting requirements

**T**imely follow-up

— Injuries

— STDs

— Birth control

— Drug and alcohol use

*Adapted from Kellogg ND, Sugarek NJ. Sexual trauma.* Atlas of Office Procedures. *1998;1(1):181-197.*

judgmental, clinically focused approach reduces anxiety in the child and facilitates information-sharing.

## Assure Normalcy of Feelings

As the interview progresses, the child may allude to feelings of shame, guilt, fear, and embarrassment regarding his or her victimization, family life, criminal behavior, and risky health lifestyle. Children and adolescents will be sensitive to the responses of health professionals as they "admit" to, and share feelings about, these circumstances. Clinicians should maintain a nonjudgmental demeanor, restate their reasons for asking such questions, and acknowledge that such feelings are "normal" among other children in similar circumstances: "I know this is hard for you to talk about. I have talked with other teens about this, and it is hard for them, too. These questions will help me decide whether I should check you for sexually transmitted diseases. If you feel more comfortable, you can write down or whisper your answers instead of saying them out loud. I really need your help before I can decide how to best help you."

## Medical Issues

The clinician should begin with past medical history including hospitalizations, gynecological examinations or conditions, injuries, psychiatric treatment, treatment for drug and alcohol use, pregnancy, menstrual history, medications, and drug allergies. If the child has had a gynecological examination or an STD or has been pregnant, the clinician should ask for details and results of tests, outcomes, and sexual history as outlined in **Table 17-2** under "Gynecological History." Though many of these details may be inaccurate or forgotten, some inportant information may be obtained. The order in which the following medical issues are discussed with the child depends on the presenting medical complaint; for example, children presenting as victims of prostitution should be questioned about sexual/physical victimization first, and those presenting with symptoms of acute inhalant abuse psychosis should be questioned about drug and alcohol use first. Regardless of the presenting complaint, all medical issues outlined here should be discussed with any adolescent or child in whom participation in prostitution or pornography is suspected.

Sexual/Physical Victimization

**Table 17-2** outlines the medical interview for victims of acute or nonacute sexual assault. Information gathered through this interview will determine the need for forensic evidence collection, testing for STDs, pregnancy testing, emergent psychiatric evaluation, and medical management for infections, drug/alcohol intoxication, pregnancy prophylaxis, and acute anxiety/depression. The clinician should begin this portion of the interview with nonleading questions: "Sometimes teens tell me that someone has hurt or touched them in a scary, uncomfortable way. Has anything like this ever happened to you?" Some victims of pornography and prostitution do not consider their victimization frightening, embarrassing, or hurtful. When a child responds "no" to this first question, a more direct follow-up question may be necessary: "Has anyone ever touched your privates with any part or parts of their body?" The child may spontaneously disclose sexual abuse when discussing their

---

**Table 17-2. Medical Interview for Sexual Victimization**

CURRENT PHYSICAL/EMOTIONAL/PSYCHOLOGICAL SYMPTOMS

— Pain/tenderness over body surfaces

— Bite marks (recent/healed)

— Genital symptoms (pain/bleeding, dysuria, discharge, abdominal pain)

— Recent drug/alcohol use; memory lapses, mental status changes

— Symptoms of shock, depression, suicide

HISTORY OF EVENT(S)

— Frequency and most recent incident

— Type(s) of sexual contact

— Condom use, lubrication

— Perpetrator identity/risk factors for sexually transmitted diseases, HIV (stranger, gang member, substance abuser)

— Bodily injuries; attack/defense injuries

GYNECOLOGICAL HISTORY

— Prior gynecological evaluations/conditions/infections/pregnancy

— Sexual history (timing and type[s] of previous sexual contact, contraceptive use, gender of partners)

— Last menstrual period

*Adapted from Kellogg ND, Sugarek NJ. Sexual trauma. Atlas of Office Procedures. 1998;1(1):181-197.*

---

presenting medical complaint or problem: "My private hurts because my uncle put his private down there." When the child spontaneously discloses abuse, details should be gathered at that point before returning to questions about physical symptoms and other medical issues.

A physical abuse or assault history should begin with discipline methods used by parents and caretakers: "When you were little and even now, when you get in trouble, how are you usually punished? Are you ever hit? With what? Where?" Severity of injuries ("Did it leave a mark or bruise? Did you ever get broken bones?"), hospitalizations, and CPS notification/intervention should also be noted. Adolescents should be asked similar questions regarding partner violence ("Have you ever lived with or dated someone who hit or hurt you?") and violence by adults that facilitate the child's participation in prostitution or pornography. The child may disclose spousal/partner abuse, drug/alcohol use, and criminal behavior among family members. Such information is important in identifying a temporary or permanent safe harbor for children.

### Drug and Alcohol Use

If a child or adolescent presents with obvious signs of intoxication or spontaneously admits to drug or alcohol use, the clinician should assess which drugs are used and the severity of use. Problem-severity assessment includes frequency and quantity of drug and alcohol use, context of use (social use only, alone, or both), dependence, and any legal difficulties resulting from alcohol or drug use. When substance use interferes with work, school, or interpersonal relationships or recurs in hazardous settings, it is considered substance abuse (American Psychiatric Association, 1994). When symptoms of drug tolerance or withdrawal occur, frequency of use escalates, or one's lifestyle centers around drug acquisition and use, then the diagnosis of substance dependence should be considered.

Some children and adolescents who use drugs or alcohol may deny use. Symptoms of drug use and withdrawal are presented in **Table 17-3**. Other less specific clinical signs of substance abuse include weight loss, persistent red eyes/nasal irritation/hoarseness, chronic cough, hemoptysis, chest pain, and wheezing (Fuller & Cavaznaugh, 1995). When substance use is suspected, the clinician may ask screening questions such as those proposed by the CRAFFT Screening Test (**Table 17-4**). This 6-question screening tool has demonstrated high sensitivity and specificity in a study population of

---

**Table 17-3. Symptoms of Drug Use and Withdrawal**

| SUBSTANCE | INTOXICATION EFFECTS | WITHDRAWAL EFFECTS |
|---|---|---|
| **Ethanol** | — Varies from impaired coordination to stupor<br>— Nausea/vomiting<br>— Hypoglycemia<br>— Gastritis | — Varies; includes headache, tremors, tachycardia, insomnia (delirium tremens are rare) |
| **Marijuana** | — Varies from euphoria to paranoia/psychosis<br>— Decreased problem-solving, memory<br>— Increased appetite<br>— Impaired coordination | — Sleep disturbances, tremors, anorexia<br>— Chronic use: decreased motivation, global cognitive impairment, mild feminization, decreased sperm count |

*(continued)*

## Table 17-3. Symptoms of Drug Use and Withdrawal *(continued)*

| Substance | Intoxication Effects | Withdrawal Effects |
|---|---|---|
| **Heroin and other opiates** | — Respiratory depressant/arrest<br>— Pupillary miosis<br>— Impaired mentation<br>— Seizures<br>— Hypotension, bradycardia, arrhythmias<br>— Chronic use: generalized pruritus, constipation, bronchospasm | — Myalgias<br>— Elevated temperature<br>— Irritability<br>— Nausea/vomiting<br>— Tremors<br>— Hypertension, tachycardia |
| **Cocaine** | — Hyperalertness, euphoria<br>— Insomnia, paranoia, psychosis<br>— Pupillary miosis<br>— Hypertension, tachycardia<br>— Elevated temperature<br>— Coronary vasospasm<br>— Rhabdomyolysis | — Depression, irritability<br>— Tremor<br>— Lethargy<br>— Nausea<br>— Chronic use: unsatisfiable craving for more |
| **Hallucinogens (LSD, PCP)** | — Altered visual/auditory sense<br>— Altered mood, sense of time/space<br>— Aggressive state (PCP)<br>— Elevated temperature<br>— Tachycardia | — No specific withdrawal symptoms |
| **Amphetamines** | — Hyperactivity<br>— Irritability, anxiety, panic<br>— Elevated temperature<br>— Hypertension, tachycardia<br>— Insomnia<br>— Anorexia<br>— Seizures, arrhythmias | — Lethargy<br>— Depression<br>— Sweats<br>— Abdominal cramps<br>— Muscle cramps<br>— Hypotension |
| **Depressants (prescription drugs including sedatives, hypnotics, tranquilizers)** | — Similar to ethanol intoxication<br>— Sedation<br>— Ataxia, slurred speech<br>— Respiratory depression | — Similar to ethanol withdrawal<br>— Irritability, tremors, elevated temperature, tachycardia, hypertension<br>— Chronic use: cognitive deficits, motor slowing, incoordination, mood lability |
| **Inhalants (toluene, paint thinner, glue, spray paint, gasoline, freon, propane)** | — Euphoria<br>— Hallucinations<br>— Nystagmus<br>— Rhinorrhea<br>— Respiratory depression/arrest | — No specific withdrawal symptoms<br>— Chronic use: tremor, ataxia, peripheral neuropathy, hyperactivity, expressive/receptive processing difficulties, dementia |
| **Other club drugs (Ecstasy, gamma-hydroxybutyrate [GHB], ketamine, Rohypnol)** | — Tachycardia<br>— Hypertension<br>— Hyperthermia<br>— Confusion/anxiety/paranoia<br>— Heart/kidney failure<br>— Respiratory depression<br>— Amnesia | — No specific withdrawal symptoms |

*Adapted from Fishman M, Bruner A, Adger H. Substance abuse among children and adolescents. Pediatr Rev. 1997;18(11):394-403; Schwartz B, Alderman EM. Substances of abuse. Pediatr Rev. 1997;18(6):204-215.*

**Table 17-4. CRAFFT Screening Test for Adolescent Substance Abuse**

**C** - Have you ever ridden in a CAR driven by someone (including yourself) who was "high" or had been using alcohol or drugs?

**R** - Do you ever use alcohol or drugs to RELAX, feel better about yourself, or fit in?

**A** - Do you ever use alcohol/drugs while you are by yourself, ALONE?

**F** - Do your family or FRIENDS ever tell you that you should cut down on your drinking or drug use?

**F** - Do you ever FORGET things you did while using alcohol or drugs?

**T** - Have you gotten into TROUBLE while you were using alcohol or drugs?

*Reprinted from CeASAR: The Center for Adolescent Substance Abuse Research. The CRAFFT questions. Available at: http://www.slp3d2.com/rwj_1027/webcast/docs/screentest.html. Accessed July 29, 2003.*

99 adolescents (Knight et al, 1999). In this study, 2 or more affirmative answers had a sensitivity of 92% and specificity of 82% for intensive substance abuse treatment need. When interviewing adolescent prostitutes who are homeless or living with friends, the clinician should be aware that one of the strongest risk factors for substance abuse is drug/alcohol use in the peer group (Fishman et al, 1997). In one study of street youth (Unger et al, 1998), the most common peer group was "gang members" (34%), followed by "druggies" (20%) and "alternatives/guardian" (20%).

In a comparison study of homeless prostituted adolescents and homeless adolescent nonprostitutes (Yates et al, 1991), 97% of the prostitutes and 78% of the nonprostitute group used drugs or alcohol. Use of hallucinogens (39%), stimulants (58%), inhalants (17%), narcotics (25%), marijuana (70%), and alcohol (78%) was approximately twice as high among the prostitute group (Yates et al, 1991).

### Psychiatric Symptoms and Diagnoses

Sexually exploited adolescents are at risk for a variety of psychological symptoms and diagnoses including depression, suicide, posttraumatic stress disorders, and aggression (Lanktree & Briere, 1995; Yates et al, 1991). Symptoms include changes in sleeping patterns, school or work functioning, and weight/ appetite. Asking questions about daily life may reveal areas of concern: "Do you ever have trouble falling asleep or with waking up at night?" "Has your appetite or weight changed?" "Are your grades going up, down, or staying the same?" "Have you ever found yourself crying for no reason?" The clinician should specifically ask about suicidal thoughts: "Have you ever felt so bad that you thought about hurting yourself?" If the child answers "yes," follow-up questions include: "When was that?" "Did you think of a way you wanted to hurt yourself?" "Did you try to hurt yourself?" "Did you tell anyone what you thought about doing (or did)?" Any adolescent with current suicidal thoughts should be referred for an emergent psychiatric evaluation.

Adolescents with substance use disorders may also have a psychiatric disorder. The most common psychiatric symptom in adolescent substance abusers is depression (Fishman et al, 1997). Contributing factors to depression include toxic effects of the drug(s) and demoralization from the losses, burdens, and chaos of addiction (Fishman et al, 1997). The substance abuse should be treated first before diagnosis of a comorbid psychiatric disorder is made (Fishman et al, 1997).

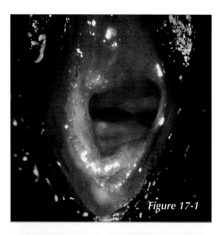

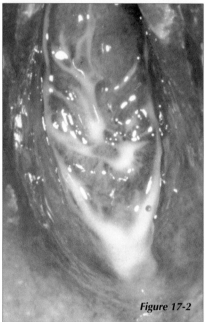

**Figure 17-1.** *Prepubertal female with gonorrhea and trichmoniasis. No apparent discharge or abnormal anatomical findings.*

**Figure 17-2.** *Thick white discharge in an adolescent with* Trichomonas vaginalis *infection.*

## SAFETY ISSUES

### Family History/Support

Adolescents or children may reveal substance use and violence among family members when discussing their own physical or sexual victimization or drug addiction. Some children fear repercussions from family members or peers if they disclose illegal activities or victimization. Children should be asked explicitly if they fear going home for any reason. If the child is a victim of prostitution, pornography, physical abuse, or sexual abuse and is accompanied by a parent, the parent's belief of and support for the child should be clearly established before the child is dismissed from the clinic.

### Runaway Tendencies

The clinician should ask the child if he or she has ever thought about running away or has run away from home. If children have run away from caretakers previously, then reasons, frequency, and outcome should be established.

## TEST AND TREAT PRESUMPTIVELY

The medical management of child and adolescent victims of prostitution or pornography should encompass testing for STDs, pregnancy, AIDS, and, under appropriate circumstances, substance and alcohol use. While presumptive treatment for gonorrhea, chlamydia, and *Trichomonas* (**Figures 17-1** and **17-2**) can be considered, testing should also be conducted so that sexual partners can also be notified and treated if an STD is identified. When appropriate, adolescents should be offered emergent postcoital contraception and long-term birth control options. Treatment protocols are discussed in detail under the section titled "Clinical Evaluation and Management."

## ACCESS APPROPRIATE PSYCHOLOGICAL AND LEGAL ASSISTANCE

When possible, crisis intervention services should be provided to the adolescent or child victim at the time of his or her medical evaluation. A clinical social worker can provide valuable assistance in locating community resources and financial assistance.

The clinician is obligated to report suspected child abuse as determined by the laws of each state. Most states require reporting within 48 hours of determining that abuse is suspected. More emergent CPS involvement may be required when (1) the child has no responsible caretaker or safe residence; (2) the parent accompanying the child appears ambivalent, nonbelieving, or nonsupportive of the child's statements of victimization; or (3) the parent accompanying the child appears incapacitated or angry toward the child.

## TIMELY FOLLOW-UP

Telephone and appointment follow-up should be attempted for all children of the night. Telephone follow-up should address psychological and physical symptoms. The goals of medical follow-up appointments include the following:

1. Access resolution of injuries from physical or sexual assault

2. Symptomatic relief of STDs

3. Appropriate use of birth control and barrier methods

4. Ongoing assessment of STDs with prolonged incubation periods

In addition, the clinician may monitor drug or alcohol abstinence with drug levels.

# MEDICAL EMERGENCIES

## SEXUAL ASSAULT EMERGENCIES

Severe injuries of sexual assault are rare. Injuries of moderate severity occur in approximately 5% of victims and include lacerations, hematomas, and fractures (Marchbanks et al, 1990) of the nongenital sites. The head and neck areas are most commonly involved, followed by the extremities and trunk (Kellogg & Sugarek, 1998). Approximately 1% of victims will have genital injuries requiring surgical repair (Geist, 1988); these include upper vaginal lacerations, intraperitoneal extension of a vaginal laceration, and deep anal lacerations.

Adolescents who present with abdominal pain, fever, dysuria, irregular vaginal bleeding, and/or vaginal discharge may have PID. A careful bimanual examination will usually reveal cervical motion tenderness or adnexal tenderness. Complications of this condition include infertility, increased risk of ectopic pregnancy, tubo-ovarian abscess, and pelvic adhesions (Marchbanks et al, 1988; Sweet, 1990). Because of the significant complications, adolescents should be treated emergently for PID; hospitalization to ensure treatment completion is recommended (AAP, 2000). Recommended inpatient treatment includes intravenous cefoxitin or cefotetan plus oral doxycycline or intravenous clindamycin and gentamicin. If adolescents refuse hospitalization or leave against medical advice, intramuscular cefoxitin (plus 1 gram oral probenecid) and ceftriaxone plus oral doxycycline can be given (AAP, 2000).

Acute sexual assault victims may require an emergent examination for forensic evidence collection. In one study of prepubertal children (Christian et al, 2000), most forensic evidence was recovered within 24 hours, but fewer than 25% of all forensic evidence collections yielded "positive" findings. In this study, most (64%) forensic evidence was recovered from clothing and linens. While 36% of forensic evidence was recovered from body surfaces or orifices, no swabs taken from the child's body more than 13 hours after the assault were positive for blood or semen (Christian et al, 2000). The recovery of forensic evidence among postpubertal patients may be higher than in prepubertal children due to physiological differences and the fact that more adolescents may present within a time frame conducive to evidence collection.

Foreign material, head hair combings/pluckings, clothing, and debris may be collected first. Debris or foreign bodies found in the mouth, vagina, or rectum may be submitted as evidence. Pubic hair combings/pluckings and swabs from the mouth, vagina, or rectum should be submitted for analysis. Patient saliva and blood samples are also required to establish the patient's blood type and whether blood group antigens were secreted into his or her bodily fluids. Evidence collection should follow protocols established by state or regional crime laboratories, and a chain of custody for collected material should be maintained.

A victim of an acute sexual assault may require emergent medical care for post-coital contraception. Emergency contraception may be given to nonpregnant females within 72 hours or up to 5 days of unprotected intercourse. A negative serum pregnancy test done at the time of the medical evaluation does not exclude an early pregnancy resulting from intercourse occurring between 5 and 10 days prior to the evaluation (Kellogg & Sugarek, 1998). Postcoital contraception is provided as follows: 2 50 mg ethinyl estradiol tablets immediately, repeat dose in 12 hours, or 3 35 mg ethinyl estradiol tablets immediately, repeat dose in 12 hours. An antiemetic should be provided with either regimen. Alternatives include Preven and Plan B, which are sometimes considered more effective. Adolescents should be told that irregular menstrual bleeding is not uncommon and does not indicate a miscarriage.

Human immunodeficiency virus infection is frequently a significant concern for victims of sexual assault and for those engaged in risky sexual behaviors, including prostitution. The risk of HIV transmission from a known infected person during a single act of vaginal intercourse is 0.1% to 0.2%; estimated risk for receptive penile-anal exposure is 0.1% to 3% (AAP, 2000). Prophylaxis with zidovudine plus lamivudine may be considered for patients presenting within 24 to 48 hours after an assault if the assault involved transfer of secretions and if the assailant is known or suspected to have HIV infection (AAP, 2000). There are no data on effectiveness or safety of HIV prophylaxis for child and adolescent victims of sexual abuse. Prophylactic treatment is given for 4 weeks; significant side effects include nephrolithiasis, pancytopenia, and hepatitis.

### SUBSTANCE ABUSE EMERGENCIES

Acute alcohol intoxication with a serum ethanol level over .4 g/dL is associated with severe respiratory depression and death. Such patients require emergent respiratory support, gastric lavage, and intravenous fluids with glucose. Effects of cocaine use that may present acutely include hypertensive crisis, coronary vasospasm with ischemia, cardiac arrhythmia, cerebral ischemia, and rhabdomyolysis (Fishman et al, 1997). Such patients may require treatment with nitroprusside, labetalol, nitrates, and calcium channel blockers. Heroin overdose may present with symptoms of hypotension, stupor, and respiratory depression requiring airway and circulatory support as well as naloxone. The most common cause of death due to inhalant overdose is arrhythmia (Fishman et al, 1997); management entails close cardiac monitoring and treatment of the arrhythmia. A high (> 10 mg) dose of phencyclidine may produce seizures, hypoventilation, arrhythmias, rhabdomyolysis, and renal failure. Respiratory and circulatory support measures as well as gastric lavage and nasogastric suction are indicated. Amphetamine and depressant overdose may also require circulatory and respiratory support measures; specific treatment regimens are available for barbiturate and for benzodiazepine overdoses.

### PSYCHIATRIC EMERGENCIES

An actively suicidal or psychotic patient requires hospitalization, observation, and an evaluation for medication. Such patients should be managed by a psychiatric consultant. A screen for substance abuse should be conducted in all suicidal, homicidal, and psychotic patients.

## CLINICAL EVALUATION AND MANAGEMENT

### CONDITIONS RELATED TO SEXUAL OR PHYSICAL VICTIMIZATION

Victims of sexual exploitation should be first assessed for nongenital injuries. Many physical injuries associated with sexual assault are minor abrasions or contusions that do not require medical treatment. Intraoral injuries may indicate forced oral-penile penetration. Bite marks to the neck or breasts may also occur during sexual assault. Suspicious areas may be swabbed during forensic evidence collection and submitted to test for the assailant's saliva (AAP & C. Henry Kempe National Center on Child Abuse and Neglect, 1994). Types and mechanisms of injuries seen in sexual assault victims are summarized in **Table 17-5**. Whenever possible, an experienced photographer should document injuries with a 35mm or digital camera. Photographs should be clearly labeled with patient identifier and date, and a ruler/color guide should be placed next to each injury. The clinician should also fully document color, location, and size of injuries on a body map. Some deep bruises may not become apparent for 2 to 3 days; areas of tenderness should be documented with follow-up photographs as bruises appear. The clinician should avoid precise dating of bruises; bruises can be described as "acute" (within 3 days) characterized by edema, a violaceous or red-blue color, and less distinct margins (AAP & C. Henry Kempe National Center on Child Abuse and Neglect, 1994). Recent or healed bite marks can be referred to a forensic odontologist for photography and forensic analysis, if such a resource is available.

After an assessment for nongenital injuries, the clinician should examine the genitalia and anus. The keys to a successful genital examination of a child or teenager are (1) adequate preparation of the child for the examination; (2) familiarity with various examination positions; and (3) a confident yet sensitive approach to the child.

**Table 17-5. Nongenital Injuries in Assailt Victims**

| Type | Mechanism |
|---|---|
| Perioral or intraoral injuries, especially erythema/petechiae near junction of hard/soft palate | Hand restraint (voice muffling), forced penile-oral penetration |
| Neck bruises, "hickies" | Choke by hand or ligature, suction/bite |
| Oval or semicircular bruises to neck, chest, breasts, extremities | Bite |
| Impact bruises to face, body, especially lips and eyes; intra-abdominal hematomas or organ rupture | Penetrating blow with fist |
| Impact bruises to extensor surfaces of upper/lower arms, knuckles | Defense injuries (victim tries to protect head with arms) |
| Traumatic alopecia, subgaleal hematoma | Hair-pulling |
| Numerous small (2-3 cm) bruises on shoulders, arms, thighs, face | Hand restraint bruises or grab marks |
| Ligature marks to wrists/ankles | Restraint with rope or wire |
| Abrasions, friction injuries to bony prominences of back | Victim struggle while restrained in supine position on firm surface |

## Adequate Preparation

The goal of preparation is to reduce anxiety and give the child some control. The child or teenager should be shown the examination room and any equipment prior to the medical evaluation. This preparation is ideally done by a nurse or other support personnel. Children may look through a colposcope (if used) to see how small objects are magnified and may like to hold their hand under the light to see that it does not hurt. It may be helpful to show them a sample cotton-tipped applicator used for cultures and to let them touch the cotton tip to appreciate how soft it feels. Preparation can be done in the presence of a parent or support person to reduce their anxiety as well. With adequate preparation, most examinations can be done without sedation.

## Familiarity With Examination Positions

There are 5 positions that may be helpful during the medical examination. Most examinations require only 2 of these positions. The following is a description of the positions and appropriate uses for each.

### Supine Frog-Leg Position

This position is used for smaller prepubertal children. The child places the soles of the feet together with the knees flexed laterally. This position provides an adequate view of the vulva, hymen, and vestibule. If abnormalities of the hymen are seen in this position, examination in the prone knee-chest position is essential to confirm these findings. In the supine position, the normal hymen may sometimes fold on itself, creating an artifactual abnormality (thickening or irregularity) that unfolds or normalizes in the prone knee-chest position.

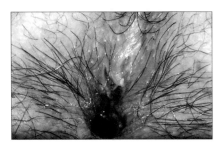

**Figure 17-3.** *Adolescent who denied anal penetration and denied any pain or bleeding in her anal area. In the prone knee-chest position, 2 tears are seen at 12 and 1 o'clock.*

### Supine Lithotomy Position

This position is used for larger female prepubertal children and all female adolescents. The feet are placed in the examination table stirrups, the patient moves the hips and buttocks to the end of the table, and flexes the knees outward "to the side." This position provides an adequate view of the vulva, hymen, and vestibule.

### Prone Knee-Chest Position

This position is used for prepubertal children and provides the best view of the perianal area (**Figure 17-3**). The child's shoulders, elbows, and forearms are placed on the table; the lower back is lordotic, extending the hips upward; and knees are placed about 18 inches apart. As discussed above, this position is also important for confirming irregularities seen in the supine position. The prone knee-chest position is also helpful in confirming healed tears or clefts in the hymen. In this position, it is possible to visualize the vagina and cervix without inserting a speculum.

### Supine Knee-Chest Position

This position is generally used for infants to examine the anus. (Lateral position may be used instead.) The knees are drawn up onto the chest to visualize perianal structures.

### Lateral Decubitus Position

This position can be used for all age groups to examine the anus. The knees should be together and drawn up on the chest such that the anus can be visualized; the examiner should avoid distortion of the tissue with minimal gluteal separtation. (**Figures 17-4** and **17-5**).

## Confident, Yet Sensitive Approach to the Child

When an examiner is nervous and anxious, the child or teenager is more likely to be nervous and anxious. Respect the child's privacy and need for control. Tell the child you will "explain everything before it happens." Raise the head of the examination table up so the child can see you and so you can gauge the child's reaction and anxiety during the examination. Allow him or her to change into the examining gown in private and keep all other areas of the body draped. Let the child choose a support person to be present during the examination. (Many teenagers prefer no one!) Touch the child's knee or arm with a sample cotton-tipped applicator before obtaining vaginal or anal cultures. Begin with labial separation (the labia majora are moved laterally and inferiorly), then progress to labial traction (the labia majora are grasped close to the posterior commissure and pulled gently in the anterior direction), and the lateral or prone knee-chest position, as appropriate and indicated. Avoid "shop talk" during the examination, moving quickly and gently through the examination. When using any of the examination techniques, apply constant, even, gentle pressure with your fingers; avoid "groping" movements. After the examination, have the child sit up or change into clothing before giving him or her the results.

**Figure 17-4.** *14-year-old girl with a history of anal penetration occurring 3 days prior. Note tear at 9 o'clock. Patient is in left lateral decubitus position.*

**Figure 17-5.** *15-year-old adolescent boy with a long-term history of anal-penile penetration. Note laxity of anal opening and scar tissue at 9 o'clock. Patient is in the lateral decubitus position.*

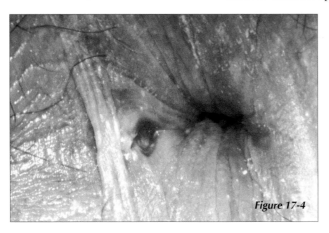

Figure 17-4

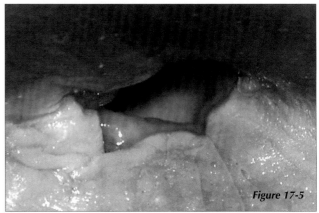

Figure 17-5

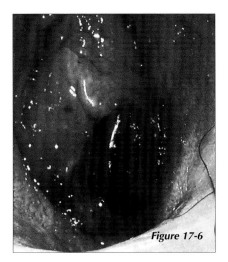

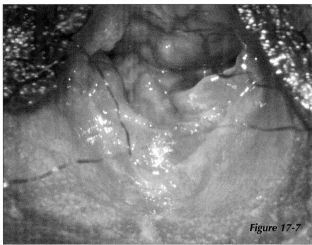

Examination findings and treatment plans should be discussed with the child or adolescent first, followed by caretakers, supportive adults, or investigators.

DOCUMENTATION OF INJURIES

During the genital examination the clinician should first follow protocols for forensic evidence collection (when indicated) and then document genital and anal findings and test for STDs (when appropriate). Forensic evidence collection is discussed previously under "Sexual Assault Emergencies."

Genital injuries can be photographed with a 35mm camera (equipped with ring flash and zoom lens) or a photocolposcope. The photocolposcope may enhance detection of injuries when victims are examined within 48 hours of vaginal-penile penetration. Photographic documentation of injuries greatly enhances the presentation of evidence in legal settings.

Most sexual trauma victims will have no visible anogenital injury. The presence and extent of injury depends on several factors (eg, the amount of force used, physical response of the victim, size of the victim, use of lubrication, the victim's prior sexual experience, intoxication state of the victim). Additionally, acute injuries may resolve completely within days (**Figures 17-6** and **17-7**). Two factors that may be associated with an increased likelihood of visible injury are vaginal bleeding and examination within 72 hours of an assault (Adams et al, 1994), yet in this study a minority of those examined within 72 hours (42%) or reporting vaginal bleeding (46%) had injuries consistent with sexual assault (Adams et al, 1994).

Injuries may be acute or healed. Injuries from acute vaginal-penile penetration include lacerations (**Figure 17-8**), edema, and submucosal hemorrhages. Most injuries occur in the posterior vestibule or posterior rim of the hymen between 3 and 9 o'clock. More severe injuries may extend to the perineum, lateral vestibule, and intravaginal area. Genital trauma may be present even when the victim is asymptomatic. Penetrating anal injuries also resolve rapidly and completely. Acute anal findings include lacerations, hematomas, edema, and anal sphincter spasms. Although most anal or genital injuries resolve within a few days, some may require weeks to heal.

Nonacute or healed injuries associated with vaginal penetration bear no legal significance in the adolescent with numerous sexual partners. An obvious exception would be a victim of in-

*Figure 17-6. Hematoma. 15-year-old victim of vaginal-penile penetration 36 hours previously.*

*Figure 17-7. Same patient as **Figure 17-6**, 5 days after initial exam.*

*Figure 17-8. 5-year-old girl victm of vaginal-penile penetration occurring 36 hours earlier. Complete hymenal tear at      6 o'clock, and posterior vestibule tear with bruising*

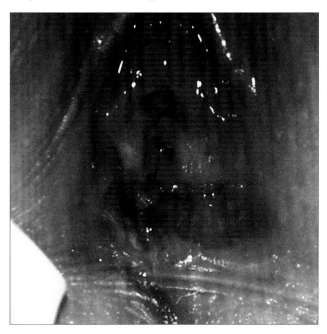

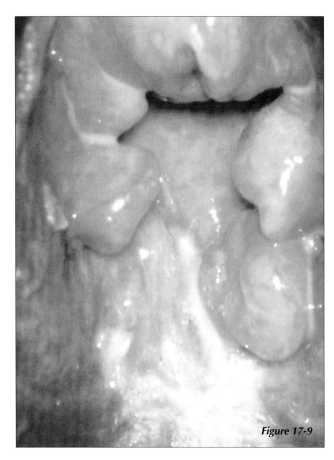

Figure 17-9

juries caused by anal-penile penetration when the victim has had no prior consensual contact of that nature. For this reason, it is important for the clinician to specifically ask whether anal-penile penetration has occurred; many adolescents are reluctant to disclose this information until they are directly questioned. Healed injuries include complete clefts of the hymen (**Figures 17-9** and **17-10**) and scarring of the posterior vestibule or anus (**Figures 17-11** and **17-12**).

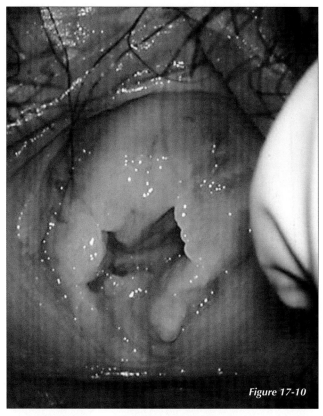

Figure 17-10

**Figure 17-9.** *Adolescent female with several hymenal clefts, resulting in isolated "clumps" of hymen (caruncles). There is no visible hymenal tissue from 4 to 8 o'clock. History of long-term sexual activity with several individuals.*

**Figure 17-10.** *Healed tear, or cleft, from 5-7 o'clock.*

**Figure 17-11.** *Posterior vestibule scar and large area from 4 to 8 o'clock of no visible hymenal tissue.*

**Figure 17-12.** *13-year-old female victim of repeated anal-penile penetration by 2 individuals over a period of 3-4 years. Extensive perianal scarring and immediate anal sphincter dilatation is noted (patient is in the prone knee-chest position). The absence of stool in the anal vault and the presence of other traumatic findings supports trauma as the cause of this dilatation. The child also reported some difficulty with fecal incontinence over the past year.*

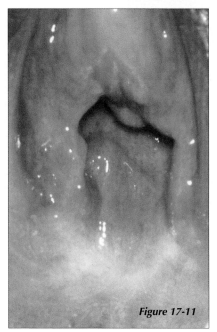

Figure 17-11

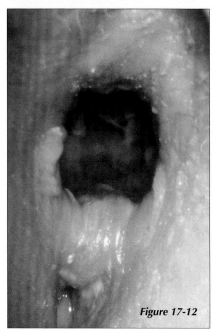

Figure 17-12

Children and adolescents infected with sexually transmitted organisms may or may not have symptoms of disease. While prepubertal children with vaginal gonorrhea tend to be symptomatic (Siegel et al, 1995), adolescents with vaginal gonorrhea or chlamydia are less likely to have symptoms. Herpes simplex virus (HSV) type 1 or 2 may occur on the genitals (see **Figure 17-13**, herpes in an asymptomatic adolescent) or perianal tissues (**Figure 17-14**). Any ulcerative or vesicular lesions should be cultured for herpes; a definitive diagnosis is critical to appropriate long-term management and treatment of the disease.

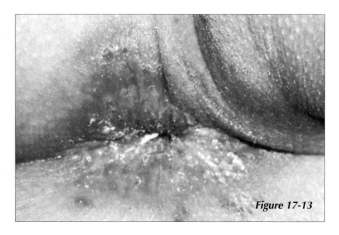

*Figure 17-13*

## DIAGNOSTIC TESTING

### Sexually Transmitted Diseases

Child victims of pornography or prostitution should be comprehensively tested for STDs. The AAP (1991) recommends the following tests for suspected victims of child or adolescent sexual abuse: serum rapid plasma regain (RPR) test; a wet mount for *Trichomonas vaginalis*; throat, rectal, and genital cultures for *Neisseria gonorrhoeae*; and rectal and genital cultures for *Chlamydia trachomatis*. While cultures are considered the legal "gold standard" due to high specificity rates, a positive test for an STD is legally relevant only when the child or adolescent has had no sexual contact outside of the abuse. On the other hand, a sexually assaulted adolescent who has had several sexual partners is at a significant risk for STDs and should be tested with the most sensitive detection techniques available to ensure adequate treatment and management of identified diseases.

The Centers for Disease Control and Prevention (CDC) (2002a) has recently recommended that nucleic acid amplification tests (NAATs), such as polymerase chain reaction (PCR) and ligase chain reaction (LCR), be used in sexually active adults to detect *N. gonorrhoeae* and *C. trachomatis*. An added benefit of NAATs is that a urine sample rather than a vaginal sample can be submitted from adolescents who refuse examinations. Other new and promising diagnostic techniques for STDs include *Trichomonas* culture utilizing InPouch TV, NAATs for HSV, and serologic glycoprotein G-based assays for HSV-1 and HSV-2 (first available in 1999, this test is the first accurate type-specific assay) (CDC, 2002b).

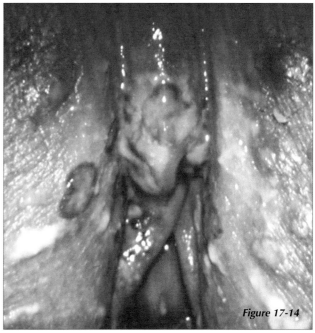

*Figure 17-14*

**Figure 17-13.** *Herpes simplex virus (HSV) type 2 lesions with secondary Group A beta hemolytic streptococcus infection (note crusted leading edge, lower half of image) in a prepubertal girl with no history of sexual contact. She also had vaginal gonorrhea and chlamydia infections.*

**Figure 17-14.** *HSV type 1 in a 10-year-old girl who initially denied sexual contact. She later admitted to oral (perpetrator)-genital (victim) contact by a relative.*

Sexually active victims, victims of high-risk assault (multiple or unknown assailants), and victims who engage in other risky health behaviors should be tested for HIV; hepatitis A (HAV), hepatitis B (HBV), and hepatitis C (HCV); and syphilis. Although HAV is generally transmissible through fecal-oral contact, it can also be transmitted during sexual activity (CDC, 2002b). HBV is most commonly transmitted through sexual contact. HCV is primarily transmitted through percutaneous exposure to blood products and sexual activity. Acute disease is diagnosed with serological confirmation of serum immunoglobulin M (IgM) antibody to HAV, IgM antibody to HBV core antigen, antibody to HCV, or HCV ribonucleic acid (RNA) (CDC, 2002b). A positive RPR or Venereal Disease Reference Laboratory (VDRL) followed by a positive treponemal-specific test such as fluorescent treponemal antibody absorbed (FTA-ABS) or *Treponema pallidum* particle agglutination (TP-PA) confirm the diagnosis of syphilis. Some laboratories are screening for syphilis with a treponemal-specific ELISA test; patients with positive reslults are then retested with RPR to confirm active, untreated disease. An HIV test begins with a highly

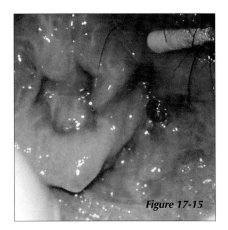

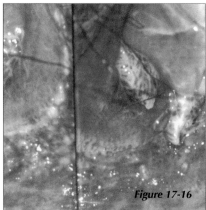

**Figure 17-15.** Human papillomavirus (HPV) (venereal warts) lesions in an adolescent. Lesions at 3 o'clock were obscured by hymenal folds. Cotton-tipped applicator used to move hymenal flaps centrally in order to examine the vestibule for lesions.

**Figure 17-16.** HPV lesions in the posterior vestibule at 3, 6, and 9 o'clock.

sensitive enzyme immunoassay, and positive screens are confirmed with either Western blot or immunofluorescence assay for HIV antibodies. HIV antibody is detectable in about 95% of patients within 3 months of infection (CDC, 2002b). Serological testing during the initial visit and 6 weeks later is recommended for HIV, syphilis, HAV, HBV, and HCV; serology for HIV should be repeated 12 and 24 weeks after the initial testing. Bacterial vaginosis (BV) is not conclusive of sexual transmission and can be diagnosed by wet mount examination ("clue cells" and leukocytosis). Human papillomavirus (HPV) infection (**Figures 17-15** and **17-16**) is usually diagnosed clinically or by Pap smear; a biopsy is necessary only when lesions are atypical or do not resolve with treatment.

## Pregnancy

A serum pregnancy test should be done prior to administering antimicrobials or pregnancy prophylaxis. Medications such as Metronidazole may be contra-indicated in pregnancy. Emergency contraception may be given to nonpregnant females. It has been suggested that oral contraceptives given during pregnancy may cause fetal abnormalities. Although this has not been proven, consideration may be given to this when prescribing estradiol and when counseling patients regarding its use.

## Substance Abuse Screening/Testing/Monitoring

As previously discussed, all suspected victims of prostitution or other forms of sexual exploitation should be questioned about drug and alcohol use. Testing of urine or

**Table 17-6. Management of Uncomplicated Sexually Transmitted Diseases in Child\* Victims of Sexual Abuse**

| Organism | Prophylactic Treatment | Treatment of Confirmed Disease |
|---|---|---|
| **Gonorrhea** | Cefixime 8 mg/kg (up to 400 mg) PO[†] x 1, or ceftriaxone 125 mg IM[†] x 1 PLUS treatment for chlamydia | Ceftriaxone 125 mg IM x 1 |
| **Chlamydia** | Azithromycin 20 mg/kg (up to 1 g) PO x 1 or erythromycin 50 mg/kg/d x 10 days PLUS treatment for gonorrhea | Same as for prophylaxis |
| **Hepatitis** | Begin or complete hepatitis A and B immunization | None |
| **Trichomonas, bacterial vaginitis** | Consider: metronidazole 15 mg/d (TID[†]) x 7 days, or 40 mg/kg (up to 2 g) PO x 1 | Same as for prophylaxis |
| **Syphilis**[‡] | (Gonorrhea prophylaxis has efficacy against incubating syphilis) | Benzathine penicillin G 50 000 U/kg IM x 1 up to 2.4 million U |
| **Herpes simplex virus type 2** | None up to 1.0 g/d x 7-10 days | Acyclovir 80 mg/kg/d PO (TID-QID[†]) |

*(continued)*

**Table 17-6.** *(continued)*

| ORGANISM | PROPHYLACTIC TREATMENT | TREATMENT OF CONFIRMED DISEASE |
|---|---|---|
| **Human papillomavirus** | None | Patient administered: podofilox; 5% solution or gel or imiquimod 5% cream Clinician administered: podophyllin, trichloracetic acid, cryotherapy, or surgical excision |
| **Human immunodeficiency virus** | No specific recommendations for children | Consult with infectious disease specialist |

*\* Preadolescent children weighing < 100 lbs.*
*† Abbreviations: PO=orally, IM=intramuscularly, TID=3 times daily, QID=4 times daily.*
*‡ Cerebrospinal fluid examination recommended prior to treating confirmed disease.*

*Adapted from American Academy of Pediatrics.* 2000 Red Book: Report of the Committee on Infectious Diseases. *25th ed. Elk Grove Village, Ill: American Academy of Pediatrics; 2000.*

**Table 17-7. Management of Uncomplicated Sexually Transmitted Diseases in Adolescent\* Victims of Sexual Abuse**

| ORGANISM | PROPHYLACTIC TREATMENT | TREATMENT OF CONFIRMED DISEASE |
|---|---|---|
| **Gonorrhea** | Cefixime 400 mg PO† x 1 or ceftriaxone 125 mg IM† x 1 PLUS treatment for chlamydia | Same as for prophylaxis |
| **Chlamydia** | Azithromycin 1 g PO x 1 PLUS treatment for gonorrhea | Azithromycin 1 g PO x 1 or doxycycline 200 mg/d (BID†) x 7 days |
| **Hepatitis** | Begin or complete hepatitis A and B immunization | None |
| **Trichomonas, bacterial vaginosis** | Metronidazole 2 g PO x 1 | Metronidazole 2 g PO x 1 or 250 mg TID† x 7 days |
| **Syphilis‡** | (Gonorrhea prophylaxis has efficacy against incubating syphilis) | Benzathine penicillin G 2.4 million U IM x 1 or doxycycline 200 mg/d (BID) PO x 14 days |
| **Herpes simplex virus type 2** | None | Acyclovir 1000-1200 mg/d (3-5 x/d) PO x 7-10 d |
| **Human papillomavirus** | None | Patient administered: podofilox .5% solution or gel or imiquimod 5% cream Clinician administered: Podophyllin, trichloracetic acid, cryotherapy, or surgical excision |
| **Human immunodeficiency virus** | Consider if high-risk contact occurs: zidovudine 150 mg (BID) x 4 weeks | Consult with infectious disease specialist |

*\* Includes preadolescents weighing > 100 lbs.*
*† Abbreviations: PO=orally, IM=intramuscularly, BID=2 times daily, TID=3 times daily.*
*‡ Cerebrospinal examination is recommended for those with central nervous system symptoms.*

*Adapted from American Academy of Pediatrics.* 2000 Red Book: Report of the Committee on Infectious Diseases. *25th ed. Elk Grove Village, Ill: American Academy of Pediatrics; 2000.*

| Table 17-8. Follow-up Considerations for Victims of Sexual Trauma |
| --- |

**2 Weeks**

1. Healing of injuries

2. Type 2 herpes simplex virus: 3-10 days incubation

3. Trichomoniasis, bacterial vaginosis, chlamydia, gonorrhea: 10-14 days incubation (if no initial prophylaxis given)

4. Pregnancy (if oral contraception is not provided at initial evaluation)

5. Psychological support/reassurance

6. Drug/alcohol monitoring/treatment (if coordinated with specialist)

**2-3 Months**

1. HIV testing: repeat at 6 weeks, 3 months, 6 months, 1 year

2. Syphilis and hepatitis: 6-8 weeks incubation

3. Human papillomavirus: 2-3 months average incubation; up to 20 months incubation in rare cases

4. Psychological support

5. Drug/alcohol monitoring (if coordinated with specialist)

*Adapted from Kellogg ND, Sugarek NJ. Sexual trauma.* Atlas of Office Procedures. *1998; 1(1):181-197.*

serum for drugs should be conducted only with the patient's knowledge and consent or when mental status is compromised (Committee on Substance Abuse, 1998). Follow-up testing may be conducted for monitoring purposes as part of a treatment protocol.

TREATMENT
Management of uncomplicated STDs in child and adolescent victims of sexual abuse is summarized in **Tables 17-6** and **17-7**.

FOLLOW-UP
**Table 17-8** outlines follow-up considerations and recommendations for STDs, pregnancy, and psychological recovery.

REFERRALS
Ideal management of child and adolescent victims of sexual exploitation involves the coordination of multidisciplinary long-term services for victim and supportive/ nonabusive caretakers. The victim's first encounter with a medical care provider will have an impact on compliance with treatment recommendations, referrals, and likelihood of returning for follow-up care.

## CONCLUSION
Medical care for the children of the night presents clinical, legal, and moral challenges for the healthcare provider. The clinician must balance legal obligations of reporting and evidentiary procedures while gaining the child's trust and compliance with a comprehensive evaluation and treatment. The clinician has a unique opportunity to help a person who has been treated with the ultimate disrespect by working with her in a caring, competent, and compassionate manner and thus helping her to begin her journey toward healing.

# REFERENCES

Adams JA, Harper K, Knudson S, Revilla J. Examination findings in legally confirmed child sexual abuse: it's normal to be normal. *Pediatrics.* 1994;94(3):310-317.

American Academy of Pediatrics, Committee on Child Abuse and Neglect, American Academy of Pediatric Dentistry, Ad Hoc Work Group on Child Abuse and Neglect. Oral and dental aspects of child abuse and neglect. *Pediatrics.* 1999a;104(2 Pt 1): 348-350.

American Academy of Pediatrics. *2000 Red Book: Report of the Committee on Infectious Diseases.* 25th ed. Elk Grove Village, Ill: American Academy of Pediatrics; 2000.

American Academy of Pediatrics Committee on Child Abuse and Neglect. Guidelines for the evaluation of sexual abuse of children. *Pediatrics.* 1991;87:254-260.

American Academy of Pediatrics Committee on Child Abuse and Neglect. Guidelines for the evaluation of sexual abuse of children. *Pediatrics.* 1999b;103(1): 186-191.

American Academy of Pediatrics, C. Henry Kempe National Center on Child Abuse and Neglect. *The Visual Diagnosis of Child Physical Abuse.* Elk Grove Village, Ill: American Academy of Pediatrics; 1994.

American Psychiatric Association. *Diagnostic and Statistical Manual of Mental Disorders.* 4th ed. Washington, DC: American Psychiatric Association; 1994.

CeASAR: The Center for Adolescent Substance Abuse Research. The CRAFFT questions. Available at:http://www.slp3d2.com/rwj_1027/webcast/docs/screentest. html. Accessed July 29, 2003.

Centers for Disease Control and Prevention. Screening tests to detect *Chlamydia trachomatis* and *Neisseria gonorrhoeae* infections. *MMWR Recomm Rep.* 2002b;51:1-38.

Centers for Disease Control and Prevention. Sexually transmitted diseases treatment guidelines. *MMWR Recomm Rep.* 2002a;51(No. RR-6):1-80.

Christian C, Lavelle J, DeJong A, Loiselle J, Brenner L, Joffe M. Forensic evidence findings in prepubertal victims of sexual assault. *Pediatrics.* 2000;106:100-104.

Committee on Substance Abuse, American Academy of Pediatrics. Tobacco, alcohol, and other drugs: the role of the pediatrician in prevention and management of substance abuse. *Pediatrics.* 1998; 101(1):125-128.

Fishman M, Bruner A, Adger H. Substance abuse among children and adolescents. *Pediatr Rev.* 1997;18(11):394-403.

Fuller PG, Cavanaugh RM. Basic assessment and screening for substance abuse in the pediatrician's office. *Pediatr Clin North Am.* 1995;42(2):295-315.

Geist RF. Sexually related trauma. *Emerg Med Clin North Am.* 1988;6:439-466.

Kellogg ND, Sugarek NJ. Sexual trauma. *Atlas of Office Procedures.* 1998;1(1):181-197.

Knight JR, Shrier LA, Bravender TD, Farrell M, Vander Bilt J, Shaffer HJ. A new brief screen for adolescent substance abuse. *Arch Pediatr Adolesc Med.* 1999;153: 591-596.

Lanktree CB, Briere J. Outcome of therapy for sexually abused children: a repeated measures study. *Child Abuse Negl.* 1995;19(9):1145-1155.

Marchbanks PA, Annegers JF, Coulam CB, Strathy JH, Kurland LT. Risk factors for ectopic pregnancy: a population-based study. *JAMA.* 1988;259:1823-1827.

Marchbanks PA, Lui KJ, Mercy JA. Risk of injury from resisting rape. *Am J Epidemiology.* 1990;132:540-549.

Schwartz B, Alderman EM. Substances of abuse. *Pediatr Rev.* 1997;18(6):204-215.

Siegel RM, Schubert CJ, Myers PA, Shapiro RA. The prevalence of sexually transmitted diseases in children and adolescents evaluated for sexual abuse in Cincinnati: rationale for limited STD testing on prepubertal girls. *Pediatrics.* 1995;96(6):1090-1094.

Sweet DL. Pelvic inflammatory disease. In: Sweet RL, Gibbs RS, eds. *Infectious Diseases of the Female Genital Tract.* 2nd ed. Baltimore, Md: Williams & Wilkins; 1990: 241-266.

Texas Penal Code § 22.011(e) (2002).

Unger JB, Simon TR, Newman TL, Montgomery SB, Kipke MD, Albornoz M. Early adolescent street youth: an overlooked population with unique problems and service needs. *J Early Adolesc.* 1998;18(4):325-349.

Yates GL, MacKenzie RG, Pennbridge J, Swofford A. A risk profile comparison of homeless youth involved in prostitution and homeless youth not involved. *J Adolesc Health.* 1991;12:545-548.

18

# THE MEDICAL IMPLICATIONS OF ANOGENITAL TRAUMA IN CHILD SEXUAL EXPLOITATION

F. Bruce Watkins, MD

## INTRODUCTION

When considering **child sexual exploitation** (CSE), the practice by which a person achieves sexual gratification or financial gain through the abuse or exploitation of a child's sexuality, genital trauma is an appropriate topic. The subsequent discussion will recognize normal anatomical findings. This analysis artificially divides childhood into 3 prominent phases:

1.  *Infant* or *toddler.* Children between birth and 5 years, during which time there normally is no endogenous estrogen effect in females.

2.  *Juvenile* or *preadolescent.* Immature and prepubescent males and females (usually prior to menarche) between the ages of 6 and 12 years.

3.  *Adolescent.* Males and postpubertal, menstruating, and childbearing females between the ages of 13 and 18 years.

While the inherent inadequacy of this synthetic classification method is accepted, it facilitates an uncomplicated analysis and discussion that will review the landmarks, gross vascularity, and neurological innervations of importance. After discussing the normal anatomical architecture of female and male genitalia in the artificial 3 stages of development, the ensuing discussion will attend to childhood genital trauma in general.

Following an outline of some suggestions of hints and highlights that should be considered in the patient history and physical examination, the focus will shift to a discussion of the commercial sexual exploitation of children (CSEC) and will consider the implications of genital trauma and subsequent genital injury within the context of CSEC. Lastly, the discussion will focus on the acute and chronic consequences of genital trauma and infective etiologies, treatment options, preemptive strategies, and fertility issues.

Although CSE is a leading cause of international concern for children, both incidence and mortality seem to be on the rise. Some hypothesize that it is because the problem has become reportable and punishable (Leventhal, 1990), indicating we have come a long way from child sexual abuse cases of decades ago, which were once virtually undocumented and barely acknowledged except anecdotally (Kempe, 1978). These reports of exploitation were occuring in foster care, group homes, shelters, and prisons. Relationships that were considered safe are now being revealed as high risk. The loving, compassionate relationships of family members as well as religious, educational, and sports mentors are now unreliable. Additionally, long-term systemic denial of the problem has resulted in a system lacking support and treatment for victims throughout the world.

# NORMAL ANATOMY

To recognize abused and injured genitalia, healthcare professionals must be fluent with normal anatomy for comparison (Cowell, 1981). Changes that occur in male and female children reflect both hormonal changes and physical growth (Berenson, 1998). This fact must be significant in the examination of a child, especially in the genital examination (Zitelli, 2002).

## EMBRYONIC DEVELOPMENT

In nature, the embryo is female first and then differentiated into a male as a result of genetic and hormonal directives at specific developmental milestones. Briefly, in the early embryo, the gonads are indifferent. Both male and female anatomy precursors exist together. The important event seems to be the gonadal differentiation into testis, which becomes visible between weeks 8 and 9 of gestation. Without the genetic impulse of the Y chromosome the gonad becomes an ovary. The embryonic Sertoli and Leydig cells give hormone signals to produce testosterone and subsequent male differentiation and virilization occurs.

## NORMAL GENITALIA

"Better understanding of anogenital anatomy in the absence of abuse is critical in order to differentiate normal from posttraumatic findings" (Heppenstall-Heger et al, 2003). Below is a brief discussion of normal genitalia in male and female children.

### Males

For the male child, several significant physical genital findings should be observed (McAleer & Kaplan, 1995). Penile length, foreskin anatomy, urethral meatus location, scrotal anatomy (ie, darkening and enlargement), presence and/or absence of testes, scrotal hair growth, and presence and/or absence of scrotal or inguinal masses are all important. Findings consistent with congenital abnormalities can often be diagnosed by imaging techniques that examine the upper urinary components (eg, intravenous pyelogram, computed tomographic [CT] scan, or ultrasound). Scrotal transillumination with a bright, cool light source may identify the lack of testicular descent. This condition requires location of the testes and potential surgical therapy. Without circumcision, foreskin retraction occurs by the age of 5 years. Careful examination may differentiate trauma from balanitis or phimosis. In male development approaching the ages of 11 and 12 years, the first sign of pubertal onset is testicular growth and/or enlargement. Pubic hair also becomes visible. Penile length, hair growth, and testicular size all increase and may continue to increase throughout puberty and adolescence. The impact of race on anatomy must also be addressed (Kadish et al, 1998).

An erection occurs as a result of simple excitation of the cavernous nerve that causes arterial filling of the corpora cavernosa. Tumescence of the corpora compresses the veins to maintain this state. When excitement of the cavernous nerve ceases, the opposite occurs.

Injuries to the male urethra that result from physical violence often mimic a straddle injury. Such injuries can cause urethral rupture near the prostate gland. This rupture can cause extravasations of urine into the perineum, which can result in swelling of the shaft of the penis and distention of the perineum in front of the anus and in the scrotal sac. The swelling can ascend into the abdominal wall.

The scrotum, testes, and penis derive their predominant nerve supply from lumbar nerves 10 and 11 and sacral nerves 2 through 4. The blood supply of the male genitalia derives from the internal and external pudendal arteries and veins, which serve as tributaries of the internal iliac artery and veins.

### Females

The neonatal female should be examined in a supine position with the legs flexed. No difference in size or texture of labia majora or minora should be evident. Separation of the labia reveals the clitoris, vaginal introitus, hymen, and urethral meatus. Clitoral enlargement or labial fusion are possible signs of virilization. Vaginal bleeding may occur secondary to estrogen withdrawal after delivery (**Table 18-1**). An analysis of colposcopic photographs of female patients between the ages of 10 months and 5 years emphasizes the visual superiority of supine labial separation and traction methods (McCann, 1990). Common findings include follicles in the fossa navicularis, periurethral bands, labial adhesions, vestibular erythema, fourchette avascularity, and urethral dilation as normal, nonabusive findings. Imperforate hymen, foul vaginal discharge, and retained foreign body should be considered before assuming potential sexual abuse (Botash & Jean-Louis, 2001).

The literature emphasizes findings of the hymen (**Figures 18-1-a, b, c, d,** and **e**). In newborn girls the hymen is redundant, thick, and estrogenized because of maternal exposure *in utero*, whereas infants lack this hormonal influence (Berenson et al, 1991). The prepubertal patient has an annular, crescentic, thin, redundant, sleeve-like, and unestrogenized hymen (Berenson et al, 1992). The pubertal girl has a thick, elastic, estrogenized hymen from an endogenous source (Heger et al, 2002). White discharge is common at all ages. Imperforate, cribriform, septate, and micro perforate

---

**Table 18-1. Differential Diagnosis of Vaginal Bleeding in the Prepubertal Girl**

Trauma
— Accidental
— Sexual abuse

Vulvovaginitis
— Irritation, pinworms
— Nonspecific vulvovaginitis
— *S. pyogenes, Shigella*

Endocrine abnormalities
— Newborn bleeding due to maternal estrogen withdrawal
— Isosexual precocious puberty
— Pseudoprecocious puberty
— Precocious menarche
— Exogenous hormone preparations
— Hypothyroidism

Dermatoses
— Lichen sclerosis

Condyloma accuminata (human papilloma virus)

Foreign body

Urethral prolapse

Blood dyscrasia

Hemangioma

Tumor
— Benign
— Malignant

---

*Reprinted with permision from Emans SJ. Vulvovaginal problems in the prepubertal child. In: Emans SJ, Laufer MR, Goldstein DP, eds.* Pediatric and Adolescent Gynecology. *4th ed. Philadelphia, Pa: Lippencott-Raven; 1998:75-107.*

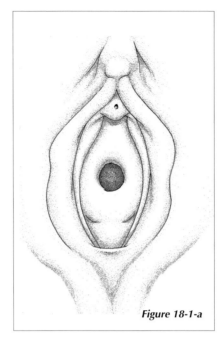

Figure 18-1-a

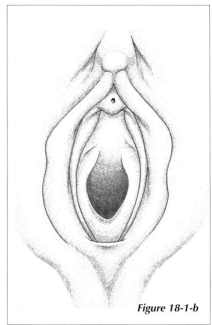

Figure 18-1-b

**Figures 18-1-a, b, c, d,** and **e.** *Types of hymen include annular (a), crescentic (b), cuff-like (c), imperforate (d), and septate (e).*

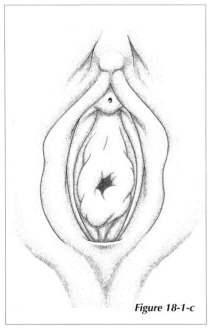

Figure 18-1-c

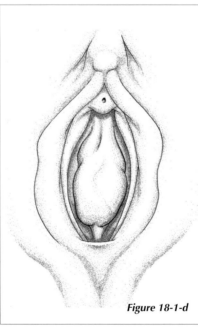

Figure 18-1-d

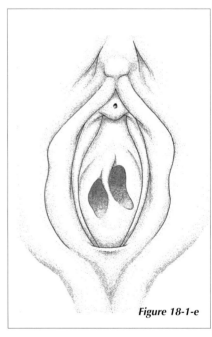

Figure 18-1-e

hymen configuration may reflect congenital abnormalities, although other etiologies should be clinically excluded.

Infants should be examined in a position similar to that of neonates, that is, with the perivaginal skin in posterolateral fashion. The examiner should increase the gentleness and sensitivity of the examination as the child becomes older and develops appropriate resistance. In an effort to help make the experience less distasteful and stressful to the child, the examiner should also have a chaperone (ie, a professional who is not a family member) present, explain the process clearly to the child, and allow for the child to gown herself privately. The positioning of the patient, sitting on the chaperone's lap with the knees of the patient spread apart (frog-leg), increases comfort and convenience.

Preadolescent patients are best examined in a frog-leg or knee-chest position. The vaginal mucosa still lacks estrogen and is, therefore, quite thin and reddened with a watery, non–foul-smelling discharge. Blood, foul discharge, or odor should elicit further investigation into etiologies. Berenson's (1998) study provides a well-documented review of normal female anatomy. Descriptions of hymenal configuration and measurements, posterior vestibule, and the perianal area are all detailed.

In rare cases, external vaginal soft-tissue masses in female children may represent urethral prolapse with eversion in young African-American females. In European-American girls, there may be an ectopic ureterocele. At puberty, breast development followed by pubic hair growth should occur. All female patients should be assessed for Tanner staging of the breasts at any age, since this may enhance the clinical diagnosis. Lichen sclerosis, a rare skin disorder that mimics abusive trauma, may manifest as ulcers, fissures, or hypertrophy of the perianal skin. This thin skin reflects trauma easily and is quite fragile. The vagina appears to be estrogen-stimulated with elasticity and thickening. Leukorhea, which is a non-foul watery discharge, is normal.

# CHILDHOOD GENITAL TRAUMA IN GENERAL

Genital trauma in adults is very similar to that of the postpubertal child. Examples incorporate a nearly innumerable list of random events, deliberate or intentional. These incidents may be overt and directed at the genitals. There may be physical evidence, which may be temporary. The genitals can be the primary or secondary site of injury. Genital trauma in adults or children can result from whole body trauma and/or straddle injuries. Whole body trauma can include lower abdominal concussion with subsequent bladder, bowel, or bone damage. It is important to understand general genital trauma to differentiate between it and trauma related to sexual abuse.

## STRADDLE INJURY

Straddle injuries are a consequence of falling onto the urogenital area with the force of the body weight. The bony margins of the pelvis, usually the ischium, compress the soft tissue, resulting in a crush injury in the majority of cases. Laceration may occur. Differentiation from sexual abuse is usually based on the relevant history and physical findings.

## Males

In males, this injury manifests as a blood collection (hematoma) or, in rare circumstances, a progressive swelling secondary to urine extravasation (urinoma). Hematuria frequently occurs. Scarring, neuromas, dysparenuia, and secondary impotence can be sequelae. Laceration may occur primarily or as a coincidental event. The degree of damage is dependent on the object that was straddled. Accidental or intentional laceration may result in superficial and/or deep injury. Total excision of either or both components of the external genitalia is another possiblility, and reattachment is complex, but an option. Accidental testicular and scrotal injury are infrequent until adequate genital growth occurs (ie, usually after becoming 12 years old). A pediatric urologist should manage significant hematomas or penetrating injury. Penile straddle injury is usually superficial and can be managed with warm soaks, absorbable suture, and/or local anesthetic.

## Females

With such injuries, significant pain is combined with anxiety. Straddle injuries are commonly unilateral, superficial, and anterior. A nonpenetrating, female genital injury in children usually causes minor trauma with labial laccrations, hcmatomas, or abrasions, depending on the object that was straddled. Anal trauma is unusual in this setting. Hematomas usually resolve spontaneously and should be treated with pressure and ice initially and then with heat after 12 to 24 hours. Possibly, urinary diversion with intermittent short-term catheterization is required. Lacerations should be allowed to heal without intervention unless suturing is necessary for hemostasis. Use of a general anesthesia is recommended in cases requiring suture repair.

A penetrating straddle injury is dangerous and represents the greatest risk of internal injury. As in other cases of CSE, the logical and unencumbered history, consistent with the physical findings, is vitally important. The child should be able to relate the elements of the accident without deep thought or hesitation. The physical findings may be unilateral and associated with hymenal disruption and vaginal laceration. Symmetrical findings with posterior hymenal disruption might infer intercourse. On photocolposcopy, the hymen and vagina may demonstrate microabrasions (Hobbs et al, 1995). When used for forensic purposes, this evidence is seldom irrefutable.

## COINCIDENTAL GENITAL TRAUMA

Coincidental genital trauma is customarily situational and can be found with consensual sex, with or without pregnancy, and in nonsexual physical assault (Jones et al, 2003). This type of trauma should not be confused with sexual assault.

### Coincidental Genital Trauma in Pregnancy

In pregnancy, hormonal alterations along with increased vascularity result in new vulvar/vaginal tenderness and easy bruising or frank bleeding. If abortion is sought, vulvar and vaginal trauma are minimal. During delivery though, the vagina is distended greatly and often beyond its limits. This may result in various forms of lacerations, episiotomies, hematomas, and contusions. The lateral sulcus, or cervix, can sustain lacerations, especially with operative vaginal deliveries (vacuum or forceps assisted). These injuries can spontaneously heal, or they can be surgically reapproximated using absorbable suture. There is a risk of fistula formation after anterior or posterior vaginal repair. The fistulas become apparent in the puerperium and are described as rectovaginal or vesicovaginal, according to their anatomical position. Postpartum, there are naturally modifications to vaginal size and volume. These changes are usually permanent without intervention. These are issues of concern in decisions made by the postpubertal patient.

## NONSEXUAL VIOLENCE AND GENITAL TRAUMA

Nonsexual violence against female children can also result in genital injury as a primary or secondary consequence. Violence that targets female children can include: gender-selective violence during armed conflict or by police and security forces, gender-selective violence against refugees and asylum seekers, violence associated with prostitution and pornography, sexual harassment, domestic violence, female circumcision, and rape. Some of these practices can also be gender-specific to males.

### Female Circumcision

Female circumcision, also called *female genital mutilation* (FGM) or *female genital cutting* (FGC), is a cross-cultural, cross-religious ritual that refers to the removal of portions of the female external genitalia (ACOG, 1999; Aziz, 1980; Female Genital Mutilation, 1997; Toubia, 1994, 1995). It is estimated to involve approximately 120 million females worldwide. Female circumcision has been practiced for thousands of years (Little, 2003) and certain areas of sub-Saharan Africa and other devoutly Muslim countries currently maintain this tradition.

**Figure 18-2** illustrates normal female genitalia. **Figures 18-3-a, b,** and **c** depict various types of FGM procedures. (For more information, see http://www.fgmnetwork.org.)

— *Type I.* Excision of the clitoral hood (prepuce) with or without part or all of the clitoris, called **sunna circumcision** (**Figure 18-3-a**)

— *Type II.* Excision of the clitoris, hood, and all or part of the labia minora and labia majora, called **clitoridectomy** (**Figure 18-3-b**)

— *Type III.* Excision of the clitoris, hood, labia majora and minora, and the joining of the scraped sides across the vagina where they are secured with thorns, suture, or thread, called **infibulation** or **pharaonic circumcision** (**Figure 18-3-c**)

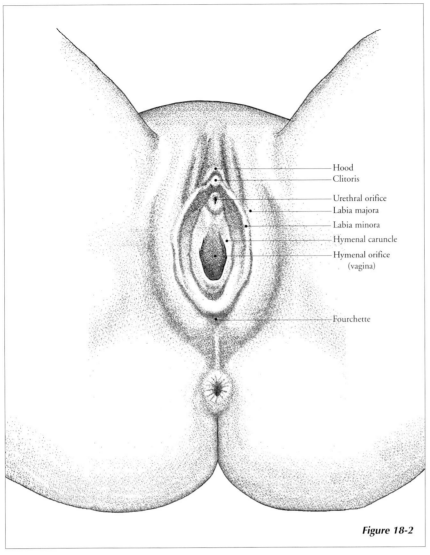

Hood
Clitoris
Urethral orifice
Labia majora
Labia minora
Hymenal caruncle
Hymenal orifice
(vagina)

Fourchette

*Figure 18-2*

*Figure 18-2.* Normal female genitalia.

*Figures 18-3-a, b,* and *c.* Type I (a), type II (b), and type III (c) procedures of female circumcision.

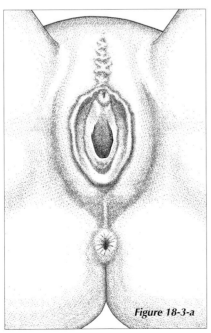

*Figure 18-3-a*

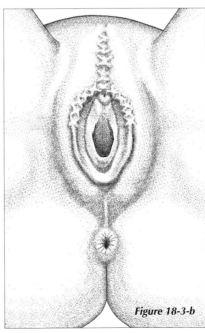

*Figure 18-3-b*

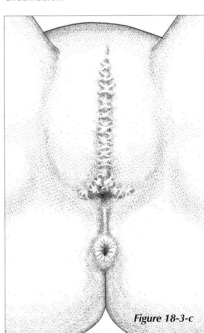

*Figure 18-3-c*

— *Type IV.* Burning, pricking, and/or scraping of the vulvar tissue

— Scraping the tissue around the vagina or cutting the vagina

— Applying corrosive substances or herbs into the vagina to incite sclerosis and narrowing

These procedures are frequently performed by practitioners who use unclean instruments in unsanitary conditions, thereby promoting the transmission of viral and bacterial infections. Antisepsis and anesthetic are frequently not used, and several girls are usually circumcised in succession. Of course, there are long-term physiological, sexual, and psychological effects. These effects may include frigidity, genital malformations, delayed menarche, recurrent urinary tract infections (UTI), pelvic inflammatory disease (PID), and obstetrical complications. The sequelae are individual since some victims experience no untoward effects or compromise in sexual function. Some victims request reestablishment of their previous anatomical status after the necessary modifications related to vaginal delivery, which may reflect a reverential regard for circumcision as a social custom.

Depending upon the local ritual and custom, girls who undergo circumcision may be as young as 3 years old. Justifications and rationalizations for the procedure include religious, hygienic, sexual, and sociological reasons, though the overriding motivation for parents is love for their daughters. "Being a wife and a mother is a woman's livelihood in these societies; thus, not circumcising one's daughter is equivalent to condemning her to a life of isolation. Infibulation protects her future" (Nour, 2003).

Multiple international organizations have expressed opposition to female circumcision. In September 1996, the United States passed the Federal Prohibition of Female Genital Mutilation Act of 1995. Other international organizations dedicated to eradicating FGC include the World Health Organization (WHO); United Nations Population Fund (UNFPA); United Nations Children's Fund (UNICEF); National Organization of Circumcision Information Resource Centers (NOCIRC); Research Action and Information Network for Bodily Integrity of Women (RAIN BO); and Amnesty International (**Table 18-2**).

---

**Table 18-2. Helpful Web Sites Related to Female Circumcision**

ORGANIZATIONS

**The Female Genital Cutting Education and Networking Project**
— http://www.fgmnetwork.org

**Amnesty International**
— http://www.amnesty.org/ailib/intcam/femgen/fgm1.htm

**United Nations Children's Fund (UNICEF)**
— http://www.unicef.org/newsline/fgm2.htm

**World Health Organization (WHO)**
— http://www.who.int

**Research Action and Information Network for the Bodily Integrity of Women (RAINBO)**
— http://www.rainbo.org

*(continued)*

---

**Table 18-2.** *(continued)*

CHILD ABUSE ORGANIZATIONS

**National Council on Child Abuse and Family Violence**

— http://www.nccafv.org

**Office for Victims of Crime (OVC)**

— http://www.ojp.usdoj.gov

**Rape, Abuse & Incest National Network**

— http://www.rainn.org

**Sexual Assault Nurse Examiner (SANE) Sexual Assault Response Team (SART)**

— http://www.sane-sart.com

## Gynecological Surgery and Genital Trauma

Gynecological surgery for congenital abnormalities, genital injury, or disease therapy can be a cause for genital trauma. Some congenital fascial abnormalities may result in vaginal cystocele in which the bladder undergoes symptomatic descent. A similar diagnosis may result in herniation of the bowel into a space between the vagina and rectum, known as *rectocele*, though this is rare. These situations are amendable with surgical repair via a vaginal approach. These problems have been reported rarely in female children; they occur most commonly in the multigravida who is older than 30 years and has torn the fascial supports during vaginal delivery. Uterine prolapse may also occur in this mature patient. Customary childhood problems may include urethral prolapse, an imperforate hymen, some neoplastic vulvar entities (ie, sarcoma botryoides), and routine skin tags of various sizes (**Tables 18-3** and **18-4**). In order to choose the correct diagnosis and rule out abuse, it is important to consider preexisting changes caused by underlying diseases.

**Table 18-3. Differential Diagnosis of the Vulvar Dermatoses**

| CONDITION | CLINICAL APPEARANCE | DIAGNOSTIC TEST | THERAPY |
|---|---|---|---|
| Psoriasis | Red plaques with silvery scale; also on knees, elbows, scalp; nail pitting | Clinical appearance; cutaneous biopsy; | Topical steroids (triamcinolone 0.1%); systemic antimetabolite Rx if severe |
| Seborrheic dermatitis | Scaling/erythema; also on eyebrows; nasolabial folds, hairline, occasional axillae | Clinical appearance; KOH preparation of scale negative | Dandruff shampoos, hydrocortisone 1% cream |
| Dermatophyte (tinea cruris) | Annular plaque with central clearing and peripheral scale | KOH preparation of scale positive | Topical imidazole creams bid until clear for 1 week |
| Chronic dermatitis (contact or irritant) | Often eczematous and oozing; may involve congruent areas; eyelids; may generalize | Careful history and patch testing if indicated | Cool compresses, Crisco or hydrocortisone 2.5% ointment, no allergens |
| Lichen simplex chronicus | Thick, furrowed vulva; other common sites are ankle, arm, or nape of neck | Cutaneous biopsy | Triamcinolone 0.1% ointment for 4-6 weeks; rule out vaginal *Candida* |

*(continued)*

**Table 18-3. Differential Diagnosis of the Vulvar Dermatoses** *(continued)*

| CONDITION | CLINICAL APPEARANCE | DIAGNOSTIC TEST | THERAPY |
|---|---|---|---|
| Lichen planus | "Purple polygonal papules and plaques," lacy white pattern or erosions on oral and vulvar mucosa, wrists, shins common | Cutaneous biopsy | Topical steroids: cream or suppositories (clobetasol x 1-2 weeks, taper to hydrocortisone 1%) |
| Lichen sclerosus | White, wrinkly; usually only vulva, anus ("keyhole" pattern); dermis thick, epidermis atrophic; occasional patchy on trunk | Clinical appearance, cutaneous biopsy | Topical steroids (clobetasol x 2 weeks, than taper, 1% hydrocortisone ointment or cream); emollients, hygiene |

*Reprinted with permission from McKay M. Vulvitis and vulvovaginitis: cutaneous considerations.* Am J Obstet Gynecol. *1991;165:1176.*

---

**Table 18-4. Etiology of Vulvovaginal Symptoms in the Prepubertal Child**

— "Nonspecific" vulvovaginitis
— Specific vulvovaginitis
　— Respiratory pathogens
　　— *Streptococcus pyogenes* (Group A ß-streptococcus)
　　— *Staphylococcus aureus*
　　— *Haemophilus influenzae*
　　— *Streptococcus pneumoniae*
　　— *Branhamella catarrhalis*
　　— *Neisseria meningitidis*
　— Enteric
　　— *Shigella*
　　— *Yersinia*
　　— Other flora
　— Candida
　— Sexually transmitted diseases
　　— *Neisseria gonorrhoeae*
　　— *Chlamydia trachomatis*
　　— Herpes simplex
　　— *Trichomonas*
　　— Condyloma accuminata (human papillomavirus)
— Pinworms, other helminths
— Foreign body
— Polyps, tumors
— Systemic illness: measles, chickenpox, scarlet fever, Stevens-Johnson's syndrome, mononucleosis, Kawasaki disease, histiocytosis, Crohn's
— Vulvar skin disease: lichen sclerosus, seborrhea, psoriasis, atopic dermatitis, scabies, contact dermatitis (nickel allergy), zinc deficiency, bullous pemphigoid
— Trauma
— Psychosomatic vaginal complaints
— Miscellaneous: draining pelvic abscess, prolapsed urethra, ectopic ureter, disposable diapers

*Reprinted with permission from Emans SJ. Vulvovaginal problems in the prepubertal child. In: Emans SJ, Laufer MR, Goldstein DP, eds.* Pediatric and Adolescent Gynecology. *4th ed. Philadelphia, Pa: Lippencott-Raven; 1998:75-107.*

## Differential Diagnosis for Childhood Genital Trauma

In general, the gross categories of vulvar disease include dermatological, infectious, inflammatory, and congenital disorders. Clinical presentations of these disorders vary but usually involve a mass effect, color change, rash, or excoriation (**Table 18-4**). In female patients, vaginal bleeding may suggest sexual abuse; however, many causes should be excluded before considering abuse or genital trauma and secondary genital injury. Additionally, the patient's age and sexual maturity define the differential diagnostic possibilities (**Tables 18-1** and **18-5**).

Every healthcare provider should be alert to potential child sexual assault as an antecedent event, be it acute or chronic. This deliberation is the primary way that the diagnosis will be routinely considered and recognized. Verification of such a diagnosis requires a complete physical examination. A focus on the genitalia should be the final component of the examination. A speculum examination with cervical visualization is

---

**Table 18-5. Differential Diagnosis of Abnormal Vaginal Bleeding in the Adolescent Girl**

**Anovulatory uterine bleeding**

**Pregnancy-related complications**
— Threatened abortion
— Spontaneous, incomplete, or missed abortion
— Ectopic pregnancy
— Gestational trophoblastic disease
— Complications of termination procedures

**Infection**
— Pelvic inflammatory disease
— Endometritis
— Cervicitis
— Vaginitis

**Blood dyscrasias**
— Thrombocytopenia (eg, idiopathic thrombocytopenic purpura, leukemia, aplastic anemia, hypersplenism, chemotherapy)
— Clotting disorders (eg, Von Willebrand's disease, other disorders of platelet function, liver dysfunction)

**Endocrine disorders**
— Hypo- or hyperthyroidism
— Adrenal disease
— Hyperprolactinemia
— Polycystic ovary syndrome
— Ovarian failure

**Vaginal abnormalities**
— Carcinoma
— Laceration

**Cervical problems**
— Cervicitis
— Polyp
— Hemangioma
— Carcinoma

**Uterine problems**
— Submucous myoma
— Congenital anomalies
— Polyp
— Carcinoma
— Use of intrauterine device
— Breakthrough bleeding associated with oral contraceptives or other hormonal contraceptives
— Ovulation bleeding

**Ovarian problems**
— Cyst
— Tumor (benign, malignant)

**Endometriosis**

**Trauma**

**Foreign body (eg, retained tampon)**

**Systemic diseases**
— Diabetes mellitus
— Renal disease
— Systemic lupus erythematosus

**Medications**
— Hormonal contraceptives
— Anticoagulants
— Platelet inhibitors
— Androgens
— Spironolactone

*Reprinted with permission from Emans SJ. Vulvovaginal problems in the prepubertal child. In: Emans SJ, Laufer MR, Goldstein DP, eds.* Pediatric and Adolescent Gynecology. *4th ed. Philadelphia, Pa: Lippencott-Raven; 1998:75-107.*

not appropriate for the prepubertal child unless the examination is done under anesthesia. The speculum examination may be appropriate based on the clinical context of the adolescent patient.

In order to successfully diagnose certain childhood conditions, the vast array of available imaging technologies has the potential to add considerably to description and diagnosis. Standard radiographs, enhanced CT scans, intravenous pyelography (IVP), ultrasound, and magnetic resonance imaging (MRI) should be considered. Interventional radiology can be used to answer chronic and emergent clinical questions. Laparoscopy, rather than laparotomy, is liberally applied to address pain syndromes and intra-abdominal injury.

# THE PATIENT HISTORY

This component of the investigation of genital trauma and possible genital injury is compromised by the influence of interpersonal interaction. Interpretation and semantics are very important in legal arguments. Knowing how to pose the questions correctly, what vital issues to address, and how to document the responses are crucial in inspiring an authentic recreation of time and events.

## THE IMPORTANCE OF OBTAINING A HISTORY

Each patient's medical history and physical examination must be customized. With sexual assault victims, healthcare providers should be especially sensitive to a victim's age, race, gender, sexual orientation, national origin, and mental status. Healthcare providers should strive to ask nonleading questions that reconstruct the history. **Table 18-6** provides some valuable tips for obtaining such histories from victims. **Table 18-7** lists further questions that can be revealing after and in reference to the patient's account of the abuse. These general questions can be modified to work with any victim, including a victim of sexual assault.

---

**Table 18-6. Obtaining a Victim's History**

When interviewing a victim, other sources, or an alleged perpetrator, an investigative team must observe the following indicators and record them in writing and on audiotape or videotape.

AVAILABLE HISTORICAL AND INFORMATIONAL SOURCES:

— The victim
— The perpetrator and/or coconspirator
— The authorities (ie, police officer, security officer, teacher)
— A witness or collateral observer
— Family member
— Outreach worker
— Friend and/or companion (ie, confidant)

THE ASSESSMENT TEAM SHOULD OBSERVE AND DOCUMENT ALL SUBTLE CLUES FROM THE SOURCE:

— Victim is emotional, afraid, or stoic
— Victim is communicative
— Victim is aggressive and/or confrontational
— Victim is under the influence of drugs or alcohol
— Victim changes details
— Victim has trigger points or issues
— Victim has mood changes

*(continued)*

---

**Table 18-6.** *(continued)*

THE ASSESSMENT TEAM SHOULD OBSERVE AND DOCUMENT ALL SUBTLE CLUES FROM THE SOURCE:

— Victim is incensed
— Victim is unclear, illogical, or incoherent
— Victim seems abrupt or hurried
— Victim seems to be protecting someone
— Victim has an inappropriate affect
— Victim is clutching something physical
— Victim is avoiding a particular subject

**Table 18-7. Revealing Questions That May Provide Further Information About Abuse**

Interviewers should avoid questions that require one-word answers. If "yes" or "no" is all the patient provides, question futher to get more in-depth answers.

HOME ENVIRONMENT

— Where do you live?
— How long have you lived there?
— With whom do you live?
— Describe your relationships with parents and siblings.
— What are your responsibilities in the home?
— Do you receive an allowance?
— Describe your daily schedule.
— Have you run away from home?

EDUCATION

— Do you attend school?
— Describe your behavior at school.
— Describe your grades.
— What subjects do you find interesting?
— What subjects do you find boring?
— Have you ever been suspended from school?
— Are you involved in any after-school activities?
— Do you have a job?
— Are you involved in sports?
— Do you plan to pursue more or advanced schooling?

ACTIVITIES

— What do you like to do for fun?
— Are you involved in out-of-school sports or teams?
— Are you involved in any organizations (eg, scouts, church, community, gangs)?
— Do you like to read? If yes, what do you like to read?
— What type of music do you prefer?
— Do you have a car available to you? If yes, who owns the car?

*(continued)*

**Table 18-7. Revealing Questions That may Provide Further Information About Abuse** *(continued)*

ACTIVITIES

— Do you have any hobbies?
— Describe your friends (eg, Who are they? What do your friends do?).
— Who is your best friend?
— How much time do you spend with friends?
— How much time do you spend watching television?
— What do you like to watch on television?
— How much time do you spend playing video games?
— What type of video games do you like to play?
— Do you have an income? If yes, what is the source of this income?
— Are you a member of any groups?

DRUGS

— Do your peers use drugs? If yes, what type of drugs do they use?
— Do members of your family use drugs? If yes, what types of drugs do they use?
— Do you or have you used drugs? If yes, what type of drugs do you use and when do you use them? How do you pay for these drugs?

SEX

— Do you date?
— Have you had previous sexual experiences? If yes, what type of experience have you had? How many sexual partners have you had all together? When was your first sexual experience?
— Are any of your friends sexually active? If yes, what type of sexual experiences do they have?
— Are you currently sexually involved with someone?
— What is your sexual preference?
— Have you ever had a sexually transmitted disease? If yes, what type have you had?
— Do you use contraception? If yes, what type do you use?
— How frequently do you have sexual intercourse?
— Have you ever been pregnant?
— Have you ever had an abortion?
— What are your feeling about intercourse?

SUICIDE

— Do you currently have any suicidal ideas or thoughts?
— Have you ever tried to commit suicide?
— Have you ever planned a suicide attempt?
— Would you ever kill yourself?
— Have any of your friends ever attempted to commit suicide or succeeded in commiting suicide?

### THE INTERVIEWER

A good medical interviewer collects information and sets the stage for subsequent interactions. This skill is ultimately perfected through practice and experience. Interviewers must be aware that their personal style, personality, biases, philosophy, sensitivity, and experiences influence the collection of evidence while obtaining a patient history. Absolute objectivity is unlikely.

Interviewers must be mature and open-minded as well as genuinely interested in the interviewee and their problems. In addition, interviewers should effectively communicate with the patient and assure confidentiality; however, the patient should be informed that absolute confidentiality can not be assured since the history, physical examination, and medical records could become court evidence. The interviewer should also be sensitive, flexible, and culturally appropriate.

No book can adequately teach the art of relating to patients and people who can provide information. **Table 18-8** does, however, provide some general guidelines for interviewers when obtaining a patient's history.

## CONCLUDING THE INTERVIEW
At the end of an interview the interviewer should summarize the proposed diagnosis and outline the next step and its purpose, that step being the physical examination.

---

### Table 18-8. Interviewer Tips for Obtaining a History

— Establish rapport with the patient; share common ground.
— Refer the patient to someone else if the situation is uncomfortable for either participant.
— Ask with whom the patient would feel most comfortable or prefer to have ask these questions.
— Select the first setting for the interview in a nonmedical environment and then move to a medical space for the physical examination.
— The interview should be conducted in a one-on-one setting.
— A repeated interview with a chaperone may provide additional information.
— If the child is mature enough and communicative, consider using the HEADSS (**H**ome, **E**ducation/employment, **A**ctivity, **D**rugs, **S**exuality, **S**uicide/depression screen) interview line of questioning for the personal history.
— Remember that the personal history provides a context for the recollection of events.
— Summarize and restate the objectives and goals of the interview and physical examination recurrently.
— Determine the immediacy of the physical examination according to the amount of time that has elapsed since an event.
— Always keep the objectives and goals in mind in selecting questions and doing tests.
— Assure confidentiality though explain what information can not be kept confidential.
— Avoid interruptions to maintain rapport.
— Take notes regarding observations; develop a timeline of events.
— Mention previous history issues.
— Avoid the role of the surrogate parent or that of a pal or friend.
— Act as an advocate.
— Circumvent power struggles.
— Listen without interruption.
— Ask open-ended questions.
— Avoid leading questions.
— Promote self-responsibility and resistance to peer pressure.
— Inquire about the patient's family, past medical history, present concerns, and the family structure and dynamics.
— Identify family members and their roles and relationships.
— Encourage family counseling.
— Ask whether the patient is in danger; this directs the thrust of the investigation.
— Inform the patient that some personal but important questions will be asked.

*Adapted from Adams, 2001; American Academy of Pediatrics, Committee on Child Abuse and Neglect, 1999; Neinstein & Ratner Kaufman, 2002; Patel & Minshall, 2001.*

Additionally, the interviewer should listen to and discuss any questions or concerns that the patient may have. The interviewer should emphasize the importance of compliance, and they should forecast future appointments, follow-up, and counseling.

# THE PHYSICAL EXAMINATION

From a medical perspective, the essential part of any therapeutic endeavor is making the correct diagnosis. The diagnosis is accomplished by establishing the history and by the physical examination of the patient and the actual collection of evidence. Once the laboratory data is collected and evaluated, a diagnosis is proposed. It is important to propose a cause of trauma, including whether it occurred spontaneously or was intentionally inflicted.

A number of protocols and methods of physical examination of victims exist. Physical examinations are intended to gather objective evidence that will corroborate and confirm the victim's accusations (**Table 18-9**). Further deductions of intentional etiologies should be reserved until the completion of the evaluation. Most importantly, the practitioner must determine whether the victim's condition requires emergency care or if it is life threatening. In the event of a trial, the data obtained from an examination is presented to the court or jury in order to verify testimony and records (Soules et al, 1978).

Examiners should recognize their role in the process and avoid inappropriate behaviors such as judging, exhibiting a negative attitude, lecturing, admonishing the patient, and using leading questions and statements. They should strive to be independent observers and be sensitive, gentle, communicative, problem-oriented, suspi-

---

**Table 18-9. A Physical Examiner's Checklist**

When performing a physical examination on a child victim of sexual assault, the physical examiner should:

— Recruit the patient for compliance.

— Describe the trauma sites.

— Describe the degree of injury.

— Describe the pattern of injury.

— Propose the mechanism of injury.

— Observe whether the injury is acute or nonacute.

— Decide whether the child is in danger.

— Always be aware of the chain of evidence.

Additionally, the physical examiner should remember the following facts:

— Many child molestations are nonviolent and do not involve visible genital injury.

— From the child's point of view, the physical examination should not be worse than the molestation.

— Being very careful, gentle, and sensitive is important.

— When genital injury is apparent, an age-appropriate, differential diagnosis should be generated.

— The motive for evidence collection, taking a history, and conducting a physical examination may change with time.

cious, intuitive, and open-minded. To promote child and family compliance, examiners act as the victim's advocate. In an effort to make the physical examination and collection of evidence less stressful for the victim, the physical examiner should allow the presence of a chaperone and/or assistant during the procedure. An example of a state's protocols for physical examinations can be found in **Table 18-10**.

When conducting a physical examination, the examiner should remember the who, when, where, how, and why of the examination.

---

**Table 18-10. Physical Examination Questions and Procedures in Illinois**

Use of a tape recording unit for audio or video record of questioning is recommended by the Illinois State Police Division of Forensic Services. Any evidence from the sexual assault kit may be used in court to prosecute sexual assault cases; therefore, it is important to follow instructions and write legibly.

THE SEXUAL ASSAULT KIT

— Collect specimens from victims of sexual assault for submission to forensic science laboratories for analysis and storage.

— May replace or supplement the medical record in sexual assault cases.

PROCEDURE CHECK LIST

— All specimens must be labeled and sealed.

— A signed patient consent for the physical examination and medical care must be obtained.

— A signed authorization must be obtained to release information and forensic findings.

— A drape should be spread on the floor to collect miscellaneous debris while the patient undresses.

— The patient's clothing should be placed in a paper bag.

— Oral specimens must be obtained.

— Penile or cervical specimens must be obtained.

— Anal specimens must be obtained.

— Miscellaneous stains and/or bite-mark evidence must be documented.

— Pubic hair combings must be collected.

— Head hair combings must be collected.

— Fingernail specimens must be obtained.

— Blood specimens on filter paper must be obtained.

— Physical injuries must be photographed.

— A receipt of information must be included.

— Patient disclosure materials must be provided.

REMINDERS

— Use paper bags, *not* plastic.

— Label and seal all envelopes.

— Complete forensic laboratory report forms.

— Do not include unused or extra components in the kit.

— Seal the kit with red evidence tape.

*Adapted from the Illinois State Police Division of Forensic Services.*

---

## WHO IS THE EXAMINER

Determining the ideal examiner for a case is often a dilemma. Examiners could be the patient's personal healthcare provider, an emergency room physician, or an assessment team trained in evaluating CSE. The interpretations and methods of the physical examination will differ according to who performs the examination, thereby impacting the results. If forensics are important for litigation purposes, then the best choice is an assessment team specializing in CSE or a healthcare provider who is certified and trained in CSE evaluation. Of utmost importance, in the hands of a CSE expert, the physical examination is customized to best serve the patient and perhaps the patient's family.

## WHERE TO EXAMINE

The examiner must consider the best location in which to conduct the physical examination (eg, ER, operating room, physician's office, off site). To determine the appropriate answer, the examiner must consider a composite of coincidental issues: the relevant history, the time that has elapsed since the alleged assault, the patient's age, the availability of evidence, and the victim's psychological state. Patients place a high value on convenience and comfort after an alleged assault (Heger & Emans, 1992).

## WHEN TO EXAMINE

The physical examiner must decide when the examination should take place. The earlier the examination takes place, the more likely evidence will be recovered and the findings will be useful in diagnosis or litigation. Sexual assaults often do not have anogenital findings; however, an immediate interview and physical examination of untouched clothing and debris may offer clues. The examination should be conducted before the victim cleans up and bathes.

## HOW TO EXAMINE

The method of an examination and the technology used are important considerations. As with any routine physical examination, the examiner should begin by checking the patient's vital signs, followed by observing and documenting the physical findings from head to toe. The examiner should always remain observant and carefully collect all physical evidence. The genital examination should occur last (Lenahan et al, 1998).

There are a number of important decisions regarding the way an examination is conducted, including the following:

— Whether to use a speculum

— Whether to obtain samples for a culture and wet mount from the vagina

— Whether and how to collect samples of specimens (eg, semen, saliva, blood, hair, skin) found on the victim; these samples can be analyzed to identify the deoxyribonucleic acid (DNA) component

— Whether to use a Wood's lamp (ie, a portable ultraviolet lamp) to reveal dried bodily secretions on the victim, which would otherwise remain invisible, so that samples can be obtained and preserved; these secretions can be used to identify the perpetrator

— Whether to test and how to conduct and follow up on a test since many cultures and serum assays may require serial studies to verify transmission, therefore encouraging a repeat examination; initial tests may assess an immediate or baseline status; appropriate tests and/or cultures should be chosen and omitted according to the victim's clinical circumstance

## WHY EXAMINE

An examiner needs to understand and determine why an examination should be conducted. There are many reasons to do the examination (Muram, 1989), and as time passes, the motive and purpose of the investigation frequently change. **Table 18-11** lists some objectives.

# LABORATORY TESTING

An examiner who is fluent in laboratory testing must be constantly updated on the evolution of testing methods and collection requirements. In CSE alleged circumstances, the examiner should evaluate for sexually transmitted disease (STD) transmission and collect DNA. Baseline liver function, thyroid status, bone growth, bone injury, and nutritional status may also be needed.

## SEXUALLY TRANSMITTED DISEASE TESTING

STD testing during evidence collection may reflect the presence of preexisting infection or exposure to certain previous infections. This testing can document the baseline status of certain disease entities in potential cases of alleged assault. In some cases, prophylaxis is provided to prevent possible exposure to human immunodeficiency virus (HIV), syphilis, gonorrhea, and *Chlamydia*. If not, repeat testing should be performed between 1 and 2 weeks and then at 3 months after the alleged assault.

## DEOXYRIBONUCLEIC ACID UPDATE

DNA evidence is critical in deciding criminal cases in the United States as well as in international jurisdictions. DNA is a genetic fingerprint that distinctly identifies an individual. It is exactly the same in every cell of a person's body, and it is found in multiple areas of every cell in the body. Only identical twins have the same DNA. Since every person's DNA is distinct, locating and identifying an individual's DNA profile on evidence found at the crime scene or on the victim can verify that an individual was at the crime scene at some point in time. Such evidence can validate or deny allegations from the victim or defendant.

The development of a DNA profile may include the collection of blood, saliva, skin, hair, and semen from the crime scene, the alleged victim, or the perpetrator. Specimens are compared to the DNA of the alleged victim and perpetrator and to the Federal Bureau of Investigation's (FBI's) Combined DNA Index System (CODIS), which enables the comparison of specimens to people who may not be suspected in these cases. This information may validate or invalidate certain assertions.

### Processing and Analysis

The processing and analysis of DNA evidence usually requires weeks or months and is expensive to the authorities who request it. An independent laboratory evaluates 13 specific loci and compares the results to the results in known specimens. Since a person's DNA is the same from all sites of that person (eg, skin, hair, saliva, sweat,

| Table 18-11. Objectives for Conducting a Physical Examination on an Assault Victim |
|---|
| — Diagnose and treat the physical, emotional, and behavioral consequences of abuse |
| — Confirm and validate statements made in the interview |
| — Establish the basic condition of the victim and recognize any underlying health problems |
| — Acquire and preserve forensic evidence |
| — Establish present baseline status in reference to sexually transmitted diseases, pregnancy, body systems and their functions since many tests require serial observations |
| — Plan prophylaxis and/or preemptive therapy |
| — Assess the amount of objective corroborating evidence |

semen), the results can be crosschecked. Crime scene DNA profiles are examined with the intent to identify the DNA from the victim or another person. If the DNA matches another person, a statistic is produced that reflects how frequently this match might occur in the general population. Much like the database of fingerprints, the FBI can compare DNA profiles to those already on file within the CODIS database.

The locations in the cell that are used for DNA analysis include the nucleus and the mitochondria. Methods of DNA analysis include:

— *Polymerase chain reaction (PCR) of nuclear DNA.* This process produces millions of copies of the DNA so that identification of the archetype becomes possible. One must be careful not to contaminate this evidence since sometimes, only minute amounts are available.

— *Restriction Fragment Length Polymorphism (RFLP).* This method analyzes mitochondrial DNA and, therefore, it requires a much larger sample.

— *PCR of mitochondrial DNA.* This process is used to identify samples not suitable for the other 2 methods either because of an inadequate amount or a degraded specimen (eg, in postmortem specimens of hair, bone, or blood).

Results from these tests may be used to identify an unrecognizable victim. The results may also be used to identify or verify an alleged perpetrator's presence at the crime scene.

The types of DNA profiles can be classified as follows:

— *Inclusive.* An **inclusive** DNA profile infers that an individual's DNA matches evidence from the crime scene. Such a finding reflects the high likelihood that a person was present at the crime scene at some point in time.

— *Exclusive.* An **exclusive** DNA profile suggests that the DNA profile generated from the crime scene does not match an individual.

— *Inconclusive.* An **inconclusive** DNA profile includes neither of the 2 aforementioned classifications, in that no determination can be assumed.

## COLLECTION AND STORAGE OF SPECIMENS

Evidence must be collected, transported, and preserved in a manner that resists contamination, intentional corruption, and degradation. For that reason, sexual assault victims should not alter the crime scene by bathing, changing clothes, douching, or even washing their hands. The authorities can examine and investigate the victim's space, but a trained sexual assault examiner must conduct the physical examination of the victim's body. This physical examination should occur as soon as possible to test the victim for STDs and to secure legitimate forensic evidence. The collection of DNA evidence usually requires a special kit that includes sterile cotton swabs.

Contamination can occur because of the extremely small volume of evidence available. Seemingly insignificant issues, such as handling evidence without gloves and sneezing or coughing over the specimen, can inoculate the specimen with foreign DNA. Also, degradation of the specimen is accelerated when exposed to heat and humidity. As a result, evidence must be packaged in paper rather than plastic to avoid wet or moist conditions optimal for bacterial growth. Biological evidence must be air-dried, packaged in paper, and labeled. This evidence must also include documentation of the chain of custody to avoid intentional corruption, loss, or theft.

# COMMERCIAL SEXUAL EXPLOITATION OF CHILDREN

The **commercial sexual exploitation of children** (CSEC) refers to the sexual manipulation of a person younger than 18 years old for monetary gain. This exploitation includes pornography, prostitution, and trafficking of children for sexual purposes. This problem exists in many countries. Exploited children may be rented, leased, or borrowed for involvement in acts that are usually depicted (eg, photos, drawings, videotapes) for the sexual stimulation of adults.

In infants, the diagnosis is rape for any established contact for sexual stimulation (Resnick et al, 2000). Rape diagnoses become more difficult to ascertain as children grow older and the reproductive organs and external genitalia develop because the demarcation that separates consent from imposition is sometimes unclear.

### CAUSES FOR GENITAL TRAUMA IN PROSTITUTED CHILDREN

Genital trauma occurs in CSEC depending on who the offender is (eg, the sponsor/pimp or the consumer/john). A colonial slavery model is an appropriate analogy for the sponsor relationship. The following list represents some of the sponsor's controlling actions:

— Traumatizing the child's face or genitalia, therefore, deeming the child unfit for exchange

— Enslaving the child by fear

— Motivating more encounters, thus ensuring more illicit revenue

— Protecting and hiding their own identity

— Inhibiting the child from keeping any part of the income

— Promoting absolute obedience

— Fulfilling their own masochistic desires

The following are some possible reasons for genital trauma to occur at the hand of the consumer:

— Conveying disgust for themselves, the child, or the sponsor

— Punishing themselves, the child, or the sponsor

— Distracting the child while refusing to pay for services

— Fulfilling the consumer's masochistic desires

### GENITAL INJURY RELATED TO THE COMMERCIAL SEXUAL EXPLOITATION OF CHILDREN

Genital injury is caused by different types of genital trauma, and it may not always produce visible physical evidence. Genital injury may not be apparent during the examination of a child's genitals if the assault occurred more than 72 hours before the examination. Injury occurs most frequently in acute circumstances, but less often in chronic cases (American Academy of Pediatrics, Committee on Child Abuse and Neglect, 1991).

Many variables (eg, age, gender, race, physical size, sexual maturity, the amount of resistance presented by the child) are related to the degree of injury to a victim. Certain perpetrator characteristics are also related to the degree of injury, such as age, motive for injury, and the relationship of the offender to the child. Family members tend to inflict less injury and use more intimidation, while unknown assailants tend to ensure a greater chance of injury and are more likely to use threats of injury or death.

Forced penetration is often evidenced by tears in and around the vagina or anus. Depending on the victim's age and previous sexual experience, such tears may be present. Tears may occur secondary to hematoma-induced expansion. Healed lacerations or tears in the introitus may manifest with hymenal changes, which are chronicled by diameters and locations of disruptions or ridges (McCann et al, 1992). Erythema is an often transient and obscure finding. The sexual assault expert will be attuned to recognize abrasions and redness. Fistula formation usually occurs after healing and may reflect chronic assault. This requires a fluent knowledge of normal age-specific anatomy (Adams et al, 1992).

The sexual maturity of a child is reflected in many body sites. Precocious puberty may result in changes of the voice, hair (eg, shape, amount, distribution), skin texture, and breasts, in addition to numerous other subtle changes. Putting the genital findings in context emphasizes the need for a well-trained and experienced sexual assault assessment team to adequately gauge the extent and impact of the genital injury.

Generally, injuries can be classified into 2 types: *visible* or *physical* (Elam & Ray, 1986) and *invisible* or *inoculation*. Determining whether an injury is invisible or inoculated routinely requires serial visits, examinations, and laboratory testing at the time of injury (Slaughter et al, 1997). Forecasting the victim's subsequent reproductive future is futile because of possible inoculation injuries. Physical and laboratory evaluation of an alleged perpetrator is an inadequate predictor of inoculation injuries in the victim (Muram, 1989).

When reevaluating a child during a follow-up examination, an examiner should first review all laboratory results from the initial postassault examination, including written medical and forensic evidence. Then the physical examination should be completed, beginning with a whole-body examination and followed by a genital examination.

# CONSEQUENCES OF GENITAL TRAUMA
## ACUTE VISIBLE INJURIES
Visible injuries, such as lacerations or tears may require suture repair. If hemorrhage is controlled, ice application and pressure will suffice (Sachs & Chu, 2002). The vagina may have first-, second-, third-, or fourth-degree lacerations. These are described ranging from simple epithelial disruption of the vagina or perineum to complete division of the rectal sphincter and a rectal mucosal tear. The estrogen mediated distensibility of the vagina influences the degree of the laceration and the bleeding. First- or second-degree injuries can be managed conservatively; third- and fourth-degree injuries require suture repair to align the structures in an anatomically correct fashion and secure function (Berenson et al, 2000). Hematomas may manifest with expansion that necessitates incision and drainage. Care must be taken not to compromise the underlying visceral blood supply to the uterus, bladder, or bowel. General anesthetic will guarantee patient compliance without compromising the appropriate resistance. Deep-vessel injury may necessitate exploration of the abdominal cavity to expunge adjacent visceral injury (Adams, 1996). Injuries to male children that require significant suturing should be handled by a general surgeon or urologist. Intervention may entail exploration, cauterization, packing for tamponade, suturing, or drainage (both active and passive).

## ACUTE INTERNAL INJURIES
The degree of injury to the internal reproductive organs is contingent on the extent of abdominal trauma. A great deal of force must be transmitted to cause internal pelvic injury. The abdominal wall absorbs much of the energy and is usually bruised or lacerated. Internal injury can occur as a result of severe physical trauma or an indolent inoculation insult. Some STDs infect only the cervix, but unabated, these diseases can attack the fallopian tubes. In this clinical scenario, the offending organism ascends from the vagina, through the cervix, out of the tubes, and into the peritoneal cavity. This syndrome is called ***pelvic inflammatory disease*** (PID), which can manifest with the involvement of the pelvic peritoneum by inflammation and pus with the development of adhesions with subsequent pelvic pain. Infertility may result from bilateral pyosalpinges or abscesses and tubal obstruction if left untreated. Subsequent pregnancies may put the patient at risk of ectopic implantation.

Laboratory testing with serial complete blood counts (CBCs), urinalysis, cervical cultures, and imaging by ultrasound and/or CT scan provides objective signs of progress or lack thereof. Laparoscopy and laparotomy are also possible treatment options for resistant cases of PID. Laparoscopy allows serial bacterial dilution with simple saline or lactated ringer's solution, thereby decreasing the infectious load, augmenting the antibiotic effect, and shortening the recovery period. Hysterectomy with the removal of the fallopian tubes and ovaries is an option for the worst-case scenarios.

The bony pelvis, or the fracture of the bony perimeter, is another internal injury that may occur when a child is struck by a vehicle, thrown from a moving vehicle or a building, or struck with a blunt object. Definitive diagnosis may require a radiograph or CT scan, though MRI offers the most reliable visualization. Immobilization is a rare treatment option since venous thrombosis is a major potential complication. Orthopedic consultation is recommended. Soft-tissue injury and damage is expected in these cases; therefore, serial general surgical evaluations are required.

## CHRONIC CONSEQUENCES

Genital trauma usually impacts the victim physically and psychologically. These consequences are both immediate and long-standing. The following lists some of these chronic consequences:

— The child's sexuality is added to the publicity implicit in prosecution. This is compounded by the alleged victim's immaturity. The resultant perspective of the victim is one of confusion. The plan must be to treat the victim's body and mind prophylactically.

— The chronicity of sexual assault in a child patient does not depend only on the child's age, gender, race, and cultural biases. Other factors might include self-image, available support system, baseline general health and immune status, relationship with and accessibility to the alleged perpetrator, proximity to the assault location, whether the alleged perpetrator is punished, and the patient's secondary punishment.

— The monetary and intangible costs of sexual abuse can not be calculated. Visits and charges for healthcare may last for years.

## COMMON SEXUALLY TRANSMITTED DISEASES

One of the potential consequences of genital trauma is the transmission of STDs. The following are some of the more common STDs that may be found:

— *Neisseria gonorrhea* can manifest with arthritis and a rash in advanced cases (Ingram et al, 1997). Both gonorrhea and *Chlamydia* may attack the cervix with cervicitis, discharge, and pain. An untreated infection may result in PID.

— *Chlamydia trachomitis* may be the etiology of PID, lymphogranuloma venerum, and mucopurulent cervicitis.

— Syphilis, caused by a *Treponema pallidum* infection, can attack the central nervous system and manifest with a wide range of diverse symptoms and findings. Condyloma lata are a late physical finding. These viruses have no cures.

— HSV-1 and HSV-2 are oversimplified classifications according to the site location of recurrence. Genital herpes is a recurrent, incurable STD that has reached epidemic proportions. Perhaps genital stimulation by the active HSV lesion can account for increased sexual activity during outbreaks, thus promoting its transmission (Munday & Mullan, 2001).

— Human papilloma virus (HPV) manifests with nearly 100 serotypes. About 30 serotypes occur in the anogenital region and about 15 of these are considered high-risk because of oncogenicity. If left untreated, only 30% of patients develop condyloma accuminata (genital warts). Nearly all patients with abnormal Papanicolaou tests have been infected with a strain of HPV, termed koilocytosis (nuclear clearing). High-risk strains of HPV can now be documented with the fluid based cytology screening method. Patients with high-risk designation are at greater risk of developing cervical or vulvar dysplasia and cancer. This development should be a cause for concern and close follow-up (Kellogg & Parra, 1995).

— HIV is frequently associated with the other viruses listed as well as all other bacterial STDs. HIV is transmitted by unprotected intercourse and exposing a victim to infected blood. HIV infection overwhelms the cell-mediated immune system and, if untreated, results in opportunistic infections, neoplasms, and a multisystem compromise that includes acquired immunodeficiency syndrome (AIDS), with associated dementia and malabsorbtion. Clincal sequelae may range from a simple recurrent monilial vaginitis to Kaposi's sarcoma or respiratory infection by *Pneumocystis carinii*.

— *Trichomonas vaginalis* causes a vaginitis that may be symptomatic.

— Sexually transmitted viral hepatitis is usually caused by the hepatitis B and C strains. Clinically it can result in active or chronic hepatic compromise.

— Molluscum contagiosum is caused by poxvirus. It is only mildly contagious and can be autoinoculated by nonsexual contact.

— Scabies and *Phthirus pubis* can be, but are not always, transmitted by sexual contact.

## PREEMPTIVE, PREVENTIVE, AND PROPHYLACTIC THERAPIES

These therapies are an attempt to avoid or prevent the results of inoculation injuries. The following sections present the potential health issues followed by a preventive therapy option.

### POSTCOITAL CONTRACEPTION

#### Plan A

Yuzpe protocol calls for the patient to ingest multiple birth control pills within 72 hours of intercourse (2 doses of oral contraception pills (OCPs), 100 mcg of ethinyl estradiol with each dose, every 12 hours) (ACOG, 2001). The estrogen and progesterone components combine to inhibit ovulation, ovum transport implantation, and fertilization. The progesterone may also elicit withdrawal bleeding.

#### Plan B

The patient receives high-dose progesterone every 12 hours (2 doses of 0.75 mg of levonorgesterel) within 8 hours of intercourse. At this time, the Food and Drug Administration is considering this regimen for nonprescription availability.

### BACTERIAL AGENT TREATMENT

*Neisseria gonorrhea* and *Chlamydia trachomatis* must be treated distinctly. The Centers for Disease Control and Prevention recommends the therapeutic dose of ceftriaxone intramuscularly. Azithromycin administered orally may provide protection, especially if it is followed by doxycycline treatment. Erythromycin and quinalones have been suggested as alternatives or if allergies are a complication (Centers for Disease Control and Prevention, 2002).

In cases of syphilis, no prophylactic treatment has been outlined. However, a weight-adjusted, once-weekly regimen of procaine penicillin given for 3 weeks should provide protection from transmission, even in early infestation.

In the case of tuberculosis, no prophylactic treatment has been specified. Therapy for cohabitants of tuberculosis-positive persons is controversial without verified conversion.

### VIRAL AGENTS

Viral etiologies include the following:

— HIV treated with a classic zidovudine treatment allows the suppression of HIV replication and may avoid any transmission as in antepartum therapy or after proven exposure in a hospital setting (Katz & Gerberding, 1997). The CDC now recommends a multidrug regimen.

— HSV does not have proven prophylaxis.

— HPV may be treated with a vaccination to induce immunity to serotype 16. This vaccine is not yet commercially available.

— Hepatitis C does not have a prophylaxis on record.

— Hepatitis B vaccine can be given to induce immunity.

Practitioners should be tenacious in order to uncover obscure etiologies that may be even more hidden by the history. Diagnosis is the foundation of any prophylactic or therapeutic regimen.

## CONCLUSION

All practitioners (eg, pediatricians, family physicians, emergency physicians, obstetricians, gynecologists, advanced practice nurses) *can* examine a child for genital trauma and *may* discover some history and physical findings, at least superficially (De Jong & Rose, 1991). The essential question is whether they *should* (Makoroff et al, 2002).

The best-case scenario for the victim, the alleged perpetrator, their families, the medical system, and the legal system is to discover the truth and act justly. Development and use of a specialized sexual assault assessment team can be an asset. The sexual assault assessment team should be available for the examination of victims and the investigation of their cases. The members should be experts who are trained, certified, and updated (Gray-Eurom et al, 2003). Optimally, members of this team are on-call and are shared as a resource for several communities. For the investigators, suspicions and intuitions are significant perceptions and, therefore, should be entertained while performing the history, physical examination, and pertinent laboratory studies. As previously mentioned, the physical exam can validate or impugn the allegation and/or history (McGregor et al, 1999). Team members should:

— Be observant.

— Be careful.

— Be sensitive.

— Remain open minded.

— Recognize that the motive for the collection of evidence may change as time passes.

## REFERENCES

Adams JA. Evolution of a classification scale: medical evaluation of suspected child sexual abuse. *Child Maltreat*. 2001;6:31-36.

Adams JA. Medical evaluation of suspected child sexual abuse. In: Pokorny SF, ed. *Pediatric and Adolescent Gynecology*. New York, NY: Chapman & Hall; 1996:1-14.

Adams JA, Harper K, Knudson S. A proposed system for the classification of anogenital findings in children with suspected sexual abuse. *Adolesc Pediatr Gynecol*. 1992; 5:73-75.

American Academy of Pediatrics, Committee on Child Abuse and Neglect. Guidelines for the evaluation of sexual abuse of children. *Pediatrics*. 1991;87:254-260.

American Academy of Pediatrics, Committee on Child Abuse and Neglect. Guidelines for the evaluation of sexual abuse of children: subject review. *Pediatrics*. 1999; 103:186-191.

American College of Obstetricians and Gynecologists (ACOG). *Emergency Oral Contraception*. Washington, DC: ACOG; 2001. *ACOG Practice Bulletin*; no 25.

American College of Obstetricians and Gynecologists (ACOG). F*emale Circumcision/ Female Genital Mutilation: Clinical Management of Circumcised Women* [slide-lecture kit]. Washington, DC: ACOG; 1999.

Aziz FA. Gynecologic and obstetric complications of female circumcision. *Int J Gynaecol Obstet*. 1980;17:560-563.

Berenson AB, Chacko MR, Wiemann CM, Mishaw CO, Friedrich WN, Grady JJ. A case control study of anatomic changes resulting from sexual abuse. *Am J Obstet Gynecol*. 2000:182:820-831.

Berenson AB, Heger AH, Andrews S. Appearance of the hymen in newborns. *Pediatrics*. 1991;87:458-465.

Berenson AB, Heger AH, Hayes JM, Bailey RK, Emans SJ. Appearance of the hymen in prepubertal girls. *Pediatrics*. 1992;89:387-394.

Berenson AB. Normal anogenital anatomy. *Child Abuse Negl*. 1998;22:589-596.

Botash AS, Jean-Louis F. Imperforate hymen: congenital or acquired from sexual abuse? *Pediatrics*. 2001;108:e53.

Centers for Disease Control and Prevention. Sexually transmitted diseases treatment guidelines. *MMWR Recomm Rep*. 2002;51(RR-6):52-53.

Cowell CA. The gynecologic examination of infants, children, and young adolescents. *Pediatr Clin North Am*. 1981;28:247-266.

De Jong AR, Rose M. Legal proof of child sexual abuse in the absence of physical evidence. *Pediatrics*. 1991;88:506-511.

Elam AL, Ray VG. Sexually related trauma: a review. *Ann Emerg Med*. 1986;15: 576-584.

Emans SJ. Vulvovaginal problems in the prepubertal child. In: Emans SJ, Laufer MR, Goldstein DP, eds. *Pediatric and Adolescent Gynecology*. 4th ed. Philadelphia, Pa: Lippencott-Raven; 1998:75-107.

*Female Genital Mutilation: A Joint WHO/UNICEF/ UNFPA Statement*. Geneva, Switzerland: World Health Organization; 1997.

Gray-Eurom K, Seaberg DC, Wears RL. The prosecution of sexual assault cases: correlation with forensic evidence. *Ann Emerg Med*. 2003;39:39-46.

Heger A, Emans SJ, eds. *Evaluation of the Sexually Abused Child: A Medical Textbook and Photographic Atlas*. New York, NY: Oxford University Press. 1992.

Heger AH, Ticson L, Guerra L, et al. Appearance of the genitalia in girls selected for nonabuse: review of hymenal morphology and nonspecific findings. *J Pediatr Adolesc Gynecol*. 2002;15:27-35.

Heppenstall-Heger A, McConnell G, Ticson L, Guerra L, Lister J, Zaragoza T. Healing patterns in anogenital injuries: a longitudinal study of injuries associated with sexual abuse, accidental injuries, or genital surgery in the preadolescent child. *Pediatrics*. 2003;112:829-837.

Hobbs CJ, Wynne JM, Thomas AJ. Colposcopic genital findings in prepubertal girls assessed for sexual abuse. *Arch Dis Child*. 1995:73(5):465-471.

Ingram DL, Everett D, Flick LA, Russell TA, White-Sims ST. Vaginal gonococcal cultures in sexual abuse evaluations: evaluation of selective criteria in pre-teenaged girls. *Pediatrics*. 1997;99:E8.

Jones JS, Rossman L, Hartman M, Alexander CC. Anogenital injuries in adolescents after consensual sexual intercourse. *Acad Emerg Med*. 2003;10:1378-1383.

Kadish HA, Schunk JE, Britton H. Pediatric male rectal and genital trauma: accidental and nonaccidental injuries. *Pediatr Emerg Care*. 1998;14:95-98.

Katz MH, Gerberding JL. Postexposure treatment of people exposed to the human immunodeficiency virus through sexual contact or injection-drug use. *N Engl J Med*. 1997;336:1097-1100.

Kellogg ND, Parra JM. The progression of human papillomavirus lesions in sexual assault victims. *Pediatrics*. 1995;96:1163-1165.

Kempe CH. Sexual abuse, another hidden pediatric problem: the 1977 C. Anderson Aldrich lecture. *Pediatrics*. 1978;62:382-389.

Lenahan LC, Ernst A, Johnson B. Colposcopy in evaluation of the adult sexual assault victim. *Am J Emerg Med*. 1998;16:183-184.

Leventhal JM. Epidemiology of child sexual abuse. In: Oates RK, ed. *Understanding and Managing Child Sexual Abuse*. Sydney, Australia: Harcourt Brace Jovanovich Group; 1990:18-42.

Little CM. Female genital circumcision: medical and cultural considerations. *J Cult Divers*. 2003;10:30-34.

Makoroff KL, Brauley JL, Brandner AM, Myers PA, Shapiro RA. Genital examinations for alleged sexual abuse of prepubertal girls: findings by pediatric emergency medicine physicians compared with child abuse trained physicians. *Child Abuse Negl*. 2002;26:1235-1242.

McAleer IM, Kaplan GW. Pediatric genitourinary trauma. *Urol Clin North* Am. 1995;22:177-188.

McCann J, Voris J, Simon M: Genital injuries resulting from sexual abuse: a longitudinal study. *Pediatrics*. 1992;89:307-317.

McCann J. Use of the colposcope in childhood sexual abuse examinations. *Pediatr Clin North Am*. 1990;37:863-880.

McGregor MJ, Le G, Marion SA, Wiebe E. Examination for sexual assault: is the documentation of physical injury associated with the laying of charges? A retrospective cohort study. *CMAJ*. 1999;160:1565-1569.

Munday PE, Mullan HM. Clinical uses of herpes simplex virus type-specific serology. *Int J STD AIDS*. 2001;12:784-788.

Muram D. Child sexual abuse: relationship between sexual acts and genital findings. *Child Abuse Negl*. 1989;13:211-216.

Neinstein LS, Ratner Kaufman F. Normal physical growth and development. In: Neinstein LS, ed. *Adolescent Health Care: A Practical Guide*. 4th ed. Philadelphia, Pa: Lippincott Williams & Wilkins; 2002:1-51.

Nour NM. Female circumcision and genital mutilation: a practical and sensitive approach. *Contemp Ob Gyn*. 2000;45:50-55.

Patel M, Minshall L. Management of sexual assault. *Emerg Med Clin North Am*. 2001;19:817-831.

Resnick H, Acierno R, Holmes M, Dammeyer M, Kilpatrick D. Emergency evaluation and intervention with female victims of rape and other violence. *J Clin Psychol*. 2000;56:1317-1333.

Sachs CJ, Chu LD. Predictors of genitorectal injury in female victims of suspected sexual assault. *Acad Emerg Med*. 2002;9:146-151.

Slaughter L, Brown CR, Crowley S, Peck R. Patterns of genital injury in female sexual assault victims. *Am J Obstet Gynecol.* 1997;176:609-616.

Soules MR, Pollard AA, Brown KM, Verma M. The forensic laboratory evaluation of evidence in alleged rape. *Am J Obstet Gynecol.* 1978;130:142-147.

Toubia N. Female circumcision as a public health issue. *N Engl J Med.* 1994;331: 712-716.

Toubia N. *Female Genital Mutilation: A Call for Global Action.* New York, NY: RAINBO;1995.

Zitelli BJ, Davis HW. *Atlas of Pediatric Physical Diagnosis.* Philadelphia, Pa: Mosby; 2002.

# COMMUNITY AND MENTAL HEALTH SUPPORT OF JUVENILE VICTIMS OF PROSTITUTION

Mary P. Alexander, MA, LPC
Nancy D. Kellogg, MD
Phyllis Thompson, LCSW

The provision of community and mental health support for child and adolescent victims of prostitution presents daunting and unique challenges. First, few providers or programs have the training and expertise to address all of the specific needs of these victims. Victims tend to be treated in a fragmented fashion that reflects the sequelae of their prostitution and victimization rather than the underlying causes. They may be treated for substance abuse, sexually transmitted diseases (STDs), or physical assault injuries, but their need for safety, education, social and trade skills, and protection are too often overlooked. Short-term therapy or treatment may be available but rarely addresses the sexual victimization. This problem is compounded by victims' reluctance to disclose abuse and the tendency to avoid treatment until their physical health and mental health are severely affected.

The second challenge to providing community and mental health services for young victims of prostitution is that many victims do not want help or are too scared to seek and/or accept it. Many have been extensively groomed to accommodate their victimization while others have been frequently threatened, blackmailed, beaten, mutilated, and tortured by their pimps or perpetrators. Some victims avoid getting help out of fear of being reported to the juvenile justice system, getting placed into foster care, or having to return to the dysfunctional or abusive family from which they ran away and entered into prostitution in order to survive in the first place (Unger et al, 1998). To avoid disclosure and discovery of their victimization, children and adolescents typically and convincingly lie about their age and circumstances. Many victims even continue to deny their experiences of abuse even after service providers share eyewitness accounts, photographic evidence, or the perpetrator's confession of their victimization.

Once victims of prostitution are identified, service providers face the challenge of gaining trust while complying with child abuse reporting laws and the need for safety plans. Many prostituted youth are generally knowledgeable about child protection and juvenile detention systems and tend to know what information is reportable and which activities are criminal. If service providers attempt to gather information that may result in police or child protective services (CPS) intervention, child or adolescent victims may recant the information they shared, refuse services, and leave quickly without returning.

## HEALTHCARE SETTINGS

Child and adolescent victims of prostitution may present for treatment in any healthcare setting. They may enter the setting with medical or psychiatric problems related to their victimization, or they may disclose their abusive experiences after sustaining physical or sexual assault injuries. Other victims may be brought to a healthcare setting after the discovery of pornographic materials or a perpetrator's confession. Once a child or adolescent is identified as a victim of abuse, protocols for physical and sexual abuse are employed, and the police and CPS agencies are immediately notified. CPS then becomes responsible for developing and enforcing an immediate safety plan as well as follow-up care and support services. Follow-up services commonly include visits to hospital emergency rooms, community child abuse centers, or specialized outpatient settings.

Due to a general reluctance to seek healthcare and fear of being reported, children and adolescent victims tend to seek services only after physical or psychological symptoms become extreme. They may present to emergency rooms, STD clinics, or detoxification units exhibiting symptoms of drug or alcohol intoxication, overdose or withdrawal, suicidal ideation, STDs, pelvic inflammatory disease, pregnancy, or physical assault injuries.

## AMBULATORY CARE CLINICS

Victims of juvenile prostitution who continue to reside with their families may present to ambulatory care clinics. In these circumstances, the family may or may not be aware of the child's victimization. Family members that are aware of, or assist in, the child's victimization will devise convincing but deceptive explanations for the child's symptoms. Family members may make attempts to deflect health professionals' concern and their need to report abuse to authorities by claiming that the child or adolescent is much older than he or she is or that he or she is consensually sexually active with other adolescents.

## EMERGENCY CARE FACILITIES

Law enforcement officers may bring victims of juvenile prostitution into the emergency room if their victimization is witnessed or if they are found on the streets with significant health problems. A healthcare professional's level of concern for victimization should increase whenever children and adolescents do not present themselves voluntarily for necessary medical care. This often indicates a need for a comprehensive assessment of risky behaviors that could affect victims' physical and mental health.

Victims who present in emergency care facilities may exhibit an array of emotions that range from inconsolable crying and shaking to a controlled response. Clinicians may also notice victims exhibiting incongruent affects, such as laughing at inappropriate times. This is common and the victim can still be traumatized by an event. Combative or intoxicated victims may claim no memory or a "black-out" after they wake up with various injuries or find their clothes gone or in disarray. While intoxication may be a factor in lapsed memory, victims frequently deflect questions about abusive experiences they recall in order to avoid discovery and the necessity of someone filing a child abuse report with authorities.

Clinicians who practice in emergency settings need to be calm and reassuring, maintain control of their emotions, give choices to victims, and provide them with developmentally appropriate information. Providing information clearly and simply will serve to prevent victims from becoming further traumatized by their own ideas of what they think might happen and help them to make sense of their surroundings and current experiences (Perry, 1998).

## MENTAL HEALTH CLINICS

Prostituted youth are known to be at increased risk for depression, suicide, posttraumatic stress disorder (PTSD), and neuroses (Gibson-Ainyetteet et al, 1988; Seng, 1989; Yates et al, 1991). They may present to emergency rooms with acute overdoses or other signs of self-injurious behaviors. As with physical symptoms, children and adolescents are unlikely to present voluntarily for mental health services unless they are in an extreme state of crisis. Clinicians who respond need to recognize that this may be the only time this child or adolescent seeks help and that his or her response may be a decisive factor for further intervention and saving his or her life. Therefore, clinicians should be trained to respond appropriately and to be knowledgeable about their community resources to assist these victims effectively.

### JUVENILE DETENTION FACILITIES

Many of the children and adolescent victims of prostitution are first identified in the juvenile justice system. About 60% of prostituted youth have had at least one justice system contact (Seng, 1989). They are often arrested for distribution or possession of an illegal substance, public intoxication, running away, prostitution, burglary, possession of an illegal weapon, aggravated assault, or aggravated robbery. While the detention facility presents an opportunity for mandated treatment, the trust and cooperation of detained children and adolescents are difficult to obtain. They are generally angry and uncooperative with the juvenile detention personnel. Many of the case studies presented in this chapter are based on the experiences of juveniles who were detained for extended periods of time. Their histories of victimization were, in many cases, revealed for the first time during their tenure in a juvenile detention facility.

## INITIAL ASSESSMENT OF VICTIMS

Within a healthcare setting, the clinician's role is to identify medical and psychiatric emergencies and to facilitate referral for a more extensive developmental, behavioral, emotional, and family history assessment. The interview approach should initially be symptom-based, and an immediate referral to the clinical therapist or social worker is recommended for a more comprehensive initial assessment and recommendations for further management.

Prostituted youth who present to mental health clinics generally have severe psychiatric and emotional problems; therefore, initial assessments tend to focus primarily on acute symptoms. Compliance with follow-up appointments and assessment is generally poor. The assessment of high-risk health behavior and emotional status should evolve from the presenting complaint. Substance abuse or intoxication leads to questions about nonconsensual sexual contact when intoxicated, home life, support systems, and how the substances are acquired. Symptoms of STDs lead to questions of sexual partners, protection, human immunodeficiency virus (HIV) risk factors, and unwanted sexual experiences. Sexual or physical victimization should lead to questions about sexual perpetrators, access to weapons, and injury mechanisms.

Every effort should be made to interview the child or adolescent alone because the accompanying adult may be a perpetrator, pimp, or nonsupportive parent. The clinician and therapist should assume nothing and ask everything. If victims begin to make vague statements about their feelings or what happened to them, they should be asked to provide concrete expressions (Crisis Connection, 1994). One 14-year-old prostitution victim incarcerated for attacking her teacher said she disclosed her prostitution simply "because someone [at juvenile detention] asked." Healthcare professionals need to inquire about the number of sexual partners, the genders of their sexual partners, prior STDs or pregnancies, and use of barrier methods. Inquiry into eating and sleeping habits, nightmares, trouble sleeping, and decreased appetite should also be conducted as these symptoms may be a result of PTSD or depression.

### ESTABLISHING COMMUNICATION AND TRUST

Most victims of child prostitution do not present in clinical settings by choice. They have not chosen to go to a juvenile detention facility and may not be in the emergency room to escape their victimization. Their belief that nothing can change the destiny of their current lifestyle perpetuates a lack of desire to change their circumstances. This subsequently leads to feelings of cynicism, alienation, and nonconformity (Gibson-Ainyette et al, 1988). This fatalistic outlook reinforces their destructive criminal behavior against others, their self-injurious coping skills, and their resistance to service providers and intervention.

Homeless prostituted youth are the most challenging clients. Their extreme survival skills do not permit dependence on others or a sense of victimization. Yet, they are still children marked by a childhood of abuse and unmet needs of proper care, love, nurturance, guidance, and protection. Therapists tend to see these children and adolescents as victims and delinquents. In order to provide effective treatment, therapists need to facilitate the victims' disclosures in a healthy manner, validate their experiences, and understand the dynamics of prostitution and sexual abuse.

Unfortunately, by the time children and adolescents are identified as victims of juvenile prostitution, many are "mad as hell" and "not going to take it anymore." They have frequently experienced getting kicked out of their homes, their school, the juvenile justice system, and mainstream society; their belief that the world is against them often leads them to justify obnoxious and violent behavior toward others. Their anger, demands, and manipulations are ineffective defenses against feelings of helplessness, anxiety, shame, and incompetence and are used to regain control (Crisis Connection, 1994).

Child and adolescent victims of prostitution readily recognize fear, disdain, frustration, and lethargy in the medical or mental health provider and they are experts at provoking alarm, frustration, and anger in others. They are cavalier in describing the dangers of their lifestyle and often challenge medical and mental health providers with "shock statements" and obscenities. Service providers must stay calm, observe nonverbal cues, appear confident, withhold their emotions and judgment, and provide assurance that they want to help (Crisis Connection, 1994). During the initial assessment, it is important to build rapport with the client. Steps for doing this are summarized in **Table 19-1** and discussed below.

---

**Table 19-1. Initial Assessment and Rapport-Building Interview**

— Introduce self

— Identify purpose

— Build rapport

— Provide choices for contextual elements of the interview

— Establish rules of confidentiality (exceptions: suicide, homicide, child abuse)

— Obtain information about family history (who they are, where they are, what they are like)

— Ask about school history (attendance, special education classes)

— Inquire about social support system

— Assess self-injurious thoughts and behaviors (suicidal ideation, written contract)

— Ask about physical abuse/sexual abuse/prostitution

— Request information about drug history (assess need for immediate medical attention, what they use, when they began to use, frequency, source, financial support, need for medical testing)

— Inquire about runaway behavior (frequency, reasons)

---

Initial Assessment and Rapport-Building Interview

*Introduce Self, Identify Purpose, and Build Rapport*

The clinician or therapist should state his or her name and purpose: "My name is Mary Smith, and my job is to check on you and make sure you are doing okay while you are here." By attempting to gather nonthreatening information, clinicians begin to build the rapport necessary for establishing a positive relationship and facilitating an atmosphere of respect, trust, and safety. The clinician can use this interaction to assess cognitive and development levels, maturity and social skills, and the child or adolescent's current mental and emotional state.

*Provide Choices for Contextual Elements of the Interview*

The clinician or therapist should give children and adolescents the opportunity to make choices about the contextual elements surrounding their interview if they are resistant to talking or sharing any information. Providing them with choices such as the time of the interview, in which room the interview will take place, or possibly, the preference for a male or female interviewer facilitates cooperation with the interviewer, is respectful, and allows children and adolescents to have some control over their current surroundings.

*Establish Rules of Confidentiality*

Two important responsibilities that clinicians have are to explain to their clients clearly what confidentiality means and to ensure that clients understand the limitations of confidentiality. For example, "Confidentiality means I will not talk to your parents, family, lawyer, probation officer, or anyone else in the facility about what you tell me. If you tell me that you are going to hurt or kill yourself, I have to tell people here so we can watch you and make sure you are okay. If you tell me you are going to kill someone, I have a legal duty to warn that person. If you tell me that you have been physically or sexually abused, I have a legal obligation to report it to the proper authorities." Once clients understand the meaning of confidentiality, the clinician should ask if they know the exceptions to the confidentiality rules.

Children and adolescents who know the exceptions should review them with the clinician to ensure their proper understanding, and the clinician should then inquire about any previous experiences with counseling. A review of previous counseling experiences should include questions of prior hospitalizations, psychiatric diagnoses, and whether or not family members participated. If the children or adolescents do not know the confidentiality exceptions, the clinician should explain them clearly and reinforce that he or she (1) will protect the child from doing harm to himself, herself, or others, (2) is interested in the child's welfare and safety, (3) will be honest about what needs to be reported, and (4) will not hurt or judge the child.

*Obtain Family History*

The clinician should establish with whom the child lives and whether they are relatives or nonrelatives. Information should be obtained about both parents, including how often the child sees his or her parents, his or her last contact with them, and his or her reasons for not seeing or living with them. Inquiries regarding the decision-makers in the family, their communication and patterns of interactions, how affection was displayed, the level of attachment between the child or adolescent and the family, and the family's community involvement lends clues to the degree of alienation between the child and male/female figures.

The stability of the home environment can be determined by establishing how long each adult has resided in the child's or adolescent's home, whether or not siblings have different sets of parents, histories of family domestic violence, incarceration of parents, or unnatural deaths. Clinicians should also explore whether any of the family members suffer from chronic mental or medical illnesses, are cognitively challenged, or abuse drugs or alcohol. The roles and responsibilities of all family members, including siblings and grandparents, may reveal a lack of role boundaries and "parentified" children, socioeconomic status, and enmeshment with criminal behavior.

Questions regarding culture and ethnicity are equally as important when the clinician or therapist assesses how victims' relationships compare to their cultural norms. This line of questioning can also lead to vital information for foreign children who have either been brought to the United States and forced into prostitution or entered the United States on their own and were later recruited (Estes & Weiner, 2002).

*Ask about School History*
The child should indicate the name of his or her school, grade, and participation in any special education classes. Reasons for truancy may include caring for younger siblings at home, selling/distributing drugs, domestic violence, physical abuse, prostitution, or working in order to support the family. Sometimes parents encourage the adolescent to drop out of school so the student will not be fined for absenteeism or get in trouble with the courts. About half of prostituted youth drop out of school (Seng, 1989).

*Inquire about Past and Present Social Support Systems*
Inquiry into the child or adolescent victim's social network system is helpful in assessing additional protective and risk factors in his or her life. Surprisingly, the prostituted youth's current social support system is often extensive. Through the systematic process of blackmailing, isolating, degrading, and dehumanizing these victims, pimps and perpetrators instill in them the notion that they are their "god" and that if they "mess up, there's a price to pay, and they know it's a heavy price" (Hofstede, 1999).

However, by assessing past support systems, clinicians may learn that the victim is actually a part of an increasing number of children and adolescents who had positive support systems but because of low self-esteem or other vulnerabilities were either lured and forced into prostitution or recruited by same-sex peers, boyfriends, family members, or pimps (Hofstede, 1999). Due to their pimps' systematic programming, their own shame, self-blame, hopelessness, fear of rejection, and the violence to which they are continuously subjected, children and teens may be too scared of the punishment their pimps may inflict on them if an attempt to contact their previous support system is discovered.

In other cases, clinicians and therapists may discover that the victim they are assessing was recruited or lured into gangs that operate juvenile prostitution businesses in order to contribute to the gang's economy. Estes & Weiner (2002) suggest that 1 out of 3 to 4 girls who are involved with male-dominated gangs contribute to the gang's economy through prostitution and point out that there is variation in female participation rates between ethnically organized gangs. For example, female prostitution is more common among Native American and African American organized gangs than in Hispanic, Asian, or Caucasian gangs. Additionally, clinicians may find themselves assessing children and teens who do not view themselves as prostitutes but acknowledge that they entered a gang by exchanging sex for shelter and drugs (Hofstede, 1999). Under any circumstance, a thorough review of current and past social network systems will provide direction on how to proceed with safe and appropriate interventions.

*Assess Self-Injurious Thoughts and Behaviors*
Clinicians need to ask children and adolescent victims of prostitution explicitly if they ever have thoughts of hurting themselves or wanting to die. Affirmative answers should be elaborated by establishing whether they have hurt themselves or attempted suicide, the frequency and most recent attempt, and the method they employed. The clinician can inquire about what was going on at the time they tried to harm themselves and what stopped them from doing so. If they have not yet attempted suicide,

ask if they have a plan and the means to do it. Assessing their coping style and capacity and any previous exposure to someone who has either attempted or committed suicide is also important. Clinicians need to talk about suicide openly, provide a supportive and caring environment, encourage them to keep options open, provide resources for support and coping, make appropriate referrals, and develop a short-term plan (Crisis Connection, 1994).

Clinicians can ask children and adolescents who have a history of harming themselves to sign a safety contract that explicitly states, "I agree not to hurt or kill myself." The safety contract should also specify that the child or adolescent agrees to inform someone at the facility if something changes and they are in danger of hurting themselves. Children and adolescents who refuse to sign a safety contract or honor an already existing signed agreement need to be placed under suicide observation or participate in an emergent psychiatric evaluation. If they become angry, the clinician should firmly restate his or her job and obligation to their safety in a caring and supportive manner.

### Ask About Physical Abuse/Sexual Abuse/Prostitution

Children and adolescents tend to appear more comfortable discussing physical abuse than sexual abuse. The clinician can inquire about patterns of discipline by asking questions such as, "What happens when you get into trouble or your parents get mad at you?" or "Are you ever hit or hurt?" Studies indicate that between 17% and 47% of prostituted youth have been physically abused (Earls & David, 1989; Seng, 1989; Yates et al, 1991).

Once victims of juvenile prostitution are brought into the business, they are frequently raped, threatened with weapons, physically abused, and tortured by their pimps, perpetrators, and customers. Some prostituted youth may also report witnessing the abuse and torture of other prostituted youth or the sudden disappearance of someone who worked under her pimp.

The Hofstede Report (1999) states that in an Oregon study, 53% of prostitutes, many of whom began prostituting as juveniles, reported being gagged, bound, burned, or hung or having their body parts mutilated by pinching, clamping, and stapling. According to Hofstede (1999), 60% to 73% of prostituted youth report a history of sexual abuse when they were young. If children or adolescents reveal sexual abuse, the clinician should find out when the last incident occurred, the type of sexual contact, the identity of the perpetrator, the abusers' current access to the victims, and whether or not the abuse was reported.

The clinician should be direct in requesting information about the victims and duration of abuse, while remaining nonjudgmental and mindful of adolescents' perspective of their victimization. If they minimize the abuse as "just touching" or "only molestation," the clinician may decide to reinforce the seriousness of the crime by referring to the incident(s) as "abuse" or "rape" but needs to remain cognizant that the victims' initial minimization may be a way to cope with the experience.

When juveniles report a history of prostitution, a detailed history should be taken that includes the following:

— How they got involved

— The length of time they have been involved

— How many people they have been with sexually and the genders of those people

— The types of sexual activity that they have engaged in

— If protection was used

— Any current or previous physical injuries

— STDs

— Pregnancies

— Abortions or miscarriages

— Any children and where they are

— If they obtained physical injuries or experienced torture

— Prior attempts to escape from their pimps

— Whom they have worked for

— Where they are from

— Where they are currently staying

— Any current fears for their safety

Not surprisingly, male victims of sexual abuse are often embarrassed and reticent to talk about their victimization; disclosure becomes even more difficult when the perpetrator was male. Often, their sexual abuse goes unreported or their sexual abuse experience is heard for the first time after a male child or adolescent victim is charged with sexually abusing another child. Educating prostituted youth about the relationship between child abuse and present maladaptive behaviors can also help enhance the clinician-client bond because many children and adolescent victims are surprised to discover a correlation.

*Request Information About Drug History*
Nearly half of prostituted youth are substance abusers (Seng, 1989). Drugs are readily provided to prostituted youth by members of organized crime units in order to increase their dependency on them (Estes & Weiner, 2002), and juveniles often use drugs to "self-medicate" in order to avoid or attenuate their pain. Juveniles are more willing to disclose information about their use of drugs if rapport is established, the limits of confidentiality are defined, and they do not fear that these activities will be reported. Histories of drug use should include the kinds of drugs used, when drug use started, frequency of use, and mechanism of use (eg, intravenous, inhaled). The clinician should establish when they last took drugs and what kind they ingested in order to assess the possibility of withdrawal and side effects so that appropriate interventions may be provided.

While questions about drug sources and financial support may reveal prostitution, children and adolescents are generally reluctant to provide such information because they are ashamed and embarrassed. Sometimes, however, they may be more willing to write down this information. Clinicians should also be ready to educate juveniles about health risks (HIV and hepatitis) associated with intravenous drug usage, assess the need of testing for infections, and make appropriate referrals.

Since many juveniles are arrested for drug-related crimes, their probation officers are aware of the problem, and drug counseling will be a condition of their release. If juveniles are arrested for other crimes, the clinician may ask permission to share information regarding their drug use with their probation officer. They may then be able to enter treatment voluntarily to obtain or maintain their freedom.

*Inquire About Runaway Behavior*
If clients have a history of running away, the clinician should establish when they first ran away, how often, and whether they are running away from something/someone or running to something/someone. Some reasons juveniles run away from home are to escape from sexual, physical, or emotional abuse in their home; parental domestic

violence; parental drug and alcohol abuse; their own drug addictions; and to be with friends. In one report, runaway or homeless youth comprised approximately 75% of all prostituted youth (Cohen, 1987). The longer runaway children or adolescents are out on the street, the more susceptible they become to hunger, malnutrition, illness, and violence. These experiences compounded with their lack of education, immaturity, drug use, and will to survive are the contributing factors that pave the way for runaways to succumb to the violent world of prostitution (Estes & Weiner, 2002).

During treatment, child and adolescent victims are sometimes encouraged to express their thoughts and feelings through writing and drawing. In **Case Study 19-1**, Richard*, an adolescent boy incarcerated in juvenile and adult jail facilities for violent crimes and murder, writes and draws about his experiences to his therapist. (See **Figures 19-1** through **19-6** for Richard's drawings.) Although Richard does not admit to pimping or prostituting, his childhood background and subsequent lifestyle embodies the loss, despair, and hatred that victims of child abuse experience.

**Case Study 19-1**

"Well ... now is as good a time as any to tell you a little about my childhood. You said that you know very little about my dad and nothing about my mother; let's see if you can figure out why.

I don't remember much from before 7. Mostly bad memories. I remember drug houses, beatings and violence, being on the run from state to state with my mom, being with my dad sometimes. My dad going to jail. Spending dreaded stints with abusive babysitters, being molested by my grandpa. All kinds of fucked-up crap. Then at 7, I remember my dad always beating my mom, then fighting literally. The cops. My dad almost killed my mom one time. He pulled out his shotgun and jammed it in her stomach; I seen his hand move back the trigger, and I just started screaming. I knew what I was about to see. That day she decided to leave. She came back for some stuff once, and Dad hit her in the head with a wrench. Split open. Then I went to live with her for a day under a bridge in a tent before I went back home. It sucked. I tried to catch us a fish to eat. I went back with my Mexican family. Then when I was at my uncle's house, my mom came to say goodbye. She came and my uncle beat her up, but she refused to leave till she seen us. Me and sis. When I seen her she had blood running down the back of her neck, and she asked if I wanted to go with mommy. Like a shitty-ass ungrateful bastard I said, No. So she walked off down the long sidewalk with nowhere to go and nothing but the clothes on her back. When I seen that she wasn't coming back, I tried to run after her, yelling till I ran out of breath, but she didn't hear me. So I sat there and cried.

After Mom left (I went back to Dad), my dad started hitting on me for everything. Also showing me the street life. I've worked since I was 8 in some form or fashion. We were always living in flea-infested project-type apartments. Life sucked after that. I was the black sheep in the family. Not even invited to birthday parties. At Christmas time, I never got many presents; got a special present one time, an SKS 7.62-mm Russian assault rifle. I accidentally killed someone with that.

At 14, I went to live with my mom for 2 months before she kicked me out for various reasons. I guess she wasn't used to having a teenager. Me and my dad hated each other. Whippins turned into fights. I lost them all. I started fucking up in school; I went from being gifted to being expelled. Eventually the courts sent me to a hospital to see if I was crazy. I was starting to hear and see things. Scary things. I took off from the hospital. I was going to find a field off in the middle of nowhere, where they have a lot of nice green grass and pretty trees around. And I was going to meet my Maker with an SKS 7.62-mm Russian assault rifle.

Instead I awaken every day in a web like hell with dreams that will stay unfulfilled, memories that haunt. And I can never seem to find God's face."

"Awaken in a web like hell

How did I reach this place

Why are they haunting me

I can't look at God's face" (Slayer, "Divine Intervention")

Richard was incarcerated by age 14 and sent to the adult prison system when he was 15. His writings and drawings capture the longing for normal childhood experiences (eg, birthday

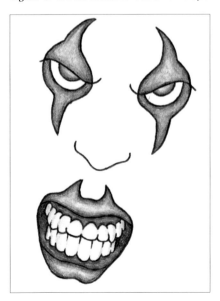

***Figure 19-1.*** *Blue demonic face on envelope.*

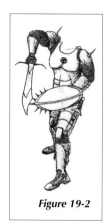

Figure 19-2

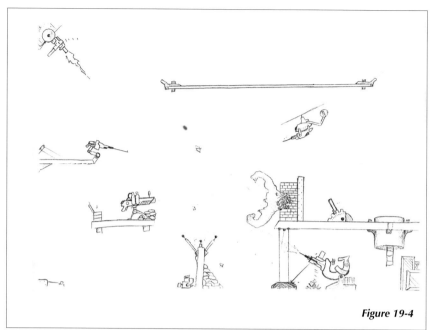

Figure 19-4

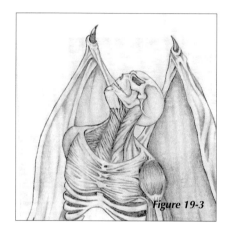

Figure 19-3

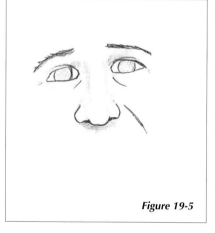

Figure 19-5

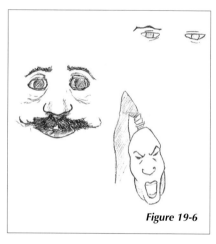

Figure 19-6

**Figure 19-2.** *Early drawing by Richard prior to incarceration: "I could not think of anything to finish this picture."*

**Figure 19-3.** *Later drawing by Richard after going to prison: "I was not thinking of anything in particular when I drew this."*

**Figure 19-4.** *Drawing demonstrating his fascination and obsession with weapons of destruction.*

**Figure 19-5.** *Drawing depicting desperation and silence.*

**Figure 19-6.** *Faces and masks.*

parties, Christmas), a parent, love, protection, nurturance, and stability. As he runs from family member to family member and from place to place, he is rejected or driven away. He does not find a safe harbor and begins to reject his parents, school, and the world while he literally arms himself with destructive weapons and manners of coping. His drawings reflect the cynicism, violence, and incompleteness of his life.

## PSYCHIATRIC ASSESSMENT

Violent, combative behavior directed against others or themselves is commonly encountered in child and adolescent victims of prostitution. Depression and suicidal ideation and behavior are particularly common among young prostitute victims (Gibson-Ainyette et al, 1988; Seng, 1989; Yates et al, 1991). During the course of assessment or therapy, some victims may become suicidal, as shown by **Case Study 19-2.**

### Case Study 19-2

Fifteen-year-old Billy entered therapy when he was incarcerated for possession and distribution of heroin and assaulting a prostitute. He was third-generation Mexican mafia. His first childhood memory was when he was 4 years old. His 2 older brothers took him for a ride. They forced another man into the car and drove to an isolated area. One brother stayed in the car with Billy while the other brother and the stranger got out. The brother in the car told Billy, "Today you are going to begin to learn about the business." The first rule was that "no matter what happens," Billy could not cry. The other brother forced the stranger to his knees, told him to put his hands behind his back, and shot him in the head. Billy began to cry. His brother punched him in the face and said, "Shut up, you little shit." He continued to punch Billy until he stopped crying.

When Billy was 11 years old, his family placed him in charge of 10 boys who were responsible for selling and distributing heroin and collecting the profits. When Billy turned 13, he acquired a new responsibility: pimping heroin-addicted prostitutes. Billy told his therapist, "This was a very big responsibility." His mother approved of these activities, and her sons were proud that they could support her so she would not have to work. Billy's last memory of having fun was when he was 12 and went to visit his father, who was not in the mafia. He recalled swimming, "playing around," and "not having to pack a gun." When Billy and his oldest brother were in detention, their sister wrote letters to them scolding them for "getting locked up" and "putting Mami (Mother) through all this." She also indicated that she would carry on the drug runs and manage the prostitution business ("take over what you got going until you get out again.")

Billy was released after one week in juvenile detention. He killed himself 2 weeks later.

The most obvious diagnostic presentations are substance-related disorders, dissociative disorders, impulse control, and antisocial personality traits, and most or all of the AXIS IV psychosocial and environment problems in the *Diagnostic and Statistical Manual of Mental Disorders*, 4th edition (DSM-IV). Emergent restraint and sedation may be required for combative clients. Immediate referral to a psychiatrist is required for clients who are homicidal or suicidal. Some develop psychoses (see **Case Study 19-1**) and require an immediate psychiatric assessment. Clinicians who are calm, appear unrushed, and are caring will be more successful at gathering the information that is needed to make an appropriate assessment for intervention (Crisis Connection, 1994).

Unless they are seen in the hospital emergency room for a suicide attempt, the less obvious and most prevalent AXIS I mood disorders such as major depressive disorder and PTSD are often missed in the initial interview. Some of the symptoms that these child and adolescent victims may exhibit include hypervigilance, difficulty concentrating, an exaggerated startle response, rage, and dissociation. Other symptoms they may describe include denial, difficulty concentrating, autonomic arousal, insomnia, nightmares, psychic numbing, and recurrent and intrusive memories of abuse. They may frequently use alcohol or drugs to self-medicate to avoid or numb their feelings and thoughts of the traumatic events. As a result, clinicians tend to overlook PTSD, and victims' drug abuse becomes the diagnostic focus (American Psychiatric Association [APA], 1994).

By the time these children and adolescents are identified as victims, they are masterful in their survival skills, and it may take months or years of therapy for them to disclose or recall the traumatic events in their lives; they do not view things with the same horror as outsiders (such as therapists) do. Illegal substances are effective numbing agents, and the most common response to the question, "Why do you do drugs?" is "To forget the pain."

One of the primary difficulties with incarceration at juvenile detention facilities is the compulsory drug withdrawal and detoxification. Incarceration may be the first time that these children or adolescents have been drug-free and sober, and the "pain" in their lives begins to seep into what they thought were impenetrable walls. This makes detention and secured placements a perfect opportunity for effective therapeutic intervention. Addressing the trauma, decreasing anxiety, and treating depression should be the first stage of treatment. If these problems are identified, acknowledged as significant in their lives, and properly treated, the substance-related disorders can be addressed more effectively with better long-term results.

Obsessive-compulsive behaviors are also commonly missed in these children. This diagnosis can be overlooked if the clinician spends only short amounts of time with the child and if family members are not interviewed. For example, other family members may provide details that would not normally be revealed in individual coun-

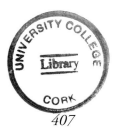

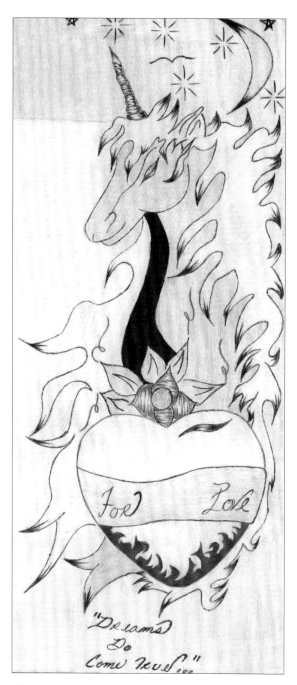

*Figure 19-7. Drawing on letter to Rhonda from the older man serving jail time for sexual assault of Rhonda. The enclosed letter was used to press charges against the defendent.*

seling. Obsessive-compulsive behavior represents extraordinary effort to control insignificant but specific events in their lives in a futile effort to counter the over-whelming barrage of destructive and demoralizing events that characterize their lives.

## DEVELOPMENTAL, BEHAVIORAL, AND EMOTIONAL ASSESSMENT

A significant proportion of adolescents and children victimized by long-term sexual abuse, physical abuse, neglect, prostitution, or pornography have physical, cognitive, emotional, and social delays. These delays may be related to a premature birth, maternal substance abuse (such as fetal alcohol syndrome), or other maternal habits harmful to the fetus. Cognitive deficits and learning disabilities may reflect either exposure to drugs while in utero or chronic substance abuse (especially of inhalants) during childhood or adolescent years. The most common conditions are attention-deficit/hyperactivity disorder (ADHD) and conduct disorder.

ADHD is "a persistent pattern of inattention and/or hyperactivity-impulsivity that is more frequent and severe than is typically observed in individuals at a comparable level of development" (APA, 1994). Common symptoms of ADHD are an inability to concentrate, distractibility, avoidance, and hyperactivity. Clinicians who evaluate children and adolescents need to be aware that there are similarities between symptoms of ADHD and PTSD. During the evaluation, clinicians need to explore the possibilities of any previous traumas, as well as the onset and duration of symptoms. This will help prevent the possibility of victims being misdiagnosed and treated for ADHD when they are actually suffering from PTSD.

Conduct disorder is a "persistent pattern of behaviors in which the basic rights of others or major age-appropriate societal norms or rules are violated" (APA, 1994). Major categories for this disorder are "aggression to people and animals, destruction of property, deceitfulness or theft and serious violations of rules" (APA, 1994). These conditions often reflect a chaotic home environment and contribute to school difficulties during preadolescence and school truancy and dropping out during adolescence. These disorders may be exacerbated when the child is in a closed or secured facility, and many are placed in isolation. Knowledge about developmental or mental health conditions may help the service provider assess the language and cognitive skills of the child and adolescent and structure interview questions and therapy plans accordingly.

Some victims may claim no behavioral or emotional problems. In some cases, this may reflect the extent of acceptance and accommodation to the victimization. For other victims, the nonchalant demeanor and denial of problems serve as a deterrent to therapists and a barrier to potential friends. **Case Study 19-3** illustrates these points.

### Case Study 19-3

Rhonda was sent to juvenile detention for possession of marijuana. She was a beautiful 14-year-old child with the sophistication and mannerisms of a 30-year-old. She admitted to feeling "silly ... being in here with all these kids." Rhonda had extremely violent outbursts during which she would attack staff members, other children, and herself. She spent most of the time in juvenile detention in security and under suicide observation.

Rhonda's mother introduced her to a 34-year-old man (**Figure 19-7**) when Rhonda was 12. The mother "allowed" Rhonda to date him and "stay with him" whenever she wanted. Rhonda knew that this man gave her mother money "whenever she needed it" and began to resent this over time. When Rhonda met a boy her own age that she liked and wanted to date, Rhonda's mother became furious and demanded that Rhonda remain faithful to the older man. This was when Rhonda began to drink a lot and use drugs. She used whatever drugs were available as often as she could. She said, "I know my mom is using me to get money."

# INTERMEDIATE AND LONG-TERM COMMUNITY AND MENTAL HEALTH SUPPORT OF VICTIMS

## CLINICAL TREATMENT SITES

The success of ongoing intervention and treatment depends on (1) the willingness of the victim to undergo therapy, (2) the support of a parent or custodial agency, and (3) the availability of shelters and resources, educational opportunities, and effective therapeutic programs in clinical and neighborhood settings. While victims of prostitution may disclose their victimization and engage in therapy with the support of their legal guardian, homeless prostituted adolescents are less likely to engage in therapy unless they are placed in prisons or lock-up treatment facilities where therapeutic treatment is mandatory.

Community and school clinics are more accessible to street youth, but long-term use of these facilities is rare. According to Hofstede (1999), the "single most determinative factor" that caused children and adolescents to turn to prostitution was being homeless for more than 30 days. Yet, interestingly, some youth may even be denied access to shelter services if they do not have a driver's license or other identification (Unger et al, 1998). Shelter is even more of a problem for lesbian, gay, bisexual, and transgender youth because they are frequently subjected to abuse from the other homeless children and adolescents staying there (Hofstede, 1999).

Community and school interventions need to focus on accessibility, safe harbor, constructive survival skills, and the provision of basic resources and child care, as well as medical, legal, and therapeutic services. For homeless youth, immediate needs for food and shelter, education regarding the dangers of substance use, gangs, HIV-risk behaviors, and assistance with the transition from street life to a stable living and work environment are top priorities (Unger et al, 1998; Yates et al, 1991).

Since service providers are mandated reporters, they must report allegations of child abuse to law enforcement and/or CPS. Even so, public social service agencies may tend to "look the other way" and not report such cases (Yates et al, 1991). While homeless youth are generally resentful and resistant to intervention by governmental agencies, secure placement may eventually facilitate intermediate and long-term change.

Another role for community programs serving prostituted youth is routine and systematic assessment of the relationship between neighborhood opportunities and recruitment into prostitution (Longres, 1991). Such programs may incorporate (1) self-help and social support networks between concerned or threatened families and youth, (2) community education regarding prostitution, recruitment into prostitution, pornography, and gang involvement, (3) community watches and efforts to remove prostitution from identified residential areas, and (4) enhancement of regional legitimate economic opportunities for adults and youths engaged in prostitution (Longres, 1991). Supportive parents of adjudicated youths may be valuable resources for such programs, and community- and school-based prevention and intervention programs may be the most effective in identifying the youth at risk for prostitution (Rickel & Hendren, 1992).

Younger victims of prostitution are more likely to live at home, are usually introduced into prostitution by a relative, and occasionally disclose their involvement in prostitution to another family member or friend (Inciardi, 1984). Younger victims may also present in clinical settings after their abuse is accidentally discovered or the child begins to exhibit symptoms of STDs, sexual assault injuries, or physical assault injuries. Young victims of prostitution may benefit most from therapy with specialized sexual abuse therapists because they may deny emotional and physical trauma (Inciardi, 1984) and are often desensitized and conditioned to respond as sexual objects (Lanning & Burgess, 1989).

**Case Study 19-4**

Laura was 9 years old when her 12-year-old friend, Nina, invited her over to play. When Nina's step-father began taking pornographic photos of Nina, he invited Laura to watch, then participate. The abuse was reported when an anonymous caller turned in one of the pornographic pictures of Nina and Laura.

Nina and Laura came to the sexual abuse clinic together. They wanted to be present for each other's examination. They giggled and hugged each other frequently. Laura's interview took place in a room with a one-way mirror. As she spoke of the pictures Nina's stepfather took, she slung her legs sideways over the arm of the chair, studied her reflection in the mirror of the interview room, and began to lift her shirt seductively. She smiled and giggled throughout the interview even when discussing her dreams of "Dad killing Mom," "me drowning in the water," and "the guy that raped me" (Nina's stepfather). She said she was sad and wanted the perpetrator killed, yet when asked how the abuse had made her feelings or body different, Laura said, "Nothing's different."

Laura was placed in her maternal grandmother's custody because her mother was in jail for drugs. The grandmother reported that Laura's mother used to have sex in front of the children, and a neighborhood policeman reported rumors of Laura's mother selling Laura and her sister for drugs or money.

Laura presented a therapeutic challenge because she had integrated her sexualized existence with her daily life. She does not yet comprehend the serious medical risks and consequences of her victimization. She has lived in an environment where sexual activity was public and normalized and has never been taught the appropriate boundaries of behavior. A therapeutic approach for this child must contrast the trauma of the abuse with the apparent lack of response by Laura to reveal her defense mechanisms and underlying lack of self-respect. Another therapeutic goal would be to show Laura that she is a victim of sexual abuse rather than a sexual person. Fortunately, Laura's grandmother is supportive and committed to helping Laura and her sister, so compliance with long-term therapy is likely.

## GOALS OF LONG-TERM THERAPY

The goals of long-term therapy vary with the victim's age, internal attributes, external supports, their victimization experiences, and level of trauma. General goals are to (1) reduce high-risk health behaviors, (2) enhance decision-making skills, (3) address gender and other identity issues, (4) establish a positive support system, (5) instill a sense of hope and positive outlook toward their future, and (6) identify a permanent safe harbor.

The most effective long-term therapy may begin with a 9- to 12-month stay in a secured environment. This ensures safety and cessation of substance abuse, runaway behavior, and prostitution while addressing issues that led to their deleterious lifestyles. Good physical health and emotional stability provide the foundation for therapeutic intervention, and juveniles who are provided with necessary medical treatment, psychiatric care, prescribed medications, exercise, relaxation skills, and proper monitoring begin to feel better physically and become motivated to maintain this new, healthier self.

Individual and group counseling should be used. A weekly individual session allows children and adolescents an opportunity to establish a trusting relationship with a responsible adult. The therapist models appropriate adult/child (parent/child) boundaries, and the children or adolescents are given an opportunity to address difficult issues in a safe environment. The children or adolescents should have some input into the development of their treatment plan, and the therapist should incorporate strategies to help them learn skills to decrease anxiety, experience small successes, detach from unhealthy relationships, and obtain ideas, suggestions, and opportunities to establish a new or different healthy support network. During individual treatment sessions, the therapist may facilitate cognitive restructuring, correct unhealthy cognitive distortions, provide clarification for issues that are confusing, employ relaxation techniques, and develop healthy relationships with the children or adolescents.

Once a treatment plan is written, it becomes an effective tool for measuring progress and can aid in the therapist's ability to recognize successes and patterns of self-defeating thoughts and behaviors. The therapist can review the plan and reinforce positive attitudes and behavior and also address thinking errors, poor judgment, rationalizations, or unhealthy avoidant behavior. Allowing children or adolescents to be a part of the evaluation process allows the therapist to assess their current thinking and feelings and gives the therapist an opportunity for further insight. By reviewing the goals and objectives and measuring progress or regression, appropriate adjustments or changes to the treatment plan can be made.

Individual therapy can also be used to gather pertinent family information and specific topics that can be explored in later group sessions. Group therapy provides vital peer feedback for inappropriate behaviors and juveniles are often more receptive to peers when they are confronted about destructive behaviors, poor decisions, and life threatening behaviors. Common themes that emerge from group sessions include substance abuse, lack of trust, promiscuous sexual behavior, family violence, anti-social behaviors, and poor problem-solving skills. The therapist's role is to guide and monitor the topics while maintaining clear boundaries and a safe environment. Despite individual differences and unique situations, family dynamics and world-views are generally similar for most adolescents. These commonalities facilitate the acceptance and participation in the group support system. Long-term group therapy provides a temporary support system and promotes the development of self-esteem and self-reliance necessary to reenter society and establish healthy, more permanent support systems.

If placement back in the home is possible, family therapy should begin about 3 months before reunification. All family members residing in the home should be encouraged to participate. The primary caregiver should be encouraged and positively reinforced for attending weekly family sessions. Juveniles and family members should not be punished if the father, stepfather, or another member will not attend the sessions. When family members do not attend sessions, the therapist may help the children or adolescents understand and cope with nonsupportive family members.

Long-term goals for children and adolescents who should not or can not return to their dysfunctional family systems should include enrollment in a general equivalency diploma (GED) program and job training. Obtaining financial, educational, and emotional independence is critical to individual positive outcomes. Having the proper tools, self-confidence, and ego strength to live independently and have hope for a positive future is the ultimate goal. Encouraging, nurturing, and providing educational opportunities are often new experiences for these adolescents and can play a vital part in their healing. Acquiring their GED and maintaining a full- or part-time job is crucial for building their self-esteem, separating from their previous life, and developing their own sense of self.

Once juveniles are placed back in the foster home, with a relative, or with an alternative caregiver, therapeutic follow-up care should be provided 2 to 4 times a month for 6 months. If they have a crisis or desire more frequent contact, services should be provided. Additionally, juveniles should be provided with legal and therapeutic support if they will be called to testify in any legal proceedings against their abusers or pimps.

During the period of reunification or alternative placement, juveniles may reassociate with their previous peer group and begin repeating problematic behaviors.

**Case Study 19-5**

Manuel requested counseling 3 months after he had been reunified with his mother. He had successfully completed an 11-month placement before reunification. He obtained his GED and worked full-time at McDonald's. Manuel then began to "hang out" with his old friends again and smoked marijuana one day. He and his mother became alarmed. They contacted the counselor and underwent 4 family sessions. The counselor discovered that Manuel stopped receiving antidepressants after leaving placement. He had asked his mother to make an appointment with a physician, but his mother wanted him to cope with his depression without medication. After Manuel acquiesced and smoked marijuana with his friend, he recognized his desire to self-medicate with illicit substances because the antidepressants were not available to him. The counselor explored Manuel's mother's reluctance to renew the medication while reinforcing her concern and compliance with counseling. The counselor reinforced Manuel's insight and recognition that he was tempted to get involved with criminal activities again. Manuel's mother realized his need for medication and agreed to take Manuel to the doctor. Manuel stopped using marijuana and, 1 year later, successfully completed boot camp and joined the army.

## Special Issues for Boys

According to Estes & Weiner (2002), more boys report in engaging in prostitution for pleasure and money than girls, many of them think of themselves as "hustlers" instead of prostitutes, and about 25% to 35% of boys identify themselves as either gay, bisexual, or transgender/transsexual. Conflicts regarding gender identity are common among male prostitutes (Boyer, 1989; Savin-Williams, 1994), and as many as 83% have had at least one negative sexual experience before becoming prostitutes (Boyer, 1989). Among males, homosexual prostitutes are twice as likely as heterosexual prostitutes to be a victim of rape (42% vs 21%) (Boyer, 1989). As victims, they confront the trauma of male-male rape and the skepticism of law enforcement authorities if the crime is reported. Because of the stigma associated with homosexuality, they rarely report the abuse (Boyer, 1989) and at times will begin to identify with their aggressors by becoming pimps themselves. Family members may further alienate victims and throw them out of the house because of sexual orientation (Savin-Williams, 1994). Little data are available regarding lesbian adolescents and prostitution (Savin-Williams, 1994).

Robert (**Case Study 19-6**) was concerned about being homosexual. By discussing his childhood sexual abuse and prostitution, the basis for his gender identity concerns was revealed.

**Case Study 19-6**

Robert, 14 years old, was arrested for aggravated assault with a deadly weapon. He abused alcohol and drugs and was extremely violent. Robert spent most of his time in security and had assaulted almost every male staff member in the juvenile detention facility before being transferred to another secured facility.

Robert did not know who his father was, and his mother never visited him during his 3-month stay at the juvenile detention facility. The night before being transferred, Robert commented that he planned to stop smoking marijuana. When the therapist asked why he had made this decision, Robert said, "When I'm high, I get paranoid, and I start thinking that all my friends think I'm a fag." This was a surprising comment considering that Robert was a masculine-appearing adolescent who was proud of being "macho" and one who "loves girls." The counselor then asked about sexual abuse.

Robert put his head in his hands and began to sob uncontrollably. When he was 5 years old, Robert became a "latchkey kid." He had an older brother who came home from school at a different time than Robert. Instead, a 19-year-old male in the neighborhood would come to his house and "make me do things to him." Two years later, Robert learned that the 19-year-old had paid Robert's brother for these sexual favors. It was this abuse that made Robert question his sexual orientation.

## Providing a Safe Environment

Identifying a permanent safe harbor for prostituted youth is problematic because family members are often perpetrators or are unable to support and protect their children. Placement in a shelter or foster home may be necessary, with longer-term options to include adoption or reunification with family members. Identifying a safe harbor for street youth is extremely challenging and dependent entirely on their willingness to cooperate.

**Case Study 19-7**

Brenda began running away from home at age 12. From ages 12 to 14, she danced at a local bar that allowed young girls to dance and leave with patrons (**Figure 19-8**). During that period, Brenda lived with several older men, using whatever drugs or alcohol they had available. Brenda had tattoos all over her body. She entered the mental health system when she was incarcerated for runaway behavior and prostitution. She was placed in a secured facility for almost 2 years and received extensive therapy during that time. Brenda was then placed back home.

Brenda's mother was "supportive" in that she wanted Brenda to live at home, but she had poor parenting skills. Having given birth to all of her daughters during her teenage years, Brenda's mother was young and more interested in being her daughter's friend than her mother. She constantly compared her physical appearance and attractiveness to that of her daughters. Brenda admitted that she had no respect for her mother.

### SPECIFIC THERAPEUTIC APPROACHES

#### Visual Cues

Children and adolescents are concrete thinkers, and many are visually oriented. While interviewing or counseling them, the therapist may provide concrete cues to demonstrate abstract concepts. For example, when working with juvenile sexual offenders, to introduce the concept that they spent an earlier part of their life as a victim and then later as a perpetrator, the clinician may spread their arms apart using one to represent the victim and the other to represent the perpetrator. Move both arms simultaneously to the middle and place hands together to demonstrate how the 2 experiences have intersected. Then show how the victim and perpetrator can be separated and resolved. Say, "I am not a victim." (Move one arm out.) "I do not allow anyone to hurt me. And I am not a perpetrator." (Move the other arm out.) "I do not hurt others." While moving both arms to the center again say, "Now I am right here. I am something else." Then ask, "Do you think it is possible for you to be something other than a victim or a perpetrator?" Children and adolescents tend to retain and understand these concepts better when visual clues are provided. For these reasons, genograms, maps, timelines, and written contracts are effective tools.

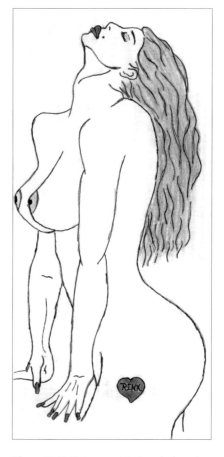

***Figure 19-8.*** *Picture sent to Brenda from her 18-year-old lover*

Visual demonstrations are also effective while addressing issues concerning victims' parents. Children can become defensive about their parents even when they are abusive, neglectful, and delinquent. It is important to differentiate mothers or fathers as individuals from their parenting skills. While extending one arm out, say, "Your mom and dad are always going to be your mom and dad, and you love them." Then extend the other arm and say, "But they don't have good parenting skills." For example: "You love your father and want the best for him." (Show left hand.) "But," (show right hand) "a good parent does not have sex with his daughter and does not sell his daughter to his friends." Using the term "parent" or "parenting skills" is preferable to "your mother" or "father" when pointing out weaknesses and prevents children from becoming defensive. Acknowledging bad parenting rather than labeling someone a bad mother or father allows clients to express anger, disappointment, or sadness without feeling disloyal or disrespectful to their mothers or fathers.

Hand visuals are also effective when discussing boundaries and the ***parentified child*** (ie, children who take on the role of caregiver). Place one hand about 12 inches above the other and say, "In a family, there are adults," (show higher hand) "and there are children" (show lower hand). "No matter how many responsibilities you have, you are still a child." Indicate that siblings also recognize that they are all "underneath" the adults. Clients may have been given the responsibilities of an adult but without the power or authority. Parentified children are often surprised to learn that counselors recognize this frustration. As it becomes apparent why their role as an adult parent has not been successful, they experience a degree of relief.

Providing the children with a small object or symbol of their progress can provide strength and guidance when they face challenges at home or in the streets. For example, after 6 weeks of group therapy for sexual abuse, participants were awarded a small plastic purple heart. This served as a reminder that they were wounded but that they were also survivors. It was awarded to them for the bravery it took to come forward and talk about their abuse and their determination to be survivors rather than victims.

### Family History and Family Genograms

When gathering information about the families of prostituted youth, several commonalities emerge. Parents of these children are likely to abuse drugs or alcohol, neglect or inappropriately supervise their children, physically abuse or assault the adults and children in their homes, and perpetuate an existence where violence is normalized in the home. Parents are likely to have been teen mothers or fathers, have no healthy family support system, and live in poverty. Mothers are often battered women, and the fathers of the children and paramours of the mother are often indiscriminate sexual offenders of women and children. One or both parents are likely to have spent time in prison, and children assume responsibility for their own care and safety early in life, often becoming parentified providers for their siblings. They often run away, leave, or get kicked out of their homes during adolescence.

Gathering information about family members in the form of a genogram can be an effective method of uncovering past childhood trauma. Victims may more effectively relate the perpetrators and abusive acts while directing their attention to the genogram rather than to their memories.

The family genogram should be obtained in the third or fourth session. This non-threatening approach of gathering information about the family reveals family patterns and behaviors. The therapist may begin the session by asking children if they would like to create a "family tree." Most people are familiar with this term and are interested in the idea.

The therapist should define "genogram" and write it at the top of the page. Begin by asking the names of the mother and father. Males are squares and females are circles. Place the father on the left side of the paper and the mother on the right. Always begin with the natural parents and fill in the stepparents and boy/girlfriends later. Use discontinuous lines to indicate nonmarital relationships and double lines crossing a solid line to indicate a divorce. A single line crossing a solid or discontinuous line indicates separation. To the extent possible, establish when relationships started and ended.

If the juveniles are female adolescents, ask if they have ever been pregnant. If so, find out about the baby's father. Ask what decision was made for going through with the pregnancy and what arrangements were made if the baby was born. At this point, adolescents may express grief that someone made them do something against their will or that they had a miscarriage or lost custody of their babies. Often, the fathers of such babies are also the pimps of the adolescents and use the babies to force the adolescents to continue working for them.

Next ask about siblings, including names and ages. Ask whether they are in school and what grade(s) they are in. If older siblings reside outside the home, ask if they have any children. Inquire about their maternal and paternal grandparents; begin with the maternal side if they reside with their mothers.

Finally, add maternal and paternal aunts and uncles to the genogram. The goal is to diagram 3 generations of family members. If children indicate that a family member is deceased, ask when and how this person died.

When diagramming the genogram, children may spontaneously begin to share details about their family and childhood. As children point and comment on the genogram, the therapist should write in their description of each family member. By placing people and problems on paper, clients begin to distance themselves from actual family experiences.

After names, ages, and relationships are established, more specific information regarding family support, behaviors, and dysfunction can be explored. Do the mother and father work, and what is their vocation? If they do not work, where do they get the money to pay the bills? Does anyone else support them? Does anyone in the family have significant health or psychiatric problems? Are any members of the family low-functioning? Is there any history of domestic violence or sexual abuse within the family?

If the client has been arrested for drugs or prostitution, list the drugs used. Ask what illegal substances other people on the genogram have used and write the name of each drug beside the user's name. Point to the genogram and ask if anyone has been to jail or prison. Looking at and pointing to the genogram keeps this interaction from becoming a personal attack on parents, siblings, grandparents, or other family members. Children generally present this information in a nonemotional, matter-of-fact manner. They are also eager to give accurate and detailed information.

When children are incarcerated for prostitution or sex-related crimes, begin with their history. What were the circumstances surrounding their initial involvement? How old were they when they started? Does anyone else in their family prostitute or participate in their involvement? Do they have a pimp? How many pimps have they had? What is their current relationship with their pimp or perpetrator? How did the pimp or perpetrator punish them or keep them under his control? Did anyone ever take any pictures or videotape them? Have they had to provide sexual services in other states and/or countries, and do they have any current fears for safety? Follow up with questions related to previous child sexual abuse, pornography, and exposure to adult sexual activity.

For children incarcerated for violent crimes, ask if anyone else in the family has a bad temper and if that person's temper ever got him or her into trouble.

If the children have no contact with their mother or father, ask what information they know or have heard about their parents and how they feel about not seeing them. Write all of this information on the genogram. If the children ask you to remove something, comply with their request.

When the genogram appears complete, ask children if anything is missing. Ask them if they notice any patterns in the family, and explain how behaviors and addictions are learned and handed down from one generation to the next. This is often new information and introduces the idea that the child is not inherently bad. The therapist should continue to focus on the overall genogram and patterns of behavior and not on specific people in the genogram. After asking about any other thoughts about the genogram, conclude the session.

The overall goal of this session should be to present information about the family, support systems, protective and risk factors, and behaviors in such a way that children can think about them in a less stressful or emotional way.

For some children, nightmares or dreams about family life resurface. Others may have visits from family members and begin to think differently about them. Children may also wish to discuss conversations they have had with others about their genograms. The genogram provides a framework built by the children and also a direction for therapy. **Case Studies 19-8** and **19-9** demonstrate this technique.

**Case Study 19-8**

Sara was first detained for possession of illegal substances at the juvenile facility when she was 13 years old. She was intelligent and articulate, but her speech was slow and sometimes slurred. She remained guarded and spoke nothing of her childhood until she was incarcer-

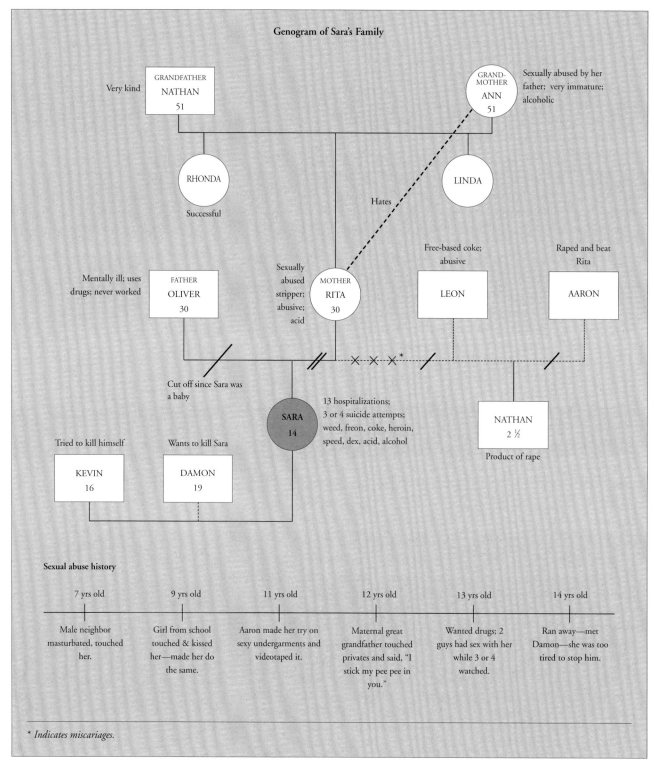

**Genogram of Sara's Family**

GRANDFATHER
NATHAN
51 — Very kind

GRAND-MOTHER
ANN
51 — Sexually abused by her father; very immature; alcoholic

RHONDA
Successful

LINDA

Hates

FATHER
OLIVER
30 — Mentally ill; uses drugs; never worked

MOTHER
RITA
30 — Sexually abused stripper; abusive; acid

LEON — Free-based coke; abusive

AARON — Raped and beat Rita

Cut off since Sara was a baby

SARA
14 — 13 hospitalizations; 3 or 4 suicide attempts; weed, freon, coke, heroin, speed, dex, acid, alcohol

NATHAN
2 ½ — Product of rape

KEVIN
16 — Tried to kill himself

DAMON
19 — Wants to kill Sara

**Sexual abuse history**

| 7 yrs old | 9 yrs old | 11 yrs old | 12 yrs old | 13 yrs old | 14 yrs old |
|---|---|---|---|---|---|
| Male neighbor masturbated, touched her. | Girl from school touched & kissed her—made her do the same. | Aaron made her try on sexy undergarments and videotaped it. | Maternal great grandfather touched privates and said, "I stick my pee pee in you." | Wanted drugs; 2 guys had sex with her while 3 or 4 watched. | Ran away—met Damon—she was too tired to stop him. |

*\* Indicates miscarriages.*

***Figure 19-9.** Sara's genogram.*

ated the second time. She admitted to abusing marijuana, freon, cocaine, heroin, speed, dexedrine, acid, and alcohol. Sara stated that she did not really care which drug she used, as long as it got her "high." She was a chronic runaway and had been hospitalized numerous times for drug use and depression. She was placed on suicide observation while she was in juvenile detention.

Only 7 months passed between her first and second detention at the juvenile facility. Sara was ordered to undergo long-term placement for drug abuse. She was in juvenile detention for 4 months awaiting court and placement. After 2 months of counseling in juvenile detention, she began to discuss her past with her therapist. During one session, Sara suddenly asked, "Do you think it's possible that a person is born knowing about sex?" Sara then began to remember her very early sexual encounters. The therapist used a genogram to facilitate Sara's discussion of her family history (**Figure 19-9**). As the sexual abuse history shows, Sara was a victim of sexual abuse by age 7, pornography by age 11, and prostitution for drugs by age 13.

Sara never understood the relationship between her childhood abuse and her desire to stay "high" through drugs. She can not remember the last time she was not depressed or suicidal. She requested a copy of her genogram when she left juvenile detention for another treatment facility. She did not have much hope of feeling better but did feel that the genogram was important in her treatment plan.

**Case Study 19-9**

Fifteen-year-old Isaac was first detained at a juvenile facility for burglary. Six months after getting out, he returned for the murder of a rival gang member. During this period Isaac was combative and angry, mostly at his 14-year-old brother who shot and killed himself in front of Isaac. Isaac was bright, artistic, and introspective.

Isaac was the product of a one-night stand and never knew his father. His family support consisted of his maternal grandmother, recently released from jail after she was incarcerated for the murder of 3 people; his mother, a drug addict and prostitute; and his 17-year-old sister, also a drug addict and prostitute. In a letter to his therapist, Isaac described how he saw his life and the undeterminable odds against him:

"Don't feel sorry for me. When sea turtles hatch from their eggs, they don't see their mom, right, because she's long gone. They go into the ocean not knowing all the dangers in front of them. If they get eaten and die, well, then they die; if they happen to live, well, then they must have been real fast swimmers. HA HA!! Nah, but the point is that they don't need anyone ... human babies will die with no one to help them so that's where our so-called God comes in."

The therapist drew Isaac's genogram after Isaac asked her if he was "born bad." The genogram introduced the concept that Isaac acquired or learned bad behaviors and could learn good behaviors if he wished to change his life. Although he was told his father was a heroin and crack addict, Isaac theorizes a "good family" on his paternal side (**Figure 19-10**).

## Example of a Treatment Program

Experientially based social development programs address multiple issues. These include but are not limited to identification of individual concerns and fears, anger management/conflict resolution, self-esteem issues, separation and grief issues, substance abuse issues, communicating effectively, and developing cooperation skills with peers and authority figures (Cavazos, 1996). The advantages of using experiential, adventure-based programs in conjunction with traditional therapy for children and adolescents are numerous. Such programs allow passive therapeutic interaction to become active and multidimensional, provide an alternative method of behavioral assessment that can enhance other traditional means of assessment, enhance the use of solution-oriented approaches in the therapeutic interaction, present an unfamiliar environment that enriches therapeutic interventions, and provide a method to bypass resistance to treatment and change (Gillis, 1995).

This program can be provided over 3 days to children and adolescents with a history of criminal behavior or victimization. According to Cavazos (1996), many of these children and adolescents feel

isolated and hopeless with little self-esteem. Often they either act out their anger or withdraw into depression. Group work is an effective means of creating changes, and experiential groups are particularly effective. The client will actually experience two separate realities simultaneously, the concrete realities of the various initiatives, as well as how these initiatives are metaphors for their lives. The key is that while being successful in the literal experiential program reality, the individual finds a way also to be successful in his or her metaphorical reality and his or her more generalized life events.

This direct link between the concrete experience and the abstraction to "real life" works particularly well in children who are by nature concrete thinkers. Trust is a predominant issue for these children. This program introduces the concept that they may be able to trust people and still be safe after years of victimization and mistrust.

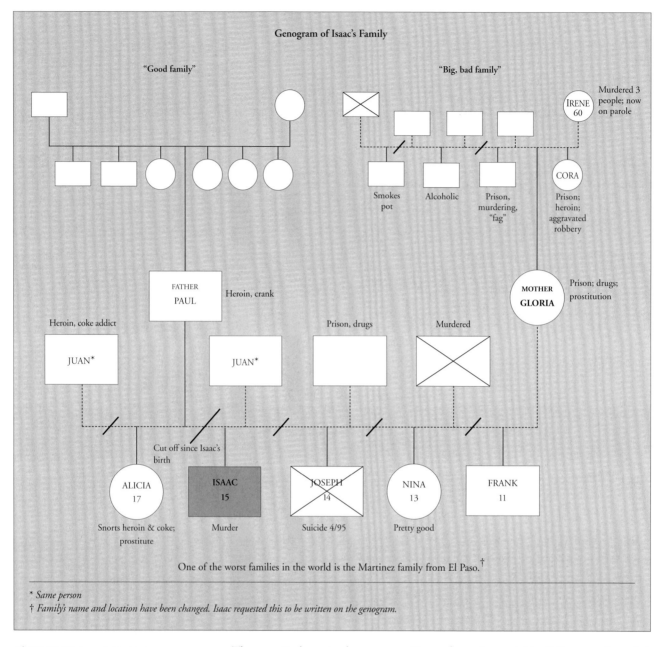

**Figure 19-10.** *Isaac's genogram.*

There are 3 phases in the program. Group formation activities "allow people to feel safe and important. The activities give the group members a sense of inclusion and ownership in the group ... as well as the freedom to invest something of themselves in the process" (Cavazos, 1996). In the next phase, establishing cohesion, rules and goals are negotiated, creating a "certain amount of conflict" and "restlessness" as boundaries are tested. During this second phase "criticism, silence, and power struggles are common experiences while establishing cohesion" (Cavazos, 1996). It is also during this phase that children begin to reveal some of their personal life experiences with abuse and neglect. In the third phase, group maintenance, more challenging tasks are provided and the group becomes most concerned with making "revisions in its structure and working toward the goals it has established. It is a time of hard work, creativity, and exploration" (Cavazos, 1996). A full day is devoted to "high initiatives" or climbing activities. The children learn that they must work as a team member for everyone to remain safe and for the group to ultimately achieve its goals. The experience during this phase has "a lasting impact on self-esteem, communication skills, decision-making, interaction with peers, and knowledge" (Cavazos, 1996).

# LONG-TERM PROGNOSIS

Long-term goals for victims of prostitution include short-term recovery from victimization and long-term resiliency. Resilience can be considered "the process of, capacity for, or outcome of successful adaptation despite challenging or threatening circumstances" (Masten et al, 1990). In their review of resilience literature, Heller et al (1999) identified protective factors associated with resilience: highly developed cognitive skills, a sense of self-worth, internal locus of control, external attribution of blame, spirituality, ego-control, family cohesion, and extrafamilial support.

Highly developed cognitive skills may lead to academic success and a sense of competence or may lead to more effective coping strategies in abused children (Cicchetti et al, 1993). A sense of self-worth may be a protective factor against depression (Moran & Eckenrode, 1992) or may moderate the numerous ongoing negative messages of his or her maladaptive or maltreating environment (Cicchetti et al, 1993). Internal locus of control refers to the understanding that an individual has power and control over certain aspects of his or her life. Research suggests that resiliency is associated with an internal locus of control for good events and that locus of control orientation for bad events is not significantly associated with depression (Moran & Eckenrode, 1992). In other words, it appears important that victims realize that some good things do happen to them because of who they are or what they do, not because of luck or factors out of their control.

External attribution of blame with regard to sexually abusive experiences appears to enhance resiliency (Valentine & Feinauer, 1993). Those with external attribution of blame accept that the abuse is not their fault and that the abuse affects them but not everything they do. Spirituality refers to a sense of purpose in life and a feeling of self-worth despite abusive experiences. Involvement in religious support groups provides an external support system and facilitates spirituality (Heller et al, 1999). Ego-control refers to one's susceptibility or vulnerability to his or her environment (Block & Block, 1980). Ego-overcontrol is associated with resilience in maltreated children (Cicchetti et al, 1993); these children are characterized as being reflective, persistent, attentive, dependable, and relaxed and may be more aware and avoidant of risk factors for maltreatment (Cicchetti et al, 1993).

Family cohesion refers to the presence of a sensitive, consistent, and safe caregiving environment (Heller et al, 1999). Research has consistently shown that such an environment, especially during early childhood years, is related to resilience after maltreatment (Egeland et al, 1993; Romans et al, 1995; Toth & Cicchetti, 1996). Family cohesion promotes other resiliency factors, including ego-control and spirituality. Extrafamilial support includes school involvement, extracurricular activities or hobbies, and religious/group involvement, all of which have been related to the development of resilience in abused children (Egeland et al, 1993; Herrenkohl et al, 1994). Positive experiences within any intrafamilial or extrafamilial support systems are likely to enhance self-esteem and feelings of self-worth.

When considering all factors that promote resilience in maltreated children, it is evident that victims of prostitution are unlikely to live within an environment conducive to the development of resiliency. Prostituted youth are more likely to be runaways, school dropouts, and nonparticipants in extracurricular or religious activities. They come from unstable, often violent, families that do not promote a feeling of mastery over their lives or a sense of self-worth. Therefore, long-term prognosis for these victims depends primarily on the identification and maintenance of a support system that is consistent and safe. This is particularly challenging among prostituted youth because family and friends often do not offer a safe harbor and because they rarely want intervention and help in identifying alternative living or working arrangements. Other resiliency factors, such as sense of self-worth, ego-control, and internal locus of control, are more likely to develop after placement in a safe environment than to be inherently present in the character and personality of prostituted children.

## PREVENTION

The prevention of prostitution depends on early identification of, and intervention for, families incapacitated by substance abuse, violence, or crime. It is also imperative that childhood abuse victims be identified and treated, given therapy, and permanently removed from the offending environment and placed in a safe one. Relapses in dysfunctional behaviors should be tracked and treated aggressively to ensure children's safety. Early detection of child and adolescent victims of abuse and gang involvement can be enhanced through public awareness and through training clinicians on child abuse dynamics and effective interview and communication skills. Once victims and gang members are identified, the goals of assessment and therapy should include family dysfunction, child safety, effects of victimization, reduction of risky health behaviors, and strategies to increase victims' positive support systems.

An increase in emergency and transitional shelters as well as community, educational, legal, and child care resources will help to prevent homeless children and teenagers from entering into prostitution in the first place. The implementation of stricter laws and enforcement of those laws and severe penalties against perpetrators, pimps, and customers of prostitutes are also necessary to protect these youth (Estes & Weiner, 2002).

## REFERENCES

American Psychiatric Association (APA). *Diagnostic and Statistical Manual of Mental Disorders.* 4th ed. Washington, DC: American Psychiatric Association; 1994.

Block JH, Block J. The role of ego control and ego-resiliency in the organization of behavior. In: Collins WA, ed. Minnesota Symposia on Child Psychology. *Development of Cognition, Affect, and Social Relations.* Hillsdale, NJ: Erlbaum; 1980;13: 39-101.

Boyer D. Male prostitution and homosexual identity. *J Homosex.* 1989;17(1-2): 151-184.

Cavazos J. *Elements of Change Group Therapy.* San Antonio, Tex; 1996.

Cicchetti D, Rogosch ML, Holt KD. Resilience in maltreated children: processes leading to adaptive outcome. *Dev Psychopathol.* 1993;5:626-647.

Cohen M. *Identifying and Combating Juvenile Prostitution.* Washington, DC: National Association of Counties Research, 1987.

Crisis Connection. *Helping People in Crisis: Basic Skills in Crisis Intervention.* Minneapolis, Minn: Crisis Connection; 1994.

Earls CM, David H. A psychosocial study of male prostitution. *Arch Sex Behav.* 1989;18(5):401-419.

Egeland B, Carlson E, Sroufe LA. Resilience as process. *Dev Psychopathol.* 1993;5: 517-528.

Estes RJ, Weiner NA. *The Commercial Sexual Exploitation of Children in the U.S., Canada and Mexico.* Philadelphia: University of Pennsylvania, School of Social Work; February 2002.

Gibson-Ainyette I, Templer DI, Brown R, Veaco L. Adolescent female prostitutes. *Arch Sex Behav.* 1988;17(5):431-438.

Gillis HL, ed. *Adventure Based Counseling Training Manual.* Hamilton, Mass: Project Adventure Inc; 1995.

Heller SS, Larrieu JA, D'Imperio R, Boris NW. Research on resilience to child maltreatment: empirical considerations. *Child Abuse Negl.* 1999;23(4):321-338.

Herrenkohl EC, Herrenkohl R, Egolf B. Resilient early school-age children from maltreating homes: outcomes in late adolescence. *Am J Orthopsychiatry.* 1994; 64: 301-309.

Hofstede A. The Hofstede Committee report: juvenile prostitution in Minnesota. Minneapolis, Minn: 1999. Available at: http://www.ag.state.mn.us/consumer/PDF/hofstede.pdf. Accessed September 16, 2003.

Inciardi JA. Little girls and sex: a glimpse at the world of the "baby pro." *Deviant Behav.* 1984;5:71-78.

Lanning K, Burgess A. Child pornography and sex rings. In: Zillmann D, Bryant J, eds. *Pornography: Research Advances and Policy Considerations.* Hillsdale, NJ: Lawrence Erlbaum Associates; 1989:235-255.

Longres JF. An ecological study of parents of adjudicated female teenage prostitutes. *J Soc Serv Res.* 1991;14(2):113-127.

Masten AS, Best KM, Garmezy N. Resilience and development: contributions from the study of children who overcome adversity. *Dev Psychopathol.* 1990;2:425-444.

Moran PB, Eckenrode J. Protective personality characteristics among adolescent victims of maltreatment. *Child Abuse Negl.* 1992;16:743-754.

Perry BD. Children's reaction to stress. Section 21 in: Foltin GL, Tunik MG, Cooper A, et al. *Teaching Resource for Instructors in Prehospital Pediatrics.* New York, NY: Center for Pediatric Emergency Medicine; 1998. Available at: http://www.childtrauma.org/ctamaterials/emt.asp. Accessed September 17, 2003.

Rickel AU, Hendren MC. Aberrant sexual experiences in adolescence. In: Gullotta TP, Adams GR, Montemayor R, eds. *Adolescent Sexuality.* Newbury Park, Calif: Sage Publications; 1992:141-160. Advances in Adolescent Development series; vol. 5.

Romans SE, Martin JL, Anderson JC, O'Shea ML, Mullen PE. Factors that mediate between child sexual abuse and adult psychological outcome. *Psychol Med.* 1995;25: 127-142.

Savin-Williams RC. Verbal and physical abuse as stressors in the lives of lesbian, gay male, and bisexual youth: associations with school problems, running away, substance abuse, prostitution, and suicide. *J Consult Clin Psychol.* 1994;62(2):261-269.

Seng MJ. Child sexual abuse and adolescent prostitution: a comparative analysis. *Adolescence.* 1989;24(95):665-675.

Slayer. Divine Intervention. *Divine Intervention*; American; 1998.

Toth SL, Cicchetti D. Patterns of relatedness, depressive symptomatology, and perceived competence in maltreated children. *J Consult Clin Psychol.* 1996;64:32-41.

Unger JB, Simon TR, Newman TL, Montgomery SB, Kipke MD, Albornoz M. Early adolescent street youth: an overlooked population with unique problems and service needs. *J Early Adolesc.* 1998;18(4):325-349.

Valentine L, Feinauer LL. Resilience factors associated with female survivors of childhood sexual abuse. *Am J Fam Ther.* 1993;21:216-224.

Yates GL, MacKenzie RG, Pennbridge J, Swofford A. A risk profile comparison of homeless youth involved in prostitution and homeless youth not involved. *J Adolesc Health.* 1991;12:545-548.

# Intimate Partner Violence in the Lives of Prostituted Adolescents

Daniel J. Sheridan, PhD, RN, FAAN
Dawn VanPelt, BSN, RN

This chapter provides clinically based recommendations on the forensic assessment, intervention, and documentation of intimate partner violence experienced by adolescent girls who are being prostituted by their pimp boyfriends. According to the Centers for Disease Control and Prevention, **intimate partner violence** (IPV) describes "physical, sexual, or psychological harm to another by a current or former partner or spouse. This type of violence can occur among heterosexual or same-sex couples and does not require sexual intimacy" (Intimate partner violence: overview, 2005). Though little research exists on this extremely vulnerable population, assessment and intervention tactics gleaned from other domestic violence studies may be clinically useful to health providers. A brief literature review of the dynamics and myths of dating violence is followed by a discussion of known health consequences of intimate partner abuse. Violence against pimp-controlled prostitutes and others in the sex trafficking industry is international in scope, with young women and adolescent girls the primary targets. Clinical signs and symptoms and risk markers for identifying IPV are summarized, followed by tips on modifying reliable and valid IPV assessment tools created to screen adult women for use with younger women and adolescent girls. The principles of written and photographic documentation in medical records are presented followed by a brief discussion of discharge safety planning.

## Dynamics of Dating Violence

IPV is a serious national problem that affects countless families across the nation (Magdol et al, 1998; Herrenkohl et al, 2004). In the past 2 decades, vast knowledge regarding the relationships of those involved in IPV has been gained. This information has led to an increased understanding of the dynamics of battered women and the reasons why they stay in abusive relationships and do not reach out for help. The focus of abusive relationships has expanded to include the adolescent and the increasing incidence of **dating violence**, violence that occurs during a "dating" relationship with an adolescent being the victim or perpetrator. Adolescents can experience dating violence in their relationships with a pimp whom the adolescent may view as a boyfriend. Longitudinal and retrospective studies show that violence inflicted or sustained during the early dating period is often a forerunner of later violence (DeKeseredy & Schwartz, 1994; Gidycz et al, 1993; Himelein, 1995; Lavoie et al, 2000; Malamuth et al, 1995; O'Leary et al, 1994). Therefore, violence learned at this stage of development can become engrained as a lifelong pattern of abuse.

An adolescent's experience with dating violence is often associated with the adolescent's exposure to physical, emotional, and/or sexual domestic violence involving their parents and having friends who are perpetrators or victims of dating violence. Arriaga & Foshee (2004) found that though friend dating violence and parental domestic violence were significant correlates of participants' own perpetration or victimization, the effect of friend dating violence was more significant. Thus, overall, friends seem to be more influential than parents in shaping standards of acceptable dating behaviors during adolescence. This information is consistent with the enormous power peers are known to exert during adolescence (Harris, 1995).

## MYTHS SURROUNDING SEXUAL VIOLENCE

A large amount of information regarding the incidence and occurrence of sexual assault is available to the general public. Unfortunately, not all of the information is factual in content. Burt (1980) termed the false beliefs surrounding sexual violence *rape myths*. Rape myths deny or minimize victim injury or blame the victims for their own victimization.

Carmody & Washington (2001), in a stratified random sample of undergraduate college students, found that the majority of respondents disagreed with most rape myths. Examples of rape myths include but are not limited to: (1) a woman who goes to the apartment of a man on the first date implies that she is willing to have sex; (2) any healthy woman can successfully resist a rapist if she really wants to; (3) in the majority of rapes, the victim is promiscuous or has a bad reputation; (4) a prostitute can not be raped; and (5) a prostituted woman can quit any time she wants. Falsely held rape myths lead to increased victimization of women and escalating violence; therefore, educational programs concerning rape myths need to be targeted toward a younger population, even elementary-age children, and should emphasize the need for respect and honesty in interpersonal relationships as well as violence prevention strategies (Wiehe & Richards, 1995).

Education regarding IPV and dating violence strongly determines nurses' response to abused women and adolescents. Nurses' beliefs surrounding violence affects what is offered to a victim or how that victim will respond to offered interventions. Myths, lack of education, and other factors including issues and dynamics, health effects, and practitioners' professional roles and responsibilities contribute to a wide variation in the healthcare provider's understanding of and response to abused women and children (Henderson, 2001).

## INTERNATIONAL SANCTIONING OF PROSTITUTION

Internationally, prostitution of women of any age is physically and psychologically dangerous and results in lifelong health consequences. When governments legalize and/or regulate prostitution, it guarantees the survival of a social system that condones violence against women, young girls, and children, and promotes illegal trafficking (Aghatise, 2004).

The Netherlands, Germany, Austria, Denmark, Greece, and Switzerland have some type of legalized prostitution (Aghatise, 2004). In Italy, where authorities unofficially condone prostitution, most women and young girls being trafficked for sex are from Nigeria, with smaller numbers from Kenya, Ghana, the Ivory Coast, Romania, Albania, Moldavia, Russia, and Bulgaria (Aghatise, 2004).

Many Nigerian women are lured with promises of higher earnings working in factories, offices, farms, and as dancers or entertainers in nightclubs. Once in Europe, the women are sold into sexual slavery to pay off immigration costs (Aghatise, 2004). It can cost between 62 000 and 124 000 euros for a trafficked woman to buy her freedom. The average "trick" in Europe pays about 10 euros. Some trafficked Nigerian women become madams who buy women and girls from the traffickers, who are predominantly men. Initially, the madams are kind and offer food, clothing, and shelter to newly trafficked women, and many of the trafficked women see the madams as their rescuers from the traffickers. Over time, they realize they are being used and this can result in more psychological trauma. Many Nigerian women have to swear during black magic juju rites to not reveal who trafficked them or for which madam they work. Breaking this oath is believed to cause curses against the woman or young girl and her family in Africa (Aghatise, 2004). In addition to the magic juju rites, exploiters use a number of other tactics to keep women controlled, including physical and emotional abuse, rape, and torture (eg, burning with hot irons) (Aghatise, 2004).

Women and young girls being trafficked from Eastern Europe have become ensnared in organized crime rings that convince their families to send their daughters to Italy with the promise of marriage and a rich life. The supposed husband sets up an apartment with his soon-to-be wife then feigns unexpected financial hardships and cajoles the woman into temporarily prostituting so they can be financially stable. For love, this woman sells her body on the roadside (Aghatise, 2004). What she does not know is her soon-to-be husband has numerous women in numerous apartments doing the same thing. If she discovers she is being used, the man will beat her and threaten to kill her if she tries to leave. If the woman tries to leave, the man calls or returns to her home country and ruins her reputation by telling her family she ran away and got involved in criminal activity. When the woman turns to her family for support, she finds none. Because of the lies of the abusive men, some families feel dishonored by their daughters to such an extent that she is told if she returns home they will kill her (Aghatise, 2004).

## PROSTITUTION RECOGNIZED AS MALE VIOLENCE AGAINST WOMEN

Sweden passed laws in 1999 recognizing prostitution as a form of male violence against women and children, thus the purchase of sexual services was criminalized. Swedish law recognizes that prostitution without male demand would markedly decrease (Ekberg, 2004; Raymond, 2004). Raymond (2004) states men buy prostituted women because they can and identifies numerous myths that are often used globally to excuse men who choose to purchase sex from prostitutes. These myths include that men who purchase sex from women (1) are basically decent men just looking for fun; (2) are men who are not getting the sex they need from the regular women in their lives; (3) are away from home for extended periods of time and need to release tension; and (4) are giving women a chance to earn an income. These myths are used to perpetuate and rationalize abuse of prostituted women. For over 20 years, women in IPV relationships have had similar myths used by men to justify abuse against them. Well-meaning health professionals still commonly say, "Why does she stay in the abusive relationship? She could leave if she wanted to!"

In Australia and New Zealand, where prostitution has been legalized, the demand for prostitutes is extremely high (Farley, 2004; Raymond, 2004) and is met with the importation of Asian women. In the Netherlands, another country with legalized prostitution, the demand is so high that sex industry lobbyists (former pimps) have lobbied the legislature to allow the importation of women from countries outside of the European Union to work as prostitutes (Raymond, 2004). Instead of calling it trafficking, the professional buyers and entrepreneurs of the sex industry call it "voluntary migration for sex work" (Raymond, 2004). The so-called volunteers are recruited from poor and uneducated developing, yet impoverished, countries (Raymond, 2004). Prostituted women in the "cheaper venues" commonly have sex with 20 to 30 men per day (Raymond, 2004). In comparison, in one US study the majority of prostitutes reported having sex with 6 to 20 men per day (Raymond, 2004).

In another US study, trafficked women and prostitutes stated condoms were used in only about half of their sexual encounters (Farley, 2004). While many brothels require condom use, sex without condoms can be negotiated for a higher fee (Farley, 2004; Raymond, 2004). Sex without condoms places high-risk women at higher risk for sexually transmitted diseases (STDs), especially human immunodeficiency virus/ acquired immunodeficiency virus (HIV/AIDS). The public health response has been aimed at the routine testing of prostitutes and not the routine testing of the men who are purchasing sex, ie, men who are willing to pay extra for unprotected sex or who threaten to harm women who insist on protected sex (Farley, 2004; Raymond, 2004).

## PIMPS AS PREDATORS

Not all prostitutes use pimps. The use of a pimp is often associated with younger girls who are runaways and lack food, clothing, and shelter (Williamson & Cluse-Tolar, 2002). Pimps can provide emotional support to younger and older women. An effective pimp develops a persuasive set of manipulation skills that get his woman to love him, capitalizing on the woman's need to feel loved. There is usually a courting or honeymoon period when the pimp and his soon-to-be prostitute spend time dating like a normal couple, going to dinner or the movies (Williamson & Cluse-Tolar, 2002). Prostitutes involved with pimps who have only a small number of prostituted women in their possession (stable) were more likely to say they were in a loving relationship with the pimp, and women involved with pimps with larger stables described feeling infatuation, admiration, and loyalty. A successful pimp becomes skilled at "arousing love and fear in his women" (Williamson & Cluse-Tolar, 2002). To endure the relationship, the woman needs to focus on the positive aspects of the relationship such as protection and security and that the pimp is not always violent. Women in abusive relationships frequently minimize the seriousness of the abuse and tend to justify and defend the severe abusive behaviors of the abusers (Sheridan, 1998, 2001).

Dutton & Painter (1981, 1993) identified ***traumatic bonding*** as a barrier to abused women leaving abusive relationships. Traumatic bonding is characterized by intermittent, unpredictable abuse and power imbalances that can result in powerful emotional attachments, even within new relationships. Isolated from the reality of caring family or friends, the woman is intermittently abused followed by a period of improved relationships with the abuser that feeds her fantasy of being loved (Dutton & Painter, 1993). Though abusive men in intimate partner relationships can feign contrition as a tactic to keep women traumatically bonded, the social norms of being a pimp would never allow the pimp to show weakness by apologizing for violent behaviors. Williamson & Cluse-Tolar (2002) state, "[a] pimp's approach is never to cow down to his woman at any time. He cannot let love cloud his judgments concerning business."

Leaving an abusive intimate partner is the most potentially dangerous, and often deadly, time in the relationship (Campbell et al, 2004). This can be especially true for pimp-controlled young prostitutes. Even threats of leaving a pimp can lead to severe beatings. A planned escape, often coupled with moving to a new location, is often the only way women can leave pimp-controlled relationships (Williamson & Cluse-Tolar, 2002).

## HEALTH CONSEQUENCES OF DATING VIOLENCE

Much is known about the negative health consequences of violence for adult women in abusive relationships. The same negative health consequences can be inherent for adolescents in a violent relationship and are potentially more detrimental to their health and well-being. Direct physical and psychological violence against a still-growing and maturing adolescent can be the precipitant of lifelong negative health consequences. Negative health consequences can occur even when the adolescent witnesses repeated violence against others. In general, most healthcare providers have had little to no training in screening and documenting most forms of family violence. Healthcare providers who identified adult abused women failed to involve the primary care physician in the patients' plan of care despite the known negative health consequences of abuse (Henderson, 2001). If trained healthcare providers do not acknowledge the full and detrimental ramifications of abuse directed toward women, others involved in the complex care of abused adolescents will find it difficult to accept and realize the consequences on the youth's future. Studies have shown that early detection of abuse and treatment leads to better outcomes for the youth (American Academy of Pediatrics [AAP], Committee on Child Abuse and Neglect, 1991). Therefore, healthcare providers caring for older adolescents and teenagers, especially those entering into dating relationships, must begin screening for teenage dating violence as soon as their patients begin to date. Dating violence, including acquaintance rape, has been reported to occur in 19% to 55% of adolescent dating relationships (Gray & Foshee, 1997). Harner (2003) emphasizes this by stating that for many of these teenagers the lessons learned in early dating relationships may serve as relationship "scripts" for the future.

Direct effects of violence such as injury and mortality are easy to identify and understand. Injuries sustained can range from minor to life threatening. Tjaden & Thoennes (2000), in an analysis of data from the National Survey of Violence Against Women (NSVAW), revealed that minor injuries (scratches, bruises, and welts) are the most common, and lacerations, knife wounds, broken bones, head injuries, sore muscles, internal injuries, broken teeth, burns, and bullet wounds occur with decreasing frequency. Results from the direct injury can lead to long-term health effects. Traumatic brain injury can be devastating, with increasing symptoms noted depending on the severity and frequency of blows to the head (Jackson et al, 2002). Violence directed at a woman or adolescent can lead to an increased risk for a disability. Many studies find self-reported disabilities in abused women to be 1.8 to 3.5 times that of women who were not abused (Plichta, 2004). A review by Plichta (2004) of several large studies found a greater prevalence of chronic pain among women who are abused.

Pregnancy can result from IPV and can be seen as a time of increased risk for escalating violence. Gazmararian et al (2000) estimate that between 4% and 8% of all women who were pregnant were abused at least once during pregnancy. A much higher rate was found to be true for adolescents (Covington et al, 1997; Curry et al, 1998; Renker, 1999).

Poor general physical health and IPV have been shown to have a consistent relationship in many different studies, despite being difficult to measure and identify (Plichta, 2004). Clinical studies of women who are abused show an increase in the number of physical symptoms (eg, poor general health, headaches, gastrointestinal disorders, and immune system functioning) compared to nonabused women. One study of 1931 women seen in primary care practices found that the number of reported symptoms increased as the severity of the violence increased (McCauley et al, 1998). Campbell et al (2002) have conducted research showing an increase in gastrointestinal disorders and headaches in women who endure IPV.

Increased sexually transmitted infections (STIs) and urinary tract infections are seen in women who are abused, especially those who experience sexual violence (Glass et al, 2003). Victims of sexual violence may be at increased risk of invasive cervical cancer or dysplasia due to the increased number of STIs (Coker et al, 2000). Menstrual problems, pelvic pain, and sexual dysfunction (painful intercourse, decreased sexual desire) are associated with IPV (Campbell, 2002).

Ainscough & Toon (1993) refer to research showing that 50% of women and 23% of men receiving psychiatric help have been sexually abused at some point in their life. Childhood sexual abuse has been linked to adult psychological problems such as anxiety, anger, depression, revictimization, self-mutilation/self-harm, sexual problems, substance abuse, suicidality, impaired self-concept, interpersonal problems, obsessions and compulsions, dissociation, posttraumatic stress disorder (PTSD), and somatization.

Not surprisingly, women who are abused are more likely to have poor concepts of self-care. Smoking, drinking, and drug use are seen at an increased rate in women who are abused compared to women who do not experience abuse. Kaukinen (2002) found that those victimized in adolescence are more likely than adult and early childhood victims and nonvictims to engage in frequent episodes of binge drinking. Adolescent victimization also predicts consequential drinking behaviors. Researchers have discovered a new consequence arising from the biological, cognitive, and social disruptions endured in adolescence: the willingness to engage in high-risk behaviors (DiClemente et al, 1996; Elliot et al, 2002). Elliot et al (2002) found that young adolescent females exposed to family violence were 3 times as likely to engage in risky sexual activity.

## HEALTH CONSEQUENCES OF PROSTITUTION

While violence to prostitutes from the men who purchase sex has been documented (Aghatise, 2004; Farley, 2004; Norton-Hawk, 2004; Raymond, 2004), Williamson & Cluse-Tolar (2002) state, "pimp-related violence remains a viable force that negatively effects some women's health and well being." Pimp-controlled prostitutes are statistically more likely to experience more violence from customers, have sex and use drugs at a younger age, and sell their bodies for sex earlier than non–pimp-controlled prostitutes (Norton-Hawk, 2004). Prostituted women have significantly higher reported health problems, and death rates are more than 40 times higher than the average population (Farley, 2004). Illnesses include STDs, vaginal infections, cervical cancer, hepatitis, viral infections, headaches, stomachaches, eating disorders, exhaustion, and depression (Farley, 2004). The leading cause of death among prostitutes in numerous countries including the United States is murder (Farley, 2004).

Rosen's (2004) qualitative study of over 30 low-income adolescent women who were either pregnant or had recently given birth found teens who were not in school were more likely to be involved in an ongoing violent relationship than teens who had left violent relationships or had never been in a violent relationship. Birth control decisions were made more often by the male partner in the abusive relationships and forced or coerced sex was described by many of the ongoing abused and formerly abused women (Rosen, 2004). Women in the study reported the decision to keep or abort the pregnancy was made by the abusive male partner. Other women reported miscarrying after being beaten while pregnant (Rosen, 2004). Escaping from abusive relationships was directly linked to having a safe social support network. The more isolated the adolescent mother, the more difficult it was to leave safely. The fear of being homeless with a baby kept some women in abusive relationships (Rosen, 2004).

## VICTIMS BECOMING VIOLENT

Repeated exposure to violence, even if not directed toward the adolescent, can lead to a propensity to commit violent acts. Russell (1998) reported that in a sample of violent street adolescents, approximately half reported witnessing violence in the home. Therefore, many believe that the adolescent perpetrates violence because it is a learned behavior from their childhood. Aggressive behavior can be seen as a coping mechanism for dealing with physical, sexual, or both forms of repeated abuse for some teenagers. However, some of the aggressive acts committed by the adolescent may be due to the adolescent confusing the current victim with a victimizer of the past. Simkins & Katz (2002) state that substance abuse is another coping mechanism that adolescents employ to help deal with the trauma of abuse. This can lead to violence with the need to continue to procure more and more drugs to medicate themselves against harsh realities of the ongoing abuse. The use of alcohol and other illicit substances can lead to the youth being kicked out of the home or seeking a life on the streets to ensure continued access to drugs.

Many adolescents leave their abuse-filled homes looking for a better existence and end up living on the streets. Living homeless on the streets may erode the youth's ties to conventional society and destroy any inhibitions restricting violent behavior while placing the adolescent in locations and situations in which violence is more likely to occur (Baron, 2003; Baron & Hartnagel, 1997). Homelessness can lead to substance abuse to help negate the feelings of isolation and loneliness. Homeless young women are prey to pimps who are looking to replenish their stables of young prostitutes.

The need for a reputation on the streets can lead to escalating violent behavior. This violent behavior can be viewed as survival of the fittest for homeless adolescents. The need for a reputation leads to the lack of fear of authority figures. Lack of fear and respect for authority figures can lead to the first of many negative contacts with the juvenile justice system. Many adolescents are diagnosed with oppositional defiant disorder when they may, in fact, be suffering from PTSD or depression. With the diagnosis of oppositional defiant disorder, many adolescents will be held in the juvenile court system without proper treatment, potentially leading to a life of escalating violent acts. Therefore, adolescents brought before the juvenile justice system need to be examined in a broader context expanding beyond the assault. This broader context is essential to determine the appropriate intervention and treatment. Early intervention is key, as Salter et al (2003) report in a longitudinal study that followed 224 male child victims of sexual abuse up to the age of 18 to 32 years to assess whether they were known by the police or social services on a national basis to have been perpetrators of sexual aggression. Overall, 11 (6%) of the victims became violent later in life.

# CLINICAL PRESENTATIONS

Prostituted adolescents seek treatment for various acute clinical symptoms including pregnancy testing, treatment of STIs, abortion services, miscarriage, drug overdose, and abscesses, especially at injection sites. Trauma presentations include facial bruising and lacerations, bruised and broken ribs, vaginal and rectal tears, bruising to the abdomen and back, cut and stab wounds, and gunshots. Though any of the above symptoms should immediately be a red flag for abuse screening, all adolescents should be routinely screened for abuse.

## SCREENING

Because of the high prevalence of violence in traditional dating relationships, all adolescent females need to be routinely screened for physical and sexual abuse. There is no screening tool unique to identifying abused prostituted adolescent women in relationships with their pimps. However, the Abuse Assessment Screen (AAS) (Soeken et al, 1998) (**Table 20-1**) has been used effectively with adult and adolescent girls. Various AAS tools are in use in clinical settings ranging from 2 questions to 6 questions. The 6-question version included in this chapter has been effective in the authors' clinical practices in screening for physical, sexual, emotional, and psychological abuse, including fear of harm. If a provider is working in a jurisdiction with any form of mandatory reporting to authorities, ethically, the patient needs to be informed of these reporting requirements. It is inappropriate to screen for abuse and then, if positive, say, "Now that you have told me about the abuse your life, I have to call the police and/or child protective services."

Screening for abuse must be conducted in a private setting. Whether it is parents abusing children, boyfriends abusing girlfriends, husbands hurting wives, or pimps beating prostitutes, abusers are abusers. They tell their victims that if they disclose the abuse to anyone, they will be more seriously hurt or killed. Whether the abuse involves the hovering (ie, always wanting to be present) parent, boyfriend, pimp, or girlfriend, young women will not disclose their abuse histories unless their privacy is assured. In many healthcare settings, privacy is an illusion since treatment areas are separated by, at best, walls, a thin cloth, or a plastic curtain.

When the patient has been placed in as private a setting as possible, preface all screening efforts with a global statement that you, as a concerned practitioner, routinely screen *all* patients for violence because it is so common throughout society. Tell the

**Table 20-1. Abuse Assessment Screen**

1. When you and your partner argue, are you ever afraid of him?

2. When you and your partner argue, do you think he is trying to emotionally hurt (abuse) you?

3. Does your partner try to control you? Who you see? Where you can go?

4. Has your partner ever hit, slapped, pushed, kicked, or otherwise physically hurt you?

5. Since you have been pregnant (or when you were pregnant), has your partner (or anyone) hit, slapped, pushed, kicked, or otherwise physically hurt you?

6. Has your partner (or anyone) forced you into sex when you did not want to participate?

With any and every answer of "yes," thank the patient for sharing the information, then ask for an example and when it last occurred.

*Adapted with permission from Daniel J. Sheridan.*

patient that young women are commonly afraid and/or ashamed to answer the questions that are about to be asked, but assure them that the healthcare setting is a safe place. Do not promise the patient complete confidentiality since mandatory reporting statutes may require the practitioner to notify the police and/or child protective services of any suspected or known abuse or crime.

Any time a patient says "yes" to an abuse screening question, the provider should first thank the patient for sharing. Next, the provider needs to ask for a specific example and when the abuse last occurred. Though it can be time-consuming, the provider needs to write a detailed history of current and past abuses in the medical record.

## Documentation

A written summary of the patient's abuse history needs to be placed in the medical record, preferably using a commonly taught documentation system called SOAP (Subjective, Objective, Assessment, and Plan) charting. The documentation needs to be as verbatim as possible (Brockmeyer & Sheridan, 1998; Sheridan, 2001, 2003, 2004). Injuries need to be documented carefully and thoroughly using correct medical terms. For example, a *laceration* (ie, splitting of skin most often from blunt impact) is different from a *cutting injury* (ie, skin opening made by a sharp object) (Sheridan, 2001, 2003, 2004). *Bruising* (ie, the direct result of rapid bleeding from trauma) is not the same as *ecchymoses* (ie, a slower leakage of blood often from medical or hematological conditions) (Sheridan, 2001, 2003, 2004). During interpretation, the provider needs to be sensitive to injuries that do not fit the history of occurrence being provided by the patient or the person(s) accompanying the patient. Young women beaten by boyfriends who are also their pimps will not likely be allowed to seek medical care unless the injuries are very severe or are not healing. Therefore, a red flag for abuse is a young woman with delayed presentation for care.

Patterned injuries such as bruises suggestive of whips, cords, belts, fists, and fingertips; burns suggestive of cigarette lighters, especially on areas of the body not easily reached by the patient; bite marks; and other injuries that suggest the offending object are often indicative of abuse.

Written documentation should include, at a minimum, a description of the size, shape, and color of the injury as well as the presence or absence of pain. Detailed body maps should be used on all patients with injury. The injuries should be drawn on the maps and appropriately labeled. Healthcare settings that do not have access to standardized body maps can easily download a plethora of body maps from Internet searches engines.

PHOTOGRAPHIC DOCUMENTATION*

Though injury maps are an effective method of visually documenting the location of injuries, photographs are more helpful. Photographs taken in medical settings can be used to communicate to other health professionals and the authorities a true and accurate visual representation of the nature of the injuries. While photographs taken for medical documentation are not necessarily taken as evidence, they can be subpoenaed and used as evidence (Brockmeyer & Sheridan, 1998; Sheridan, 2001, 2003, 2004). Various photographic systems are available to providers. One of the easiest to use is the Polaroid Spectra Law Enforcement camera that can take images as close as 2 feet without adaptor lenses. With the adapter lenses that come with the kit, close-ups can be taken 10 inches and 4 inches away from the injury. This system usually costs a few hundred dollars and is easy to learn. The film develops quickly and if the image is substandard, the provider can immediately take another picture. Another option is the Polaroid Macro 5 system, a larger camera that has 5 built in lenses that can enlarge the injury to 3 times its original size. The Macro 5 costs $700 to $900 and uses the same film as the Spectra camera. The Macro 5 usually produces images far superior to the images from the Spectra system. While Polaroid cameras are easy to use, they do not allow for easy duplication and/or enlargements.

The 35 mm SLR film camera is currently widely used because it has many advantages. With the explosion of interest in digital cameras, good 35 mm SLR cameras can be purchased for a few hundred dollars. Advantages of 35 mm cameras include markedly improved quality prints and negatives from which one can make unlimited copies and enlargements. Most providers are comfortable using 35 mm SLR cameras and the courts readily accept images from these cameras into evidence. Disadvantages of using these cameras for injury documentation include: (1) concerns as to where to develop sensitive images; (2) not knowing if the image captured the injury until the image is developed; and (3) underexposure and overexposure potential.

Digital cameras are rapidly becoming the camera of choice for health professionals as well as law enforcement investigators. Using a digital camera, a provider knows within a few seconds if he or she captured the image (injury) of interest. For medical documentation of injury, the provider should use a digital camera with at least 4 megapixels of resolution (Shaw, 2002). Quality digital cameras for everyday use can range from $500 to $1000. Digital cameras require the provider to develop a system of storing the images, usually to a mainframe and/or compact disc, and printing the images on a quality color printer on special digital image paper. Before a provider uses digital camera imaging on reported or suspected abuse patients, he or she should call the county prosecutor to ask if the judges in the county allow digital images to be introduced as evidence. Since it is easier to manipulate and alter digital images compared to other photodocumentation systems, some judges in some jurisdictions do not allow digital images to be used as evidence. Ultimately, it is the prosecutor's responsibility to convince the court to allow digital images as evidence, and it is the provider's responsibility to assure the court the digital images have not been altered.

# SAFETY PLANNING AND REFERRALS

As with abused women in general, young women in abusive relationships with their pimps are often at various stages of leaving the relationship. Some young women are so convinced their pimp boyfriend loves them and that they are going to be rescued from the streets that they may see no need for any intervention by the healthcare provider.

---

*\* All product recommendations and descriptions listed herein are those of the authors.*

Unless a mandatory reporting requirement pertains to an individual type or age of patient who has been victimized, the provider can do little except offer education, resources, and referrals. All patients need to hear from the provider that they can return to the healthcare setting at any time for any reason. All known or suspected abuse patients need to hear that the healthcare setting is a temporary safe zone that can be used as a base to conduct more in-depth safety planning.

Posters containing crisis numbers for substance abuse, sexual assault, and domestic violence should hang on the walls in the treatment area. Bathrooms can be an especially private location to provide wallet-sized referral cards or tear-off help-line numbers. Local resources are always appropriate; however, many mid- to small-sized communities lack the social referral networks found in larger communities. Therefore, national numbers such as the National Youth Crisis Hotline (800-442-4673) or the National Domestic Violence Hotline (800-799-SAFE) need to be readily available.

Though police officers are increasingly better trained in appropriate interviewing of crime victims, many battered women and sexual assault survivors have not had positive experiences when they have turned to the police for help. Runaways, drug addicts, and prostitutes have found the police to be especially unhelpful if they report a physical and/or sexual assault. The healthcare provider, as a respected professional, can be a patient advocate to help ensure law enforcement officers interact with the victim in a professional manner, regardless of the victim's background.

Creative safety planning that provides the victim options to safely leave IPV relationships can be time consuming. Having a team approach to safety planning that includes (if available) on-site social workers, forensically trained nurses, and community-based advocates is most effective. If in-person advocacy and referral services are unavailable, the provider needs to provide the victim access to a telephone in a private setting and connect the patient to 24-hour help-line experts. In addition to being the right thing to do, providers need to realize that screening for physical and sexual abuse is a standard of care as well as forensic documentation (Sheridan, 2001, 2003, 2004). Failure to screen, document, and refer places the provider at a liability risk and at risk for noncompliance with federal healthcare regulatory guidelines such as those established by the Joint Commission on the Accreditation of Healthcare Organizations and the Centers for Medicaid and Medicare Services.

Health providers should have available on all clinical units local resources as well as texts written specifically to address assessment, documentation, and referrals of all forms of family violence. Among the classics used frequently by the authors are Humphreys & Campbell's (2003) *Family Violence in Nursing Practice* and Campbell's (1998) *Empowering Survivors of Abuse: Health Care for Battered Women and Their Children.*

## CONCLUSION

Many similarities exist between the plight of young women in abusive relationships with boyfriends or husbands and the plight of young women and girls in relationships with their pimps. If the healthcare provider does not ask or is uncomfortable asking about emotional, verbal, physical, and sexual abuse, it is very unlikely the patient will volunteer such information. There is no quick fix or cure to ending abuse. The medical intervention model of diagnose and treat does not fit well with the patient/victim population. A public health model of repeated information, empowerment, and support can be effective in providing patients with options to make safer life choices.

## REFERENCES

Aghatise E. Trafficking for prostitution in Italy: possible effects of government proposals for legalization of brothels. *Violence Against Women.* 2004;10:1126-1155.

Ainscough C, Toon K. *Breaking Free: Help for Survivors of Child Sexual Abuse.* London, England: Sheldon Press; 1993.

American Academy of Pediatrics (AAP), Committee on Child Abuse and Neglect. Guidelines for the evaluation of sexual abuse of children. *Pediatrics.* 1991;87:254-260.

Arriaga XB, Foshee VA. Adolescent dating violence: do adolescents follow in their friends', or their parents', footsteps? *J Interpers Violence.* 2004;19:162-184.

Baron SW. Street youth violence and victimization. *Trauma Violence Abuse.* 2003;4: 22-44.

Baron SW, Hartnagel TF. Attributions, affect and crime: street youths' reaction to unemployment. *Criminology.* 1997;35:409-434.

Brockmeyer DM, Sheridan DJ. Domestic violence: a practical guide to the use of forensic evaluation in clinical examination and documentation of injuries. In: Campbell JC, ed. *Empowering Survivors of Abuse: Health Care for Battered Women and Their Children.* Thousand Oaks, Calif: Sage Publications; 1998:23-31.

Burt M. Cultural myths and supports for rape. *J Pers Soc Psychol.* 1980;38:217-230.

Campbell JC. Health consequences of intimate partner violence. *Lancet.* 2002;359: 1331-1336.

Campbell JC, ed. *Empowering Survivors of Abuse: Health Care for Battered Women and Their Children.* Thousand Oaks, Calif: Sage Publications; 1998.

Campbell JC, Jones AS, Dienemann J, et al. Intimate partner violence and physical health consequences. *Arch Intern Med.* 2002;162:1157-1163.

Campbell JC, Torres S, McKenna LS, Sheridan DJ, Landenburger K. Nursing care of survivors of intimate partner violence. In: Humphreys J, Campbell JC, eds. *Family Violence and Nursing Practice.* Philadelphia, Pa: Lippincott, Williams, & Wilkins; 2004:307-360.

Carmody DC, Washington LM. Rape myth acceptance among college women: the impact of race and prior victimization. *J Interpers Violence.* 2001;16:424-436.

Coker AL, Sanderson M, Fadden MK, Pirisi L. Intimate partner violence and cervical neoplasia. *J Womens Health Gend Based Med.* 2000;10:861-866.

Covington DL, Dalton VK, Diehl SJ, Wright BD, Piner MH. Improving detection of violence among pregnant adolescents. *J Adolesc Health.* 1997;21:18-24.

Curry MA, Perrin N, Wall E. Effects of abuse on maternal complications and birth weight in adult and adolescent women. *Obstet Gynecol.* 1998;92:530-534.

DeKeseredy WS, Schwartz MD. Locating a history of some Canadian woman abuse in elementary and high school dating relationships. *Humanity Soc.* 1994;18:43-63.

DiClemente RJ, Hansen WB, Ponton LE, eds. *Handbook of Adolescent Health Risk Behavior.* New York, NY: Plenum Press; 1996.

Dutton DG, Painter SL. Traumatic bonding: the development of emotional attachments in battered women and other relationships of intermittent abuse. *Victimology.* 1981;1:139-155.

Dutton DG, Painter SL. Emotional attachments in abusive relationships: a test of traumatic bonding theory. *Violence Vict.* 1993;8:105-120.

Ekberg G. The Swedish law that prohibits the purchase of sexual services: best practices for prevention of prostitution and trafficking in human beings. *Violence Against Women.* 2004;10:1187-1218.

Elliot GC, Avery R, Fishman E, Hoshiko B. The encounter with family violence and risky sexual activity among young adolescent females. *Violence Vict.* 2002;17:569-592.

Farley M. "Bad for the body, bad for the heart": prostitution harms women even if legalized or decriminalized. *Violence Against Women.* 2004;10:1087-1125.

Gazmararian JA, Petersen R, Spitz AM, Goodwin MM, Saltzman LE, Marks JS. Violence and reproductive health: current knowledge and future research directions. *Matern Child Health J.* 2000;4:85-92.

Gidycz CA, Coble C, Latham L, Layman MJ. Sexual assault experience in adulthood and prior victimization experiences. *Psychol Women Q.* 1993;17:151-168.

Glass NE, Campbell JC, Kub J, Sharps PW, Fredland N, Yonas M. Adolescent dating violence: prevalence, risk factors, health outcomes, and implications for clinical practice. *J Obstet Gynecol Neonatal Nurs.* 2003;32:2-12.

Gray H, Foshee VA. Adolescent dating violence: differences between one-sided and mutually violent profiles. *J Interpers Violence.* 1997;12:126-141.

Harner HM. The relationship between domestic violence and child maltreatment. In: Giardino ER, Giardino AP, eds. *Nursing Approach to the Evaluation of Child Maltreatment.* St. Louis, Mo: GW Medical Publishing; 2003:411-428.

Harris JR. Where is the child's environment? A group socialization theory of development. *Psychol Rev.* 1995;102:458-489.

Henderson A. Factors influencing nurses' responses to abused women. What they say they do and why they say they do it. *J Interpers Violence.* 2001;16:1284-1306.

Herrenkohl TI, Mason WA, Kosterman R, Lengua LJ, Hawkins JD, Abbott RD. Pathways from physical childhood abuse to partner violence in young adulthood. *Violence Vict.* 2004;19:123-136.

Himelein MJ. Risk factors for sexual victimization in dating: a longitudinal study of college women. *Psychol Women Q.* 1995;19:31-48.

Humphreys JC, Campbell JC, eds. *Family Violence in Nursing Practice.* Philadelphia, Pa: Lippincott, Williams, & Wilkins; 2003.

Intimate partner violence: overview. Centers for Disease Control and Prevention Web site. Available at: http://www.cdc.gov/ncipc/factsheets/ipvoverview.htm. Accessed February 9, 2005.

Jackson H, Philp E, Nuttall RL, Diller L. Traumatic brain injury: a hidden consequence for battered women. *Prof Psychol Res Pr.* 2002;33:1, 39-45.

Kaukinen C. Adolescent victimization and problem drinking. *Violence Vict.* 2002;17:669-689.

Lavoie F, Robitaille L, Hebert M. Teen dating relationships and aggression. *Violence Against Women.* 2000;6:6-36.

Magdol L, Moffitt TE, Caspi A, Silva PA. Development antecedents of partner abuse: a prospective-longitudinal study. *J Abnorm Psychol.* 1998;107:375-389.

Malamuth NM, Linz D, Heavey CL, Barnes G, Acker M. Using the confluence of sexual aggression to predict men's conflicts with women: a 10-year follow-up study. *J Pers Soc Psychol.* 1995;60:353-369.

McCauley J, Kern DE, Kolodner K, Derogatis LR, Bass EB. Relation of low-severity violence to women's health. *J Gen Intern Med.* 1998;13:687-691.

Norton-Hawk M. A comparison of pimp- and non–pimp-controlled women. *Violence Against Women.* 2004;10:189-194.

O'Leary KD, Malone J, Tyree A. Physical aggression in early marriage: prerelationship and relationship effects. *J Consult Clin Psychol*. 1994;62:594-602.

Plichta SB. Intimate partner violence and physical health consequences: policy and practice implications. *J Interpers Violence*. 2004;19:1296-1323.

Raymond JG. Prostitution on demand: legalizing the buyers as sexual consumers. *Violence Against Women*. 2004;10:1156-1186.

Renker PR. Physical abuse, social support, self-care, and pregnancy outcomes of older adolescents. *J Obstet Gynecol Neonatal Nurs*. 1999;28:377-388.

Rosen D. "I just let him have his way": partner violence in the lives of low-income, teenage mothers. *Violence Against Women*. 2004;10:6-28.

Russell LA. *Child Maltreatment and Psychological Distress Among Urban Homeless Youth*. New York, NY: Garland; 1998.

Salter D, McMillan D, Richards M, et al. Development of sexually abusive behavior in sexually victimized males: a longitudinal study. *Lancet*. 2003;361:471-476.

Shaw C. Admissibility of digital photographic evidence: should it be any different than traditional photography? *Update*. 2002;15(10). Available at: http://www.ndaa-apri.org/publications/newsletters/update_volume_15_number_10_2002.html. Accessed February 9, 2005.

Sheridan DJ. Forensic identification and documentation of patients experiencing intimate partner violence. *Clin Fam Pract*. 2003;5:113-143.

Sheridan DJ. Legal and forensic nursing responses to family violence. In: Humphreys J, Campbell JC, eds. *Family Violence and Nursing Practice*. Philadelphia, Pa: Lippincott, Williams, & Wilkins; 2004:385-406.

Sheridan DJ. *Measuring Harassment of Abused Women: A Nursing Concern* [doctoral dissertation]. Portland: Oregon Health Services University; 1998.

Sheridan DJ. Treating survivors of intimate partner abuse: forensic identification and documentation. In: Olshaker JS, Jackson MC, Smock WS, eds. *Forensic Emerg Med*. Philadelphia, Pa: Lippincott, Williams, & Wilkins; 2001:203-228.

Simkins S, Katz S. Criminalizing abused girls. *Violence Against Women*. 2002;8: 1474-1499.

Soeken KL, McFarlane J, Parker B, Lominak MC. The abuse assessment screen: measuring frequency, severity, and perpetrator abuse against women. In: Campbell JC, ed. *Empowering Survivors of Abuse: Health Care for Battered Women and Their Children*. Thousand Oaks, Calif: Sage Publications; 1998:195-203.

Tjaden P, Thoennes N. *Full Report of the Prevalence, Incidence, and Consequences of Violence Against Women: Findings From the National Violence Against Women Survey*. Washington DC: US Depart of Justice; 2000.

Wiehe VR, Richards AL. *Intimate Betrayal: Understanding and Responding to the Trauma of Acquaintance Rape*. Thousand Oaks, Calif: Sage Publications; 1995.

Williamson C, Cluse-Tolar T. Pimp-controlled prostitution: still an integral part of street life. *Violence Against Women*. 2002;8:1074-1092.

# ONLINE VICTIMIZATION: WHAT YOUTH TELL US*

David Finkelhor, PhD
Kimberly Mitchell, PhD
Janis Wolak, JD

In the analysis of crime, the perspectives of victims and potential victims often yield different and complementary insights to the perspective of law enforcement officials for conventional crime; the victim perspective is represented, for example, by the National Crime Victimization Survey, which has been an important complement to the law enforcement perspective obtained from police records. To understand ways to prevent and intervene in the problem of Internet offenses, this victim-level perspective is equally important and was the impulse behind the Youth Internet Safety Survey described in this chapter.

This national study, funded by the US Congress through a grant to the National Center for Missing & Exploited Children (NCMEC), confirms some of the reality portrayed by other chapters in these volumes. Large numbers of young people who use the Internet are encountering unwanted sexual solicitations, sexual material they do not seek, and people who threaten and harass them in various ways. The study also presents a complementary picture of the many kinds of situations young people experience that tend to escape official detection. Further, it shows that some youth are able to glide past unwelcome online encounters as mere litter on the information superhighway, but others experience them as real collisions with a reality they did not expect and are distressed to find.

This chapter describes the variety of disconcerting experiences young Internet users have online and the variety of ways they react. It provides a window into the ways families and young people are addressing matters of danger and protection on the Internet. Some of the news is reassuring. At the same time, these results suggest that the seamy side of the Internet spills into the lives of an uncomfortably large number of children, and relatively few families or young people do much about it. The findings highlight a great need for private and public initiatives to raise awareness and provide solutions.

Nothing in this chapter contradicts the increasingly well-documented fact that children and their families are excited about the Internet and its possibilities. They are, in effect, voting for the Internet with their fingers and pocket books even though they are aware of some of its drawbacks. Since the Internet is destined to play such an

* This chapter is adapted with permission from Finkelhor D, Mitchell KJ, Wolak J. Online Victimization: A Report on the Nation's Youth. University of New Hampshire Crimes Against Children Research Center. Alexandria, Va: NCMEC; 2000. NCMEC Order No. 62. Available at: http://www.missingkids.com/en_US /publications/NC62.pdf.

The report was funded by the US Congress through a grant to the National Center for Missing & Exploited Children, which is the national clearinghouse and resource center funded under Cooperative Agreement #98-MC-CX-K002 from the Office of Juvenile Justice and Delinquency Prevention, US Department of Justice. Study findings can also be found at the aforementioned Web site.

important role in the lives of young people growing up today, the question of how to temper some of the drawbacks of this revolutionary medium is worthy of serious consideration now at the dawn of the Internet's development.

# METHODS

## PARTICIPANTS

The Youth Internet Safety Survey used telephone interviews to gather information from a national sample of 1501 young people between the ages of 10 and 17 who were regular Internet users. **Table 21-1** presents the demographic characteristics of the sample. "Regular" Internet use was defined as using the Internet at least once a month for the past 6 months on a computer at home, school, library, someone else's home, or some other place. This definition was chosen to exclude occasional Internet users while including a range of "heavy" and "light" users. Prior to the youth interview, a short interview was conducted with a parent or guardian in the household. Regular Internet use by a youth was determined initially by questions to the parent or guardian and then confirmed during the youth interview. (Further details about the methodology of the survey are found in **Appendix 21-1**.)

| Table 21-1. Youth and Household Characteristics* (n = 1501) | |
| --- | --- |
| CHARACTERISTIC | % ALL YOUTH |
| **Age of youth (in years)** | |
| 10 | 4% |
| 11 | 8% |
| 12 | 11% |
| 13 | 15% |
| 14 | 16% |
| 15 | 18% |
| 16 | 17% |
| 17 | 13% |
| **Gender of youth** | |
| Male | 53% |
| Female | 47% |
| **Race of youth** | |
| Non-Hispanic White | 73% |
| Black or African American | 10% |
| American Indian or Alaska Native | 3% |
| Asian | 3% |
| Hispanic White | 2% |
| Other | 7% |
| Unknown/Refused to answer | 2% |
| **Marital status of parent/guardian** | |
| Married | 79% |
| Divorced | 10% |
| Single/Never married | 5% |
| Living with partner | 1% |
| Separated | 2% |
| Widowed | 2% |
| **Youth lives with both biological parents** | 64% |

*(continued)*

**Table 21-1.** *(continued)*

| Characteristic | % All Youth |
|---|---|
| **Highest level of completed education in household** | |
| Not a high school graduate | 2% |
| High school graduate | 21% |
| Some college education | 22% |
| College graduate | 31% |
| Post-college degree | 22% |
| **Annual household income** | |
| Less than $20 000 | 8% |
| $20 000 to $50 000 | 38% |
| $50 000 to $75 000 | 23% |
| More than $75 000 | 23% |
| **Type of community** | |
| Small town | 28% |
| Suburb of large city | 21% |
| Rural area | 20% |
| Large town (25 000 to 100 000) | 15% |
| Large city | 14% |

*\* All the data in this table are based on questions asked of the parent and/or guardian, with the exception of the information regarding race.*

*NOTE: Categories that do not add up to 100% are due to rounding and/or missing data.*

*Reprinted with permission from the NCMEC.*

## PATTERNS OF YOUTH INTERNET USE

Most of the youth who were interviewed (74%) had access to the Internet at home. They used the Internet in a number of other locations, including school (73%), other households (68%), and public libraries (32%). The majority of youth (86%) used the Internet in more than one location. At the time of the interview, most youth had last used the Internet during the past week (76%), with 10% reporting Internet use in the last 2 weeks and 14% in the past month or longer. In a typical week, 40% used the Internet 2 to 4 days a week, 31% went online 5 to 7 days a week, and 29% went online once a week or less. When they used the Internet, 61% of youth spent 1 hour or less online during a typical day; 26% spent 1 to 2 hours; and 13% spent more than 2 hours online during a typical day.

## OVERALL INCIDENCE OF ONLINE VICTIMIZATION

We asked youth about unwanted sexual solicitations or approaches, unwanted exposure to sexual material, and harassment during the year before the interview. **Table 21-2** provides definitions for the types of online victimization measured in this survey. More detailed information about the measures and limitations of the study can be found in **Appendixes 21-2** and **21-3**.

## SEXUAL SOLICITATIONS AND APPROACHES

Approximately 1 in 5 of the youth interviewed (19%) received an unwanted sexual solicitation or approach during the previous year (**Figure 21-1**). Not all of these episodes were disturbing to the recipients; however, 5% of the total number of youth (1 in 4 of those solicited) reported a solicitation that left them feeling very or extremely upset or afraid, cases that we called ***distressing incidents***. In addition, for 3% of the total number of youth (1 in 7 of all the solicitations), the sexual solic-

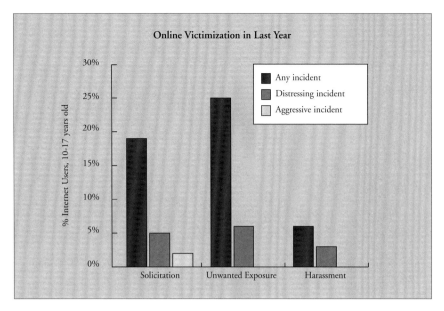

**Figure 21-1.** *Online victimization (including solicitation, unwanted exposure, and harassment) of youth ages 10 to 17 years old during 1999-2000.* Reprinted with permission from the NCMEC.

itation included an attempt at offline contact in person, over the telephone, or by regular mail. We called these ***aggressive sexual solicitations***.

## Unwanted Exposure to Sexual Material

Twenty-five percent of the youth experienced at least one unwanted exposure to pictorial sexual material in the last year. Seventy-one percent of these exposures occurred while youth were searching or surfing the Internet; 28% happened while they were opening e-mail or clicking on links in e-mail or instant messages. Because exposure to sexual images, even when unwanted, is not necessarily offensive, we designated a category of ***distressing exposures*** to identify situations in which youth found an exposure very or extremely upsetting. Six percent of youth reported distressing exposures to sexual material on the Internet in the last year.

## Harassment

Six percent of youth were the targets of threats or other kinds of offensive behavior, which we called ***harassment***. One third of these youth reported distressing incidents,

---

**Table 21-2. What is Online Victimization?**

People can be victimized online in many ways. In the Youth Internet Safety Survey, we asked about 3 kinds of victimization that have been prominent in discussions of youth and the Internet—sexual solicitation and approaches, unwanted exposure to sexual material, and harassment. (See **Appendix 21-2** for a complete explanation of these variables.)

**Sexual solicitation and approaches**
Requests to engage in sexual activities or sexual talk or give personal sexual information that were *unwanted* or, whether wanted or not, *made by an adult*.

**Aggressive sexual solicitation**
Sexual solicitations involving *offline contact* with the perpetrator through regular mail, by telephone, or in person, as well as attempts or requests for offline contact.

**Unwanted exposure to sexual material**
Without seeking or expecting sexual material, being exposed to pictures of naked people or people having sex when conducting online searches, surfing the Web, and opening e-mail or e-mail links.

**Harassment**
Threats or other offensive behavior (not sexual solicitations) sent online to the youth or posted online for others to see. Not all such incidents were distressing to the youth who experienced them. *Distressing incidents* were episodes during which the youth rated themselves as very or extremely upset or afraid as a result of the incident.

*Reprinted with permission from the NCMEC.*

---

that is, harassment that left them feeling very or extremely upset or afraid. What follows are more detailed descriptions of our findings.

# Sexual Solicitations and Approaches

With so many young people socializing on the Internet, a key law enforcement concern has been the access and anonymity that the Internet affords to persons who might want to exploit youth sexually. The Youth Internet Safety Survey confirms that large numbers of youth get sexually propositioned online although not always in the form of the most frightening law enforcement stereotypes.

To assess the problem of sexual exploitation, the survey asked youth about 4 kinds of incidents:

1. Sexual approaches, that is, when someone online tried to get them to talk about sex when they did not want to or asked unwanted, intimate questions

2. Sexual solicitations from people online who asked them to do sexual things they did not want to do

3. Close friendships formed online with adults, including whether these involved sexual overtures

4. Encouragement from people they met online to run away, a ploy apparently favored by some individuals looking for vulnerable youth

## Youth Targets for Sexual Solicitations

Girls were targeted for sexual solicitation at almost twice the rate of boys (66% versus 34%), but given that girls are often thought to be the exclusive targets of sexual solicitation, the sizable percentage of boys solicited is important. More than three quarters of targeted youth (77%) were 14 years old or older (**Figure 21-2** and **Table 21-3**). Only 22% of the youth were between the ages of 10 and 13 years of age, but this younger group reported 37% of the distressing episodes, thereby suggesting that younger youth have a harder time shrugging off such solicitations.

## Perpetrators of Sexual Solicitations

Virtually all perpetrators (97%) were persons the youth originally met online (**Table 21-3**). Adults were responsible for 24% of sexual solicitations and 34% of the aggressive solicitations. Most of the adult solicitors were reported to be between the ages of 18 and 25. About 4% of all solicitors were known to be older than 25.

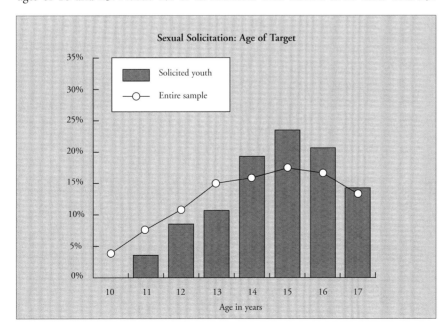

**Figure 21-2.** Youth as targets of online sexual solicitation, ages 10 to 17 years old. (NOTE: Adds up to less than 100% due to rounding and/or missing data.) Reprinted with permission from the NCMEC.

| Table 21-3. Internet Sexual Solicitation of Youth (n = 1501) | | | |
|---|---|---|---|
| INDIVIDUAL CHARACTERISTICS | ALL INCIDENTS (N = 286) 19% OF YOUTH | AGGRESSIVE INCIDENTS (N = 43) 3% OF YOUTH | DISTRESSING INCIDENTS (N = 72) 5% OF YOUTH |
| **Age of youth (in years)** | | | |
| 10 | <1% | — | — |
| 11 | 3% | 5% | 10% |
| 12 | 8% | 2% | 14% |
| 13 | 11% | 14% | 13% |
| 14 | 19% | 12% | 8% |
| 15 | 23% | 28% | 24% |
| 16 | 21% | 25% | 15% |
| 17 | 14% | 14% | 17% |
| **Gender of youth** | | | |
| Male | 34% | 33% | 25% |
| Female | 66% | 67% | 75% |
| EPISODE CHARACTERISTICS | ALL (N = 293) | AGGRESSIVE (N = 44) | DISTRESSING (N = 72) |
| **Gender of solicitor** | | | |
| Male | 67% | 64% | 72% |
| Female | 19% | 25% | 13% |
| Unknown | 13% | 11% | 14% |
| **Age of solicitor** | | | |
| Younger than 18 years | 48% | 48% | 54% |
| 18 to 25 years | 20% | 27% | 17% |
| Older than 25 years | 4% | 7% | 8% |
| Unknown | 27% | 18% | 19% |
| **Relation to solicitor** | | | |
| Met online | 97% | 100% | 96% |
| Knew in person before incident | 3% | — | 3% |
| **Location of solicitor** | | | |
| Youth knew where person lived | 13% | 29% | 17% |
| Person lived near youth (1-hour drive or less) | 4% | 11% | 7% |
| **Location of computer when incident occurred** | | | |
| Home | 70% | 66% | 51% |
| Someone else's home | 22% | 27% | 36% |
| School | 4% | 2% | 5% |
| Library | 3% | 5% | 4% |
| Another place | 1% | — | 1% |
| **Place on Internet where incident first happened** | | | |
| Chat room | 65% | 52% | 60% |
| Using instant messages | 24% | 36% | 26% |
| Specific web page | 4% | 7% | 7% |
| E-mail | 2% | 2% | 1% |
| Game room, message board, newsgroup, or other | 3% | — | 2% |
| Do not know/Refused to answer | 2% | 2% | 1% |

*(continued)*

**Table 21-3.** *(continued)*

| EPISODE CHARACTERISTICS | (N = 293) | (N = 44) | (N = 72) |
|---|---|---|---|
| **Forms of offline contact**[*][†] | | | |
| Asked to meet somewhere | 10% | 66% | 20% |
| Sent regular mail | 6% | 39% | 9% |
| Called on telephone | 2% | 14% | 4% |
| Came to house | <1% | 2% | — |
| Gave money, gifts, or other things | 1% | 5% | 1% |
| Bought plane, train, or bus ticket | <1% | 2% | — |
| None of the above | 84% | — | 70% |
| **How situation ended** | | | |
| Logged off computer | 28% | 25% | 35% |
| Left site | 24% | 16% | 22% |
| Blocked perpetrator | 14% | 25% | 17% |
| Told them to stop | 13% | 11% | 5% |
| Changed screen name, profile, or e-mail address | 5% | 13% | 13% |
| Stopped without youth doing anything | 4% | 9% | 5% |
| Called police or other authorities | 1% | 2% | 3% |
| Other | 20% | 20% | 18% |
| **Incident known or disclosed to**[*] | | | |
| Friend/Sibling | 29% | 41% | 32% |
| Parent | 24% | 32% | 33% |
| Another adult | 4% | 7% | 7% |
| Teacher or school person | 1% | 2% | 3% |
| Internet Service Provider/CyberTipline | 9% | 14% | 11% |
| Police or other authority | <1% | 2% | 1% |
| Someone else | 1% | — | 1% |
| No one | 49% | 36% | 37% |
| **Youth with no/low levels of upset and being afraid** | 75% | 55% | — |
| **Youth was very/extremely embarrassed about the incident** | 17% | 32% | 50% |
| **Stress symptoms (more than a little or all the time)**[*][‡] | | | |
| At least one of following: | 25% | 43% | 60% |
| Stayed away from Internet | 20% | 32% | 44% |
| Thought about it and could not stop | 11% | 27% | 35% |
| Felt jumpy or irritable | 5% | 20% | 21% |
| Lost interest in things | 3% | 5% | 10% |
| **Presence of five or more depression symptoms**[§][‖] | 17% | 30% | 24% |

[*] *Multiple responses possible.*

[†] *Only youth who did not know the solicitor before the incident were asked this question (n = 284 for all incidents, n = 44 for aggressive incidents, and n = 70 for distressing incidents).*

[‡] *These items were adapted from a psychiatric inventory of stress responses and represent avoidance behaviors, intrusive thoughts, and physical symptoms.*

[§] *In the entire sample, 8% of youth (n = 117) reported 5 or more symptoms of depression.*

[‖] *The values for this category are based on individual characteristics rather than episode characteristics.*

*NOTE: Categories that do not add to 100% are due to rounding and/or missing data.*

*Reprinted with permission from the NCMEC.*

Juveniles made 48% of the overall and 48% of the aggressive solicitations. Slightly more than two thirds of the solicitations and approaches came from males. One quarter of the aggressive episodes came from females. In 13% of instances, the youth knew where the solicitor lived. Youth stated that the solicitor lived nearby (ie, within a 1 hour drive of the youth's home) in only 4% of incidents.

Thus, not all of the sexual trawlers on the Internet fit the media stereotype of an older, male predator. Many are young, and some are women. It must be kept in mind, given the anonymity provided by the Internet, that individuals may easily hide or misrepresent themselves. In a large percentage of cases (27%), the youth did not know the age of the person making the overture. In 13% of cases, the gender was unknown. In almost all of the cases in which the youth gave an age or gender for a perpetrator, the youth had never met the perpetrator in person, thereby leaving the accuracy of the identifying information in question.

### SOLICITATION INCIDENT CHARACTERISTICS
Based on the descriptions given to interviewers, many of the sexual propositions appear to be solicitations for ***cybersex***—a form of fantasy sex that involves interactive chat room sessions during which the participants describe sexual acts and sometimes disrobe and masturbate. In 70% of incidents, the youth were at home when they were solicited; in 22% of incidents, the youth were at someone else's home (**Table 21-3**). In 65% of incidents, the youth met the person who solicited them in a chat room; in 24% of episodes, the meeting occurred through instant messages. In 10% of incidents, the perpetrators asked to meet the youth somewhere; in 6% of incidents, the youth received regular mail; in 2% of incidents, the youth received a telephone call; and in 1% of incidents, the youth received money or gifts. In 1 instance, the youth received a travel ticket. We labeled these incidents ***aggressive solicitations***. In most incidents, the youth ended the solicitations by using various strategies: logging off the computer, leaving the site, and/or blocking the person. **Table 21-4** describes some of these experiences.

### YOUTH RESPONSE TO ONLINE SEXUAL SOLICITATIONS
In almost half of the incidents (49%), the youth did not tell anyone about the episode, and even when the episode was aggressive, the youth did not tell anyone in 36% of incidents (**Table 21-3**). Some youth disclosed the incident to a parent (24%) or to a friend or sibling (29%). Only 10% of incidents were reported to an authority, such as a teacher, an Internet Service Provider, or law enforcement officer. Even with aggressive episodes, only 18% were reported to an authority.

It is remarkable that so few of the sexual solicitation episodes, even those that were quite distressing, prompted the youth to confide in someone or make a report to an authority. Some of this probably reflects that, in some cases, the youth were not that alarmed. Many probably did not know or doubted whether anything could be done. But some of it may reflect embarrassment or shame, because the youth may have believed they had gone places on the Internet where parents, law enforcement officers, or even friends would disapprove. Some may have been concerned that their access to the Internet would be restricted if they told a parent about an incident.

### IMPACT OF SOLICITATIONS ON YOUTH
In 75% of incidents, youth had no reaction or only a minor reaction, saying they were not very upset or afraid in the wake of the solicitation (**Table 21-3**); however, in 20% of incidents, youth were very or extremely upset, and in 13% of incidents, they were very or extremely afraid. In 36% of the aggressive solicitations, youth were very or extremely upset, and in 25% of incidents, they were very or extremely afraid. In 17% of incidents, youth were very or extremely embarrassed. This was true in 32% of aggressive incidents. In one quarter of incidents, youth reported at least one

**Table 21-4. Testimony From Youth Regarding Sexual Solicitations**

— A 13-year-old girl said that someone asked her about her bra size.

— A 17-year-old boy said someone asked him to "cyber" (ie, have cybersex). The first time this happened, he did not know what cybersex was. The second time it happened, he "just said, 'no.'"

— A 14-year-old girl said that men who claimed to be 18 or 20 would send her instant messages asking for her measurements and other questions about what she looked like. She said she was 13 years old when this happened, and the men knew her age.

— A 12-year-old girl said people told her sexual things they were doing and asked her to play with herself.

— A 15-year-old girl said an older man kept "bothering" her. He asked her if she was a virgin and wanted to meet her.

— A 16-year-old girl said a man would talk to her about sexual things he wanted to do to her and suggest places he would like to meet her.

— A 13-year-old boy said a girl asked him how big his privates were and wanted him to "jack off."

— Another 13-year-old boy said that a man had sent him a drawing of a man having sex with a dog. The man said it was a picture of himself.

*Reprinted with permission from the NCMEC.*

symptom of stress (eg, staying away from the Internet, not being able to stop thinking about the incident, feeling jumpy or irritable, losing interest in things) "more than a little" or "all the time." The aggressive episodes were more distressing, with at least one symptom of stress reported in 43% of episodes. Seventeen percent of the youth who were solicited experienced 5 or more symptoms of depression at the time we interviewed them, which is twice the rate of depressive symptoms in the overall sample.

Most of the youth who were solicited appeared to brush off the encounters and treat them as minor annoyances. Nonetheless, there was a core group of youth who experienced high levels of upset and/or fear. For these youth, the experience may have provoked stress responses. It is reassuring that most solicited youth are not affected, but given the large proportions of youth who are solicited, the group with the strongly negative reaction is quite substantial.

YOUTH AT RISK FOR SEXUAL SOLICITATION

Identifying the vulnerable population of youth is an important first step in the development of effective prevention and intervention programs surrounding online sexual solicitations. Logistic regression findings from these data suggest youth at risk tend to be older (ie, between 14 and 17 years), female, troubled, have high rates of Internet use, use chat rooms, talk with strangers online, engage in high online risk behavior, and use the Internet in households other than their own (Mitchell et al, 2001) (**Table 21-5**). These findings suggest that troubled youth and youth with high Internet use and risk behavior may be at increased risk for victimization and are worth targeting for prevention efforts. Yet, caution needs to be taken not to focus exclusively on these youth, because 42% of youth reporting sexual solicitations were not troubled or high or risky Internet users.

**Table 21-5. Composite Variable Characteristics**

— *Troubled* is a composite variable that includes items from a negative life event scale (eg, a death in the family, a move to a new home, divorced or separated parents, the loss of a parent's job), the physical and sexual assault items on a victimization scale, and a depression scale, or more depression symptoms in the past month. Those with a composite value 1 standard deviation above the mean or higher were coded as having this characteristic while the rest were coded as 0.

— *High Internet use* is a composite variable consisting of high experience with the Internet (ie, 4 or 5 on a scale of 1 to 5), high importance of Internet in the child's life (ie, 4 or 5 on a scale of 1 to 5), spending 4 or more days online in a typical week, and spending 2 or more hours online in a typical day. Youth with a composite value 1 standard deviation above the mean or higher were considered high Internet users.

— *High online risk behavior* is a composite variable of the following dichotomous variables pertaining to behavior online: posting personal information, making rude or nasty comments, playing a joke on or annoying someone, harassing or embarrassing someone, talking about sex with someone the youth never met in person, and going to X-rated sites on purpose. Youth with a composite value 2 standard deviations above the mean or higher were considered high online risk takers.

## ARE YOUTH FORMING RISKY INTERNET FRIENDSHIPS WITH ADULTS?

A key law enforcement concern is that many adults are using the Internet to form friendships with youth for purposes of sexual exploitation. To assess this question, we asked youth about the friendships they had formed through the Internet.

Sixteen percent of youth reported forming close friendships with someone they had met online. ***Close friendship*** was defined as "someone you could talk to online about things that were real important to you." These close friendships were predominantly with other youth. Just 3% of youth had formed a close friendship with an adult they met on the Internet. The youth involved in friendships with adults (defined as people older than 18) were almost exclusively between the ages of 15 and 17 years old. Girls were somewhat more likely than boys (ie, 59% of girls versus 41% of boys) to have formed close online friendships with adults.

The adult Internet friends were male and female and were usually young adults (between the ages 18 and 25). The youth typically met them in chat rooms, where they shared similar interests. In most of these friendships (69%), there had been some contact between the adult and youth outside of the Internet, that is, mostly by the telephone or regular mail. Parents knew about approximately three quarters of these friendships with adults. In almost one third of the youth-adult friendships, the youth actually met the adult in person. Usually this meeting took place in a public place with a friend present. Parents knew about one third of these meetings.

Regarding the key question of interest to parents and law enforcement officials, 2 of the total number of close friendships with adults were reported as having sexual aspects. One was a romantic relationship between a 17-year-old male and a woman in her late twenties; his parents knew about the relationship. The second friendship involved a man in his thirties who traveled to meet a 16-year-old girl. Although she stated that the relationship was not sexual, he did want to spend the night with her.

The study presents a complex picture about Internet relationships. Many young people are forming close friendships through the Internet, and some are forming close friendships with adults. Most such relationships appear to have no taint of sexual exploitation. The fact that our survey found few sexually oriented relationships between youth and adults does not mean they do not occur. They certainly do occur but probably at a level too infrequent to be detected by a survey of this size. These relationships seem to be few in a much larger set of seemingly benign friendships.

Young people may come to consider Internet friendships as one of the great resources the Internet provides. Prevention educators should acknowledge this as they try to become credible sources of useful information about safety practices.

From a prevention point of view, the survey found that many simple cautions (ie, do not form friendships with people you do not know, do not form relationships with adults, or do not have lunch with people you meet on the Internet) are unlikely to be seen as realistic, particularly by older teenagers. Though telling teenagers to inform their parents about Internet friends seems sound advice, for many older teenagers, this is also not likely to be practiced. Probably the best approach, based on findings here, is to remind youth that people they meet may have ulterior motives and hidden agendas. The caution to first meet someone from the Internet in a safe, public, or supervised place, as well as to alert others (eg, family, friends) about such a meeting, seems something that teenagers may be more likely to put into practice.

## Are Youth Being Solicited to Run Away by Potentially Predatory Adults?

Another situation of concern to law enforcement authorities has been youth who are encouraged to run away from home by persons they meet over the Internet. Seven youth (0.4% of the sample) revealed such an episode. In 2 instances, the episodes involved communications from teenaged friends or acquaintances. Five instances involved encouragement to run away from people unknown to the youth. Of these, 2 were identified as teenagers, 2 were identified as adults in their thirties, and in one instance, the person's age was unknown. Some descriptions of these incidents follow.

A 12-year-old girl reported an incident with a person identified as a young teenage boy. The boy encouraged her to run away and said it would make things "better." In another incident, a 16-year-old boy said he was talking to a man in his thirties about problems the boy was having with his family. The man suggested he run away and offered him a place to stay. Four of the 7 runaway incidents were not disclosed to parents or authorities. Three were disclosed to parents. Both of the episodes detailed here were disclosed to parents and reported either to law enforcement officials or an Internet Service Provider.

## Summary

Sexual solicitations and approaches occur to approximately 1 in 5 regular Internet-using youth during the course of a year. Most incidents are brief and easily deflected, but some turn out to be distressing to the recipients; some become more aggressive, including offline contact or attempts at offline contact.

While some of the perpetrators of these solicitations are the older, adult men depicted in recent media stories, many of the solicitors, when their age is known, appear to be other youth and younger adults and even some women. Even among the aggressive solicitors, a surprising number appear to be young and female. The diversity of those making sexual solicitations is an important point to recognize for those planning prevention. For example, too narrow characterization of the threat was a problem that hampered prevention efforts in regard to child molestation a generation ago. Those responding to Internet hazards should be careful not to make the same mistake. Not all of the sexual aggression on the Internet fits the image of the sexual predator or the wily child molester. A lot of it looks and sounds like the hallways of our high schools.

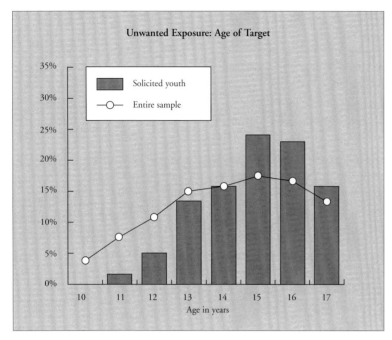

**Unwanted Exposure: Age of Target**

*Figure 21-3. Unwanted exposure to sexual material online to youth ages 10 to 17 years old. (NOTE: Adds to less than 100% due to rounding and/or missing data.) Reprinted with permission from NCMEC.*

Perhaps the most discouraging finding about sexual solicitations is that parents and reporting authorities do not seem to be hearing about the majority of these episodes. Youth may be embarrassed, may not know what to do, and may simply have accepted this unpleasant reality of the Internet. Obviously any attempt to address this problem would benefit from a more open climate of discussion and reporting.

## UNWANTED EXPOSURE TO SEXUAL MATERIAL

While it is easy to access pornography on the Internet, what makes the Internet appear particularly risky to many parents is the impression that young people can encounter pornography there inadvertently. It is common to hear stories about children researching school reports or looking up movie stars and finding themselves subjected to offensive depictions or descriptions.

To assess the problem of unwanted exposure to sexual material, the survey asked youth about 2 kinds of online experiences: (1) while conducting an online search or surfing the Web, seeing pictures of naked people or of people having sex when they did not want to be in that kind of site and (2) opening an e-mail, instant message, or a link in a message that showed them actual pictures of naked people or people having sex that they did not want to receive.

### YOUTH WITH UNWANTED EXPOSURES TO SEXUAL MATERIAL

Boys were slightly more likely than girls to have experienced an unwanted exposure (57% to 42%). More than 60% of the unwanted exposures occurred to youth who were 15 years of age or older (**Figure 21-3** and **Table 21-6**). Seven percent of the

| Table 21-6. Unwanted Exposure to Sexual Material (n = 1501) | | |
| --- | --- | --- |
| INDIVIDUAL CHARACTERISTICS | ALL INCIDENTS (N = 376) 25% OF YOUTH | DISTRESSING INCIDENTS (N = 91) 6% OF YOUTH |
| **Age of youth** | | |
| 10 | — | — |
| 11 | 2% | 1% |
| 12 | 5% | 5% |
| 13 | 13% | 21% |
| 14 | 16% | 18% |
| 15 | 24% | 22% |
| 16 | 23% | 15% |
| 17 | 16% | 18% |
| **Gender of youth** | | |
| Male | 57% | 55% |
| Female | 42% | 45% |
| | | *(continued)* |

**Table 21-6.** *(continued)*

| Episode Characteristics | All (N = 393) | Distressing (N = 92) |
|---|---|---|
| **Location of computer** | | |
| Home | 67% | 61% |
| School | 15% | 16% |
| Someone else's home | 13% | 16% |
| Library | 3% | 3% |
| Some other place | 2% | 3% |
| **Type of material youth saw or heard*** | | |
| Pictures of naked person(s) | 94% | 92% |
| Pictures of people having sex | 38% | 42% |
| Pictures that also included violence | 8% | 9% |
| **How youth was exposed** | | |
| Surfing the Web | 71% | 72% |
| Opening e-mail or clicking on e-mail link | 28% | 30% |
| Youth could tell site was X-rated before entering | 17% | 12% |

| Surfing Exposure | All (N = 281) | Distressing (N = 66) |
|---|---|---|
| **How Web site came up** | | |
| Link came up as the result of a search | 47% | 36% |
| Misspelled Web address | 17% | 18% |
| Clicked on the link when in other site | 17% | 24% |
| Other | 15% | 18% |
| Do not know | 3% | 3% |
| **Youth has gone back to Web site** | 2% | — |
| **Youth was taken into another X-rated site when exiting the first one** | 26% | 33% |

| E-mail Exposure | All (N = 112) | Distressing (N = 26) |
|---|---|---|
| **Youth received e-mail at a personal address** | 63% | 58% |
| **E-mail sender unknown** | 93% | 96% |

| Episode Characteristics (Surfing and E-mail) | All (N = 393) | Distressing (N = 92) |
|---|---|---|
| **Incident known or disclosed to*** | | |
| Parent | 39% | 43% |
| Friend/Sibling | 30% | 33% |
| Another adult | 2% | 2% |
| Teacher or school person | 3% | 9% |
| Internet Service Provider/CyberTipline | 3% | 4% |
| Police or other authority | — | — |
| Someone else | 1% | — |
| No one | 44% | 39% |

*(continued)*

| Table 21-6. Unwanted Exposure to Sexual Material (n=1501) *(continued)* | | |
|---|---|---|
| EPISODE CHARACTERISTICS (SURFING AND E-MAIL) | (N=393) | (N=92) |
| **Youth was very/extremely upset** | 23% | 100%[†] |
| **Youth with no/low levels of upset** | 76% | — |
| **Youth was very/extremely embarrassed about the incident** | 20% | 48% |
| **Stress Symptoms*** [‡]<br>Felt jumpy or irritable<br>Lost interest in things | <br>2%<br>1% | <br>7%<br>7% |
| **Presence of five or more depression symptoms**[§] [‖] | 11% | 15% |

\* *Multiple responses possible.*

† *Degree of upset was used to define this category of youth.*

‡ *These items were adapted from a psychiatric inventory of stress responses and represent avoidance behaviors, intrusive thoughts, and physical symptoms.*

§ *In the entire sample, 8% of youth (n=117) reported 5 or more symptoms of depression.*

‖ *The values for this category are based on individual characteristics rather than episode characteristics.*

NOTE: *Categories that do not add to 100% are due to rounding and/or missing data.*

*Reprinted with permission from the NCMEC.*

unwanted exposures were to 11- and 12-year-old youth. None of the 10-year-olds reported unwanted exposures. The somewhat greater exposure of boys may reflect that boys tend to allow their curiosity to draw them closer to such encounters. But the relatively small difference should not be overemphasized. Nearly a quarter of boys and girls had such exposures. Boys were slightly more likely than girls to say the exposure was distressing.

## EXPOSURE INCIDENT CHARACTERISTICS

Ninety-four percent of the unwanted images were of naked persons (**Table 21-6**). Thirty-eight percent showed people having sex. Eight percent involved violence, in addition to nudity and/or sex. Most of the unwanted exposures (67%) happened at home, but 15% happened at school. Three percent happened in libraries. Unfortunately, we do not know how many of the exposures involved child pornography. Important as this question is, we had decided that our youth respondents could not be reliable informants about the ages of individuals appearing in the pictures they viewed.

For the youth who encountered the material while surfing, the pornography came up as a result of searches (47%), misspelled addresses (17%), and links in Web sites (17%). For youth who encountered the material through e-mail, 63% of unwanted exposures came to an address used solely by the youth. In 93% of instances, the sender was unknown to the youth.

In 17% of all unwanted exposure incidents, the youth said they *did* know the site was X-rated before entering. (These were all encounters described earlier as unwanted or unexpected.) This group of episodes was not distinguishable in any fashion from the other 83% of episodes, including the likelihood of being distressing. Almost half of these incidents (48%) were disclosed to parents. It is not clear to what extent curiosity or navigational naïveté resulted in the opening of the sites in spite of the prior knowledge.

Pornography sites are sometimes programmed to make them difficult to exit. In fact, in some sites the exit buttons take a viewer into other sexually explicit sites. In 26% of unwanted exposure incidents, youth reported they were brought to another sex site when they tried to exit the original site. This happened in one third of distressing incidents. **Table 21-7** gives some examples of what youth said they encountered.

### Youth Response to Unwanted Exposure to Sexual Material

Parents found out or were told in 39% of the episodes (**Table 21-6**). Youth disclosed the incidents to no one in 44% of incidents. Authority figures were notified in a few cases; most frequently, youth disclosed to a teacher or school official (3% of incidents) and to Internet Service Providers (ie, 3% of incidents). None of these incidents were reported to law enforcement. Only 2% of youth encountering unwanted exposures said that they later returned to the site of the exposure. None of the youth with distressing exposures returned.

That so many youth did not mention their exposure to anyone (even to a friend to laugh about the experience or talk about it as an adventure) is noteworthy. It probably reflects some degree of guilt on the part of many youth. Perhaps if youth were talking about these experiences more, it might be healthier and helpful.

### Impact of Exposure

Twenty-three percent of youth were very or extremely upset by the exposure (**Table 21-6**). This amounts to 6% of regular Internet users. Twenty percent of youth were very or extremely embarrassed. Twenty percent reported at least 1 symptom of stress (staying away from the Internet; not being able to stop thinking about the incident; feeling jumpy or irritable; and/or losing interest in things) "more than a little" or "all the time" after the incident.

### Youth at Risk for Unwanted Exposure to Sexual Material

An important step necessary to inform the national debate about polices regarding youth and Internet pornography is to identify youth at risk for unwanted exposure to

---

**Table 21-7. Testimony From Youth Regarding Unwanted Exposure to Sexual Material**

— An 11-year-old boy and a friend were searching for game sites. They typed in "fun.com" and a pornography site came up.

— A 15-year-old boy looking for information about his family's Ford Escort typed "escort" into a search engine and found unwanted material.

— Another 15-year-old boy was writing a paper about wolves for school. He came across a bestiality site and saw a picture of a woman having sex with a wolf.

— A 16-year-old girl came upon a pornography site when she mistyped "teen.com." She had typed "teeen" instead.

— A 13-year-old boy who loved wrestling got an e-mail message with a subject line that said it was about wrestling. When he opened the message, it contained pornography.

— A 12-year-old girl received an e-mail message with a subject line that said "Free Beanie Babies." When she opened it, she saw a picture of naked people.

*Reprinted with permission from the NCMEC.*

sexual material on the Internet. Findings from a logistic regression analysis reveal at-risk youth to be older (14-17 years old), troubled, have high rates of Internet use, use e-mail and chat rooms, use the Internet at households other than their own, talk with strangers online, and engage in high online risk behavior (Mitchell et al, 2003) (**Table 21-5**). Again, as is the case with youth at risk for online sexual solicitation, caution needs to be taken not to create too narrow a focus on youth who are troubled and exhibit high and risky Internet use. In the cases of unwanted exposure, nearly half (45%) of youth reporting exposure were *not* troubled, high Internet users, or high online risk takers.

## SUMMARY

Unwanted exposure to sexual material appears to be widespread, occurring to a quarter of all youth who used the Internet regularly during the last year. While it is not a new thing for young people to be exposed to sexual material, the degree of sudden, unexpected, and unwanted exposure may be made more common by the widespread use of the Internet. Such exposure occurs primarily to older youth, but some youth as young as 11 years old reported exposure. Even in the older group, the exposure does not merely evoke laughs or mild discomfort. About a quarter of the exposed youth, 6% of all regular users, said they were very or extremely upset by an exposure. As with sexual solicitations, most exposure incidents, even the distressing ones, do not get reported to adults or other people in authority although a proportion of these incidents are disclosed to friends and siblings.

The experiences reported in our survey conform quite readily to anecdotal accounts from youth and adult users. Unwanted exposures mostly occur when doing Internet searches, misspelling addresses, or clicking on links. More than one third of the imagery was of sexual acts rather than simply naked people, perhaps more than people would guess, and 8% involved some violence in addition to nudity and sex.

From a social science view, the issues about youth exposure to unwanted sexual imagery are difficult to evaluate, in part, because there is almost no previous research on the matter. No one knows the actual effects. The research regarding exposure to advertising and media violence makes it clear that media exposure can affect attitudes, engender fears, and model behaviors (ie, pro- and anti-social).

Previous research about exposure to pornography is not relevant to the many issues of concern here. This research has been conducted with adults and is based on an assumption of voluntary exposure. The present study shows that in the case of unwanted exposure there are strong negative, subjective feelings for certain youth and certain youth who manifest symptoms of stress. We do not know how long these feelings or symptoms last or what ramifications they have, but these symptoms and feelings should be cause for concern. Questions of particular interest that need priority attention for future investigation are the following:

— Do any of the children so exposed have full-fledged, clinical-level traumatic reactions or other highly disturbed reactions?

— Is there any influence, traumatic or otherwise, on children's developing attitudes and feelings about sex?

— Do children with unwanted exposure relate to future Internet sexual material in different ways, that is, either more avoidant or more attracted?

— Do Internet exposures to sexual material figure negatively in family dynamics, thereby creating conflicts or barriers in any way?

Nonetheless, for many people, the issues about youth exposure are more basic than its effects. Whatever the effects, they would argue that people in general, and young people in particular, have a right to be free from unwanted intrusion of sexually oriented material in a public forum such as the Internet. On this point, some of the constitutional debate about the Internet has concerned what kind of forum the Internet is. Is it a forum like a bookstore, where if it is signposted, people can readily stay away from the sexually explicit material if they so choose? Or is it more like a television channel, where people are much more captive of the material that is projected at them? Clearly, the Internet has aspects of both; however, the present research does suggest that, in its current form, it is not simple for those who want to avoid sexual material on the Internet to do so.

## HARASSMENT

Although less publicized than sexual solicitation and unwanted exposure to sexual material, youth have reported other threatening and offensive behavior directed to them on the Internet, including threats to assault or harm the youth, their friends, family, or property as well as efforts to embarrass or humiliate them. Once again, the concern of parents and other officials is that the anonymity of the Internet may make it a fertile territory for such behaviors.

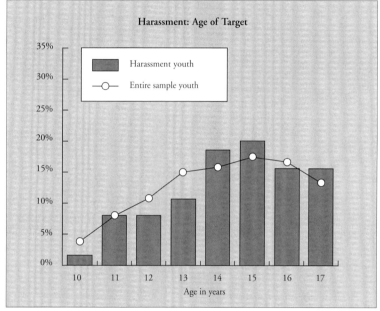

To assess the problem of harassment on the Internet, the study asked youth about 2 kinds of incidents: feeling worried or threatened because someone was bothering or harassing them online and having someone using the Internet to threaten or embarrass them by posting or sending messages about them for other people to see.

### YOUTH TARGETS FOR HARASSMENT

Boys and girls were targeted about equally for harassment (ie, 51% and 48% respectively). Seventy percent of the episodes occurred to youth 14 years old and older (**Figure 21-4** and **Table 21-8**). Eighteen percent of targeted youth were between the ages of 10 and 12.

*Figure 21-4. Youth as targets for harassment, ages 10 to 17 years old. (NOTE: Adds up to less than 100% due to rounding and/or missing data.) Reprinted with permission from NCMEC.*

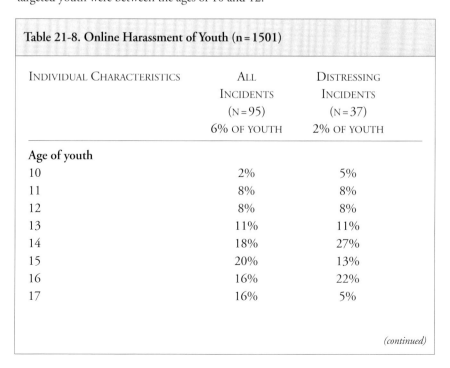

| INDIVIDUAL CHARACTERISTICS | ALL INCIDENTS (N = 95) 6% OF YOUTH | DISTRESSING INCIDENTS (N = 37) 2% OF YOUTH |
|---|---|---|
| **Age of youth** | | |
| 10 | 2% | 5% |
| 11 | 8% | 8% |
| 12 | 8% | 8% |
| 13 | 11% | 11% |
| 14 | 18% | 27% |
| 15 | 20% | 13% |
| 16 | 16% | 22% |
| 17 | 16% | 5% |

**Table 21-8. Online Harassment of Youth (n = 1501)**

*(continued)*

**Table 21-8. Online Harassment of Youth (n = 1501)** *(continued)*

| INDIVIDUAL CHARACTERISTICS | (N = 95) | (N = 37) |
|---|---|---|
| **Gender of youth** | | |
| Male | 51% | 43% |
| Female | 48% | 57% |

| EPISODE CHARACTERISTICS | ALL (N = 96) | DISTRESSING (N = 37) |
|---|---|---|
| **Gender of harasser** | | |
| Male | 54% | 51% |
| Female | 20% | 24% |
| Unknown | 26% | 24% |
| **Age of harasser** | | |
| Younger than 18 years old | 63% | 65% |
| 18 to 25 years old | 13% | 16% |
| Older than 25 years old | 1% | — |
| Unknown | 23% | 19% |
| **Relation to harasser** | | |
| Met online | 72% | 65% |
| Knew in person before incident | 28% | 35% |
| Youth knew where person lived | 35% | 24% |
| Person lived near youth (1 hour drive or less) | 43% | 35% |
| **Location of computer*** | | |
| Home | 76% | 81% |
| Someone else's home | 13% | 5% |
| School | 6% | 5% |
| Library | 1% | 3% |
| Some other place | 2% | 3% |
| Was not using a computer[†] | 2% | 3% |
| **Place on Internet incident first happened** | | |
| Using instant messages | 33% | 41% |
| Chat room | 32% | 22% |
| E-mail | 19% | 22% |
| Specific Web page | 7% | 8% |
| Game room, message board, newsgroup, or other | 6% | 5% |
| Do not know | 2% | 3% |
| **Forms of offline contact[† ‡]** | | |
| Sent regular mail | 9% | 4% |
| Asked to meet somewhere | 6% | 4% |
| Called on telephone | 4% | — |
| Came to house | 1% | — |
| Gave money, gifts, or other things | 1% | — |

*(continued)*

**Table 21-8.** *(continued)*

| Episode Characteristics | (N = 96) | (N = 37) |
|---|---|---|
| Bought plane, train, or bus ticket | — | — |
| None of the above | 88% | 96% |
| **How situation ended** | | |
| Logged off | 19% | 22% |
| Blocked that person | 17% | 11% |
| Left site | 13% | 16% |
| Told the person to stop | 11% | 16% |
| Stopped without youth doing anything | 10% | 11% |
| Changed screen name, profile, or e-mail address | 3% | 3% |
| Called police or other authorities | 2% | — |
| Other | 27% | 22% |
| **Incident known or disclosed to**[†] | | |
| Parent | 50% | 51% |
| Friend or sibling | 36% | 38% |
| Internet Service Provider/CyberTipline | 21% | 24% |
| Teacher or school person | 6% | 11% |
| Another adult | 1% | 3% |
| Police or other authority | 1% | — |
| Someone else | 4% | 8% |
| No one | 24% | 22% |
| **Distress: Very/extremely**[†] | | |
| Upset | 31% | 81% |
| Afraid | 19% | 49% |
| **Youth with no/low levels of upset, embarrassment, and fear** | 69% | — |
| **Youth were very/extremely embarrassed about the incident** | 18% | 35% |
| **Stress symptoms (more than a little or all the time)**[†] [§] | | |
| At least one of following: | 32% | 49% |
| Stayed away from Internet | 23% | 30% |
| Thought about it and could not stop | 20% | 38% |
| Felt jumpy or irritable | 6% | 16% |
| Lost interest in things | 3% | 5% |
| **Presence of five or more depression symptoms**[||] [¶] | 18% | 22% |

*\* These youth had information posted about them online by other people.*

*† Multiple responses possible.*

*‡ Only youth who did not know the harasser prior to the incident were asked this question (ie, n = 69 for all incidents and n = 24 for distressing incidents).*

*§ These items were adapted from a psychiatric inventory of stress responses and represent avoidance behaviors, intrusive thoughts, and physical symptoms.*

*|| In the entire sample, 8% of youth (ie, n = 117) reported 5 or more symptoms of depression.*

*¶ The values for this category are based on individual characteristics rather than episode characteristics.*

*NOTE: Categories that do not add to 100% are due to rounding and/or missing data.*

*Reprinted with permission from the NCMEC.*

## Perpetrators of the Harassment

More than one quarter of the perpetrators (28%) were offline friends or acquaintances of the youth (**Table 21-8**). A majority (54%) were reported to be male, but 20% were reportedly female, and in 26% of instances, the perpetrator's gender was unknown. Nearly two thirds (63%) of harassment perpetrators were other juveniles. Almost a quarter of harassment perpetrators (24%) lived near the youth (within 1 a hour drive). In distressing episodes, 35% of perpetrators lived near the youth. In contrast to the sexual solicitation episodes in which only 3% of perpetrators were known to the youth offline, approximately one quarter of the harassment episodes involved known persons and persons living relatively close to the youth.

## Harassment Incident Characteristics

Slightly more than three quarters of the youth were logged onto their computers at home when the harassment occurred (**Table 21-8**). The harassment primarily took the form of instant messages (33%), chat room exchanges (32%), and e-mails (19%). Twelve percent of the harassment episodes involving perpetrators who were not face-to-face acquaintances of the youth included attempts at offline contact by telephone, regular mail, or in person. **Table 21-9** provides some examples of the ways youth described their harassment incidents.

## Youth Response to Harassment

Parents found out or were told about these episodes half the time (**Table 21-8**). Slightly more than one third of the youth told their friends. Twenty-one percent of the episodes were reported to Internet Service Providers, 6% to teachers, and 1% to a law enforcement agency. Twenty-four percent of harassment incidents were undisclosed. It is noteworthy that, compared to sexual solicitations and exposures, a larger proportion of the harassment episodes were reported to parents and authority figures.

## Impact of Harassment

Thirty-one percent of the harassment episodes were very or extremely upsetting, and 19% were very or extremely frightening (**Table 21-8**). Eighteen percent were very or extremely embarrassing. Almost one third of the harassed youth (32%) reported at least 1 symptom of stress (staying away from the Internet; not being able to stop thinking about the incident; feeling jumpy or irritable; and/or losing interest in things) "more than a little" or "all the time" after the incident. Almost half of the youth with distressing experiences had at least one symptom of stress. Eighteen percent of the harassed youth were depressed at the time of their interview, which was more than twice the rate for the overall sample. Most of the harassed youth described the episode as mildly distressing, but an important subgroup was quite distressed.

## Summary

Sexual offenses against youth on the Internet have received the most attention, but this study suggests harassment deserves concern as well. Harassment does not occur as frequently as sexual solicitation or unwanted exposure to sexual material, but it is a problem encountered by a significant group of youth. The dark side of the Internet is not all about sex; it includes hostility and maliciousness as well.

An important feature of the harassment is that, more than sexual solicitation, it involves people known to the youth and people known to live nearby. Certainly, some of the threatening character of these episodes entails targets do not feel completely protected by distance and anonymity. The harasser could actually carry out his or her threats.

Importantly, the harassed youth were substantially more likely than the sexually solicited youth to tell someone and report the episode to an authority. Nonetheless, the percentage of youth reporting harassment to people in authority is quite low, thereby pointing to a need to publicize and educate families about available help sources.

| Table 21-9. Testimony From Youth Regarding Harassment |
| --- |
| — A 17-year-old girl said people who were mad at her made a "hate page" about her. |
| — A 14-year-old boy said he received instant messages from someone who said he was hiding in the boy's house with a laptop. The boy was home alone at the time and was very frightened. |
| — A 14-year-old girl said people at school found a note from her boyfriend, scanned it, posted it on the Web, and sent it by e-mail throughout her school. |
| — A 12-year-old girl said someone posted a note about her on the Web. The note swore at her and called her sexual names. |

# RISKS AND REMEDIES

Our lack of knowledge about the dimensions and dynamics of the problems this new technology has created for young people is a barrier to devising effective solutions. Even in the absence of knowledge, however, there has been no dearth of suggestions about things to do. Parents have been urged to supervise their children and talk with them about the perils and dangers of the Internet, and organizations have been established to monitor and investigate suspicious episodes. Have any of these remedies been taken to heart?

The survey asked various questions to find out more about the prospects for prevention. We wanted to determine to what degree parents were monitoring and advising their children about Internet activities. We asked about parents' and youth's knowledge about what remedies or information sources are available for them when they do run into problems.

## PARENTAL CONCERN

Parents and youth believed that adults should be concerned about the problem of young people being exposed to sexual material on the Internet. As might be expected, parents thought adults should be more concerned than youth thought adults should be, with 84% of parents saying adults should be extremely concerned compared to only 46% of the youth. Some inflation of concern might be expected in a survey with this topic, but other surveys confirm that this is an issue of substantial immediacy for parents and youth.

## USE OF FILTERING AND BLOCKING SOFTWARE

Thirty-three percent of households were using filtering or blocking software at the time of the interview. By far the most common option used was the access control offered by America Online (AOL) to its subscribers, used by 12% of the households with home Internet access or 35% of households using filtering or blocking software. Interestingly, another 5% of the households in our sample had used some kind of filtering or blocking software during the year, but were no longer doing so, thereby suggesting some possible dissatisfaction with its use.

## KNOWLEDGE OF HELP SOURCES

We noted earlier that few of the Internet episodes youth reported (ie, solicitation, unwanted exposure to sexual material, or harassment) were reported to official sources. One possibility is that youth and their families are not all that familiar with places interested in or receptive to such reports. Almost one third of parents or guardians said they had heard of places where troublesome Internet episodes could be reported, but only approximately 10% of them could cite a specific name or authority. Only 24% of youth stated they had heard of places to report; only 17% could actually name a place. Reporting the episode to the Internet Service Provider (most often AOL) was the option most often remembered.

## STUDY CONCLUSIONS

By providing more texture and details to our picture of the cyber hazards facing youth, the national Youth Internet Safety Survey has much to contribute to current public policy discussions about what to do to improve the safety of young people. **Table 21-10** lists some key conclusions and recommendations based on the important findings from the study, and more detail is provided within the text that follows.

### MANY YOUTH ENCOUNTER OFFENSIVE EXPERIENCES ON THE INTERNET

The percentage of youth who encounter offensive experiences (19% sexually solicited, 25% exposed to unwanted sexual material, 6% harassed) are figures for 1 year only. The number of youth encountering such experiences from the time they start using the Internet until they are 17 years old, which might include 5 or more years of Internet activity, would be higher.

The level of offensive behavior reported in this study might be placed in this perspective. Any workplace or commercial establishment in which one fifth of all employees or clients were sexually solicited annually would be in serious trouble. What if a quarter of all young visitors to the local supermarket were exposed to unwanted pornography? Would this be tolerated? Suppose 1 in 17 subway riders were threatened and harassed each year. There would certainly be a strong law enforcement presence in the subway as a result. We consider these levels of offensiveness unacceptable in most contexts. But on the Internet, will we simply accept it as the price for this new technology because it is anonymous? It certainly does confirm people's concerns about the coarseness and crudeness of the Internet experience. Sadly, the Internet is not always the nice, safe, educational, and recreational environment that we might have hoped for our young people.

### THE OFFENSES AND OFFENDERS ARE MORE DIVERSE THAN PREVIOUSLY THOUGHT

The problem highlighted in this study is not just adult males trolling for sex. Much of the offending behavior comes from other youth. There is also a substantial amount

---

**Table 21-10. Major Findings and Conclusions**

— Many youth encounter offensive experiences on the Internet.

— The offenses and offenders are more diverse that previously thought.

— Most sexual solicitations fail, but their quantity remains alarming.

— Teenagers are the primary vulnerable population.

— Sexually explicit material on the Internet is intrusive.

— Most youth brush off these offenses, but some become distressed.

— Many youth do not tell anyone about the experience.

— Youth and parents do not report these experiences and do not know where to report them.

— Internet friendships between teenagers and adults are common and seem to usually be benign.

---

from females. The nonsexual offenses are numerous and quite serious, too. We need to keep this diversity in mind. Sexual victimization on the Internet should not be the only thing that grabs public attention.

## MOST SEXUAL SOLICITATIONS FAIL, BUT THEIR QUANTITY REMAINS ALARMING

Based on current Internet use statistics, we estimate that 4.5 million young people between the ages of 10 and 17 years old are propositioned on the Internet every year. Even if only a small percentage of these encounters results in offline sexual assault or illegal sexual contact, which is a percentage smaller than we could detect in this survey, it would amount to several thousand incidents. The good news is that most young people seem to know what to do to deflect these sexual "come-ons." But there are youth who may be especially vulnerable through ignorance, neediness, disability, or poor judgment. The wholesale solicitation for sex on the Internet is worrisome for that reason.

## TEENAGERS ARE THE PRIMARY VULNERABLE POPULATION

For solicitations, as well as unwanted exposures to sexual material and harassment, most of the targets were teenagers, especially teenagers who were 14 years of age and older. Thus, it is misleading to say that child molesters are moving from the play-ground to the living room, trading in their trench coats for digicams, as some have characterized the situation. Children and teenagers are different victim populations. Preteen children use the Internet less, in more limited ways (US Department of Commerce, 2002; Roberts et al, 1999), and are less independent. It does not appear that much predatory behavior over the Internet involves conventional pedophiles targeting 8-year-old children with their modems, at least not yet. Teenagers are the target population for this Internet victimization, and that makes prevention and intervention a different sort of challenge since teenagers are more independent and do not necessarily listen to what parents and other "authorities" tell them.

## SEXUALLY EXPLICIT MATERIAL ON THE INTERNET IS INTRUSIVE

A large percentage of youthful Internet users are exposed to sexually explicit material when they are not looking for it. This occurs most often through largely innocent misspellings as well as the opening of e-mail, Web sites, and other documents. Sex found on the Internet is not nicely segregated and signposted like in a bookstore, and it is not easily avoidable. Some heavy-duty imagery is incredibly easy to stumble upon. Apparently many people who do not know this yet are inclined to think, "I don't see it, so it must be something you only get if you go looking." But youth do not have to be all that active in exploring the Internet to run across this material inadvertently.

## MOST YOUTH BRUSH OFF THESE OFFENSES, BUT SOME BECOME DISTRESSED

Most youth are not bothered much by what they encounter on the Internet, but there is an important subgroup of youth who are quite distressed by the exposure as well as the threats and solicitations. We can not assume that these are just transient effects. When youth report stress symptoms like intrusive thoughts and physical discomfort, these are warning signs. Some of this could be the psychological equivalent of a concussion rather than a slight bump on the head. It may be hard to predict exactly who will get hurt. It may depend partly on things like age, previous experience (with the Internet and sexual matters), family attitudes, the degree of surprise, and the kind of exposure. Anticipating and responding to negative impacts is something that needs more consideration.

## MANY YOUTH DO NOT TELL ANYONE ABOUT THE EXPERIENCE

Nearly half of the solicitations were not disclosed. Some of this nondisclosure certainly results from feelings of embarrassment and guilt. The higher disclosure rates for the nonsexual offenses point to that. Parents are not being informed about a lot of these episodes, and they would want to know. Some youth are not even telling their friends. Thus, they are not getting a chance to reflect about what happened, process it, and obtain ideas about ways to deal with the episodes and ways to put these episodes in perspective. Ironically, the Internet is providing places to discuss difficult topics, while at the same time may be increasing the number of difficult topics to discuss.

### YOUTH AND PARENTS DO NOT REPORT THESE EXPERIENCES AND DO NOT KNOW WHERE TO REPORT THEM

Most parents and youth did not know where to report the incidents or obtain help for Internet offenses. The low rate of reporting for actual offenses confirms this lack of awareness. Even the most serious episodes were rarely reported. The Internet is a new "country" and people do not yet know who the "cops" or authority figures are. In fact, this seems to be part of the attraction of this territory for many, that is, that there are not obvious cops or authority figures. People do, however, need to know ways to obtain help, and people with antisocial tendencies need to know that there are consequences. The choice is not between anarchy and "Big Brother," just as in regular politics the choice is not between anarchy and dictatorship.

### INTERNET FRIENDSHIPS BETWEEN TEENAGERS AND ADULTS ARE COMMON AND USUALLY SEEM TO BE BENIGN

It would make prevention easier if Internet relationships between youth and adults were uniformly sinister, and we could simply say, "Don't do it." But one of the positive things about the Internet is that it allows people of diverse social statuses to congregate around common interests.

We want young people to develop their skills and talents. We want them to find mentors. The existence of coaches who molest does not deter parents from signing their kids up for Little League. It will be a similarly complicated challenge to protect kids from the dangerous Internet relationships without squelching the positive ones. We need to learn more about the signs and symptoms of adult-youth relationships that are potentially exploitative, not just on the Internet, but in face-to-face relationships, too.

## IMPLICATIONS AND RECOMMENDATIONS

Some recommendations follow from these major findings and conclusions. They are listed in **Table 21-11** and more fully described in the following sections.

### CREATE MATERIALS SPECIFICALLY DESCRIBING DIVERSE HAZARDS

Those concerned about preventing sexual exploitation on the Internet need to mention the diversity of hazards, including threats from youthful and female offenders, in their materials. A stereotype of the adult Internet predator or pedophile has come to dominate much of the discussion about Internet victimization. While such figures exist and may be among the most dangerous of Internet threats, this survey has revealed a more diverse array of individuals making offensive and potentially exploitative online overtures. We should not ignore these offenders. We must remember that in a previous generation, campaigns to prevent child molestation characterized the threat as "playground predators," so for years the problem of youthful, acquaintance, and intrafamily perpetrators went unrecognized. Today, those doing prevention work concerning the Internet need to be careful not to make a characterization of the threat that fails to encompass all its forms whether consciously or inadvertently. One of the reasons for the mistaken characterization of child molesters in an earlier era was that people extrapolated the problem entirely from what came to the attention of law enforcement officials. A similar process could currently be underway in the case of Internet victimization, but it is probably early enough to reverse. Therefore, we need to publicize the full variety of Internet offensive behavior.

| Table 21-11. Recommendations |
|---|
| — Those concerned about preventing sexual exploitation on the Internet need to specifically mention the diversity of hazards, including threats from youthful and female offenders, in their materials. |
| — Prevention planners and law enforcement officials need to address the problem of non-sexual as well as sexual victimization on the Internet. |
| — More of the Internet-using public needs to know about the existence of help sources for Internet offenses, and the reporting of offensive Internet behavior needs to be made even easier, more immediate, and more important. |
| — Different prevention and intervention strategies need to be developed for youth of different ages. |
| — Youth need to be mobilized in a campaign to help "clean up" the standards of Internet behavior and take responsibility for youth-oriented parts of the Internet. |
| — We need to train mental health, school, and family counselors about these new Internet hazards and the ways these hazards contribute to personal distress and other psychological and interpersonal problems. |
| — Much more research is needed on the developmental impact of unwanted exposure to pornographic images among children of differing ages. |
| — More understanding is needed about families' knowledge of, attitudes about, and experience with filtering and blocking software. |
| — Laws are needed to ensure that offensive acts that are illegal in other contexts will also be illegal on the Internet. |
| — Concern about Internet victimization should not eclipse prevention and intervention efforts to combat other conventional forms of youth victimization. |

## ADDRESS BOTH SEXUAL AND NONSEXUAL INTERNET VICTIMIZATION

Prevention planners and law enforcement officials need to address the problem of nonsexual as well as sexual victimization on the Internet. An additional problem with the "Internet predator" stereotype just mentioned is that it does not give enough focus to nonsexual forms of Internet victimization. The current study shows that nonsexual threats and harassment constitute another common peril for youth that can be as or more distressing than sexual overtures. Experience in crime prevention has shown that concerns about sexual threats often eclipse other equally serious crimes. Concerted efforts should be made to ensure that nonsexual threats and harassment are included on the agendas of educators, practitioners, legislators, and law enforcement officials regarding Internet safety.

## INFORM THE PUBLIC OF HELP RESOURCES AND MAKE REPORTING OF OFFENSIVE INTERNET BEHAVIOR EASIER

More of the Internet-using public needs to know about the existence of help sources for Internet offenses, and the reporting of offensive Internet behavior needs to be made even easier, more immediate, and more important. Multiple strategies are needed to increase reporting. The Internet-using public needs to be aware of reporting options in as many ways as possible, that is, through the Internet as well as through other avenues. The public needs to be briefed on the reasons they should make such reports, including the importance of keeping the Internet a safe and enjoyable place for everyone to use. Smokey the Bear and McGruff the Crime Dog campaigns come to mind as approaches to emulate. People balk at being tattle-tales, but citizen vigilance and community involvement have traditionally been the keys to maintaining community safety.

## DEVELOPMENT OF PREVENTION AND INTERVENTION STRATEGIES FOR YOUTH OF VARYING AGES

Different prevention and intervention strategies need to be developed for youth of different ages. Most of the encounters reported to our study occurred to teenagers, specifically older teenagers. The messages that will make sense and be taken seriously by this group and their parents differ significantly from those that make sense for younger youth. This is a different problem from conventional child molestation, where we try to target and protect 7- to 13-year-olds. Older teenagers presumably have more independence, more experience, and a different relationship with adults and their families. For example, advice to tell parents to check the Internet and e-mail activity of older teenagers may be tantamount to saying parents should read their children's mail, a privacy invasion that seems unrealistic in many families. Good protection strategies, especially for the teenage group, can not be heavy on the control dimension and need to be tied to youth aspirations, values, and culture. This requires the input of youth. If young people are becoming millionaires with their Internet ingenuity, it is likely that some of that creativity could hit the jackpot in the field of Internet safety as well. It is time to involve a cadre of young people in the development of Internet victimization prevention in order to craft messages to which youth will be receptive.

## MOBILIZE YOUTH TO HELP "CLEAN UP" INTERNET BEHAVIOR STANDARDS

Youth need to be mobilized in a campaign to help "clean up" the standards of Internet behavior and take responsibility for youth-oriented parts of the Internet. Like face-to-face sexual offenses, which run the gamut from rape to harassment, Internet sexual offenses have been shown in this study to cover a spectrum of behaviors. The less serious end of the spectrum should not be ignored, since it can be the fertile soil in which more serious offenses grow. Much has been learned over the years about reducing crime, social deviance, and public disorder in communities. Many of those lessons are adaptable to the Internet, which is a community, albeit one with special properties. In the crime field, for example, success in reducing crime has been achieved through more community policing and cleaning up minor kinds of neighborhood disorder and decay. Crime-watch campaigns that deputize and empower community members to watch for crime have worked to reduce theft. In the education field, school revitalization campaigns have helped improve decorum and reduce antisocial behaviors in the schools. Thought should be given to applying such lessons to the Internet community. For example, the experience of those wanting to prevent real-world sexual harassment has been that campaigns, particularly campaigns involving whole schools, can be successful if they raise awareness about the problem and its effects and if they help youth enforce proper conduct among the peers themselves. Such youth-oriented campaigns might have some success with at least some forms of Internet victimization as well, and these campaigns may be worth a try.

## EDUCATE HEALTH, SCHOOL, AND FAMILY COUNSELORS ABOUT THE NEW INTERNET HAZARDS

We need to train mental health, school, and family counselors about these new Internet hazards and the ways these hazards contribute to personal distress and other psychological and interpersonal problems. This study reveals that substantial numbers of young people do experience distress because of Internet encounters, and they are not getting help. Mental health and other counselors need to learn to be alert and ask questions to get young people to talk about such encounters. These counselors need to know the ways that young people use the Internet so they can understand the problems of these young people. Counselors also need to be trained to treat the kinds of distress and conflicts that have a connection with negative Internet experiences. We need educational packages for schools and various youth workers for their own professional development and to use with the kids. Unfortunately, at the training conferences being offered today, most Internet education seems directed at law enforcement officials. We need to develop workshops for the educators, practitioners, psychologists, and social workers as well.

## More Research Is Needed

More research is needed on the developmental impact of unwanted exposure to pornographic images among children of different ages. The Internet is almost certainly increasing the frequency and the explicitness of such exposures, but even more important, the Internet is increasing the number of youth exposed involuntarily and suddenly. Although this topic has commanded some public attention, little research has been conducted. Even if the vast majority of such encounters are trivial or benign, however, it would be important to know under what conditions such encounters can be influential or stressful and what kinds of interventions are useful to prevent negative influence. The domain of influences could be broad and could include attitudes about sex, attitudes about the Internet, and matters of family dynamics. These are not easy matters to study in an ethical and dispassionate way; however, it can be done and should be made a priority.

## Better Understanding Is Needed About Families' Ideas About and Use of Filtering and Blocking Software

More understanding is needed about families' knowledge of, attitudes about, and experience with filtering and blocking software. This study found that only a minority of families with children were using blocking or filtering software even though most parents said adults should be very or extremely concerned about the problem of Internet victimization. Blocking and filtering software is one main line of defense available to families who are concerned about the problem. It is the defense being strongly advocated by people opposed to legislative solutions. Why is it not being used more often?

The lack of use of such software may reflect a lack of knowledge about its availability, suspicions about its utility, or a lack of suitability of such software in the context of real family dynamics and Internet use practices. For example, the introduction of such software may provoke conflicts between adults and youth or at least create fears about such conflicts. It is interesting that 5% of the families we interviewed had used filtering or blocking software in the past year and then discontinued its use.

Before recommending that more families use such software, it is important to know more about its operation. If a lack of knowledge is the problem, then education and awareness can be the answer. If the software does not suit the concerns of families or is difficult to use in real family contexts, then new designs or approaches to this software may be needed. We need detailed, real-life evaluation research about available Internet blocking and filtering technologies.

## Enact Laws to Make Offensive Acts Illegal on the Internet

Laws are needed to ensure that offensive acts that are illegal in other contexts will also be illegal on the Internet. Some of the offensive behaviors revealed in this study (especially sexual solicitations by adults of minors and some of the threatening harassment) are probably illegal under current law. Because most law was written prior to the development of the Internet, questions have been raised about whether and how various criminal statutes apply to Internet behavior. Although it is a daunting task, criminal statutes need to be reviewed systematically with the Internet in mind to make sure that relevant statutes cover Internet behaviors.

## CONVENTIONAL FORMS OF YOUTH VICTIMIZATION NEED OUR CONTINUED ATTENTION

Concern about Internet victimization should not eclipse prevention and intervention efforts to combat other conventional forms of youth victimization. This study has revealed how many offensive and distressing experiences youth encounter on the Internet. Internet victimization has not become, nor is it threatening to become, the most serious crime peril in children's lives; rather, it is just the newest. Among regular Internet users in our survey, 30% had been physically attacked in real life by other youth in the last year, 1% had been physically abused by an adult, and 1% had been sexually assaulted. None of these serious offenses had any connection, as far as we can tell, to the Internet. None of the Internet threats we documented actually materialized into a face-to-face violent offense. We need to mobilize about Internet victimization because it is new, causes distress, could mushroom, and could otherwise escape attention. But the conventional crime perils in the lives of children and youth are all too real and continuing. As reported from the National Crime Victimization Survey, youth the age of the respondents in this survey have conventional violent crime victimization rates (eg, rape, robbery, aggravated assault) that are twice that of the adult population (Hashima & Finkelhor, 1999). Children and adolescents are the most criminally victimized segment in our society. So, as much as possible, efforts to address Internet victimization should combine with and not displace efforts to prevent youth crime victimization in general.

## CONCLUSION

The study suggests that youth encounter a substantial quantity of offensive episodes, some of which are distressing and most of which are unreported. A comprehensive strategy to respond to the problem would aim to reduce the quantity of offensive behavior, better shield young people from its likely occurrence, increase the level of reporting, and provide more help to youth and families to protect them from any consequences.

## RECOMMENDED RESEARCH MATERIALS

1. The National Center for Missing & Exploited Children at: http://www.missingkids.org. Provides materials and maintains an online reporting system.

2. The CyperTipline at: http://www.cybertipline.org. For reporting online victimizations.

3. Federal Bureau of Investigation's Innocent Images Program at: http://www.fbi.gov/hq /cid/cac/innocent.htm.

4. Information and Resources about the Commission on Online Child Protection (COPA) at: http://www.COPAcommission.org.

5. National Resource Council Project on Tools and Strategies for Protecting Kids from Pornography at: http://www7.nationalacademies.org/itas.

6. Internet Safety Education for Parents and Youth at: http://www.getnetwise.com.

7. CyberAngels at: http://www.cyberangels.org. Internet safety organization.

8. Digital chaperones for kids. *Consumer Reports.* March 2001;66:20-23.

## REFERENCES

Hashima P, Finkelhor D. Violent victimization of youth versus adults in the National Crime Victimization Survey. *J Interpers Violence.* 1999;14:799-819.

Mitchell KJ, Finkelhor D, Wolak J. Risk factors for and impact of online sexual solicitation of youth. *JAMA.* 2001;285:3011-3014.

Mitchell KJ, Finkelhor D, Wolak J. The exposure of youth to unwanted sexual material on the Internet: A national survey of risk, impact and prevention. *Youth & Society.* 2003;34(3):330-358.

National Public Radio. NPR/Kaiser/Kennedy School Kids and Technology Survey. Available at: http://www.npr.org/programs/specials/poll/technology/technology.kids. html. Accessed August 26, 2004.

Roberts DF, Foehr UG, Rideout VJ, Brodie M. Kids and Media at the New Millennium: A Kaiser Family Foundation Report. Menlo Park, Calif: Henry J. Kaiser Foundation; 1999. Available at: http://www.kff.org/entmedia/loader.cfm?url=/commonspot/ security/getfile.cfm&PageID=13267. Accessed August 26, 2004.

US Department of Commerce. A nation online: how americans are expanding their use of the Internet. 2002. Available at: http://www.ntia.doc.gov/ntiahome/dn/. Accessed August 26, 2004.

# APPENDIX 21-1: METHODOLOGICAL DETAILS

The final Youth Internet Safety Survey sample consisted of 796 boys and 705 girls between the ages of 10 and 17 (**Table 21-1**). The interviews were conducted between August 1999 and February 2000. This was not a representative sample of all youth within the United States because Internet use was not evenly distributed among the population during that time period. Internet users tended to have higher incomes and more education than non-Internet users; among lower-income groups, Internet users were more likely to be white although racial difference was disappearing at higher-income levels (NPR Report, 2000). While boys were somewhat more likely than girls to use the Internet, the difference was small and attributable to boys' propensity for computer games (Roberts et al, 1999). The sample for the Youth Internet Safety Survey generally matched other representative samples of youth Internet users at the time these interviews were conducted.

Households with children in the target age group were identified through another large household survey, the *Second National Incidence Study of Missing, Abducted, Runaway, and Thrownaway Children* (NISMART-2), which was conducted by the Institute of Survey Research at Temple University between February 1999 and December 1999. NISMART-2 interviewers screened more than 180 000 telephone numbers to identify 16 000 households with children who were 18 years old and younger. Telephone numbers for households including young people between the ages of 9 and 17 were then forwarded to and dialed by interviewers for the Youth Internet Safety Survey.

Interviews for the Youth Internet Safety Survey were conducted by the staff members of an experienced national survey research firm, Schulman, Ronca, and Bucuvalas, Inc. Upon reaching a household, interviewers screened for regular Internet use by a child living in the household who was between the ages of 10 and 17. Internet use was defined as "connecting a computer or a TV to a phone or cable line to use things like the World Wide Web and e-mail." Interviewers identified the child in the household who used the Internet most often and then asked to speak with the parent who knew the most about the child's Internet use. Interviewers then conducted a short interview about household rules and parental concerns about Internet use, as well as demographic characteristics. At the end of the parent interview, the interviewer requested permission to speak with the previously identified youth. Parents were assured of the confidentiality of the interview, told that young participants would receive a $10 check, and informed that the interview would include questions about "sexual material your child may have seen."

With parental consent, interviewers described the study to the child and obtained his or her verbal consent. Youth interviews lasted about half an hour. They were scheduled at the convenience of youth participants and arranged for times when they could talk freely and confidentially. Questions were constructed so that youth responses were mostly short, one-word answers that would not reveal anything meaningful to persons overhearing any portion of the conversation. Where longer answers were required, questions were phrased, "This may be something private. If you feel you can talk freely, or move to a place where you can talk freely, please tell me what happened." Youth were not pressed for answers. They were promised complete confidentiality and told they could skip any questions they did not want to answer and stop the interview at any time. The survey was conducted under the supervision of the University of New Hampshire's Institutional Review Board and conformed to the rules mandated by research projects funded by the US Department of Justice. Youth respondents received brochures about Internet safety as well a $10 check.

## PARTICIPATION RATE
Based on standard calculations of participation rate, 75% of the households approached completed the screening necessary to determine their eligibility for participation in the survey. The completion rate among households with eligible respondents was 82%. Five percent of parents in eligible households refused the adult interview. Another 11% of parents completed the adult interview but refused permission for their child to participate in the youth interview. In 2% of eligible households, parents consented to the youth interview, but youth refused to participate. An additional 1% of eligible households was in "call-back" status when 1501 interviews were completed. (NOTE: As a result of rounding, these numbers add up to 101%.)

# APPENDIX 21-2: DEFINITIONS AND INSTRUMENTATION
The aspects of youth online victimization on which this study focused included sexual solicitations and approaches, unwanted exposure to sexual material, and harassment. (See **Table 21-2** for a list of definitions.) The incidence rates for sexual solicitation, unwanted exposure to sexual material, and harassment were estimated based on a series of screener questions about unwanted experiences while using the Internet. Two of the screeners concerned harassment, 4 involved unwanted exposure to sexual material, 3 focused on sexual solicitation, and 1 question asked if anyone online had encouraged the youth to run away from home. More extensive follow-up questions were asked about up to 2 of the unwanted incidents per youth; these follow-up questions were used to further classify the reported episodes into the categories reported on in this chapter.

Follow-up questions were limited to only 2 reported incidents because of time constraints. Consequently, some incidents reported by young people were not followed up, and these were omitted from incidence rates. If a youth reported more than one incident in a particular category, the follow-up questions referred to the "most bothersome" incident or, if none was "most bothersome," the most recent incident. The limits on follow-up questions probably led to some undercounting of incidents, particularly episodes of unwanted exposure to sexual material.

## SEXUAL SOLICITATION ITEMS
To assess the problem of sexual exploitation, the study asked several questions, the results of which were aggregated under the category of sexual solicitations and approaches. Questions were asked about:

1. Sexual approaches made to them in the past year—situations during which someone on the Internet attempted to get them to talk about sex when they did not want to or asked them unwanted intimate questions.

2. Sexual solicitations they had received in the last year from persons over the Internet who had asked them to do sexual things they did not want to do.

3. Invitations from Internet sources to help them run away, a ploy apparently favored by some individuals looking for vulnerable youth.

## UNWANTED EXPOSURE TO SEXUAL MATERIAL ITEMS

We were also interested in *unwanted* exposures to sexual material, that is, those that occurred when the youth were not looking for or expecting to receive or see sexual material. We were interested in the following:

1. Encounters with sexual material appearing while doing searches online and surfing the Web

2. When a youth was opening an e-mail or clicking on message links

In the section on sexually explicit material, we focused on unwanted exposure to pictorial images of naked people or people having sex.

## HARASSMENT ITEMS

The survey asked about the following kinds of situations that may have occurred in the last year:

1. Feeling worried or threatened because someone was bothering or harassing them online

2. Someone using the Internet to threaten or embarrass them by posting or sending messages about them for other people to see

# APPENDIX 21-3: LIMITATIONS OF THE STUDY

Every scientific study has limitations and defects. Readers should keep some of these important things in mind when considering the findings and conclusions of this study.

1. We can not be certain how candid our respondents were with us. Although we used widely accepted social science procedures, our interviews involved telephone conversations with young people regarding a sensitive subject, factors that could easily result in less than complete candor.

2. The young people to whom we did not talk may be different from the youth to whom we did speak. There were parents who refused to participate or refused to allow us to talk to their children; there were youth who refused to participate and those we could never reach. Our results might have been different if we had been able to talk of all these people.

# The Use of the Internet for Child Sexual Exploitation

L. Alvin Malesky, Jr, PhD

The predecessor of the Internet dates back to 1969 when the Advanced Research Projects Agency (ARPA) of the US Department of Defense created an experimental computer network called ARPAnet to facilitate communication among research scientists. By 1971, roughly 2 dozen computers at 15 different locations throughout the United States were connected via this system. During the 1980s, private companies began emulating the government's network by building their own private networks. In 1989, many of these private, governmental, and scientific networks were connected to create a "network of networks" or "inter" "net" (Internet). Around this time, the United States government eased restrictions on accessing the Internet, thereby facilitating its popularity and growth.

Internet usage has exploded over the past decade. By the year 2000, more than 40% of US households were connected to the Internet (US Department of Commerce [USDOC], 2001). A large number of young people are part of the Internet user population. Approximately 24 million individuals between the ages of 10 and 17 were online regularly in 1999 (Finkelhor et al, 2000). Furthermore, the growth in user popularity by this age group does not appear to be slowing down. In the year 2005, it is estimated that approximately 77 million minors will be accessing the Internet (US Department of Justice [USDOJ], 2001).

The Internet, with its large user base, has facilitated education and research, expedited communication and the flow of information, helped businesses grow and expand, and aided cultural and artistic expression. However, this technology comes with a dark side. Concerns about Internet usage include cyber addictions, where individuals spend an inordinate amount of time online (Brody, 2000; Cooper et al, 2000; Putnam & Maheu, 2000); online infidelity, where online usage causes relationship and marital discord (Young et al, 2000); advancement of extremist ideologies (eg, racism) (Schafer, 2002); and criminal activity (Conly, 1989). The focus of this chapter is on illegal Internet usage such as the distribution and acquisition of ***child pornography*** (ie, images of individuals under the age of 18 engaged in sexually explicit conduct) as well as Internet usage that is sexually deviant but not necessarily illegal (eg, supportive online communication regarding the molestation of children). This chapter also discusses the potential impact of this behavior on those who engage in this type of Internet usage.

## Why Do Individuals Use the Internet for Sexually Deviant and Illegal Purposes?

Cooper (1998) listed 3 reasons why the Internet is used for sexual gratification. He referred to them as the "Triple A": accessibility, affordability, and anonymity. Although Cooper's model was not designed specifically for sexually exploitive online activity targeting minors, it serves as a useful foundation to explain this type of behavior.

## ACCESSIBILITY

Cooper (1998) stated that the accessibility prong of the "Triple A" makes the Internet an attractive tool to fulfill one's sexual desires. Virtually any sexual material ranging from soft-core pornography to extreme pictures and video clips of bestiality, torture, and pedophilia can be found and accessed online (Durkin, 1997; Durkin & Bryant, 1995; Garreau, 1993; Kim & Bailey, 1997; Leiblum, 1997). With regard to online sexual topics, Leiblum (1997) stated, "unconventional appetites pose no problem; indeed, it is difficult to find an appetite that is not only catered to, but shared (by more people than one might have imagined)." If one considers that individuals with paraphilias, such as pedophilia, often have multiple paraphilias (Abel et al, 1987), it is logical that some individuals would use the Internet, with its abundance of sexual topics, as a "one-stop shop" for their deviant sexual desires. Thus, the Internet allows access to a wide range of sexual topics including those that many would consider aberrant (eg, sex with minors).

Regarding accessing the Internet itself, millions of American homes have Internet access (USDOC, 2001). In addition, Internet access is also available at a variety of public venues such as libraries, universities, and cyber coffee shops. Consequently, anyone with a strong desire to access the Internet will have little difficulty getting online.

An accessibility issue specific to child sex offenders is access to potential victims. Some of the more predatory, child sex offenders frequent places where there are children. Currently, a large number of children are accessing the Internet and, thus, so are offenders (Kantrowitz et al, 1994). Some offenders have proven to be quite predatory in their online behavior and appear to "troll" cyberspace searching for potential victims (LA Malesky, PhD & GV Malesky, unpublished data, 2003). This type of behavior will be discussed in more detail later in the chapter.

## AFFORDABILITY

Affordability is also an attractive feature of the Internet. The cost for Internet access from a private company such as America Online (AOL) is approximately $20 a month for unlimited usage. Other companies offer similar rates. If one uses a computer at work, school, or the library, then there is usually minimal charge or no charge to access the Internet. Once online, one can access a wide variety of free sexual material. Given that the distribution of child pornography does not appear to be a profit-driven venture (Taylor, 1999), one can acquire a large number of images and even video clips depicting this type of pornography at relatively no cost.

## ANONYMITY

Given the ease at which individuals can create anonymous e-mail addresses and fake online personas, it is not surprising that the Internet provides a sense of anonymity for its users. Typically, individuals like to keep their online sexual activity hidden from others (Cooper et al, 1999; Leiblum, 1997). The desire for secrecy is increased when the sexual conduct is illegal or socially unacceptable, such as the collection and distribution of child pornography (Lanning, 1992). Thus, the Internet is an ideal tool to engage in sexual behavior (especially illegal sexual behavior) when individuals are concerned about revealing their identities.

In addition to the inherent sense of anonymity provided by the Internet, some child sex offenders employ extra precautions to protect their identity while online (Sussman, 1995). **Remailers**, programs that strip header information from e-mails (Kopelev, 1999), electronic encryption software (Cusack, 1996), and passwords (Nordland & Bartholet, 2001) have all been used to help conceal individual' identities. In addition, online communities advocating adult/minor "relationships" also recognize the benefit of increased security to protect their members from law enforcement. One such online community actually posted links to Web sites that offered free encryption and remailer software.

Fortunately for law enforcement officials, not all individuals who engage in illegal online activity employ these additional security precautions. In his study, Malesky (2002) found that only 17% (n=17) of the incarcerated offenders, who admitted using the Internet for sexually deviant and illegal purposes (ie, receiving/distributing child pornography), also admitted using encryption software or remailers to protect computer documents or images that dealt with children and were sexual in nature. However, given that his sample consisted entirely of individuals who were eventually apprehended, Malesky cautioned against generalizing these results to all Internet users engaged in illegal online sexual activity. Perhaps unapprehended sex offenders do not come to the attention of law enforcement because they use this technology at higher rates than the participants in Malesky's study. Regardless, the Internet provides a degree of anonymity that many individuals likely find appealing when engaging in online sexual activity. Encryption software, remailers, and passwords are also employed by some Internet users to increase their online anonymity.

In addition to providing a sense of security, the anonymity of the Internet enables its users to assume multiple online personas and identities. This is important considering that some child sex offenders gain the trust of minors by portraying themselves as peers of the intended victims, a task easily accomplished over the Internet (Armagh, 1998; Durkin, 1997; Thomas, 1997). In fact, Malesky & Malesky (unpublished data, 2003) found that almost a third of the participants in the study represented themselves as children while having online conversations with actual children and adolescents. This is salient given that all of the individuals in his study used the Internet to identify potential contact victims. Furthermore, Lamb (1998) found that fewer than 10% of the individuals who accessed certain chat rooms geared for youth were actually minors. In fact, he found that two thirds of these individuals in the chat rooms were actually adults masquerading as children seeking *cybersex* (ie, online communication concerning sexual fantasies or other sexual topics, often accompanied with sexual self-stimulation) with individuals they believed to be minors.

In conclusion, the Internet is available, affordable, and relatively anonymous. This makes it an attractive tool for individuals desiring to participate in illegal or deviant sexual activity. The next section addresses how the Internet and its related technologies are used to engage in this type of behavior.

## COMPONENTS OF THE INTERNET USED FOR SEXUALLY DEVIANT AND ILLEGAL ACTIVITY

Using computers and the Internet to facilitate illegal and sexually deviant behavior is not a new phenomenon. In fact, pedophiles have used computer modems to communicate, create networks, and exchange victim information since the 1980s (Lesce, 1999). Although this online activity has existed for some time, sexually deviant and illegal Internet usage has evolved and changed as a result of multiple factors including new legislation, improved law enforcement tactics, and enhanced technology.

Kim & Bailey (1997) cited newsgroups, e-mail, Web sites, and chat rooms as facets of the Internet employed for sexually deviant and/or illegal purposes. These components are used to traffic child pornography (Huycke, 1997; Kantrowitz et al, 1994; Thompson, 2002), locate children to molest (Armagh, 1998; Booth, 1999; Durkin & Bryant, 1995; Jackson, 1989; Levy et al, 1995; McLaughlin, 2000), and assist in communication between pedophiles (Durkin, 1997; Kopelev, 1999). As an aside, the Internet is used by individuals throughout the world. Although it is beyond the scope of this chapter to go into detail about the unique issues related to technological globalization, this type of Internet usage does not appear to be unique to the United States.

## NEWSGROUPS

*Newsgroups* are sites on the Internet where electronic messages on the same general topic are collected. Once a message is read, the reader can respond to the "post" publicly (so the entire newsgroup can read the response) or, in some cases, can privately e-mail the original poster. Online newsgroups cater to a variety of topics, including extreme sexual subjects such as bondage, "snuff" stories (stories where individuals are murdered), and adult/minor sexual contact. The title of the newsgroup often provides an indication of the topics discussed, such as alt.sex.bestiality and alt. sex.paedophile; however, seemingly benign newsgroup titles have also been used to camouflage deviant topics. For example, pedophilic newsgroups have used titles dealing with gardening to conceal their true focus. The activity level of newsgroups varies greatly, with postings fluctuating from just a couple every few days to literally hundreds in a single day (Kim & Bailey, 1997).

Newsgroups can serve various functions. Some newsgroups provide peer support to individuals struggling with their pedophilic desires as well as validatation of pedophilic urges (Armagh, 1998; Durkin, 1997). Whereas most members of society believe that sex with children is wrong, the message from some online pedophile groups is that there is nothing aberrant about these desires or behaviors (Durkin, 1997). Information is also disseminated via newsgroups. For example, contact information for the North American Man/Boy Love Association (NAMBLA) has been provided as well as instructions on how to obtain books with pedophilic themes (Durkin, 1997). Thus, newsgroups consolidate and bring individuals with similar deviant interests together as well as provide support for deviant and illegal sexual desires and activities.

## E-MAIL

*E-mail,* an abbreviation of "electronic mail," is the most commonly used facet of the Internet (USDOC, 2001). This feature allows for rapid and inexpensive correspondence by transmitting electronic messages from one computer to another over the Internet. Still images, video clips, and audio clips can be sent as attachments in e-mail or in the body of the message itself. In addition to its benign uses, e-mail has been used in sexually deviant and illegal activity. For example, Operation Candyman, a recent FBI probe of a child pornography ring, investigated 7000 individuals who allegedly exchanged child pornography via e-mail (Thompson, 2002).

Groups advocating adult/child "relationships" also use e-mail to advance their agenda. An article that appeared in a NAMBLA bulletin stated the following:

There are several Usenet newsgroups and an e-mail mailing list where boy-lovers can make cyberspace contact with others who feel as they do; new resources can also be developed as the needs crystallize. The information superhighway can be a great way for boy-lovers to share and retrieve information and build interpersonal support around the world; the potential is certainly there (Man/boy love on the Internet, 1995).

Anonymity and security from detection are often concerns, but computer programs can be used to mask the e-mail user's identity (Kim & Bailey, 1997). Thus, one can solicit others for child pornography and not be overly concerned about his or her identity being discovered. It is logical that this sense of anonymity likely increases the possibility that one would use the Internet as opposed to traditional and less anonymous modes of communication (eg, US Postal Service, telephone) when conducting illegal activity such as requesting child pornography.

## WEB SITES

*Web sites*, often comprised of multiple Web pages, are electronic locations on the World Wide Web (WWW). Essentially, Web pages are computer files encoded in hypertext markup language (HTML) that can be accessed by Internet users. These sites provide information on numerous subjects, including a broad range of sexual topics, using photographs, video clips, text, sound clips, and even live images. In addition to providing information, these sites have directly facilitated the victimization of children. For example, one child sex ring, the Orchid Club, used a live Internet broadcast for its members to witness a 5-year-old girl being abused. The members of this closed online group actually posted requests regarding the types of abuse they wanted to view (Cusack, 1996).

As with e-mail, pro-pedophile groups recognize the benefits of using Web sites to advance their ideology. A 1995 newsletter published by NAMBLA listed and reviewed sites catering to topics that were of interest to its members (Man/boy love on the Internet, 1995). As disconcerting as it may be, numerous sites on the Web are devoted entirely to adult/child sexual issues and topics. At least some of these sites appear to be very popular. A site titled "Boys in the Real World," showing nude and seminude pictures of prepubescent boys and teens, received a quarter of a million visits within 3 months of operation (Armagh, 1998).

Some Web masters (individuals who maintain Web sites) employ deception in an attempt to increase online visitation to their Web site. An example of this, although not specifically related to child pornography, is that at one time, the unwary would find a pornographic Web site if he or she typed the Web address www.whitehouse.com instead of the official address, www.whitehouse.gov, to access the Web site of the US government's White House. This online deception is particularly salient when one considers that children may access pornographic sites or newsgroups when attempting to find information on seemingly innocuous topics such as the White House.

Finally, a disconcerting practice that some online pedophile groups engage in is including hyperlinks to legitimate child organizations on their Web sites. *Hyperlinks* are means of accessing other Web sites simply by clicking on a certain word, phrase, or picture. For example, online communities advocating "man-boy relationships" have hyperlinks to the Boy Scouts of America's official Web site as well as Web sites for several child adoption agencies. Thus, one could read posts about seducing children and then, with a simple click of a mouse, start the process of volunteering with the Boy Scouts or acquire information on adopting a child.

## Chat Rooms

Internet *chat rooms*, sites on the Internet where individuals communicate in real time by typing text, cater to a variety of interests and age groups. Since the Internet allows considerable anonymity, child sex offenders can present themselves as children or adolescents online. The anonymity of cyberspace makes it difficult to discern if an individual is a child communicating with other children for benign reasons or an adult masquerading as a child for nefarious purposes. Thus, adults can interact with children in chat rooms for extended periods of time without their presence being considered suspicious.

Although many chat rooms cater to children, chat rooms also exist that advocate the sexual exploitation of children. There are even chat rooms designated for individuals with specific interests in children of particular age groups and ethnic backgrounds (McLaughlin, 2000). These chat rooms bring pedophiles together and act as a consolidating mechanism to facilitate the exchange of child pornography and to reinforce deviant views pertaining to adult/minor sexual contact (USDOJ, Equality and Law Reform, 1998). The implications of participating in these chat rooms will be discussed in greater detail later in the chapter.

Evidence clearly indicates the Internet is being used as a tool in the sexual exploitation of children. Newsgroups, e-mail, Web sites, and chat rooms have all been used for sexually deviant or illegal purposes related to the sexual victimization of children. The next section will address in more detail how these components of the Internet have been used, as well as how their usage may impact sex offender treatment.

# SEXUALLY DEVIANT AND ILLEGAL INTERNET USAGE

## CHILD PORNOGRAPHY

Any discussion regarding child pornography should include the United States Supreme Court ruling *Ashcroft v Free Speech Coalition* (2002). This decision up-held the 9th US Circuit Court of Appeals' objection to the Child Pornography Prevention Act (CPPA) of 1996. One of the original purposes of this act was to make pornographic images of individuals who appeared to be, but were not actually under the age of 18, illegal. The recent Supreme Court's ruling negated the "appeared" portion of the act and effectively legalized digitally created images of child pornography. These images can be morphed (altered) pictures of adults made to appear to be under the age of 18 or digitally created images that appear to be of an actual child. Given the recentness of the ruling, it is as yet unclear what impact, if any, it will have on the amount of virtual child pornography on the Internet. Regardless of the change in legal statutes of virtual child pornography, distributing pornographic images of actual individuals under the age of 18 is still illegal. This section focuses on images that currently fall under the courts' definition of "actual" and, thus, illegal child pornography.

Child pornography on the Internet has received tremendous attention over the past several years. Articles abound in the popular press concerning law enforcement sting operations apprehending distributors of child pornography, as well as stories about pop culture icons and other popular figures who have been arrested for downloading these types of images (**Figure 22-1**). Although child pornography was available before the advent of the Internet, this technology has facilitated its resurgence in popularity as well as its availability.

As previously discussed, individuals have used the Internet to collect/trade child pornography for several reasons. In addition to the availability and anonymity that the Internet provides, this technology also allows for the rapid and inexpensive reproduction and exchange of these images. Child pornography can be duplicated simply by using the "copy" feature available on most computer programs, thereby eliminating the need for specialized reproduction equipment. It can also be rapidly transmitted around the world. O'Connell & Taylor (1998) reported that, in 1996, a colleague tracked a marked image from computers in Australia to Europe as well as from computers in Europe to North America within a 24-hour time period.

In addition, the Internet appears to foster a sense of cognitive dissonance where individuals do not believe they are doing anything wrong or are harming anyone by "simply" downloading these images from the Web. Although individuals arrested for viewing child pornography via the Internet may initially dispute that their actions have harmed children, the reality is that downloading child pornography perpetuates child sexual abuse on multiple levels. One of the ways this occurs is through a process referred to as habituation (Taylor, 1999). Most individuals who download images of child pornography do so for sexual arousal (Quayle & Taylor, 2002a). However, they tire of viewing and masturbating to the same set of images and are, thus, continually searching for more stimulating/arousing material to fuel their sexual fantasies. This desire for novel material is one of the mechanisms that drives the production of child pornography.

Given the ease of duplicating images, it is difficult to tell how many children have been victimized by online pornography; however, one study examining more than 50 000 images of child pornography downloaded from the Internet identified more than 2000 boys and girls in sexually explicit pictures (Taylor, 1999). Many of the images appeared to be 10 to 15 years old (Taylor, 1999). This suggests that numerous children are sexually exploited and, in many cases, the exploitation via pictures appearing on the Web has occurred for years.

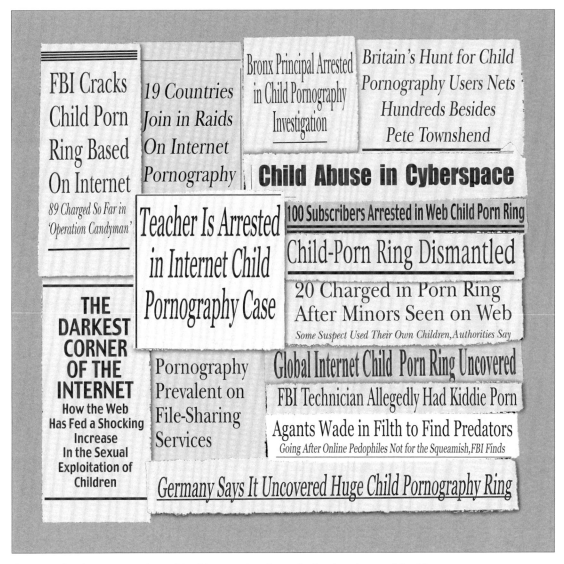

**Figure 22-1.** *Child sexually exploitative Internet usage is gaining increased media attention.*

An issue that has generated considerable attention from the legal and mental health communities is the relationship between downloading online child pornography and committing contact sex offenses. Regarding viewing child pornography over the Internet and its relationship to hands-on sex offenses, Medaris & Girouard (2002), wrote

[m]any in the law enforcement community believe that the validation and nearly constant stimulation afforded to sex offenders by the Internet put minors at greater risk for sexual exploitation. By creating a demand for new material, the Internet also creates a demand for more victims, and it may cause some individuals to move from voyeuristic activities to acting out their fantasies with live victims.

Unfortunately, research focusing on this area is limited and the results are somewhat inconsistent. Hernandez (2000) found that sex offenders who were convicted of possession of child pornography or ***traveling*** (crossing state lines to engage a minor in sex) charges committed contact sexual offenses at a higher rate (30.5 victims per offender) than sex offenders convicted specifically of contact sex crimes (9.6 victims per offender). However, Malesky (2002), who used a sample similar to the one used by Hernandez (2000), did not find a significant difference in the number of contact victims between Internet-related offenders and convicted contact sex offenders who denied viewing online child pornography. In addition, Darren Brookes, a detective inspector with the Hi-Tec Crime Unit in the United Kingdom and Internet sex offender researcher, has not found a significant difference in the number of contact victims between individuals with Internet-related convictions and those with contact convictions (D. Brookes, oral, written, and electronic communication, August 20, 2003).

Although somewhat inconsistent, the results of all 3 studies suggest that many adjudicated Internet offenders have at least as many contact victims as individuals convicted of contact sex crimes.

Although research projects are underway to assess dangerousness in pedophiles through their collection of child pornography (Taylor et al, 2001), assessment procedures do not currently exist to determine an individual's risk for contact offenses based solely on his or her online behavior. Internet offenders, like child sex offenders in general, comprise a heterogeneous group. Some of these individuals use computer programs to search out and download images of child pornography automatically whereas others spend hours a day downloading and categorizing images. For other offenders, pornographic images of children make up only a small percentage of their overall pornographic collection, and some individuals engage in a cycle of downloading and then deleting images. It is yet unknown what, if any, predictors for contact offenses can be gleaned from one's online behavior. This is obviously an area that is in need of additional research from a therapeutic and evaluative standpoint.

Although sexual gratification is likely the primary reason most individuals collect child pornography, it does not appear to be the sole motivation for engaging in this online activity (O'Connell & Taylor, 1998; Quayle & Taylor, 2002a). In fact, pictures may be collected for a variety of reasons. Images of child pornography are often part of a larger collection or series. In many instances, these series come with their own names such as the "Amy" or "Kevin" series (supposedly named after the victim in the pictures) (Lee, 2003). Offenders may attempt to complete an entire series much like a baseball card collector tries to complete sets of cards from a ball player's rookie year through his final season. Requests are routinely made on pedophile bulletin boards for specific images such as "amy173" or "kevin049" to complete a particular series or set of photographs (Lee, 2003).

Offenders also exchange images as a way to increase their social status and credibility in virtual pedophile communities (O'Connell & Taylor, 1998). In fact, some individuals collect images of child pornography that they do not find sexually arousing with the intent of "helping" others complete a series. This is done with the anticipation that these individuals will reciprocate in the future (O'Connell & Taylor, 1998). It has even been suggested that there is a "collector syndrome," that is, the compulsive acquisition of pictures for its own sake (Taylor, 1999). Although there is an expanding body of research literature regarding "cyber addiction," little attention has been given to compulsive collecting of child pornography. In short, there may be multiple reasons beyond simple sexual gratification for why individuals download images of child pornography from the Internet. It is important, however, to remember that sexual motivation appears to be the primary impetus of most individuals seeking out and collecting child pornography (Quayle & Taylor, 2002a).

## LOCATING CHILDREN TO MOLEST
In approximately 60% of the child sexual abuse cases reported to law enforcement, the offenders were nonrelative acquaintances of the victims (USDOJ, 2000). This statistic indicates that the majority of offenders know their victims prior to offending. One way sex offenders get acquainted with their victims is by communicating with them over the Internet (Booth, 1999; Durkin & Bryant, 1995; Jackson, 1989; Kopelev, 1999; Lamb, 1998; Lambert, 2003; Lanning, 1998; Levy et al, 1995; McLaughlin, 2000). These exploitative online relationships can take months to develop and may involve the offender spending literally hundreds of hours communicating with his or her intended victims before establishing face-to-face contact.

Online chat rooms appear to be a common forum used by offenders to contact potential victims (Armagh, 1998; Kantrowitz et al, 1994; Kopelev, 1999; Lamb, 1998; McLaughlin, 2000; Thomas, 1997). Malesky & Malesky (unpublished data, 2003) found that nearly three quarters of the 31 offenders in their study who used the Internet to meet children for sex indicated that chat room dialogue, specifically comments of a sexual nature, were used to identify potential victims. These authors also found that minors mentioning sex in any fashion (eg, in a child's online profile, screen name, posting, e-mail) prompted some offenders to contact these individuals. Several offenders in this study also indicated that minors who appeared needy or submissive online were targeted as potential victims. For example, one participant in the Malesky & Malesky (unpublished date, 2003) study stated, "neediness is very apparent when a child will do anything to keep talking to you. Also, that they are always online shows a low sense of parental contact or interest in the child."

In addition, the minor's screen name, especially if it sounds young, motivates some individuals to contact the child/adolescent. In response to the question in Malesky & Malesky's (unpublished data, 2003) study, "What initially attracted you to a particular child/adolescent online?" one participant wrote, "They usually had their age as pat [sic] of their id. eg. LINDA14." Thus, mentioning sex in any fashion, neediness, and readily apparent age are information or behaviors that have attracted some online predators to specific minors.

After establishing online contact with children or adolescents, many offenders attempt to set up in-person meetings with their potential victims. Adults traveling specifically for sex with minors is not a new phenomenon. Although not dealing with the Internet, a European study conducted in 1975 of self-identified pedophiles found that 51% of the participants reported traveling abroad for sexual contact with minors at least once a year (Bernard, 1975). As in the 1970s, sex offenders today are willing to travel significant distances to victimize children or adolescents that they have befriended over the Internet (Booth, 1999; Durkin, 1997; McLaughlin, 2000).

In summary, offenders have used the Internet to access potential victims. Given that many children's and adolescents' online activity is unsupervised, cyberspace has become a prime venue for predatory sex offenders to meet potential victims.

## COMMUNICATION WITH OTHER CHILD SEX OFFENDERS
Child sex offenders use the Internet not only to access potential victims but also communicate with likeminded individuals who advocate the sexual exploitation of minors (Armagh, 1998; Durkin, 1996; Jackson, 1989; Malesky & Ennis, 2004). A chilling example of this involved 2 Virginia men who met online and attempted to use a computer bulletin board to locate a 12-year-old boy for a pornographic snuff film. They planned to videotape themselves molesting and then murdering the adolescent (Jackson, 1989). Fortunately, a San Jose police officer became aware of these 2 men as they sought other individuals online with a sexual interest in children and was able to stop them before a child was victimized. In another case, a law enforcement agent posing online as the father of an 8-year-old girl stated that he was having sadomasochistic fantasies about his daughter and wondered what others thought he should do about his fantasies. The responses to his online inquiry included advice on how to torture his daughter and a suggestion that he use a date rape drug to sedate her (Masland, 2000). More common than these dramatic examples are the daily online exchange of pedophilic information. Malesky & Ennis (2004) found that providing information on pedophilia, such as links to related Web sites, occurred in more than 12% of a sample of the posts to an online pedophile message board. In addition, more than half (53%) of the posts in this study contained pictures, drawings, poetry, and/or stories related to boy love.

Another study examining the postings on a man/boy love newsgroup found that almost one quarter of the posts were attempts to set up contact with other members (Durkin, 1996). One post quoted by Durkin (1996) read as follows:

I am missing one thing: somebody I can talk to who has the same feelings as I have. It is great to know Manni and others from the Net, but I need somebody I can see, hear, smell, and feel if I talk to him. So please, if there is somebody from Vienna lurking around, try to contact me via e-mail. If you have doubts that I am a cop—and I bet you have because I had those too when I wrote my first mail—use an anonymous remailer or something like that. Maybe we learn to trust each other after a while. In short: is there a boy lover from Vienna, Austria: please e-mail me!

Additional postings indicated that individuals had already met in person as a result of the newsgroup (Durkin, 1996).

Even if offenders do not meet face to face, their cyber exchanges serve to support, encourage, and ultimately reinforce their deviant ideologies. Malesky & Ennis (2004) hypothesized that participation on pro-pedophile newsgroups provides individuals with a sense of community that may be lacking in other aspects of their lives. The fact that individuals are able to communicate with others who not only share their pedophilic interests but also listen to similar music, read the same books, and have the same hobbies likely has a tremendous normalizing effect on their deviant interests.

Unfortunately, research addressing the effects of Internet communication between pedophiles is sparse. However, one study conducted with participants in a sex offender treatment program in a federal prison found that more than half of the participants who admitted engaging in sexually deviant Internet usage engaged in online communication with other individuals who supported adult/minor sexual contact (Malesky, 2002). Results from this study are summarized in **Table 22-1**. It should be noted that only 2% of this sample reported being members of a formal organization that advocated this type of sexual contact (eg, NAMBLA). Although it is unknown how many participants in this study would have been affiliated with formal organizations such as NAMBLA if the Internet did not exist, it makes intuitive sense that virtual communities and online correspondence have assumed some of the functions previously offered by these organizations. With this said, it should be noted

**Table 22-1. Online Communication With Supporters of Adult/Minor Sexual Contact by Sexually Deviant Internet Users**

|  | Yes n (%) | No n (%) |
| --- | --- | --- |
| Visited a chat room/bulletin board that supports sexual contact between adults and children | 62 (61.4) | 39 (38.6) |
| Posted to a chat room/bulletin board that supports sexual contact between adults and children | 32 (31.7) | 69 (68.3) |
| Exchanged information online for the purpose of sharing victims | 9 (9.5) | 86 (90.5) |
| Corresponded online with individuals who support adult/minor sexual relationships | 53 (52.5) | 48 (47.5) |
| Had membership in an organization that advocates for adult/minor sexual contact (eg, NAMBLA) | 2 (2) | 99 (98) |

*Reprinted from Malesky LA. Sexually Deviant Internet Usage by Child Sex Offenders [unpublished doctoral dissertation]. Memphis, Tenn: University of Memphis; 2002.*

that some formal organizations use the Internet to perpetuate their agenda as evidenced by the existence of NAMBLA's own Web site.

Finally, it should be noted that some offenders use the Internet frequently (several times a week, if not daily) to correspond with individuals advocating "sexual relationships" between minors and adults (Malesky, 2002). This routine and frequent communication likely strengthens and validates an already entrenched belief system regarding adult/minor sexual contact for some offenders. These supportive exchanges, as well as their effects on sex offender treatment, are discussed in detail in the following section.

## THE INTERNET ROLE IN THE ETIOLOGY OF CHILD SEXUAL ABUSE

*Social Learning Theory*, by Albert Bandura, is helpful in conceptualizing the Internet's role in the etiology of some sexually abusive behaviors directed toward children. Bandura (1977) stated that learning occurs through observing and interacting with others. According to this theory, the individuals with whom one has the most contact and interaction will likely have the greatest influence on the person's learning process (Bandura, 1977). Applying the tenets of *Social Learning Theory* to deviant behavior, Akers (1977) wrote that "most of the learning relevant to deviant behavior is the result of social interactions or exchange in which the words, responses, presence, and behavior of other persons make reinforcers available."

Regarding deviant behavior, Bandura (1977) also stated, "opportunities for learning aggressive conduct, for example, differ markedly for members of assaultive gangs and for members of groups exemplifying pacific lifestyles." It follows from Akers' (1977) and Bandura's (1977) statements that if individuals spend a great deal of time interacting in pro-pedophile chat rooms, visiting pro-pedophile Web sites, and communicating with individuals advocating for the sexual exploitation of minors, the behaviors and attitudes observed in these online exchanges will likely be adopted and/or reinforced. The following post on a pro-man/boy love newsgroup, cited by Durkin (1996), supports this position:

Because of this newsgroup, I realized only one and a half months ago that I am a boy lover. I laughed, I cried, and I shared all your beautiful, sad, and funny postings. It was the first time in my life that someone showed feelings which seemed to be mine. Even I have to admit that I never was in love with a boy until now. Last week I found him and I want to be with him all the time … His name is Lukas (not his real name). He is 13 years old and he is the son of a friend I know from the university … I fell in love with him the first second I saw him … I look at him and imagine what we could do if we were alone.

Taking this posting at face value, it appears that communication via the Internet can strengthen some individuals' pro-pedophilic attitudes as well as facilitate fantasies of molesting children. It should also be noted that direct peer validation is quite common among certain virtual communities. Malesky & Ennis (2004) found validation of pedophilic ideologies in more than 21% of the posts made to a pro-pedophile online message board.

Modeling or observing others can serve a disinhibatory function and affect changes in moral judgment. Bandura (1977) stated that "seeing others engage in threatening or prohibited activities without adverse consequences can reduce inhibitions in observers." Thus, individuals who have engaged in deviant or illegal behavior online with apparent impunity may be indirectly encouraging others to act in a similar fashion. This is especially salient considering that only a small percentage of those who commit illegal activity online get caught (Armagh, 1998; McLaughlin, 2000).

## COGNITIVE DISTORTIONS

In conjunction with modeling behavior, a variety of cognitive beliefs also contribute to the perpetration of child sexual abuse. Bandura (1977) proposed that individuals use cognitive restructuring to engage in inappropriate behavior and avoid negative feelings associated with their actions. The view that cognitive restructuring (or *cognitive distortions*) influences sexual abusive behavior has substantial support in the research literature (Abel et al, 1989; Bumby, 1996; DeYoung, 1988; Durkin, 1996, 1997; Durkin & Bryant, 1999; Hayashino et al, 1995; Murphy, 1990; Neidigh & Krop, 1992; Pollock & Hashmall, 1991; Scully & Marolla, 1984; Stermac & Segal, 1989; Veach, 1999).

One way offenders employ erroneous thinking is by portraying reprehensible conduct as being in the service of a greater good and thus morally justifiable (Bandura, 1977). For example, some individuals who advocate adult/child sexual "relationships" state that they are striving for the sexual emancipation of children (De Young, 1988; Durkin & Bryant, 1999). These offenders believe they are helping children by fighting for their rights and sexual liberation. Moral justifications are extremely powerful cognitive distortions because, in addition to eliminating self-generated deterrents, they also reward deviant behavior by making it a source of self-pride (Bandura, 1977). An example of this type of distortion is the belief that active members of online pedophilic communities are similar to civil rights leaders in that they are both fighting for the rights of disenfranchised groups.

Contrasting reprehensible acts with even more deplorable conduct is also used to diminish the negative consequences of the abuse (Bandura, 1977). For example, child sex offenders may admit to fondling a child but believe that this act is acceptable when compared to the sexual penetration of a minor. Similarly, euphemistic language is used to mask the severity of reprehensible conduct (Bandura, 1977) and may occur when an offender uses an inoffensive statement in place of one that carries negative connotations. Examples of euphemistic language frequently found on the Internet include terms such as "boy lover" and "girl lover." Although it is unlikely that the general public equates love with the expressed feelings, thoughts, and behaviors of these individuals, the terms likely serve to relieve the cognitive dissonance associated with these individuals' thoughts and behaviors. By conceptualizing themselves in such fashion, offenders avoid the pejorative designation of terms such as child molester or pervert and are able to conceptualize themselves as individuals with romantic interests in children (Durkin & Bryant, 1999).

The cognitive distortions of minimizing, ignoring, or misconstruing the consequences of one's actions are also employed to excuse deplorable behavior (Bandura, 1977; Durkin & Bryant, 1999; Scully & Marolla, 1984; Veach, 1999). Bandura (1977) stated that as long as individuals "disregard the detrimental effects of their conduct, there is little likelihood that self-censuring reactions will be activated." Consistent with these distortions, many sex offenders view their crimes as less serious than do other members of society (Stermac & Segal, 1989; Veach, 1999). These errors can also be found online. For example, 39% of the identified pedophiles on a newsgroup exhibited the distorted view that sexual contact between adults and children does not harm the child (Durkin & Bryant, 1999). Some child sex offenders go beyond denying that sexual abuse harms children and actually claim that this type of sexual behavior is beneficial for the minors (De Young, 1988; Stermac & Segal, 1989). Almost 10% of admitted pedophiles using a boy-lover newsgroup asserted that children benefit from having sexual "relationships" with adults. One pedophile was quoted as posting, "[i]n all cases, the boys had a noticeable improvement in their self-esteem, their grades in school went up, they became more stable emotionally" (Durkin & Bryant, 1999).

Individuals apprehended for possession of child pornography also demonstrate cognitive distortions such as "contrasting reprehensible acts with even more deplorable conduct" and "minimizing, ignoring, or misconstruing the consequences of one's actions." For example, one offender who was incarcerated for possession of child pornography informed this author that he initially expected his parole officer (he was on parole for committing contact sexual offenses against minors) to "congratulate" him for viewing child pornography as opposed to "actually offending against a child."

This case demonstrates the inability or unwillingness of some offenders to recognize that the children in these images are actual people who have been victimized. Likewise, Internet offenders commonly state they do not understand what the "big deal is" regarding child pornography. After all, they are "only pictures" and the viewers never "actually harmed" anyone. As with the example above, these offenders do not realize, as stated in a bulletin by the US Department of Justice, that "the Internet provides a source for repeated long-term victimization of a child that can last for years, often without the victim's knowledge. Once a child's picture is displayed on the Internet, it can remain there forever" (USDOJ, 2001). In part to counter the cognitive distortions employed by offenders regarding these images, a move is underway in Europe to refer to child pornography as child abuse images, thereby placing more attention on the victims and eliminating the commercial connotation associated with the term pornography (Lee, 2003).

Distorted thinking is also exhibited when child sex offenders attempt to shift the responsibility for their actions from themselves to those who condemn them (eg, parents, law enforcement, psychologists) (De Young, 1988). Regarding a group of self-admitted pedophiles on a boy-lover Usenet group, Durkin & Bryant (1999) found that almost a third of the pedophiles used "condemnation of the condemners" as a cognitive defense mechanism. These individuals targeted law enforcement officers, social workers, mental health professionals, and parents for condemnation and often accused them of draconian persecution of pedophiles. Particularly illustrative examples of this distortion are apparent in a post on a pedophile newsgroup. This post is in response to several posts by gay men stating that pedophilia is aberrant and has nothing to do with homosexuality. The response is as follows (Durkin & Bryant, 1999):

Oh wow, you're a good homosexual. You should be accepted by society. And in many countries you will indeed. You might even find yourself integrated in society as being a homosexual. No, you don't want to be classified in the same category as those nasty, tasteless, and horrible pedophiles. You don't like the young boys so you don't even want to think about those pedophile bastards. Come on you guys! What was the situation about half a century ago? Homosexuals were in the same position as pedophiles are nowadays. People looked upon homosexuals as being nasty, tasteless, and horrible bastards. Now YOU are doing the same toward another group. You're right: pedophiles aren't in the same group, but a little bit of understanding is the least pedophiles could expect from a previously repressed group.

It is evident from the tone of this posting that the writer is condemning the gay men who took exception with pedophilia for not being open-minded and accepting of his sexual choices. By condemning these individuals and focusing on their statements, posters are able to avoid examining harmful beliefs and behaviors.

An additional example of the condemnation of the condemners appeared in the glossary of the frequently asked questions section of a boy-love Web site. In this example, the Web masters defined a "child advocate" as:

person or persons who claim to stand up for the rights of children and "protect" them from "child molestors" [sic] with whom we are ignorantly—and sometimes knowingly—lumped together. Some CA's work in government positions, some work for private organizations, and some work on their own ("vigilantes"). They watch this board, so it is important that you be careful with personal details.

Both of the preceding examples attempt to shift the negative focus from boy lovers to those whom most would consider child advocates.

Child sex offenders also employ the cognitive processes of blaming and dehumanizing the victim to avoid feeling guilty about their actions (Bandura, 1977; Scully & Marolla, 1984; Veach, 1999). Stermac & Segal (1989) found that child sex offenders attributed more responsibility to children and less responsibility to adults for the occurrence of sexual abuse than did rapists, clinicians, lawyers, police, or a group of "laypersons." By displacing responsibility, offenders avoided viewing themselves as accountable for their actions and were spared self-prohibiting reactions (Bandura, 1977). "Blaming the victim" is exhibited when offenders attribute their illegal behavior (eg, sending child pornography) to the children (or even undercover law enforcement agents) who received the images. These offenders commonly argue that the minors (or law enforcement) should be held accountable for the offenders' conduct because they were the ones who initially requested the child pornography. By taking this stance, offenders externalize the impetus for their behavior and avoid accepting responsibility for their actions.

A final point worthy of mention is the Internet's ability to introduce deviant fantasies to individuals who, before accessing the Internet, may have never explored their pedophilic desires. Regarding these individuals, McGrath & Casey (2002) stated, "by reducing disincentives, the Internet effectively dissolves the boundaries between fantasy and reality, enabling individuals to explore and realize their fantasies. A man who would never approach a child in the real world may make such contact in cyberspace just to see what might happen." If this individual's online interaction is reinforced through communicating with an actual child or even an adult masquerading as a child, then he or she may become more brazen in his or her online interactions. Furthermore, if this individual begins masturbating while interacting with children (or adults who he believes are children) online, it is likely that his deviant sexual fantasies will be further reinforced. The physical reinforcement associated with masturbation coupled with the cognitive distortions that are introduced and subsequently strengthened through online interactions may move the individual closer to actually offending against a child than if he or she had never accessed the Internet. With this said, however, a warning must also be issued. Given the dearth of research in this area, the effects of Internet usage on sex offenders are still largely speculative in nature at this time. However, Internet sex offenders possess unique issues for treatment providers and evaluators.

## RECOMMENDATIONS FOR EVALUATING AND TREATING INTERNET-RELATED SEX OFFENDERS

In addition to the points and recommendations made throughout this chapter, a few additional suggestions warrant mention. One of the goals of sex offender treatment is to enable offenders to identify situations that place them at risk to reoffend (Nelson & Jackson, 1989). For many Internet offenders, the Internet itself is a high-risk situation to be avoided. As discussed in the previous section, cognitive distortions are employed by some Internet sex offenders to justify and rationalize their online behavior. Continued participation in pro-pedophile online communication will likely strengthen offenders' distorted schemata, thereby making them more resistant to treatment. Thus, professionals involved in treatment and/or community monitoring of Internet sex offenders should prohibit Internet usage or at least closely monitor the type of online activity the offender engages in.

Some Internet offenders spend an exorbitant amount of time online. Malesky (2002) found that more than 25% of the incarcerated Internet offenders in his study were online 40 or more hours a week prior to their arrest. It is unlikely that these participants spent all of their online time engaged in sexually deviant or illegal activity, especially since several of them were employed in the computer and Internet fields. However, for at least some of these offenders, their time online may have interfered with forming or maintaining adaptive interpersonal relationships (Moody, 2001). Given that the establishment and maintenance of healthy adult relationships is often a goal of sex offender treatment, a clinical recommendation is that offenders focus on developing and strengthening "real life" pro-social adult relationships instead of spending excessive amounts of time online.

Ensuring complete compliance with Internet restriction for all offenders would be virtually impossible; however, several steps can be taken to minimize the possibility that these individuals will engage in deviant or illegal Internet usage. First, Internet offenders who were employed in the computer/Internet fields should be encouraged to pursue employment opportunities where they are not required to work extensively with computers or on the Internet. Even in cases where offenders spend minimal time online, their online activity should be actively monitored. Second, Internet offenders should not be allowed to have Internet access in their homes. If the presence of other family members or roommates makes this suggestion unrealistic, then the offender should be closely monitored to ensure that there is no misuse of the Internet. Finally, probation and parole officers working with this population should receive specialized training focusing on computer usage and the Internet to assist them in monitoring these offenders. Although these suggestions are not a panacea to prevent offenders from accessing the Internet, they do make it more difficult for offenders to engage in illegal or sexually inappropriate online behavior.

Forensic evaluators and treatment providers involved with Internet-related sex offender cases should become educated about Internet technology as well as become familiar with its unique lexicon. It has even been suggested that evaluators actively monitor newsgroups that may contain information related to their case (McGrath & Casey, 2002). Unfortunately, it appears that many individuals are unprepared to handle the unique challenges that Internet sex offenders present (Buttell & Carney, 2001; Quayle & Taylor, 2002b). Consequently, additional research is needed to focus on the unique treatment and evaluative issues specific to this population. In addition to research, however, it is also imperative that training be conducted to impart this information to those professionals who work with this population.

## CONCLUSION

As indicated by the information presented in this chapter, individuals have used the Internet and its related technologies to engage in a variety of sexually deviant and illegal activities directed toward children. In addition to the direct victimization of children perpetrated via the Internet (ie, disseminating child pornography), this technology has also facilitated the introduction and reinforcement of deviant beliefs regarding adult/minor sexual contact. This type of Internet usage likely hampers sex offender treatment efficacy by enabling individuals to become more resilient to therapeutic interventions.

Although cases involving individuals downloading child pornography from the Internet have received tremendous attention over the past several years, this behavior's relationship to committing contact offenses is still unclear. Some have suggested that viewing child pornography over the Internet as well as engaging in sexually deviant communication may act as gateway behaviors to committing hands-on offenses (Lanning, 1998; Medaris & Girouard, 2002), whereas others have suggested that this technology is simply used as an additional tool to satisfy individuals' deviant sexual desires (D. Brookes, oral, written, and electronic communication, August 20, 2003).

The ambiguity of this relationship coupled with the increasing number of individuals who are accessing this material via the Internet necessitates the development of accurate psychometric instruments assessing risk for contact offenses based on individuals' Internet usage. Treatment providers and evaluators who work with Internet-related sex offenders must educate themselves about the unique issues of this population as well as about the Internet and its related technologies. Hopefully, this increased awareness coupled with more extensive research will expedite the development and implementation of effective treatment strategies, evaluation procedures, and supervision techniques to curtail these maladaptive behaviors and consequently lower the number of children who are sexually victimized.

# REFERENCES

Abel GG, Becker JV, Mittelman MS, Cunningham-Rathner J, Rouleau JL, Murphy WD. Self-reported sex crimes of nonincarcerated paraphiliacs. *J Interpers Violence*. 1987;2(1):3-25.

Abel GG, Gore DK, Holland CL, Camp N, Becker JV, Rathner J. The measurement of the cognitive distortions of child molesters. *Ann Sex Research*. 1989;2:135-153.

Ahlmeyer S, Heil P, McKee B, English K. The impact of polygraphy on admissions and victims of offenses in adult sexual offenders. *Sex Abuse*. 2000;12(2):123-138.

Akers RL. *Deviant Behavior: A Social Learning Approach*. 2nd ed. Belmont, Calif: Wasworth Publishing Co; 1977.

Armagh G. A safety net for the Internet: protecting our children. *Juvenile Justice*. 1998;5(1):9-15.

*Ashcroft v Free Speech Coalition*, 535 US 234 (9th Cir 2002).

Bandura A. *Social Learning Theory*. Englewood Cliffs, NJ: Prentice Hall; 1977.

Bernard F. An enquiry among a group of pedophiles. *J Sex Research*. 1975;11(3): 242-255.

Booth W. Internet target: sexual predators. *Washington Post*. December 7, 1999:A29.

Brody JE. Cybersex gives birth to a psychological disorder. *New York Times*. May 16, 2000:7, 12.

Bumby KM. Assessing the cognitive distortions of child molesters and rapists: development and validation of the MOLEST and RAPE scales. *Sex Abuse*. 1996;8(1): 37-54.

Buttell FP, Carney MM. Treatment provider awareness of the possible impact of the Internet on the treatment of sex offenders: an alert to a problem. *J Child Sex Abuse*. 2001;10(3):117-125.

Conly CH. *Organizing for Computer Crime Investigation and Prosecution*. Washington, DC: US Dept of Justice; 1989.

Cooper A. Sexuality and the Internet: surfing into the new millennium. *Cyberpsychol Behav*. 1998;1(2):187-193.

Cooper A, Delmonico DL, Burg R. Cybersex users, abusers, and compulsives: new findings and implications. *Sex Addict Compulsivity*. 2000;7:5-29.

Cooper A, Scherer CR, Boies SC, Gordon BL. Sexuality on the Internet: from sexual exploration to pathological expression. *Prof Psychol Res Pr*. 1999;30(2):154-164.

Cusack J. The murky world of Internet porn: the 'Orchid Club' shakes up the law. *World Press Review*. 1996;43:8-10.

De Young M. The indignant page: techniques of neutralization in the publications of pedophile organizations. *Child Abuse Negl*. 1988;12:583-591.

Durkin KF. *Accounts and Sexual Deviance in Cyberspace: The Case of Pedophilia* [unpublished doctoral dissertation]. Blacksburg, Va: Virginia Polytechnic Institute and State University; 1996.

Durkin KF. Misuse of the Internet by pedophiles: implications for law enforcement and probation practice. *Fed Probat*. 1997;61(3):14-18.

Durkin KF, Bryant CD. Log on to sex: some notes on the carnal computer and erotic cyberspace as an emerging research frontier. *Deviant Behav*. 1995;16(3):179-200.

Durkin KF, Bryant CD. Propagandizing pederasty: a thematic analysis of the online exculpatory accounts of unrepentant pedophiles. *Deviant Behav.* 1999;20:103-127.

Finkelhor D, Mitchell KJ, Wolak J. *Online Victimization: A Report on the Nation's Youth.* Alexandria, Va: National Center for Missing & Exploited Children; 2000.

Free Spirits: BoyChat. http://www.boychat.org/faq.html#teens. Accessed August 24, 2003.

Garreau J. Bawdy bytes: the growing world of cybersex. *Washington Post.* November 29, 1993:A1, A10.

Hayashino DS, Wurtele SK, Klebe KJ. Child molesters: an examination of cognitive factors. *J Interpers Violence.* 1995;10(1):106-116.

Hernandez AE. Self-reported contact sexual offenses by participants in the Federal Bureau of Prisons' sex offender treatment program: implications for Internet sex offenders. Poster session presented at: 19th Annual Research and Treatment Conference of the Association for the Treatment of Sexual Abusers; November 2000; San Diego, Calif.

Huycke DF. Protecting our children: the US customs service child pornography enforcement program. *The Police Chief.* 1997;34:34-35.

Jackson RL. Child molesters use electronic networks: computer-crime sleuths go undercover. *Los Angeles Times.* October 1, 1989:20, 21.

Kantrowitz B, King P, Rosenberg D. Child abuse in cyberspace. *Newsweek.* April 18, 1994:40.

Kim PY, Bailey JM. Sidestreets on the information highway: paraphilias and sexual variations on the Internet. *J Sex Educ Ther.* 1997;22(1):35-43.

Kopelev SD. Cyber sex offenders: how to proactively investigate Internet crimes against children. *Law Enforcement Technology.* 1999;26(11):46-50.

Lamb M. Cybersex: research notes on the characteristics of the visitors to online chat rooms. *Deviant Behav.* 1998;19:121-135.

Lambert B. Odd call for a cab leads to charges alleging sex crimes. *New York Times* [electronic version]. Available at: http://www.nytimes.com/2003/03/01nyregion/01 TAXI.html. Accessed March 1, 2003.

Lanning KV. *Child Molesters: A Behavioral Analysis.* 3rd ed. Washington, DC: National Center for Missing & Exploited Children; 1992.

Lanning KV. Cyber pedophiles: a behavioral perspective. *The APSAC Advisor.* 1998; 11(4):12-18.

Lee J. High tech helps child pornographers and their pursuers. *New York Times* [electronic version]. February 2003. Available at: http://www.nytimes.com/2003/02/ 09technology/09PORN.html. Accessed February 9, 2003.

Leiblum SR. Sex and the Net: clinical implications. *J Sex Educ Ther.* 1997;22(1): 21-27.

Lesce T. Pedophiles on the Internet: law enforcement investigates abuse. *Law and Order.* 1999;47(5):74-78.

Levy S, Hafner K, Rosenstiel T, et al. No place for kids? *Newsweek.* July 3, 1995;126: 47-50.

Malesky LA. *Sexually Deviant Internet Usage by Child Sex Offenders* [unpublished doctoral dissertation]. Memphis, Tenn: University of Memphis; 2002.

Malesky LA, Ennis LP. Supportive distortions: an analysis of postings on a pedophile Internet message board. *J Addict Offender Couns.* 2004;24(2):92-100.

Man/boy love on the Internet. *NAMBLA Bulletin.* 1995;16(2):6-10.

Masland M. Stalking child molesters on the net. Available at:http://www.msnbc.com/news/192795.asp. Accessed September 4, 2000.

McGrath MG, Casey E. Forensic psychiatry and the Internet: practical perspectives on sexual predators and obsessional harassers in cyberspace. *J Am Acad Psychiatry Law.* 2002;30(1):81-94.

McLaughlin JF. Cyber child sex offender typology. Available at:http://www.ci.keene.nh.us/police/Typology.htm. Accessed June 15, 2000.

Medaris M, Girouard C. *Protecting Children in Cyberspace: The ICAC Task Force Program.* Washington, DC: Office of Juvenile Justice and Delinquency Prevention, Government Printing Office; January 2002. NCJ 191213. 2-3.

Moody RJ. Internet use and its relationship to loneliness. *Cyberpsychol Behav.* 2001; 4 (3):393-397.

Murphy WD. Assessment and modification of cognitive distortions in sex offenders. In: Marshall W, Laws DR, Barbaree HE, eds. *Handbook of Sexual Assault: Issues, Theories, and Treatment of the Offender.* New York, NY: Plenum Press; 1990: 331-342.

Neidigh L, Krop H. Cognitive distortions among child sexual offenders. *J Sex Educ Ther.* 1992;18(3):208-215.

Nelson C, Jackson P. High-risk recognition: the cognitive-behavioral chain. In: Laws DR, ed. *Relapse Prevention With Sex Offenders.* New York, NY: The Guilford Press; 1989:167-177.

Nordland R, Bartholet J. The web's dark secret. *Newsweek.* March 19, 2001;44-51.

O'Connell R, Taylor M. Paedophile networks on the Internet: the evidential implications of paedophile picture posting on the Internet. Paper presented at: Combating Paedophile Information Networks in Europe (COPINE) Project Conference; January 1998; Dublin Castle, Ireland.

Pollock NL, Hashmall JM. The excuses of child molesters. *Behav Sci Law.* 1991;9: 53-59.

Putnam DE, Maheu MM. Online sexual addiction and compulsivity: integrating web resources and behavioral telehealth in treatment. *Sex Addict Compulsivity.* 2000; 7:91-112.

Quayle E, Taylor M. Child pornography and the Internet: perpetuating a cycle of abuse. *Deviant Behav.* 2002a;23(4):331-362.

Quayle E, Taylor M. Paedophiles, pornography and the Internet: assessment issues. *Br J Soc Work.* 2002b;32:863-875.

Schafer JA. Spinning the web of hate: web-based hate propagation by extremist organizations. *J Crim Justice Pop Cult.* 2002;9(2):69-88.

Scully D, Marolla J. Convicted rapists' vocabulary of motive: excuses and justifications. *Soc Probl.* 1984;31(5):530-544.

Stermac LE, Segal ZV. Adult sexual contact with children: an examination of cognitive factors. *Behav Ther.* 1989;20:573-584.

Sussman V. Policing cyberspace. *US News & World Report.* January 23, 1995:55-60.

Taylor M. The nature and dimensions of child pornography on the Internet. Paper presented at: International Conference Combating Child Pornography on the Internet; September 1999; Vienna, Austria.

Taylor M, Quayle E, Holland G. Child pornography, the Internet and offending. *Can J Policy Res.* 2001;2(2):94-100.

Thomas DS. Cyberspace pornography: problems with enforcement. *Internet Res: Electron Networking Appl Policy.* 1997;7(3):201-207.

Thompson CW. FBI cracks child porn ring based on Internet. *Washington Post.* March 19, 2002:A2.

US Department of Commerce. *Home Computers and Internet Use in the United States: August 2000.* Washington, DC: Government Printing Office; September 2001. P23-207.

US Department of Justice (USDOJ), Equality and Law Reform. *Illegal and Harmful Use of the Internet.* Dublin, Ireland: The Stationery Office; 1998.

US Department of Justice (USDOJ). *Internet Crimes Against Children.* Washington, DC: Government Printing Office; December 2001. NCJ 184931. 3.

US Department of Justice. *Sexual Assault of Young Children as Reported to Law Enforcement: Victim, Incident, and Offender Characteristics.* Washington, DC: Government Printing Office; July 2000. NCJ 182990.

Veach TA. Child sexual offenders' attitudes toward punishment, sexual contact, and blame. *J Child Sex Abuse.* 1999;7(4):43-58.

Young KS, Griffin-Shelley E, Cooper A, O'Mara J, Buchanan J. Online infidelity: a new dimension in couple relationships with implications for evaluation and treatment. *Sex Addict Compulsivity.* 2000;7:59-74.

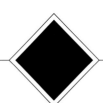

# INDEX

## A

AACAP. *See* American Association of Child and Adolescent Psychiatrists

AAP. *See* American Academy of Pediatrics

AAS, 429, 430t

Abduction. *See* Attempted nonfamily abduction; Infants; Teenagers

    involvement, 534

Abel, Gene, 279, 722

Abel VT, 284

Abercrombie ad. *See* Elementary school children mannequins

Abuse

    cases, comparison, 559t

    clergy reports, 948

    definition, 715

    images, offending process (relationship), 265–273

    medical evidence, 822

    method, 825

    pornographic evidence, 827

    questions, usage, 381t–382t

Abuse Assessment Screen (AAS), 429, 430t

Abused girls/women, criminal behavior

    frequency, 704

    questions, 704–705

    sexual characteristic, 704–705

Abused/neglected girls

    antisocial/delinquent lifestyle development, 705

    derailment mechanisms, 705–707

Abused/neglected women, derailment mechanisms, 705–707

Abused-status offenders, escalation. *See* Criminal offenders

Abusive Images Unit (AIU), investigations, 795–797

Accidental disclosure, 820

Accidental touching, 728

Acquaintance child exploitation cases, 590

Acquaintance child molestation, 532–535

Acquaintance child molesters, behavioral analysis

    caution, 529–530

    definitions, 535–542

        need, 535–536

    introduction, 529–535

    overview, 530–535

Acquaintance child molesters, determination, 533

Acquaintance sexual exploitation

    assessment/evaluation, 575–581

    big picture approach, 571

    disclosure/reporting continuum, 572–573

    emotion, reason (contrast), 570–571

    interview, 571–575

    investigation, 568–593

        perspective, 569–570

    law enforcement role, 572

    rapport, establishment, 573

    terms, clarification, 573

    videotaping, 573–574

Acquaintance-exploitation cases, 556–568

    assessment/evaluation, 575–581

    behavior patterns, documentation, 582–584

    corroboration, 581–588

    disclosure continuum status, 557–558

    dynamics, 556–558

    experts, usage, 557

    high-risk situations, 566–567

    investigation, 566–567

    medical evidence, 584

    parents, role, 557

Acquaintance-seduction preferential offender, 588

Acquired immunodeficiency syndrome (AIDS), 141, 148

    compromise, 392

    contraction, 73, 76, 747

    risk, 425, 804

    transmission, 1030

    vulnerability, 968

Acute internal injuries. *See* Genital trauma

Acute visible injuries. *See* Genital trauma

Addiction, 197. *See also* Cyber addiction; Drugs

*Admirable Discourses of the Plain Girl, The*, 6

Adolescents

    advertising guidelines, status, 45–46

    boy, anal-penile penetration (history), 360f

    female, hymenal clefts, 362f

    girls

        abnormal vaginal bleeding, differential diagnosis, 379t

        anal penetration, denial, 360f

    intimate partner violence. *See* Prostituted adolescents

    offenders, 555–556

    online contact, 477

    substance abuse, CRAFFT Screening test, 355t

    *Trichomonas vaginalis* discharge, 356f

    victims, uncomplicated STDs (management). *See* Sexual abuse

Adult/minor sexual contact, 473